Fluoropyrimidines in Cancer Therapy

Cancer Drug Discovery and Development

Beverly A. Teicher, Series Editor

Oncogene-Directed Therapies, edited by *Janusz Rak,* 2003
Cell Cycle Inhibitors in Cancer Therapy: *Current Strategies,* edited by *Antonio Giordano and Kenneth J. Soprano,* 2003
Chemoradiation in Cancer Therapy, edited by *Hak Choy,* 2003
Fluoropyrimidines in Cancer Therapy, edited by *Youcef M. Rustum,* 2003
Targets for Cancer Chemotherapy: *Transcription Factors and Other Nuclear Proteins,* edited by *Nicholas B. La Thangue and Lan R. Bandara,* 2002
Tumor Targeting in Cancer Therapy, edited by *Michel Pagé,* 2002
Hormone Therapy in Breast and Prostate Cancer, edited by *V. Craig Jordan and Barrington J. A. Furr,* 2002
Tumor Models in Cancer Research, edited by *Beverly A. Teicher,* 2002
Tumor Suppressor Genes in Human Cancer, edited by *David E. Fisher,* 2001
Matrix Metalloproteinase Inhibitors in Cancer Therapy, edited by *Neil J. Clendeninn and Krzysztof Appelt,* 2001
Farnesyltransferase Inhibitors in Cancer, edited by *Saïd M. Sebti and Andrew D. Hamilton,* 2001
Platinum-Based Drugs in Cancer Therapy, edited by *Lloyd R. Kelland and Nicholas P. Farrell,* 2000
Apoptosis and Cancer Chemotherapy, edited by *John A. Hickman and Caroline Dive,* 1999
Signaling Networks and Cell Cycle Control: *The Molecular Basis of Cancer and Other Diseases,* edited by *J. Silvio Gutkind,* 1999
Antifolate Drugs in Cancer Therapy, edited by *Ann L. Jackman,* 1999
Antiangiogenic Agents in Cancer Therapy, edited by *Beverly A. Teicher,* 1999
Anticancer Drug Development Guide: *Preclinical Screening, Clinical Trials, and Approval,* edited by *Beverly A. Teicher,* 1997
Cancer Therapeutics: *Experimental and Clinical Agents,* edited by *Beverly A. Teicher,* 1997

Fluoropyrimidines in Cancer Therapy

Edited by

Youcef M. Rustum

Roswell Park Cancer Institute
Buffalo, NY

Humana Press
Totowa, New Jersey

© 2003 Humana Press Inc.
999 Riverview Drive, Suite 208
Totowa, New Jersey 07512
www.humanapress.com

Production Editor: Adrienne Howell.
Cover design by Patricia F. Cleary.

This publication is printed on acid-free paper. ∞
ANSI Z39.48-1984 (American National Standards Institute)
Permanence of Paper for Printed Library Materials

For additional copies, pricing for bulk purchases, and/or information about other Humana titles, contact Humana at the above address or at any of the following numbers: Tel.:973-256-1699; Fax: 973-256-8341; Email: humanapr.com; or visit our Website: http://humanapress.com

Printed in the United States of America. 10 9 8 7 6 5 4 3 2 1

Library of Congress Cataloging-in-Publication Data

Fluoropyrimidines in cancer therapy / edited by Youcef M. Rustum.
p.; cm.—(Cancer drug discovery and development)
Includes bibliographical references and index.
ISBN 0-89603-956-0 (alk. paper) e-ISBN 1-59259-337-2
1. Fluoropyrimidines—Therapeutic use. 2. Cancer—Chemotherapy. I. Rustum, Youcef M. II. Series.
[DNLM: 1. Colorectal neoplasms—drug therapy. 2.Fluorouacil—therapeutic use.
3. Antimetabolites, Antineoplastic—therapeutic use. 4. Immunosuppressive Agents—therapeutic use. WI 529 F646 2002]
RC271.F55 F58 2002
616.99'4061—dc21 2002017289

PREFACE

Knowledge gained concerning mechanisms of action of 5-fluorouracil (5-FU) alone, in combination with leucovorin (LV) in in vitro and in vivo preclinical model systems, provided the basis for clinical evaluation and validation of the therapeutic efficacy and selectivity of this modulation in the early 1980s.

For more than two decades, the therapeutic options for patients with advanced colorectal cancer have been 5-fluorouracil/leucovorin modulation (5-FU/LV) based therapy. Although significant improvement in overall response rate was achieved, there has been no significant benefit as far as overall survival. With this treatment modality, diarrhea, mucositis, and neutropenia are the dose-limiting toxicities. In contrast to bolus 5-FU/LV, protracted continuous infusion of 5-FU yielded similar overall response rates with hand and foot syndrome as the dose-limiting toxicity.

In attempts to improve further on the therapeutic selectivity and efficacy of 5-FU/LV modulation, new and more specific thymidylate synthase (TS) inhibitors such as Tomudex (ZD-1694) are under extensive preclinical and clinical evaluation. However, the response rate in colorectal cancer and the toxicity profile from this drug were similar to those observed with 5-FU/LV therapy.

In clinical and preclinical model systems, 5-FU is eliminated rapidly from the plasma with a $t_{1/2}a$ of less than 10 min, and more than 85% of the injected dose of 5-FU is inactivated by dihydropyrimidine dehydrogenase (DPD) in normal and tumor tissues. The remaining 15% of 5-FU is activated via the anabolic pathways with a major fraction incorporated into cellular RNA. Preclinical results indicate that GI toxicity was associated with increased drug incorporation into cellular RNA. This suggests that the therapeutic selectivity of 5-FU may be improved by selective inhibition of PRPP transferase (PRPPT) in normal tissue, the enzyme responsible for phosphorylation of 5-FU into 5-fluorouracil-monophosphate (FUMP).

Several new treatment modalities are under evaluation: (1) the combination of 5-FU or its prodrug with an inhibitor of DPD (e.g., uracil and eniluracil) to prevent 5-FU degradation; (2) the use of PRPP inhibitor to reduce 5-FU incorporation into RNA of normal tissue (e.g., potassium oxonate); and(3) capitalizing on the differential expression of enzymes responsible for the activation of 5-FU prodrug, in normal vs tumor tissues (e.g., capecitabine).

S-1 is a new oral pyrimidine fluoride-based anticancer agent in which Ftorafur (FT) is combined with two classes of modulators, 5-chlorodihydropyrimidine (CDHP) and potassium oxonate, at a molar ratio of 1.0/0.4/1.0 for FT/CDHP/Oxo, respectively. FT is inactive until it is metabolized to 5-FU by thymidine/uridine phosphorylase. CDHP is a potent inhibitor of DPD, the enzyme responsible for degradation of 5-FU into therapeutically inactive but toxic 5-fluorodihydrouracil; CDHP is about 180 times more effective than uracil in inhibition of DPD in vitro. Oxo is a potent inhibitor of PRPPT. S-1 is in phase I and II clinical trials in patients with advanced colorectal cancer in Europe, Japan, and in the United States.

Capecitabine is an oral, inactive 5-FU prodrug that requires three-step activation to 5-FU with the final step of activation to 5-FU by thymidine/uridine phosphorylase.

Capecitabine has been approved by US FDA in patients with breast carcinoma and advanced colorectal cancer. In contrast, UFT is activated by thymidine/uridine phosphorylase to 5-FU with uracil as a DPD inhibitor.

Improving therapeutic selectivity is a major goal of anticancer drug development. The success of 5-FU/LV therapy in patients with advanced colorectal cancer demonstrated the important role of thymidylate synthase (TS) as a predictive marker for response to 5-FU-based therapy. The therapeutic roles of the other markers associated with metabolism of 5-FU and its prodrugs are under evaluation in preclinical and clinical settings.

Fluoropyrimidines in Cancer Therapy updates and reviews the mechanisms of action and therapeutic selectivity and efficacy of 5-FU, with and without leucovorin and its prodrugs in colorectal cancer therapy. The potential advantages and disadvantages of these agents and the role of predictive markers are reviewed here. Drawing on the knowledge gained to date with these agents when used individually, they are now being evaluated in combination with other drugs (e.g., irinotecan, oxaliplatin, and EGF inhibitors).

Youcef M. Rustum

Contents

Contributors

Albert Abad • *University Hospital Germans Trias I Pujol, Barcelona, Spain*
Ornella Belvedere • *University of Udine, Udine, Italy*
Giordano D. Beretta • *Unit Medical Oncology of Ospedali Riuniti, Bergamo, Italy*
Geert H. Blijham • *Department of Internal Medicine, University Hospital, Utrecht, The Netherlands*
Daniel R. Budman • *Division of Oncology, North Shore University Hospital, Manhasset, NY*
Marc E. Buyse • *International Institute for Drug Development, Brussels, Belgium*
Shousong Cao • *Roswell Park Cancer Institute, Buffalo, NY*
Edward Chu • *Yale Cancer Center, Yale University School of Medicine, and VA Connecticut Healthcare System, West Haven, CT*
Aimery de Gramont • *Service de Medecine Interne-oncologie, Hospital Saint Antoine, Paris, France*
Bruce J. Dolnick • *Department of Pharmacology and Therapeutics, Roswell Park Cancer Institute, Buffalo, NY*
Charles Erlichman • *Department of Oncology, Mayo Clinic, Rochester, MN*
Marina Garassino • *Medical Oncology Unit of Casa di Cura Igea, Milano, Italy*
Richard M. Goldberg • *Department of Oncology, Mayo Clinic, Rochester, MN*
Ashwin Gollerkeri • *Yale Cancer Center, Yale University School of Medicine, New Haven, CT*
Gunnar Hapke • *Roswell Park Cancer Institute, Buffalo, NY*
Paulo M. Hoff • *University of Texas M.D. Anderson Cancer Center, Houston, TX*
Janet A. Houghton • *Department of Hematology-Oncology, St. Jude Children's Research Hospital, Memphis, TN*
Hideo Ishitsuka • *Nippon Roche Research Center, Kanagawa, Japan*
Hedy L. Kindler • *University of Chicago Medical Center, Chicago, IL*
Roberto Labianca • *Unit Medical Oncology of Ospedali Riuniti, Bergamo, Italy*
Francis Lévi • *ICIG-Hospital Paul Brousse, Villejuif, France*
Xiukun Lin • *Yale Cancer Center, Yale University School of Medicine, New Haven, CT*
Jun Liu • *Yale Cancer Center, Yale University School of Medicine, New Haven, CT*
Christophe Louvet • *Hospital Saint Antoine, Paris, France*
Eleftherios P. Mamounas • *National Surgical Adjuvant Breast and Bowel Project, Pittsburgh, PA*
José Luis Manzano • *University Hospital Germans Trias I Pujol, Barcelona, Spain*
Marinella Mastore • *Medical Oncology Unit of Casa di Cura Igea, Milano, Italy*
Gérard Milano • *Oncopharmacology Laboratory, Centre A. Lacassagne, Nice, France*
Richard G. Moran • *Department of Pharmacology and Toxicology, Medical College of Virginia, Richmond, VA*
Gianfranco Pancera • *Medical Oncology Unit of Casa di Cura Igea, Ospedali Riuniti, Bergam, Italy*

M. ADELAIDE PESSI • *Unit Medical Oncology of Ospedali Riuniti, Bergamo, Italy*
G. J. PETERS • *Department of Medical Oncology, Vrije University Medical Center, Amsterdam, The Netherlands*
PASCAL PIEDBOIS • *Department of Oncology, Chu Henri Mondor Hospital, Creteil, France*
PAOLA POLETTI • *Unit Medical Oncology of Ospedali Riuniti, Bergam, Italy*
CARY A. PRESANT • *California Cancer Medical Center, West Covina, CA*
YOUCEF M. RUSTUM • *Roswell Park Cancer Institute, Buffalo, NY*
EVERARDO D. SAAD • *University of Texas M.D. Anderson Cancer Center, Houston, TX*
DVORIT SAMID • *Department of Oncology, Roche Laboratories, Nutley, NJ*
DANIEL J. SARGENT • *Department of Health Services Research, Mayo Clinic, Rochester, MN*
RICHARD L. SCHILSKY • *Division of Biological Sciences, Cancer Research Center, University of Chicago Medical Center, Chicago, IL*
JOHN C. SCHMITZ • *Yale Cancer Center, Yale University School of Medicine, New Haven, CT*
TETSUHIKO SHIRASAKA • *Taiho Pharmaceutical Co., Ltd., Tokyo, Japan*
ROY E. SMITH • *National Surgical Adjuvant Breast and Bowel Project, Pittsburgh, PA*
ALBERTO F. SOBRERO • *Medical Oncology, University of Udine, Udine, Italy*
TETSUO TAGUCHI • *Japan Society for Cancer Chemotherapy, Osaka, Japan*
AKIHITO TSUJI • *Kochi Municipal Center Hospital, Kochi, Japan*
VICTOR WALUCH • *University of Southern California, Los Angeles, CA*
WALTER WOLF • *School of Pharmacy, University of Southern California, Los Angeles, CA*
NORMAN WOLMARK • *National Surgical Adjuvant Breast and Bowel Project, Pittsburgh, PA*
SUSUMU YAMAMITSU • *Sapporo Tsukisamu Hospital, Sapporo, Japan*

INTRODUCTION

For years 5-fluorouracil (5-FU) was the only chemotherapeutic agent for the treatment of patients with advanced colorectal cancer. Recent advances based on delineation of the mechanism of action of 5-FU demonstrated that leucovorin (LV) can significantly potentiate the response rate to 5-FU from approximately 10% to 30%. With no major impact on survival, these important advances, however, were associated with significant toxicities, namely diarrhea, leucopenia, and mucosites, independent of the dose of LV but highly dependent on the schedule of 5-FU/LV. With the daily X 5 schedule, grade 3 and 4 mucositis (25%), diarrhea (15%), and leukopenia (15%) were clearly documented in patients with colorectal cancer. In contrast, with the weekly X 6 schedule of 5-FU/LV, the dose-limiting toxicity is diarrhea, grade 3 and 4, in approximately 30% of patients. These toxicities, especially in the adjuvant setting, could have a significant impact on patient quality of life, cost, and the ability to be used in combination with other active chemotherapeutic agents.

To date, 5-FU/LV, CPT-11 (irinotecan, a topoisomerase I inhibitor), capecitabine, and oxaliplatin are the only drugs approved by the Food and Drug Administration for treatment of patients with advanced colorectal cancer. New drugs in clinical trials include folate-based thymidylate synthase (TS) inhibitors (Tomudex [raltitrexed, ZD-1694], ZD9331, YW1843U89, AG337), a synthetic dihydrofolate reductase inhibitor (trimetrexate glucuronate), new platinum compounds (oxaliplatin and JM-216 [an oral form]), and orally bioavailable fluoropyrimidine prodrugs, including capecitabine (Xeloda), Orzel (UFT/LV), and S-1 as well as FU/EU. With the 5-FU prodrugs, the overall aim is to improve the therapeutic efficacy, selectivity, survival, and quality of life of 5-FU-based therapy and to provide an orally bioavailable form of 5-FU.

Three recognized mechanisms of action of fluoropyrimidine agents are (1) inhibition of TS by 5-fluorodeoxyuridine monophosphylate (FdUMP); (2) incorporation of fluorouridine triphosphate (UTP) into cellular RNA; and (3) degradation of 5-FU by dihydropyrimidine dehydrogenase (DPD). DPD inhibitors (e.g., uracil, 5-eniluracil [EU]), 5-chloro-2,4-dihydropyridine [CDHP]), in combination with 5-FU or ftorafur (FT) provided strong evidence for the therapeutic importance of DPD in the outcome of therapy with 5-FU and its prodrugs .

Thymidine phosphorylase (TP) catalyzes the activation of 5-FU prodrugs (5-d-FUR) and the metabolism of 5-FU into FdUrd. This enzyme is identical to platelet-derived endothelial growth factors and acts as a promoter of angiogenesis. In preclinical model systems in colorectal cancer, high levels of TP, and low levels of DPD and TS, are predictive markers for response to 5-FU and its prodrugs. High levels of TP and TS predict resistance to 5-FU.

Future studies should seek to determine whether the therapeutic efficacy of 5-FU and its prodrugs can be enhanced without increasing toxicity by the combination with agents with different mechanisms of action (e.g., platinum compounds, topoisomerase I inhibitors, and EGF/VGEF inhibitors). Studies should continue to assess the therapeutic role of dual modulation of 5-FU and its prodrugs in terms of their interfering with the anabolic and catabolic pathways of 5-FU. Future work should also attempt to determine the level and activity of metabolic enzymes (TP, DPD, and TS), in order to select patients for different treatment modalities. Finally, the predictive values of molecular markers altered by flouropyrimidine prodrugs as a consequence of sustained inhibition of TS should also receive high priority.

Future studies should aim to confirm the predictive values of TP, DPD, and TS in a well-controlled clinical trial. With this knowledge, it should be possible to design treatment on the basis of the biochemical profile of tumors prior to initiation of therapy. Furthermore, in tumors with effective and sustained inhibition of TS, the molecular markers that are being altered downstream and the therapeutic consequences of such an alterations need to be investigated.

1 Relative Role of 5-Fluorouracil Activation and Inactivation Pathways on Its Cytotoxic Effects

Preclinical and Clinical Modulation

G. J. Peters, PhD

CONTENTS

1. INTRODUCTION

5-Fluorouracil (5-FU) is an analog of uracil (Fig. 1) but, owing to its additional resemblance to orotic acid and thymine, the drug uses the same pathways as these natural substrates. 5-FU is transported into the cell either by a high-affinity nucleobase carrier or by passive diffusion *(1)*. There is increasing evidence that the dypiridamole-sensitive nucleoside transporter ENT2 also contributes to nucleobase transport. In order to be active, 5-FU has to be converted to one of its nucleotides (Fig. 2). These are

- FUTP, which can be incorporated into RNA.
- FdUTP, which can be incorporated into DNA.
- FUDP-sugars, which may interfere with glycosylation of proteins and lipids.
- FdUMP, which is an inhibitor of thymidylate synthase (TS), a key enzyme in the *de novo* synthesis of the pyrimidine deoxynucleotide deoxythymidine triphosphate (dTTP), a direct precursor for the synthesis of DNA.

Disturbances in one of these conversions can lead to resistance to 5-FU *(2,3)*. Thus the activities of the anabolic pathways (either directly via orotate phosphoribosyltransferase [OPRT] or indirectly via the pyrimidine nucleoside phosphorylase and kinase) have been associated with the cytotoxic effects of 5-FU, both the side effects and the antitumor activity.

From: *Fluoropyrimidines in Cancer Therapy*
Edited by: Y. M. Rustum © Humana Press Inc., Totowa, NJ

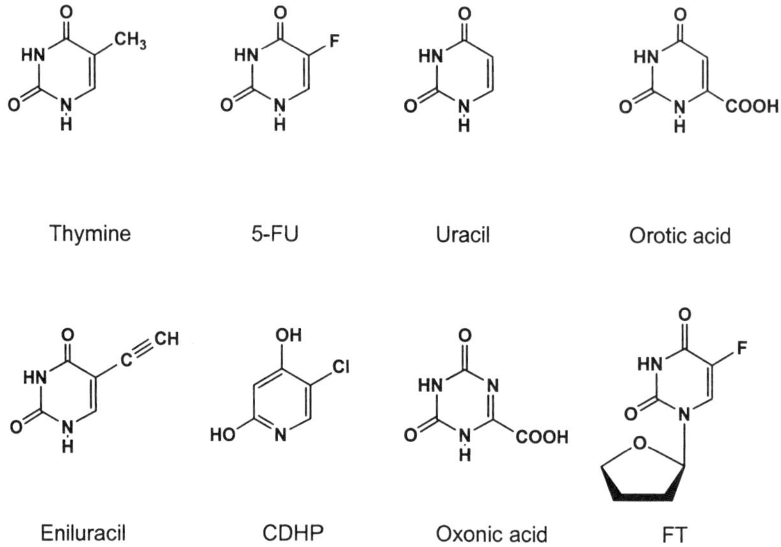

Fig. 1. Structural formulas of thymine, 5-FU, uracil, orotic acid, the DPD inhibitors Eniluracil and CDHP, the 5-FU prodrug Ftorafur, and the OPRT inhibitor oxonic acid.

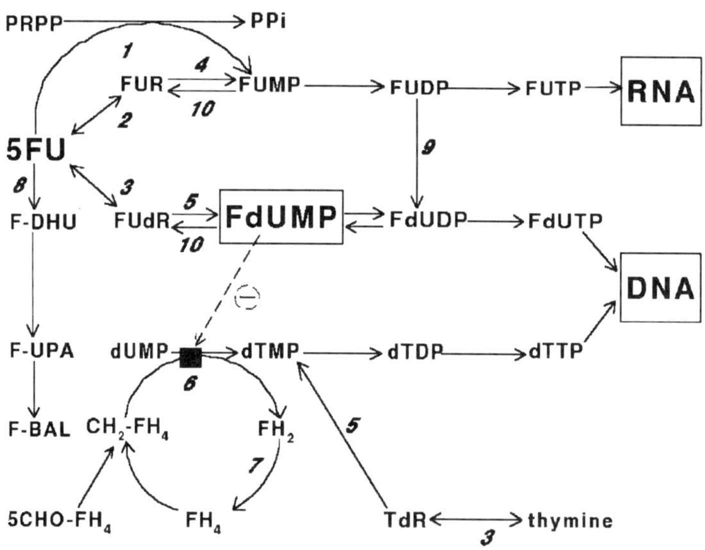

Fig. 2. Schematic representation of 5-FU metabolism with possible sites responsible for resistance. Resistance can be due to an increase of the target enzyme (thymidilate synthase), a decrease in activation, or an increased inactivation (of 5-FU itself to F-DHU or of the 5-FU nucleotides FUMP of FdUMP to the nucleosides FUR and FUdR). Inhibition of thymidylate synthase by FdUMP is represented by a Θ and a bar. The boxes indicate that a low accumulation (FdUMP) or decreased incorporation (RNA, DNA) can limit the action of 5-FU. Enzymes catalyzing these reactions are 1, orotate phosphoribosyltransferase; 2, uridine phosphorylase; 3, thymidine phosphorylase; 4, uridine kinase; 5, thymidine kinase; 6, thymidylate synthase; 7, dihydrofolate reductase; 8, dihydropyrimidine dehydrogenase; 9, ribonucleotide reductase; 10, 5′-nucleotidases and phosphatases. F-DHU, 5-fluorodihydrouracil; F-UPA, fluoroureido-propionate; F-BAL, α-fluoro-β-alanine; PRPP, 5-phosphoribosyl-1-pyrophosphate; TdR, thymidine.

Cellular transport of 5-FU itself has not been shown to limit its cytotoxicity but it has been demonstrated that transport deficiency of its nucleoside analog 5-fluorodeoxyuridine (FUdR) can lead to resistance. This chapter focuses on the relative role of the various activation and inactivation pathways in mediating the cytotoxic effects of 5-FU and whether modulation of these pathways will cause a change in the mechanism of cytotoxicity, either toward the tumor cells or against normal tissues.

2. ACTIVATION AND INACTIVATION

2.1. Activation

Initial studies on 5-FU resistance concentrated on its activation pathways (Table 1). In several model systems a low activity of uridine kinase (UK) and phosphorylase (UP) (and the channeled UP-UK) *(4–6)* and OPRT *(7,8)* were related to resistance to 5-FU. In in vivo models both high UP activity and high OPRT activity *(9,10)* were related to 5-FU sensitivity. However, Ardalan et al. *(11)* observed low 5-phosphoribosyl-1-pyrophosphate (PRPP) levels in 5-FU-resistant tumors and a higher activity of PRPP synthetase in the sensitive tumor, indicating an important role for OPRT, since PRPP is the cosubstrate for this enzyme in activation of 5-FU. Activation of 5-FU via UP also requires the action of UK, which may be limiting *(12–14)*. More evidence for the importance of the OPRT pathway was obtained by Holland et al. *(15)* who showed that injection of the UP inhibitor, benzylacyclouridine (BAU), together with 5-FU resulted in the accumulation of 5-fluorouridine (FUR) in the tumor, whereas no FUR was observed when 5-FU was injected as a single agent. This means that FUR should be formed as a degradation product of FUMP, and indicates the existence of a futile cycle 5-FU → FUMP → FUR → 5-FU. This can be considered as some "hidden" depot of 5-FU in the tumor responsible for the long retention of 5-FU in tissues *(16)*. A high activity of the OPRT pathway is essential for 5-FU activation *(14)*. Shani and Danenberg *(17)* provided evidence that activation of 5-FU may be compartmentalized. The use of various labeled fluoropyrimidines resulted in two separate phosphorylated fluorinated nucleotide pools in the cells, which do not easily mix. The UK pathway would favor incorporation into RNA, whereas 5-FU activation would favor direct conversion of 5-FU to FUMP. Thus, 5-FU activation is most likely via the direct phosphoribosylation pathway. Hence resistance may be due to a decreased activity of this pathway, but it is most likely determined by a combination of several factors also including increased breakdown of 5-FU, its nucleosides, and its nucleotides and aberrations in TS activity (*see* refs. *18,3,19*). These factors may be different for each cell or tumor type.

The role of thymidine phosphorylase (TP) in the conversion of 5-FU to FUdR and subsequently to FdUMP is unclear. The only source for the essential substrate for this reaction, deoxyribose-1-phosphate (dRib-1-P), is by degradation of purine and pyrimidine deoxynucleosides, catalyzed either by purine nucleoside phosphorylase or one of the pyrimidine nucleoside phosphorylases, uridine and thymidine phosphorylase. In addition the only source for deoxynucleosides is reduction of ribonucleotides to deoxyribonucleotides by ribonucleotide reductase, followed by dephosphorylation. Hence the physiological concentration of dRib-1-P in cells and tissues is low, usually below the detection limit of the assays used for this compound *(13,20)*, although methodological problems may have limited the reliable detection of dRib-1-P *(20)*. Indirect evidence for a role of TP in the activation of 5-FU follows from the fact that formation of FdUMP and inhibition of TS can be enhanced by providing an alternative source for dRib-1-P such as deoxyinosine, which can be degraded to hypoxanthine and dRib-1-P *(13,21–23)*. Also in vivo deoxyinosine could increase the antitu-

Table 1
Resistance to 5-FU

Mechanisms of resistance to 5-FU
A. **Decreased accumulation of activated metabolites**
a. Decreased activation
b. Increased inactivation
c. Increased inactivation of 5FU-nucleotides
B. **Target-associated resistance**
a. Decreased RNA effect
b. Altered effect on thymidylate synthase
– Aberrant enzyme kinetics
– Increased dUMP levels
– Decreased FdUMP accumulation
– Decreased stability of ternary complex
– Depletion of intracellular folates
– Decreased polyglutamylation of folates
– Recovery and enhanced enzyme synthesis
– Gene amplification
– Enzyme induction
C. **Pharmacokinetic resistance**
a. The drug does not reach the tumor
b. Disease state affects drug distribution
c. Increased elimination

Modified from ref. *3, 19.*

mor activity of 5-FU *(24)*. These latter effects were most pronounced in cells that were transfected with human TP and displayed nonphysiologically high TP levels. In in vitro studies evidence for a role of TP in direct activation of 5-FU to FUdR was only observed in cells with very high TP levels (usually achieved by transfection) *(25–28)*. Administration of FUdR to mice resulted in a rapid degradation to 5-FU *(29),* although this may be the result of a uridine phosphorylase mediated degradation of FUDR *(30)*. However, in patients TP may degrade FUdR, since it is an excellent substrate, whereas the equilibrium is likely to be in the degradative direction due to the relatively high phosphate levels and low bioavailability of dRib-1-P. It may be concluded that at physiological levels TP is unlikely to play a significant role in direct activation of 5-FU to FUDR, although it should be recognized that only very low amounts of FdUMP are necessary to inhibit TS.

2.2. 5-FU inactivation

5-FU can be inactivated by degradation to 5-fluoro-dihydrouracil (F-DHU) in a reaction catalyzed by dihydropyrimidine dehydrogenase (DPD) with NADPH as the cosubstrate. F-DHU is degraded further to FUPA (fluoroureidopropionate) and subsequently to fluoro-β-alanine, (F-BAL) NH_3, and CO_2 Conversion of F-BAL to fluoroacetate has been related to neurotoxicity *(31)*. However, F-BAL itself was shown to cause neurotoxicity manifested by a direct action on myelin inducing vacuole formation and a necrosis/softening-like change of the brain stem *(32)*. F-BAL itself can also form conjugates with bile acids such as cholate and chenodeoxycholate *(33–35)*. These conjugates may have a role in the hepatic and biliary toxicity that develop in patients receiving hepatic arterial infusions of fluoropyrimidines. 5-FU degradation occurs in all tissues, including tumors *(36),* but is most abundant in the liver and to a lesser extent in the kidney *(37)*. Thus, the liver plays an important role in 5-FU degradation and elimination. In patients, large amounts of the breakdown products have been demonstrated in plasma and urine. Breakdown products were also demonstrated in the liver with[19] F-NMR *(38)*.

3. TARGETS FOR FLUOROPYRIMIDINES

3.1. Inhibition of TS

Inhibition of TS by FdUMP is considered to be the main mechanism for the action of 5-FU (Fig. 2). Several mechanisms of resistance to 5-FU have been attributed to alterations in TS *(3)*. Characteristics of the TS enzyme have been described in detail by others *(39,40)*. TS catalyses the conversion of dUMP to dTMP, for which 5,10-methylene-tetrahydrofolate (CH_2-THF) serves as a methyl donor. FdUMP acts as a potent competitive inhibitor of TS with dUMP. The inhibition by FdUMP is mediated by the formation of a covalent ternary complex between FdUMP, TS, and CH_2-THF, whereas the retention of inhibition is also dependent on the ratio between free dUMP and FdUMP levels *(41,42)*. A low sensitivity to 5-FU has been related to a rapid disappearance of FdUMP. A high dUMP concentration or a limited FdUMP binding to TS may reduce retention of the inhibition of TS.

The stability of the ternary complex is highly dependent on the availability of CH_2-THF or one of its polyglutamates *(42)*. Leucovorin (LV) can increase the availability of CH_2-THF (Fig. 2). After transfer across the membrane, mediated by the reduced folate carrier *(43)*, LV will be metabolized to CH_2-THF *(44)*, which will be polyglutamylated and enhance inhibition of TS *(45)*. A decreased activity of folylpolyglutamate synthetase (FPGS) *(46)* and altered binding of FdUMP to TS *(41,47–49)* have been associated with 5-FU resistance. In the absence of CH_2-THF or one of its polyglutamates *(41,49–51)*, FdUMP forms an unstable binary complex, which results in poor inhibition. Also, disturbed folate pools *(51)* lead to intrinsic resistance as well as a high level of enzyme before treatment *(41,48,52)*. Gene amplification of TS and mutations in the gene *(49)* lead to acquired resistance *(53–55)*. Thus, changes in the TS gene at the DNA level (e.g., mutations or gene amplification) are clearly associated with acquired resistance to fluoropyrimidines.

Expression of TS under physiological conditions is related to the cell cycle, with a high activity during the S-phase *(56)*, which decreases when the cells do not proliferate *(57)*. The translation of the TS mRNA appears to be controlled by its end product, the TS protein, in an autoregulatory manner. However, when TS is bound to a ternary complex, the protein can no longer regulate its synthesis, leading to the observed increase. Thus, inhibition of TS in vitro either by the formation of the ternary complex between FdUMP, the enzyme, and 5,10-CH_2-THF *(58,59)* or by specific TS inhibitors such as ZD1694 *(60)* disrupt the regulation of enzyme synthesis, manifested as an increase in TS protein expression. An increase in the TS mRNA or a change in the stability of the enzyme did not accompany this increase. The increase in TS protein, however, may also be due to stabilization of the protein owing to decreased degradation of the ternary complex *(61)*. p53–mRNA translation can also be regulated by TS protein *(62)*, although wild-type p53 protein can also inhibit TS promoter activity *(63)*. Thus, regulation of induction of TS is a very complicated process, which may be even more disrupted (more induction) in cells with mutated p53 than with wild-type p53 (low induction). The 5-FU-induced increase could be prevented by interferon-γ *(64)*. A similar increase in TS was also observed in vivo in murine tumors *(29,65,66)*. This increase could be prevented by LV or by the use of a high dose of 5-FU *(67)*. These mechanisms probably play a role in the observed enhancement of the sensitivity to 5-FU and may reverse resistance to 5-FU.

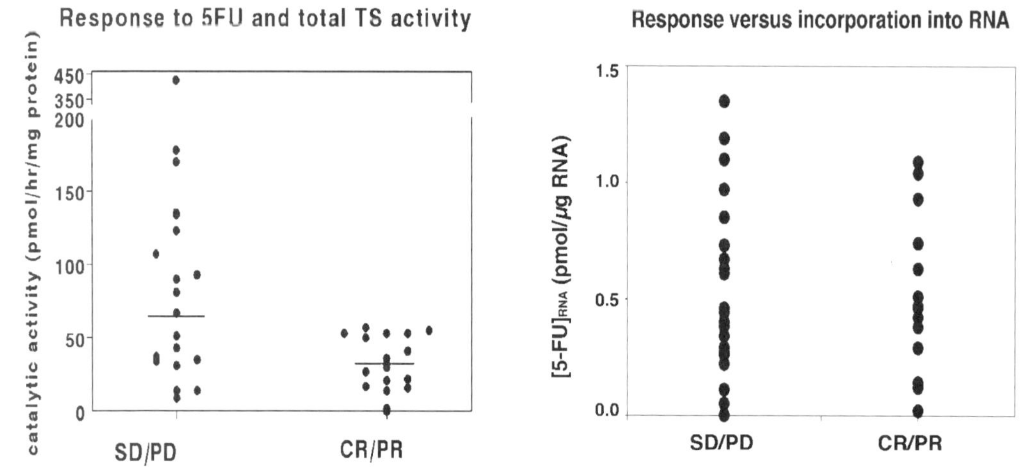

Fig. 3. Relation between response to 5-FU-based treatment and TS levels (A) and 5-FU incorporation into RNA (B) (modified from refs. *52* and *68*)

TS inhibition in primary human colon tumors and in liver metastases is retained for at least 48–72 h after a bolus injection of 500 mg/m^2 5-FU *(52,68);* in 19 patients responding to 5-FU hepatic artery infusion, TS inhibition was 2–3-fold higher and enzyme levels were 2–3-fold lower than in 21 patients not responding (Fig. 3A). Also in breast cancer patients binding of FdUMP and the effect of CH_2-THF decreased during development of resistance *(69).* These results demonstrate that analysis of biochemical parameters in tumor biopsies obtained at both short and longer time periods after 5-FU administration gives valuable information about the in vivo mechanism of action of the drug in the tumors of patients.

3.2. FU Incorporation into RNA

In most cells and tissues 5-FU will also be incorporated into all classes of RNA, including ribosomal, transfer, and messenger RNA, but in tumor cells particularly in nuclear RNA *(70).* In several model systems in vitro the amount of 5-FU in RNA correlated with the sensitivity to 5-FU *(71)* and in vivo the antitumor effect of 5-FU *(72),* together with the gastrointestinal cytotoxicity were also related to the amount of 5-FU in RNA *(73).* The cytotoxicity due to incorporation of 5-FU into RNA is mainly determined by the incorporation of 5-FU into nuclear RNA *(74).* At drug concentrations, which do not impair transcription, methylation of 4S-nuclear-RNA appeared to be impaired *(74),* possibly associated with an impaired processing of nuclear RNA to cytoplasmic RNA *(71,75,76).* A major point of discussion is whether 5-FU incorporation into RNA or inhibition of TS is the major factor responsible for antitumor activity. Because both in vitro and in vivo 5-FU incorporation into RNA are concentration- and dose-dependent, respectively, it was postulated that 5-FU RNA incorporation was related to the antitumor effect, since the antineoplastic activity was also dose-dependent *(77,78).* However, the extent and duration of in vivo TS inhibition was also dose-dependent *(29).* A higher dose of 5-FU (enabled by uridine protection) enhanced antitumor activity, and was associated with a longer duration of inhibition of TS than the lower dose, but not with an increase in the 5-FU incorporation into RNA *(67).* Similar to these in vivo studies, in vitro studies also indicated that uridine did not influence 5-FU incorporation into RNA, whereas withdrawal of 5-FU did not diminish 5-FU incorporated into RNA *(79).* Thus TS inhibition, and its downstream effects, seem the most important factors for the antineoplastic activity.

Similar findings have been obtained in samples from patients. In patients who received either 5-FU alone, or 5-FU with LV, the RNA incorporation was similar but the inhibition of TS was significantly increased in the LV group (Fig. 3B). Furthermore the RNA incorporation of 5-FU in patients with a partial or complete response was not significantly different from nonresponders, but the extent of TS inhibition was significantly different *(52,68)* (Fig. 3). There is, on the other hand, substantial evidence that the side effects of 5-FU are related to its incorporation into RNA, since a decrease of the 5-FU incorporation into RNA by uridine was associated with a decreased extent of side effects of 5-FU *(80,81)*. In summary, evidence is accumulating that the antitumor activity of 5-FU is predominantly related to the inhibition of TS, rather than to its incorporation into RNA.

3.3. DNA Directed Effects of 5-FU

5-FU can exert an effect on DNA either by its incorporation or by inducing a deoxynucleotide imbalance (decrease of dTTP and increase of dUTP, Fig. 2). 5-FU incorporation into DNA has long been considered as a very unlikely event, not contributing to 5-FU cytotoxicity. FdUTP can be formed intracellularly but its concentration remains very low, since it is hydrolyzed by dUTPase, although FdUTP incorporated into DNA may be removed by uracil-DNA glycosylase in a similar manner to the removal of uracil from DNA *(82,83)*. Owing to the inhibition of TS, the dTTP concentration is usually depleted *(12)* whereas the concentration of dUTP increases *(79,84)*. These conditions cause an imbalance in deoxyribonucleotides and may favor incorporation of both dUTP and FdUTP into DNA. The importance of dUTPase in cytotoxicity of 5-FU has been demonstrated by comparison of cell lines with high and low dUTPase and by transfection of the gene in cells with a low dUTPase. It was evident from these studies *(85–87)* that a high level of expression of dUTPase can prevent cytotoxicity of 5-FU. Despite the action of dUTPase, 5-FU can be incorporated into DNA and a relationship between 5-FU incorporation and cytotoxicity has indeed been postulated *(81)*. However, in the same group of patients in which we could relate response to 5-FU with TS levels, the extent of incorporation of 5-FU into DNA was similar in the responding and nonresponding patients *(88)*.

It seems that both misincorporation of 5-FU into DNA and the excision of these residues can be responsible for cell death. 5-FU can induce DNA strand breaks through its misincorporation, but also because of inefficient DNA repair (due to the lack of dTTP and imbalance of other deoxynucleotides) of normally occurring defects in purine and pyrimidine residues *(89)*. Thymidine depletion due to TS deficiency *(90–92)* also leads to a dTTP depletion and an increase in dATP, resulting in a G1-S arrest. Cells with a p53 wt phenotype died by apoptosis, whereas mt p53 cells along with a relatively high Bax and Fas (Apo-1, CD95) expression went in cytostasis *(91)*. Because an anti-Fas antibody could induce apoptosis, colon cancer cells seem to have a functional Fas-mediated apoptosis pathway, which may be regulated by wt p53 *(92–95)*. However, other factors may also play a role, because in wt p53 cells transfected with mt p53 apoptosis could also be induced with an anti-Fas antibody *(95)*, whereas a blockade of the Fas-receptor did not affect antifolate-induced apoptosis. Expression of the Fas-receptor possibly has clinical implication, because 5-FU administration to patients increased the expression of the Fas-receptor on tumor cells *(96)*.

More insight into the role of DNA damage caused by 5-FU treatment was obtained by analysis of the effect of interferon-α on the formation of both single- and double-strand breaks *(97,98)*. Interferon-α increased both types of strand breaks, a mechanism, which was possibly responsible for the enhanced cytotoxic effect of the combination compared to 5-FU alone.

Table 2
Pharmacokinetic Parameters of 5-Fluorouracil

Bolus injection at 400–900 mg/m²		
Half-life	$t_{1/2}\beta$	9–20 min
	$t_{1/2}\gamma$	2–7 h
Volume of distribution		14–54 l
Clearance from plasma		50–140 l/h
Peak levels		1 m*M*
Continuous infusion		
Steady-state levels		1–71 μM
Clearance from plasma		54–420 l/h
Oral admininstration		
Steady-state levels		0.5–10 μM
$t_{1/2}\beta$ (dependent on DPD inhibitor)		2–4 h

4. ROLE OF 5-FU DEGRADATION IN 5FU PHARMACOKINETICS

4.1. 5-FU Pharmacokinetics and DPD Activity

Pharmacokinetics of single dose 5-FU administered as an iv bolus injection in doses varying between 300 and 600 mg/m² have been studied most extensively *(2,99–101)*. Peak levels of 5-FU can reach the millimolar range, with a subsequent rapid decline. 5-FU is rapidly distributed over all tissues (Table 2). The total clearance was rather high, comparable to the flow through the liver, but hepatic extraction has been estimated at 50% *(102)*. The kidneys contribute to elimination by both DPD-mediated degradation and active renal secretion with about 20% of 5-FU being excreted as the parent drug *(103)*. In addition, the lungs may also contribute significantly to 5-FU clearance *(99,103)*. Collins et al. *(104)* have shown that a saturable two-compartment model can be used to describe the disappearance kinetics of 5-FU for the first hour. However, in a third compartment plasma levels fluctuated from 3 n*M* to 0.1 μ*M* between 4 and at least 24 h *(105)*. It is most likely that this 5-FU represents efflux from the tissues; 5-FU tumor levels vary from 2 to 10 μ*M* between 2 and 48 h after administration of a bolus 5-FU injection of 500 mg/m² *(16)*, while 5-FU is retained for a long period in RNA *(29,67,106)*, which may form a depot for 5-FU. Wolf et al. *(38)* demonstrated with ^{19}F-NMR that the half-life in tumors (0.5–2.1 h) was considerably longer than that in plasma (9–20 min).

This nonlinearity of 5-FU kinetics *(99,102–105,107)* is related to the saturation of 5-FU catabolism. Peak plasma levels of the first catabolite F-DHU were between 20 and 40 μM with a terminal half-life of 40–60 min *(108,109)*. With ^{19}F-NMR the other catabolites could be demonstrated in human plasma *(34)*. Cumulative urinary excretion of the catabolites showed that F-BAL was the major one followed by FUPA, while F-DHU excretion was minimal. Sweeny et al. *(33)* and Malet-Martino et al. *(34)* observed that one of the major breakdown products of 5-FU was a bile acid conjugate of fluoro-β-alanine. This conjugate may contribute to liver toxicity after intrahepatic treatment of liver metastasis with fluoropyrimidines *(35)*.

Circadian variations in DPD activity may (at least partially) be responsible for the circadian pattern in the plasma 5-FU concentration during protracted continuous infusion with 5-FU *(108,109)*, with the peak in the 5-FU concentration at 11 AM and the trough at 11 PM The ratio peak/trough was about 5. In mice a reversed circadian pattern was observed *(66)*. The concen-

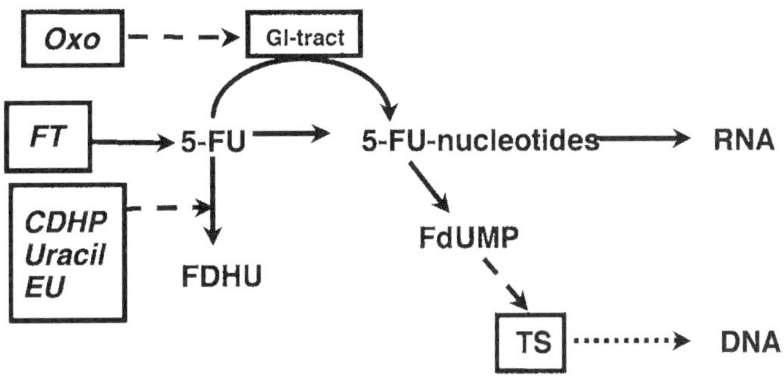

Fig. 4. Mechanism of action of various DPD inhibitors. Inhibition of DPD will lead to a higher bioavailability of 5-FU in plasma and tissues, which will enhance metabolism to active metabolites. F-DHU, 5-fluorodihydrouracil.

trations were the inverse of the circadian pattern of the catabolic enzyme dihydrouracil dehydrogenase. Circadian rhythms of metabolism have been described in mice *(110,111)*. However, recent data indicated that, under less controlled conditions (the majority of cancer patients), the circadian pattern of DPD is less consistent *(112,113),* although a circadian pattern of 5-FU plasma concentrations was still present. These data suggest that continuous infusion of 5-FU should not be given at a constant rate, but according to a circadian pattern *(114),* using programmable pumps in order to minimize host toxicity. Programmed 5-FU and LV administration with the peak at 4 AM combined with oxaliplatin (peak afternoon) showed a clear advantage compared to flat administration, with response rates of 51% compared to 29% *(115)*.

A large variability in bioavailability for orally administered 5-FU, between 28 and 100%, has been observed *(99,103),* which may be related to a saturable hepatic catabolism *(104),* but also to an additional first-pass effect. Because of these variabilities 5-FU alone should not be given via the oral route. However, in the last decade the development of orally administered drugs, including 5-FU (pro)drugs, has progressed rapidly. Currently, various forms of oral formulations are being evaluated in the clinic; these formulations are either based on a prodrug selectively activated in the tumor or on a combination of 5-FU (or prodrug) with a DPD inhibitor. Capecitabine is a prodrug of Doxifluridine *(116),* which is activated by thymidine phosphorylase, which has a higher activity in tumor tissues *(14,117)*. Capecitabine causes the hand–foot syndrome, typical for continuous infusions. Since plasma levels are in the same range, this indicates that degradation products of 5-FU (absent in the combinations with DPD inhibitors) may be responsible for this specific type of toxicity.

4.2. The Use of DPD Inhibitors to Increase Bioavailability of 5-FU and Increase its Efficacy

DPD is the first enzyme in the pathway of 5-FU catabolism and is responsible for more than 80% of 5-FUs elimination. Therefore, inhibition of 5-FU degradation would enhance the bioavailability of 5-FU to other tissues, including the tumor. Initial studies used the ability of natural substrates of DPD to modulate 5-FU. Thymidine, a precursor of thymine, however, did not improve the therapeutic index of 5-FU *(118),* while in rats toxicity was increased *(119)*. Thymidine, however, also interferes at other sites of 5-FU metabolism and may form an alternative source for dTMP, bypassing its depletion caused by TS inhibition. Uracil, the other natural substrate of DPD, has been developed more successfully as a modulator of 5-FU catabolism.

The use of inhibitors of DPD enables the use of 5-FU (or one of its prodrugs) as an oral formulation, since degradation of 5-FU in the gastrointestinal tract and other tissues is almost completely prevented (Fig. 4). Plasma concentrations of the formulations with a DPD inhibitor are generally comparable to that of continuous infusions *(120–124)* and vary depending on the drug combination and the frequency by which the drug is given. The formulations with a DPD inhibitor include 5-FU with ethynyluracil, UFT (ftorafur with uracil), S-1 (ftorafur with a CDHP and oxonic acid), *(125)*. The only combination in which 5-FU is given orally is that with ethynyluracil (776C85; EU). EU is a 5-substituted uracil analog and a potent mechanism-based irreversible inactivator of DPD *(126),* which produces an enzyme-deficient state *(127)* and thereby prevents degradation of 5-FU *(128)*. Injection of EU into mice led to rapid inactivation of the enzyme; within 25 min rat liver DPD was completely inhibited *(127)* resulting in increased plasma uracil levels to 60 μ*M,* as well as increased thymine levels *(127)*. EU increased the bioavailability of orally administered 5-FU from <5% *(128)* to 85% in mice and 100% in rats, resulting in an increased therapeutic efficacy of oral 5-FU in rats *(129)*.

Formulations of oral 5-FU with a DPD inhibitor result in plasma 5-FU concentrations in the micromolar range. The most widely used formulation at this moment is UFT in which uracil is combined with Ftorafur (FT) in a 4:1 molar ratio *(130)*. Ftorafur (1-2-tetrahydrofurany1-5-FU) acts as a depot form for 5-FU and as a single agent produced little myelosuppression, but significant gastrointestinal toxicity and neurotoxicity. The drug is well absorbed orally in contrast to 5-FU itself. Conversion to 5-FU may occur predominantly in tumor cells and the liver and is predominantly catalyzed by cytochrome P450 2A6 *(131),* although a role for thymidine phosphorylase has also been postulated. Ftorafur is not given anymore as a single agent but only in biochemical modulation regimens, which enable oral formulation forms, such as UFT (uracil with ftorafur) and S-1 (ftorafur with CDHP and oxonic acid).

Combination of uracil with 5-FU serves several purposes. First, uracil is a weak competitive inhibitor of DPD, preventing degradation of 5-FU *(132,133),* but it has no direct effect on 5-FU anabolism *(133)*. Second, in combination with FT, uracil will enhance the bioavailability of orally administered 5-FU. It was observed that coadministration of uracil with FT enhanced the 5-FU concentrations in the tumor 5–10 times compared to FT alone or 5-FU itself *(134–136)*. In a rat colon tumor model it was demonstrated that the antitumor activity could be enhanced by LV, which was associated with an increased TS inhibition (from 70% to 100% inhibition) *(137)*. Considerable differences are seen in 5-FU plasma pharmacokinetics for FT administered alone (150 mg/kg/d) compared to UFT (60 mg/kg/d of FT). The peak concentration increased from 2.8 to 19.4 μM, the area under the curve (AUC) increased 7–8-fold, and the terminal half-life about two-fold, from 4 to 7.5 h. A steady-state plasma 5-FU concentration of 10 μ*M* was maintained for about 24 h after an oral dose of UFT.

Further refinement of the strategy that led to UFT has resulted in a new mixture called S-1, which is a combination of FT, CDHP, and oxonic acid in a molar ratio of 1:0.4:1 *(138)*. CDHP is a potent reversible inhibitor of DPD *(139)* and oxonic acid is an inhibitor of OPRT (Figs. 1 and 4). Because oxonic acid accumulates specifically in normal gut *(140)* and will prevent accumulation of toxic 5-FU nucleotides *(141,142),* this will reduce the gastrointestinal toxicity of FT *(138)*. Oxonic acid can be degraded to cyanuric acid by direct conversion by the microflora in the gut and by xanthine oxidase and aldehyde oxidase. In rats and mice, 5-FU administration will lead to substantial inhibition of TS in gut tissue *(143,144),* but after treatment with S-1, inhibition of TS in gut tissue was significantly decreased compared to control tissue *(145)*. This was associated with a decreased histopathological-confirmed damage to the gut. After administration of S-1 to mice, plasma levels of 5-FU were substantially higher, with a 12- and 32-fold higher AUC for 5-FU derived from S-1 compared to that of

Table 3
Antitumor Activity of S-1

Tumor	*Phase I/II*	*N Pat*	*Response (CR/PR)*	*Median Survival (days; range)*	*Reference*
Gastric	Early II	28	53.6%	298 (29–232)	*159*
Gastric	II	50	44.2%	207 (153–334)	*160*
Gastric	Late II	51	48.1%	250 (171–376)	*162*
Colon	Early II	30	16.7%	120 (40–272)	*159*
Colon	II	62	35%	378	*161*
Breast	Early II	27	40.7%	–	*163*
Head & Neck	Early II	26	46.2%	–	*164*
Colon	II	26	23%	–	*155*
Gastric	II	19	32%	–	*156*

Refs. 155 and 156 describe European studies; the other references refer to Japanese studies.

UFT and FT, respectively *(146)*. Plasma C_{max} of 5-FU was about 15–30 μ*M* after 1 h. Although the oral formulations aim to achieve prolonged 5-FU levels in plasma and tissues, the incidence of toxicities at a similar antitumor effect of continuous infusion or S-1 was much more pronounced at the continuous-infusion schedule *(142)*. In several in vivo models (human gastric, breast, head and neck, and colon cancer; rat and mouse colon tumors) S-1 showed a better antitumor activity than UFT or 5-FU given at various schedules, either continuous infusion or as a bolus *(142,147–151)*. In a rat colon tumor the increased therapeutic efficacy of S-1 compared to Ftorafur alone and continuous infusion of 5-FU at their MTDs was associated with clearly increased induction of apoptosis and prolonged inhibition of TS in tumors from S-1-treated mice *(152)*. All these findings demonstrate that the postulated biochemical modulation was indeed effective; inhibition of DPD prolonged 5-FU plasma half-life, while accumulation of oxonic acid inhibited 5-FU activation specifically in the gut.

Based on the encouraging preclinical studies of inhibition of DPD, these formulations have been translated to the clinic. Schilsky et al. describe the combination with EU *(153)*. UFT has undergone extensive clinical evaluation and is registered in several countries for use in a variety of cancers, including colorectal and breast cancer. S-1 is registered in Japan and has also shown clinical activity in European studies (Phase II) (Table 3). 5-FU formed from tegafur in the S-1 formulation reached levels up 10 μ*M* (Fig. 5). 5-FU showed linear pharmacokinetics and its AUC was related to the dose of S-1 *(124)*. The dose-limiting toxicity in the European study was diarrhea, which was related to the AUC of plasma 5-FU (Fig. 6); at the highest dose of 45 mg/m^2 four out of five patients developed diarrhea, at the lower dose of 40 mg/m^2 severe toxicity was observed in those patients who had received severe prior chemotherapy *(124)*. It seems that exposure, especially the length of it, is responsible for the toxicity. This finding was confirmed in the Phase II study, during which limiting pharmacokinetic sampling was applied and Grade $^3/_4$ toxicity was found in colorectal cancer patients with a high AUC for 5-FU (> 400 μM · min) *(154)*. In contrast to the Phase I study 40 mg/m^2 could not be given to these patients and the dose had to be lowered to 35 mg/m^2. Also at this dose severe diarrhea was observed in colon cancer patients *(155,156)*. Hematologic toxicity was mild, with Grade 3 leukopenia and neutropenia in only one patient. Also, other toxicities were mild. In the Japanese studies, hematological toxicity was considered as dose-limiting *(123)*, but no Grade $^3/_4$ toxicity was observed. In addition to the difference in toxicity, Japanese and Caucasian patients differed in the 5-FU pharmacokinetics. Europeans

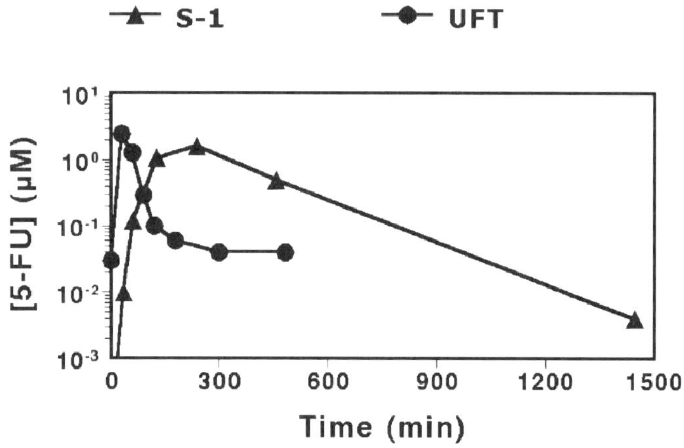

Fig. 5. Example of 5-FU pharmacokinetics after administration of S-1 or UFT (from ref. *124*).

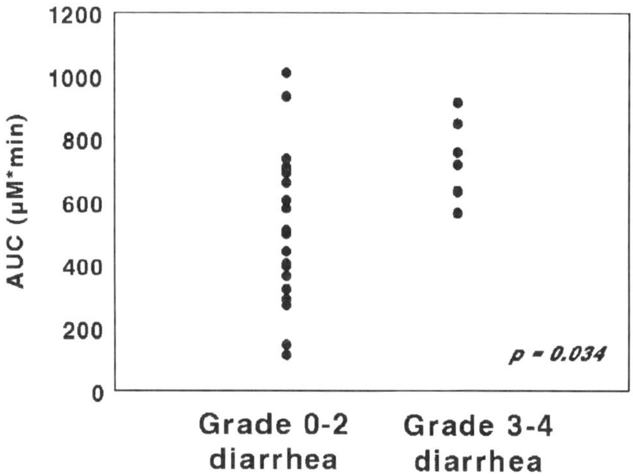

Fig. 6. Relation of between 5-FU AUC and diarrhea (from ref. *124*).

had a higher C_{max} and AUC for 5-FU than Japanese patients, which may be related to the higher levels of CYP 2A6 in Caucasians compared to Japanese *(157)*. Whether this difference is responsible for a potential different handling of the drug remains to be established. Food intake did not significantly affect the absorption of Ftorafur and subsequent conversion to 5-FU *(158)*. The activity of S-1 is comparable or better than that of UFT. The compounds show encouraging activity in gastric cancer and colorectal cancer, both in Japanese and European patients *(155,156,159–164)* despite the difference in drug handling. In general, the clinical activity of these formulations is comparable to that found with modulated 5-FU bolus schedules and continuous infusions. The main advantage is the convenient oral administration of these formulations. Further enhancement of therapeutic efficacy is being sought by other combinations with UFT, or S-1 such as with the platinum analogs cisplatin and oxaliplatin, the taxane paclitaxel, the topoisomerase I inhibitor irinotecan, and radiation.

6. MODULATION OF 5-FU ACTIVATION PATHWAYS

6.1. PALA and 5-FU

The combination of phosphonoacetyl-L-aspartate (PALA) and 5-FU is an example of the combination of an inactive drug with an active drug. Only a low dose of PALA is required to obtain the biochemical effect necessary for increased anabolism of 5-FU. By inhibition of the pyrimidine *de novo* synthesis PALA can enhance the availability of PRPP (Fig. 2), thus increasing the anabolism of 5-FU and the incorporation into RNA *(165)*. In several Phase II clinical trials, the response rate for this combination varied from 33 to 43% *(166–168)*, but in larger and randomized studies these effects were not confirmed *(169)*. PALA combinations with 5-FU are not being pursued actively.

6.2. Trimetrexate, 5-FU, and LV

Combinations of 5-FU with MTX gave controversial results in the clinic *(19)*, which is possibly due to a neutralization of the MTX effects by LV, resulting in a net modulation by LV *(170)* or a competition of MTX uptake by LV. Trimetrexate (TMQ) is a lipophilic DHFR inhibitor *(171)*, which does not use the reduced folate transport system *(172)*, cannot be polyglutamated, and does not compete with LV for cellular uptake and metabolism *(43)*. Romanini et al. *(173)* showed that LV can enhance the cytotoxicity of TMQ and 5-FU metabolism intracellularly (increased 5-FU activation) whereas LV can enhance TS inhibition. These results formed the basis for clinical studies on the combination of TMQ with 5-FU and LV. This combination had activity in previously pretreated patients with a response rate of approx 20% *(174)*, and about 50% in untreated patients *(175)*. These studies are an elegant example how a rational combination can be based on preclinical studies, combining increased 5-FU activation to enhance TS inhibition.

6.3. 5FU and uridine

In the beginning of the 1980s it was proposed that the antitumor activity of 5-FU could be increased by enhancing its incorporation into RNA *(72,176)*. For this purpose 5-FU was combined with uridine, which enabled an increase in the 5-FU dose leading to an improved therapeutic efficacy *(72,80,176,177)*. Uridine did not affect the 5-FU-induced inhibition of TS in cell culture *(80)* and murine tumors *(177)*. The effect of the 5-FU–uridine combination could be increased even more by combination with LV *(178)*. Further studies explored the possibility to use a precursor of uridine to modulate 5-FU toxicity. In mice uridine-diphosphoglucose (UDPG) can increase the concentration of UTP in liver and in intestine, but not in tumors *(179)*. The therapeutic index of 5-FU could be improved by rescue with UDPG; the dose of 5-FU could be increased from 100 to 150 mg/kg in mice, and this produced a better antitumor activity in several tumors *(180)*. Mechanistic studies in murine tumors using UDPG demonstrated that the higher dose of 5-FU did not increase the extent of TS inhibition but prolonged the retention of TS inhibition *(67)*; thus in mice treated with standard dose 5-FU, TS inhibition was retained until 7 d with a 2–3-fold induction after 10 d, while in mice treated with the high dose of 5-FU (UDPG) TS inhibition was retained until 10 d; the TS induction could be prevented by injection of the next dose of 5-FU. Incorporation of 5-FU into RNA was, however, decreased by UDPG although the antitumor effect was increased.

Clinical studies have shown that uridine can be used effectively in patients to reduce the 5-FU-induced myelotoxicity. Pharmacokinetics of short-term infusions of uridine in patients resulted in plasma levels of uridine around 2 m*M* *(181)*, but the rapid catabolism prevented an effective protection from 5-FU toxic effects. In following studies uridine has been administered continuously using a central venous catheter, but fever appeared to be the dose-limiting toxicity *(182,183),* similar to animal studies. This side effect was effectively controlled using an intermittent-infusion scheme consisting of alternating 3 h of infusion with 3 h of treatment-free period over a total of 72 h *(184).* Using this schedule in combination with a weekly injection of 5-FU, starting the uridine infusion 3 h after the injection of 5-FU, an effective reduction of myelosuppression was obtained in patients. Interestingly, the protective effect of uridine on myelosuppression was observed also during the following courses of 5-FU, which were not combined with uridine infusion. Also, in other studies the dose of 5-FU could be increased even when 5-FU was combined with different modulating agents such as PALA or methotrexate and doxorubicin (FAMTX regimen) *(185,186).* There was a marked reduction in mucositis and myelosuppression. Also in animal model systems uridine administration could reduce gastrointestinal toxicity of 5-FU *(180,187).*

Intravenous infusions of uridine must be performed via a central venous catheter in order to avoid phlebitis at the site of administration. Therefore more convenient ways of administering the drug have been explored. Preclinical data showed that with oral administration of uridine to mice it was possible to obtain plasma concentrations of approx 100 μ*M (188)* that are sufficient to reduce 5-FU toxicity *(189).* Similar pharmacokinetic data have been obtained in humans *(190);* when uridine was administered repeatedly, the dose had to be lowered to 5 g/m^2 every 6 h due to the occurrence of diarrhea. Using this schedule the myelosuppression of 5-FU was reduced *(191).* Initial studies have been performed with UDPG administration to patients; plasma uridine peak values were 40–60 μ*M,* and a concentration of 20–25 μ*M* was still present 8 h after the second dose (unpublished results). The studies could however not be continued. Another prodrug, PN401 (an acytelated prodrug of uridine), has also been tested (pre-)clinically to increase the uridine levels of 5-FU. In mice plasma concentrations of PN401 resulted in 8-fold higher plasma concentrations than equimolar uridine administrations, while in patients 6 g PN401 gave plasma levels of about 160 μ*M* and 5-FU doses could be escalated from 600 to 1000 mg/m^2 *(192),* which is somewhat higher than with uridine *(183,190).* Studies determining the effective dose of 5-FU (with or without LV) with PN401 protection are ongoing. It is expected that PN401 will protect both against myelosuppression and mucositis and that the use of higher 5-FU doses will enable TS inhibition to be prolonged and thus enhance the antitumor effect of 5-FU-LV bolus regimens.

Further evidence for a role of uridine in modulation of 5-FU and for a difference with the specific TS inhibitor ZD1694 (Tomudex, Raltitrexed) was obtained from studies using wild-type p53 and p53 knockout mice. In these mice cell death was measured as the apoptotic index in crypts of the intestine BDF-1 mice. 5-FU administration induced cell death in p53 wild-type mice but not in knockout mice, while p53 was also upregulated in wild-type mice. Uridine administration could prevent 5-FU-induced apoptosis in p53 wild-type mice, indicating an RNA-dependent mechanism of toxicity in gut tissue. Thymidine prevented ZD1694 induced toxicity in wild-type and p53 knockout mice *(193),* indicating a TS-dependent mechanism of cell death.

7. MODULATION OF TS INHIBITION

7.1. Biochemical Modulation with LV

The combination of 5-FU with LV is based on the stabilization of the ternary complex between FdUMP, TS, and CH_2-THF (Fig. 2). The bioavailability of the latter is increased by LV administration. After transfer across the membrane mediated by the reduced folate carrier

Table 4
Results of Meta-Analyses and Randomized Studies in Colorectal Cancer Using Several 5-FU Schedules

	N *Trials*	N *Patients*	*Response (CR/PR)*	p-*value*	*Median Survival (mo)*	p-*value*	*Reference*
5-FU			11%		11.0		*199*
5-FU/LV	9	1381	23%	<0.001	11.5	0.57	
Systemic 5-FU or FUDR			14%		12.2		*203*
HAI FUDR	5	391	41%	<0.001	16.0	0.14	
5-FU bolus			14%		11.3		*204*
5-FU CI	6	1219	22%	<0.001	12.1	0.04	
5-FU_{24h} + LV	A[a]	91	44%		16.2		*205*
5-FU_{24h} + IFN	B	90	18%	<0.05	12.7	<0.04	
5-FU_{24h} IFN + LV	C	49	27%		19.6		

[a] A 5-FU_{24h} 2600 mg/m^2 + LV 500 mg/m^2 2h, weekly × 6; B FU_{24h} 2600 mg/m^2 + IFN 3 MU s.c 3 ×/w, weekly ×6; C 5-FU_{24h} 2600 mg/m^2 + LV + IFN, weekly ×6;

CI, continuous infusion; IFN, interferon-α; HAI, hepatic arterial infusion Modified from Peters and Köhne *(19)*.

(43), LV will be metabolized to CH_2-THF. Although intermediates of the metabolic pathway of LV to CH_2-THF can also support the formation of the ternary complex, CH_2-THF is the most active substrate *(44)*. Polyglutamates of CH_2-THF *(45)*, which are formed by the action of FPGS, will enhance inhibition of TS. In general, prolonged exposure of cells also led to a 1.5–2-fold increased enhancement of the cytotoxicity of 5-FU and FUdR by LV 1–10 μ*M* (reviewed in refs. *19 and 194*). Lower concentrations of LV are generally not sufficient to potentiate the effects of 5-FU or FUdR, while higher concentrations generally do not enhance the effect *(195)*. There are fewer in vivo studies on 5-FU modulation by LV, usually limited to the description of the antitumor effect *(194)* but do not include mechanistic studies. 5-FU alone shows a clear tumor-dependent TS inhibition *(196,197)*, followed by a 2–3-fold induction after 2–3 wk *(29,66)*. The potentiation of the antitumor activity of 5-FU by LV given before 5-FU in several murine tumors was associated with a prevention of the induction of TS and with a more pronounced inhibition of TS by LV plus 5-FU compared to 5-FU alone *(65)*. Thus, in vivo modulation of 5-FU with LV seems to be related to prolonged TS inhibition and prevention of TS induction.

A number of different schedules have been used successfully in Phase III trials in which a clear benefit for LV–5-FU compared to 5FU alone was observed in terms of response rate, but a benefit in view of increased survival was not always evident *(198–200)*, biweekly, weekly, and daily administrations, as well as 24 h, 48 h, and continuous infusions (Table 4). LV has to be administered at a certain threshold dose allowing sufficient accumulation of LV. Although low-dose LV seems to be better than high-dose LV *(201)*, it has to be noted that the 5-FU dose was lower in the high-dose LV regimen. Altogether, it may be concluded that the best way to administer LV is as an infusion, thus allowing accumulation of folates and folylpolyglutamates in the tissues: 5-FU has to be administered either immediately after LV or during the infusion of LV. Administration of 5-FU weekly or daily times five every 4 or 5 wk generally gave the same results. Toxicity of the combination LV and 5-FU is more severe than that of 5-FU. In particular, diarrhea and stomatitis are increased. The pure active isomer, L-LV, demonstrated a similar activity *(202)* and both forms can be used interexchangeable.

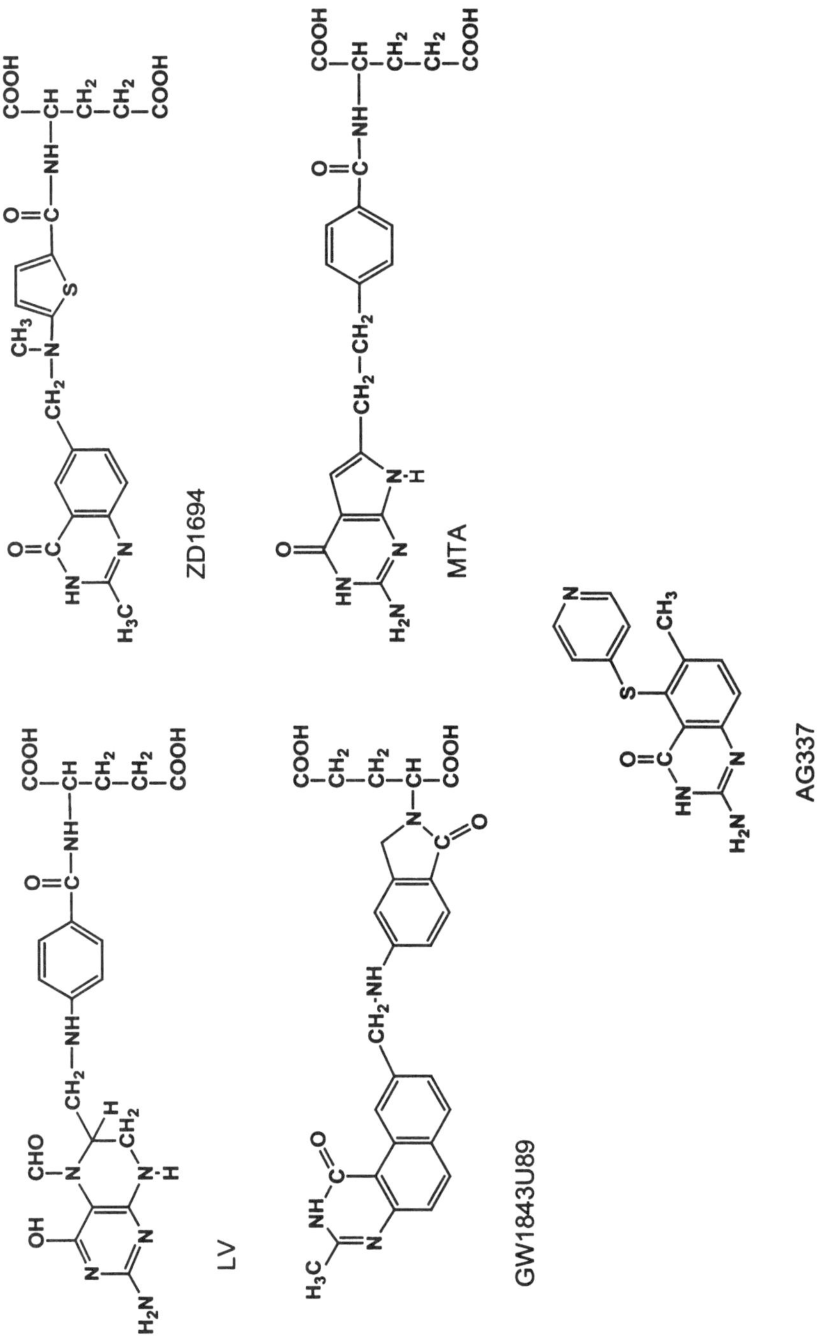

Fig. 7. Structural formulas of leucovorin (LV) and several new antifolates that inhibit TS: GW1843U89, AG337 (Nolatrexed), ZD1694 (Tomudex, Raltirexed), and MTA (LY231514, ALIMTA, Pemetrexed).

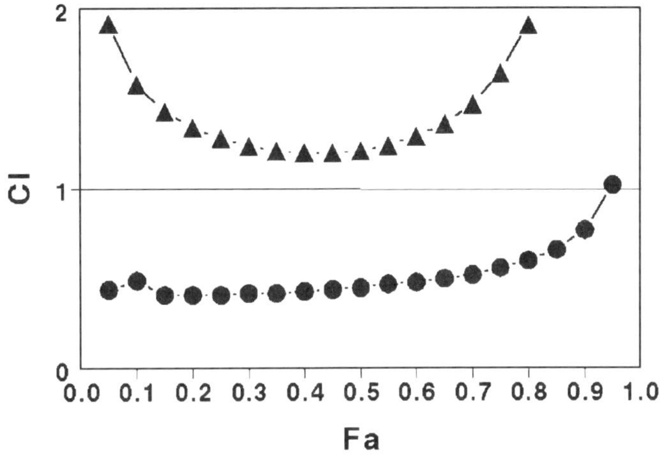

Fig. 8. Interaction between 5-FU and the TS inhibitor AG337 in SW116 (●) and LS174T (▲) colon cancer cells. Synergism was evaluated using the median-drug effect analysis *(208)*. A Cl (combination index) value above 1 indicates antagonism, below 1 synergism. *FA* is the fraction affected *(210)*.

7.2. 5-FU Combinations with Antifolate TS Inhibitors

Because FdUMP and the new antifolates (Fig. 7) bind at different sites of the enzyme, a synergistic interaction of 5-FU with new antifolate TS inhibitors was expected and combination studies were initiated. At the molecular level, Van der Wilt et al. *(206)* demonstrated that ZD1694, LY231514, AG337, and GW1843 appeared to enhance the binding of FdUMP to TS, although to different extents. With some of these drugs the extent of binding was dependent on the presence of a glutamate moiety; ZD1694-Glu4 and LY231514-Glu4 supported binding of FdUMP to TS to a similar extent as CH_2-THF. There was, however, a major difference; in contrast to the natural substrate all antifolates showed nonlinear binding with a plateau at about 1 μ*M*. Data using double labeling (^{14}C-AG337 and ^{3}H-FdUMP) indicated that the antifolates possibly induce a structural modification of the enzyme, which affects the binding of FdUMP. The binding of GW1843 is maximal at a much lower concentration than for the other antifolates, possibly related to the fact that it binds to different amino acids in the enzyme *(207)*. The concentration-dependent binding of antifolates and FdUMP to TS is possibly a major factor that should be taken into consideration when 5-FU is combined with any of these antifolates. These factors were considered in initial studies of the combination. Indeed in vitro cytotoxicity experiments revealed a concentration dependence; when 5-FU concentrations were kept constant, and the antifolate concentration varied, a synergistic effect was observed at low antifolate concentrations (Fig. 8), but only additivity at higher concentrations *(208)*. Changes in *in situ* TS inhibition paralleled these effects. The extent of *in situ* TS inhibition (5-FU alone, 15%; AG337, LY231514, or ZD1694 alone, 10–15% inhibition; GW1843, no inhibition) was more than additive for the combinations (all combinations of 5-FU with antifolates produced 30–35% inhibition) in WiDr colon cancer cells, but mostly additive in other cell lines. Furthermore, the induction of DNA damage was at least additive (5-FU, AG337, or ZD1694 alone, 25–30%; LY231514 and GW1843 alone, 10–15%; combinations of antifolate with 5-FU, 40–60% DNA damage; additive to synergistic for LY231514, ZD1694, and GW1843). In HCT-8 human colon cancer cells, exposure to ZD1694 for 24 h, followed by 4 h 5-FU exposure, resulted in a downregulation of thymidine kinase activity and mRNA level, and increased 5-FU incorporation into RNA compared to 5-

FU exposure alone *(209)*. It was postulated that this enhancement was related to the ZD1694-induced increase in dUMP, leading to an increase in the incorporation of 5-FU into RNA. These studies indicate a complex biochemical interaction. Based on the additive/synergistic interaction clinical combination studies have been initiated.

8. CONCLUSIONS

Although initial research on 5-FU in the 1960s already revealed the importance of the various metabolic pathways, their relative role in achievement of antitumor activity or toxic side effects remains a matter of debate. The interpretation of several of these studies is hampered by the use of various model systems and different conditions used in these studies. However, the use of various modulators of one of the activation or inactivation pathways (or both) has given more substantial evidence on the relative role of each pathway. Thus it can be concluded that degradation of 5-FU by DPD is the major elimination pathway, since inhibition of this pathway either naturally in patients with a DPD deficiency or by the use of DPD inhibitors necessitated a drastic decrease of the dose, because otherwise toxic side effects such as diarrhea and myelosuppression would be lethal. Under these conditions urinary excretion of 5-FU is more important than in the classical bolus and continuous-infusion schedules. For the activation pathway, most evidence supports the crucial role of the direct phosphoribosylation of 5-FU to FUMP. However, depending on substrate availability and enzyme levels, the pathway via FUR may contribute to nucleotide formation, which may proceed to a different compartment. The contribution of the TP-mediated pathway is minimal under physiological conditions; this pathway may play a role only at very high TP levels with a sufficient supply of dRib-1-P. The various pathways may also play a role in the targets, which may be affected by 5-FU. However, considering the overwhelming evidence of a relation between response to 5-FU and both TS levels and TS inhibition, it may be concluded that TS is a major determinant in the antitumor effect of 5-FU. Various modulation studies have provided substantial evidence that 5-FU incorporation into RNA contributes to the toxic side effects of 5-FU, although TS inhibition in normal gut may cause additive toxicity, probably more important under conditions of modulation of TS inhibition. Future modulation studies with nonpurine or pyrimidine compounds should ideally attempt to increase the TS-mediated effects in the tumors, not only the direct inhibition of TS but also its regulation (to prevent induction) and the downstream events leading to either apoptotic or necrotic cell death. The relative role of the various caspases and the Fas-R remains to be elucidated. Altogether, these modulation studies provided a strong basis to include 5-FU in various novel combination regimens *(210)*, which can still be improved based on a proper translation of preclinical studies to the clinic, and subsequently feedback this information.

REFERENCES

1. Griffith DA, Jarvis SM. Nucleoside and nucleobase transport systems of mammalian cells. *Biochimica Et Biophysica Acta* 1996; 1286:153–181.
2. Pinedo HM, Peters GJ. 5-Fluorouracil: biochemistry and pharmacology. *J Clin Oncol* 1988; 6:1653–1664.
3. Peters GJ, Jansen G. Resistance to antimetabolites. In: Principles of Antineoplastic Drug Development and Pharmacology (R.L. Schilsky, G.A. Milano, M.J. Ratain, eds.), Marcel Dekker, New York, 1996, pp. 543–585.
4. Sköld O. Studies on resistance against 5-fluorouracil. IV Evidence for an altered uridine kinase in resistant cells. *Biochimica Et Biophysica Acta* 1963; 73:160–162.
5. Reichard P, Sköld O, Klein G, Revesz L, Magnussen P-H. Studies on resistance against 5-fluorouracil. I Enzymes of the uracil pathway during development of resistance. *Cancer Research* 1962; 22:235–243.

6. Tezuka M, Sugiyama H, Tamemasa O, Inara M. Biochemical characteristics of a 5-fluorouracil-resistant subline of P388 leukemia. *Japn J Cancer Res (GANN)* 1982; 73:70–76.
7. Reyes P, Hall TC. Synthesis of 5-fluorouridine 5′-phosphate by a pyrimidine phosphoribosyltransferase of mammalian origin. II. Correlation between the tumor levels of the enzyme and the 5-fluorouracil-promoted increase in survival of tumor-bearing mice. *Biochem Pharmacol* 1969; 18:2587–90.
8. Kessel D, Hall TC. Wodinsky I. Nucleotide formation as a determinant in 5-fluorouracil response in mouse leukemias. *Science* 1966; 145:911–913.
9. Schwartz PM. Moir RD, Hyde CM, Turek PJ, and Handschumacher RE. Role of uridine phosphorylase in the anabolism of 5-fluorouracil. *Biochemical Pharmacology* 1985; 34:3585–3589.
10. Houghton JA, Houghton PJ. Elucidation of pathways of 5-fluorouracil metabolism in xenografts of human colorectal adenocarcinoma. *Eur J Cancer and Clin Oncol* 1983; 19:807–815.
11. Ardalan B, Villacorte D, Heck D, Corbett T. Phosphoribosyl pyrophosphate, pool size and tissue levels as a determinant of 5-fluorouracil response in murine colonic adenocarcinomas. *Biochem Pharmacol* 1982; 31:1989–1992.
12. Peters GJ, Laurensse E, Leyva A, Lankelma J, and Pinedo HM. Sensitivity of human, murine and rat cells to 5-fluorouracil and 5′-deoxy-5-fluorouridine in relation to drug-metabolizing enzymes. *Cancer Res* 1986; 46:20–28.
13. Peters GJ, Laurensse E, Leyva A, and Pinedo HM. Purine nucleosides as cell-specific modulators of 5-fluorouracil metabolism and cytotoxicity. *Eur J Cancer and Clin Oncol* 1987; 23:1869–1881.
14. Peters GJ, Van Groeningen CJ, Laurensse EJ, and Pinedo HM. A comparison of 5-fluorouracil metabolism in human colorectal cancer and colon mucosa. *Cancer* 1991; 68:1903–1909.
15. Holland SK, Bergman AM, Zhao Y, Adams ER, Pizzorno G. ^{19}F NMR monitoring of in vitro tumor metabolism after biochemical modulation of 5-fluorouracil by the uridine phosphorylase inhibitor 5-benzylacyclouridine. *MRM* 1997; 38:907–916.
16. Peters GJ, Lankelma J, Kok RM, et al. Prolonged retention of high concentrations of 5-fluorouracil in human and murine tumors as compared with plasma. *Cancer Chemotherapy and Pharmacology* 1993; 31:269–276.
17. Shani J, and Danenberg PV. Evidence that intracellular synthesis of 5-fluoroururidine – 5′-phosphate from 5-fluorouracil and 5-fluorouridine is compartmentalized. *Biochem Biophys Res Comm* 1984; 122:439–445.
18. Schmitz JC, Gollerkeri A, Lin X, Liu J, and Chu E. Molecular mechanisms regulating the expression of thymidylate synthase. In: Fluoropyrimidines in Cancer Therapy (Y.M. Rustum, ed.). Humana Press Inc., Totowa, 2002, pp. 67–82.
19. Peters GJ, and Köhne CH. Fluoropyrimidines as antifolate drugs. In: Antifolate Drugs in Cancer Therapy (A.L. Jackman, ed.), Humana Press Inc., Totowa, 1999, pp. 101–145.
20. Ipata PL, and Tozzi MG. Deoxyribose-1-phosphate: radioenzymatic and spectrophotometric assay. *J Biochem Biophys Meth* 1984; 9:343–350.
21. Evans RM, Laskin JD, and Hakala MT. Effect of excess folates and deoxyinosine on the activity and site of action of 5-fluorouracil. *Cancer Res* 1984; 41:3288–3295.
22. Schwartz EL, Baptiste N, O'Connor CJ, Wadler S, and Otter BA. Potentiation of the antitumor activity of 5-fluorouracil in colon carcinoma cells by the combination of interferon and deoxyribonucleosides results from complementary effects on thymidine phosphorylase. *Cancer Res* 1994; 54:1472–1476.
23. Ciccolini J, Peillard L, Aubert C, Formento P, Milano G, and Catalin J. Monitoring of the intracellular activation of 5-fluorouracil to deoxyribonucleotides in HT29 human colon cell line: application to modulation of metabolism and cytotoxicity study. *Fundam Clin Pharmacol* 2000; 14:147–154.
24. Ciccolini J, Peillard L, Evrard A, et al. Enhanced antitumor activity of 5-fluorouracil in combination with 2′-deoxyinosine in human colorectal cell lines and human colon tumor xenografts. *Clin Cancer Res* 2000; 6:1529–1535.
25. Patterson AV, Zhang H, Moghaddam A, et al. Increased sensitivity to the prodrug 5′-deoxy-5-fluorouridine and modulation of 5-fluoro-2′-deoxyuridine sensitivity in MCF-7 cells transfected with thymidine phosphorylase. *Br J Cancer* 1995; 72:669–675.
26. Evrard A, Cuq P, Ciccolini J, Vian L, and Cano JP. Increased cytotoxicity and bystander effect of 5-fluorouracil and 5′-deoxy-5-fluorouridine in human colorectal cancer cells transfected with thymidine phosphorylase *Br J Cancer.* 1999; 80:1726–1733.
27. Eda H, Fujimoto K, Watanabe S, et al. Cytokines induce uridine phosphorylase in mouse colon 26 carcinoma cells and make the cells more susceptible to 5′-deoxy-5-fluorouridine. *Jpn J Cancer Res* 1993; 84:341–347.
28. De Bruin, M, Pinedo, HM, Van Capel T, et al. Role of Platelet Derived Endothelial Cell Growth Factor/Thymidine Phosphorylase (PD-ECGF/TP) in Fluoropyrimidine Sensitivity. *Proc Am Assoc Cancer Res* 2001; 42:295 (Abstract 1587).

29. Van Laar JAM, Van der Wilt CL, Smid K, et al. Therapeutic efficacy of fluoropyrimidines depends on the duration of thymidylate synthase inhibition in the murine Colon 26-b carcinoma tumor model. *Clin Cancer Res* 1996; 2:1327–1333.
30. Ashour OM, Naguib FNM, Goudgaon NM, Shinazi RF, El Kouhni MH. Effect of administration of 5-(phenylselenyl)acyclouridine, an inhibitor of uridine phosphorylase on the antitumor efficacy of 5-fluoro-2′-deoxyuridine against murine colon tumor 26-10. *Biochem Pharmacol* 2000; 60:687–692.
31. Koenig H, Patel A. Biochemical basis for fluorouracil neurotoxicity. *Arch Neurology* 1970; 23:155–160.
32. Okeda R, Shibutani M, Matsuo T, Kuroiwa T, Shimokawa R, Tajima T. Experimental neurotoxicity of 5-fluorouracil and its derivatives is due to poisoning by the monofluorinated organic metabolites, monofluoroacetic acid and α-fluoro-β-alanine. *Acta Neuropathologica* 1990; 81:66–73.
33. Sweeny DJ, Barnes S, Heggie G, Diasio RB. Metabolism of 5-fluorouracil to an *N*-cholyl-2-fluoro-β-alanine conjugate: previously unrecognized role for bile acids in drug conjugation. *Proc Nat Acad Sci USA* 1987; 84:5439–5443.
34. Malet-Martino M-C, Bernadou J, Martino R, Armand JP. ^{19}F NMR spectrometry evidence for bile acid conjugates of α-fluoro-β-alanine as the main bilary metabolites of antineoplastic fluoropyrimidines in humans. *Drug Metab Dispos* 1987; 16:78–84.
35. Zhang R, Barnes S, Diasio R. Disposition and Metabolism of 2-Fluoro-beta-Alanine Conjugates of Bile Acids Following Secretion into Bile. *Biochimica et Biophysica Acta* 1991; 1096:179–186.
36. Naguib FNM, El Kouni MH, Cha S. Enzymes of uracil catabolism in normal and neoplastic human tissues. *Cancer Res* 1985; 45:5405–5412.
37. Ho DH, Townsend L, Luna ML, et al. Distribution and inhibition of dihydrouracil dehydrogenase activities in human tissues using 5-fluorouracil as a substrate. *Anticancer Res* 1986; 6:781–784.
38. Wolf W, Presant CA, Servis KL, et al. Tumor trapping of 5-fluorouracil: *in vivo* ^{19}F-NMR spectroscopic pharmacokinetics in tumor-bearing humans and rabbits. *Proc Natl Acad Sci USA* 1990; 87:492–496.
39. Danenberg PV. Thymidylate synthetase – a target enzyme in cancer chemotherapy. *Biochimica et Biophysica Acta* 1977; 473:73–92.
40. Carreras CW, Santi DV. The catalytic mechanism and structure of thymidylate synthase. *Ann Rev Biochem* 1995; 64:721–762.
41. Berger SH, Hakala MT. Relationship of dUMP and FdUMP pools to inhibition of thymidylate synthase by 5-fluorouracil. *Mol Pharmacol* 1984; 25:303–309.
42. Houghton JA, Houghton PJ. Elucidation of pathways of 5-fluorouracil metabolism in xenografts of human colorectal adenocarcinoma. *Eur J Cancer Clin Oncol* 1983; 19:807–815.
43. Jansen G. Receptor- and carrier-mediated transport systems for folates and antifolates. In: Antifolate Drugs in Cancer Therapy. (Jackman, AL, ed,) Humana Press Inc. Totowa, NJ, 1999; pp. 293–321.
44. Van der Wilt CL, Pinedo HM, De Jong M Peters GJ. Effect of folate diastereoisomers on the binding of 5-fluoro-2′-deoxyuridine-5′-monophosphate to thymidylate synthase. *Biochem Pharmacol* 1993; 45:1177–1179.
45. Radparvar S, Houghton PJ, Houghton JA. Effect of polyglutamylation of 5,10-methylenetetrahydrofolate on the binding of 5-fluoro-2′-deoxyuridylate to thymidylate synthase purified from a human colon adenocarcinoma xenograft. *Biochem Pharmacol* 1989; 38:335–342.
46. Wang FS, Aschele C, Sobrero A, Chang YM, Bertino JR. Decreased folylpolyglutamate synthetase expression: a novel mechanism of fluorouracil resistance. *Cancer Res.* 1993; 53:3677–3680.
47. Bapat AR, Zarov C, Danenberg PV. Human leukemic cells resistant to 5-fluoro-2′deoxyuridine contain a thymidylate synthase with lower affinity for nucleotides. *J Biological Chem* 1983; 258:4130–4136.
48. Priest DG, Ledford SE, Doig MT. Increased thymidylate synthetase in 5-fluorodeoxy-uridine resistant cultured hepatoma cells. *Biochem Pharmacol* 1980; 29:1549–1553.
49. Berger SH, Barbour KW, Berger FG. A naturally occurring variation in thymidylate synthase structure is associated with a reduced response to 5-fluoro-2′-deoxyuridine in a human colon tumor cell line. *Mol Pharmacol* 1988; 34:480–484.
50. Spears CP, Gustavsson BG, Berne M, Frosing R, Bernstein L, Hayes AA. Mechanisms of innate resistance to thymidylate synthase inhibition after 5-fluorouracil. *Cancer Res* 1988; 48:5894–5900.
51. Yin MB, Zakrzewski SF, Hakala MT. Relationship of cellular folate cofactor pools to the activity of 5-fluorouracil. *Mol Pharmacol* 1983; 23:190–197.
52. Peters GJ, Van der Wilt CL, Van Groeningen CJ, Meijer S, Smid K, Pinedo HM. Thymidylate synthase inhibition after administration of 5-fluorouracil with or without leucovorin; implications for treatment with 5-fluorouracil. *J Clin Oncol* 1994; 12:2035–2042.
53. Jenh CH, Geyer PK, Baskin F, Johnson LF. Thymidylate synthase gene amplification in fluorodeoxyuridine-resistant mouse cell lines. *Mol Pharmacol* 1985; 28:80–84.

54. Berger SH, Jenh CH, Johnson LF, Berger FG. Thymidylate synthase overproduction and gene amplification in fluorodeoxyuridine-resistant human cells. *Mol Pharmacol* 1985; 28:461–467.
55. Clark JL, Berger SH, Mittelman A, Berger FG. Thymidylate synthase overproduction gene amplification in a colon tumor resistant to fluoropyrimidine chemotherapy. *Cancer Treatment Rep* 1987; 71:261–265.
56. Navelgund LG, Rossana C, Muench AJ, Johnson LF. Cell cycle regulation of thymidylate synthetase gene expression in cultured mouse fibroblasts. *J Biol Chem* 1980; 255:7386–7390.
57. Peters GJ, Smitskamp-Wilms E, Smid K, Pinedo HM, Jansen G. Determinants of activity of the antifolate thymidylate synthase inhibitors Tomudex (ZD1694) and GW1843U89 against mono- and multilayered colon cancer cell lines under folate-restricted conditions. *Cancer Res* 1999; 59:5529–5535.
58. Chu E, Koeller D, Casey J, et al. Autoregulation of Human Thymidylate Synthase Messenger RNA Translation by Thymidylate Synthase. *Proc Natl Acad Sci USA* 1991; 88:8977–8981.
59. Chu E, Voeller DM, Jones KL. Identification of a thymidylate synthase ribonucleoprotein complex in human colon cancer cells. *Mol Cell Biol.* 1993; 14:207–213.
60. Keyomarsi K, Samet J, Molnar G, Pardee AB. The thymidylate synthase inhibitor, ICI-D1694, overcomes translational detainment of the enzyme. *J Biol Chem* 1993; 268:15142–15149.
61. Kitchens ME, Forsthoefel AM, Barbour KW, Rafique Z, Spencer HT, Berger FG. Ligand-mediated induction of thymidylate synthase occurs by enzyme stabilization. Implications for autoregulation of translation. *J. Biol. Chem.* 1999; 274:12544–12547.
62. Chu E, Allegra CJ. The role of thymidylate synthase as an RNA binding protein. *Bioassays* 1996; 18:191–198.
63. Lee Y, Johnson LF, Chang LS, Chen Y. Inhibition of mouse thymidylate synthase promoter activity wild-type p53 tumor suppressor protein. *Exper Cell Res* 1997; 234:270–276.
64. Chu E, Koeller D M, Johnston PG, Zinn S, Allegra CJ. Regulation of Thymidylate Synthase in Human Colon Cancer Cells Treated with 5-Fluorouracil and Interferon-gamma. *Mol Pharmacol* 1993; 43:527–533.
65. Van der Wilt CL, Pinedo HM, Smid K, Peters GJ. Elevation of thymidylate synthase following 5-fluorouracil treatment is prevented by the addition of leucovorin in murine colon tumors. *Cancer Res* 1992; 52:4922–4928.
66. Codacci-Pisanelli G, Van der Wilt CL, Pinedo HM, et al. Antitumor activity, toxicity and inhibition of thymidylate synthase of prolonged administration of 5-fluorouracil in mice. *Eur J Cancer* 1995; 31A:1517–1525.
67. Codacci-Pisanelli G, Van der Wilt CL, Smid K, et al. High-dose 5-fluorouracil with uridine-diphosphoglucose rescue increases thymidylate synthase inhibition but not 5-fluorouracil incorporation into RNA in murine tumors. *Oncology* 2002; 62:363–370.
68. Peters GJ, Van der Wilt CL, Van Groeningen CJ, et al. Effect of different leucovorin formulations on 5-fluorouracil induced thymidylate synthase inhibition in colon tumors and normal tissues from patients in relation to response to 5-fluorouracil. In: Chemistry and Biology of Pteridines and Folates (Proc. 11th International Symposium; W. Pfleiderer and H. Rokos eds.), Blackwell Science, Berlin, 1997; pp. 145–150.
69. Swain SM, Lippman ME, Egan EF, Drake JC, Steinberg SM, Allegra CJ. Fluorouracil and high-dose leucovorin in previously treated patients with metastatic breast cancer. *J Clin Oncol* 1989; 7:890–899.
70. Mandel HG. The target cell determinants of the antitumor actions of 5-FU: does FU incorporation into RNA play a role. *Cancer Treatment Rep* 1981; 65:63–71.
71. Cory JG, Breland JC, Carter GL. Effect of 5-fluorouracil on RNA metabolism in Novikoff hepatoma cells. *Cancer Res* 1979; 39:4905–4913.
72. Spiegelman S, Sawyer R, Nayak R, Ritzi E, Stolfi R, Martin DS Improving the antitumor activity of 5-fluorouracil by increasing its incorporation into RNA via metabolic modulation. *Proc Natl Acad Sci USA* 1980; 77:4966–4970.
73. Houghton JA, Houghton PJ, Wooten RS. Mechanism of induction of the gastrointestinal toxicity in the mouse by 5-fluorouracil, 5-fluorouridine and 5-fluoro-2'-deoxyuridine. *Cancer Res* 1979; 39:2406–2413.
74. Glazer RI, Hartman KD. The effect of 5-fluorouracil on the synthesis and methylation of low molecular weight RNA in L1210 cells. *Mol Pharmacol* 1980; 17:245–249.
75. Will CL, Dolnick BJ. 5-fluorouracil augmentation of dihydrofolate reductase gene transcripts containing intervening sequences in methotrexate-resistant KB cells. *Mol Pharmacol* 1986; 29:643–648.
76. Ghosal K, Jacob ST. An alternative molecular mechanism of action of 5-fluorouracil, a potent anticancer drug. *Biochem Pharmacol* 1997; 53:1569–1575.
77. Hryniuk WM, Figueredo A, Goodyear M. Applications of dose intensity to problems in chemotherapy of breast and colorectal cancer. *Semin Oncol* 1987; 14 (supp.14):3–11.
78. Gamelin E, Boisdron-Celle M, Delva R, et al. Long-term weekly treatment of colorectal metastatic cancer with fluorouracil and leucovorin: results of a multicentric prospective trial of fluorouracil dosage optimization by pharmacokinetic monitoring in 152 patients. *J Clin Oncol* 1998; 16:1470–1478.

79. Ren Q, Van Groeningen CJ, Hardcastle A, et al. Determinants of cytotoxicity with prolonged exposure to fluorouracil in human colon cancer cells. *Oncol Res* 1997; 9:77–88.
80. Peters GJ, Van Dijk J, Laurensse E, et al. *In vitro* biochemical and *in vivo* biological studies of uridne "rescue" of 5-fluorouracil. *Br J Cancer* 1988; 57:259–265.
81. Sawyer RC, Stolfi RL, Martin DS, Spiegelman S. Incorporation of 5-fluorouracil into murine bone marrow DNA in vivo. *Cancer Res* 1984; 44:1847–1851.
82. Aherne GW, and Brown S. The role of uracil misincorporation in thymineless death. In: Antifolate Drugs in Cancer Therapy. (Jackman, AL, ed.), Humana Press Inc. Totowa, NJ, 1999; pp.409–421.
83. Curtin NJ, Harris AL, Aherne GW Mechanism of cell death following thymidylate synthase inhibition: 2′-deoxyuridine-5′-triphosphate accumulation, DNA damage, and growth inhibition following exposure to CB3717 and dipyridamole. *Cancer Res* 1991; 51:2346–2352.
84. Aherne GW, Hardcastle A, Raynaud F, Jackman AL. Immunoreactive dUMP and TTP pools as an index of thymidylate synthase inhibition; effect of tomudex (ZD1694) and a nonpolyglutamated quinazoline antifolate (CB30900) in L1210 mouse leukaemia cells. *Biochem Pharmacol* 1996; 51:1293–1301.
85. Canman CE, Lawrence TS, Shewach DS, Tang HY, Maybaum J. Resistance to Fluorodeoxyuridine-Induced DNA Damage and Cytotoxicity Correlates with an Elevation of Deoxyuridine Triphosphatase Activity and Failure to Accumulate Deoxyuridine Triphosphate. *Cancer Res* 1993; 53:5219–5224.
86. Canman CE, Radany EH, Parsels LA, Davis MA, Lawrence TS, Maybaum J. Induction of resistance to fluorodeoxyuridine cytotoxicity and DNA damage in human tumor cells by expression of Escherichia coli deoxyuridinetriphosphatase. *Cancer Res* 1994; 54:2296–2298.
87. Webley SD, Hardcastle A, Ladner RD, Jackman AL, Aherne GW. Deoxyuridine triphosphatase (dUTPase) expression and sensitivity to the thymidylate synthase (TS) inhibitor ZD9331. *Br J Cancer* 2000; 83:792–799.
88. Noordhuis P, Van Groeningen CJ, Holwerda U, et al. Potential Role of 5-Fluorouracil (5-FU) Incorporation into RNA and DNA of Murine and Human Colon Tumors. Proc. *Am Soc Cancer Res* 2001; 42:295 (Abstract 1586)
89. Shuetz JD, Diasio RB. The effect of 5-fluourouracil on DNA chain elongation in intact bone marrow cells. *Biochem Biophys Res Commun* 1985; 133:361–367.
90. Ayasawa D, Shimizu K, Koyama H, Takeishi K, Seno T. Accumulation of DNA strand breaks during thymineless death in thymidylate synthase-negative mutants of mouse FM3A cells. *J Biol Chem* 1988; 258:12448–12454.
91. Houghton JA, Harwood FG, Houghton PG. Cell cycle control processes determine cytostasis or cytotoxicity in thymineless death of colon cancer cells. *Cancer Res* 1994; 54:4967–4973.
92. Houghton JA, Harwood FG, Tillman DM. Thymineless death in colon carcinoma cels is mediated via Fas signalling. *Proc Nat Acad Sci USA* 1997; 94:8144–8149.
93. Houghton JA, Harwood FG, Bibson AA, Tillman DM. The Fas signaling pathway is functional in colon carcinoma cells and induces apoptosis. *Clin Cancer Res* 1997; 3:2205–2209.
94. Tamura T, Aoyama N, Saya H, et al. Induction of Fas-mediated apoptosis in p53-transfected human colon carcinoma cells. *Oncogene* 1995; 11:1939–1946.
95. Backus HHJ, Wouters D, Koudijs M, et al. Regulation of thymidylate synthase (TS) and the Fas receptor (Fas-R)-Fas ligand (Fas-L) pathway in p53 transfected colon cancer cell lines. *Proc Am Assoc Cancer Res* 2000; 41:853 (Abstract 5421)
96. Backus HHJ, Dukers DF, Vos W, et al. 5-Fluorouracil induced Fas upregulation associated with apoptosis in liver metastases of colorectal cancer patients. *Ann Oncol* 2001; 12:209–216.
97. Houghton JA, Morton CL, Adkins DA, et al. Locus of the Interaction Among 5-Fluorouracil, Leucovorin, and Interferon-alpha-2A in Colon Carcinoma Cells. *Cancer Res* 1993; 53:4243–4250.
98. Van der Wilt CL, Smid K, Noordhuis P, Aherne GW, and Peters GJ. Biochemical mechanisms of interferon modulation of 5-fluorouracil activity in colon cancer cells. *Eur J Cancer* 1997; 33:471–478.
99. Myers CE. The pharmacology of fluoropyrimidines. *Pharmacol Reviews* 1981; 33:1–15.
100. Diasio TL, Harris BE. Clinical pharmacology of 5-fluorouracil. *Clin Pharma* 1989; 6:215–237.
101. Peters GJ, Schornagel J, Milano GA. Clinical pharmacokinetics of antimetabolites. *Cancer Surveys* 1993; 17:123–1156.
102. Ensminger WD, Rosowsky A, Raso V, et al. A clinical pharmacologic evaluation of hepatic arterial infusion of 5-fluoro-2′-deoxyuridine and 5-fluorouracil. *Cancer Res* 1978; 38:3784–3792.
103. El Sayed YM, Sadée W. The fluoropyrimidines. In: pharmacokinetics of anticancer agents in humans (MM Ames, G. Powis, Js Kovach eds.) Elsevier Science Publishers BV, Amsterdam, The Netherlands, 1983; 209–227.

104. Collins JM, Dedrick RL, King FG, Speyer JL, Myers CE. Non-linear pharmacokinetic models for 5-fluorouracil in man. *Clin Pharmacol Therap* 1980; 28:235–246.
105. Van Groeningen CJ, Pinedo HM, Heddes J, et al. Pharmacokinetics of 5-fluorouracil assessed with a sensitive mass spectrometric method in patients during a dose escalation schedule. *Cancer Research* 1988; 48:6956–6961.
106. Peters GJ, Noordhuis P, Komissarov A, et al. Quantification of 5-fluorouracil incorporation into RNA of human and murine tumors as measured with a sensitive gas-chromatography-mass spectrometry assay. *Anal. Biochem.* 1995; 231:157–163.
107. De Bruijn EA, Van Oosterom AT, Tjaden UR, Reeuwijk HJEM, Pinedo HM. Pharmacology of 5′-deoxy-5-fluorouridine in patients with resistant ovarian cancer. *Cancer Res* 1985; 45:5931–5935.
108. Harris BE, Song R, Soong S-J, Diasio RB. Relationship between dihydropyrimidine dehydrogenase activity and plasma 5-fluorouracil levels with evidence for circadian variation of enzyme activity and plasma drug levels in cancer patients receiving 5-fluorouracil by protracted continuous infusion. *Cancer Res* 1990; 50:197–201.
109. Fleming RA, Milano G, Thyss A, et al. Correlation between dihydropyrimidine dehydrogenase activity in peripheral mononuclear cells and systemic clearance of fluorouracil in cancer patients. *Cancer Res* 1992; 52:2899–2902.
110. El Kouni MH, Naguib FNM, Park KS, et al. Circadian Rhythm of Hepatic Uridine Phosphorylase Activity and Plasma Concentration of Uridine in Mice. *Biochem Pharmacol* 1990; 40:2479–2485.
111. Naguib FNM, Soong S-J, El Kouni MH. Circadian rhythm of orotate phosphoribosyltransferase, pyrimidine nucleoside phosphorylases and dihydrouracil dehydrogenase in mouse liver: possible relevance to chemotherapy with 5-fluoropyrimidines. *Biochem Pharmacol* 1993; 45:667–673.
112. Grem JL, Yee LK, Venzon DJ, et al. Inter- and intrainvidual variation in dihydropyrimidine dehydrogenase activity in peripheral blood mononuclear cells. *Cancer Chemother Pharmacol* 1997; 40:117–125.
113. Van Kuilenburg ABP, Poorter RL, Peters GJ, et al. No circadian variation of dihydropyrimidine dehydrogenase, uridine phosphorylase, β-alanine and 5-fluorouracil during continuous infusion of 5-fluoruoracil. *Adv Exp Med Biol* 1998; 431:811–816.
114. Roemeling RV, Hrushesky WJM. Circadian pattern of continuous FUDR infusion reduces toxicities. In: *Adv Chronobiology* 1987; Part B:357–373.
115. Lévi F, Zidani R, Misset J-L, for the International Organization for Cancer Chronotherapy Randomised multicentre trial of chronotherapy with oxaliplatin, fluorouracil, and folinic acid in metastatic colorectal cancer. *Lancet* 1997; 350:681–686.
116. Miwa M, Ura M, Nishida M, et al. Design of a novel oral fluoropyrimidine carbamate, capecitabine, which generates 5-fluorouracil selectively in tumours by enzymes concentrated in human liver and cancer tissue. *Eur J Cancer* 1998; 34:1274–1281.
117. Ackland SP, Peters GJ. Thymidine phosphorylase: Its role in sensitivity and resistance to anticancer drugs. *Drug Resistance Updates* 1999; 2:205–214.
118. Woodcock TM, Martin DS, Damin LAM, et al. Combination clinical trials with thymidine and fluorouracil: a phase I and clinical pharmacological evaluation. *Cancer* 1980; 45:1135–1143.
119. Engelbrecht C, Lungquist I, Lewan L, et al. Modulation of 5-fluorouracil metabolism by thymidine in vivo and in vitro studies on RNA-directed effects in rat liver and rat hepatoma. *Biochem Pharmacol* 1984; 33:745–750.
120. Humerickhouse RA, Dolan ME, Haraf DJ, et al. Phase I study of eniluracil, a dihydropyrimidine dehydrogenase inactivator, and oral 5-fluorouracil with radiation therapy in patients with recurrent or advanced head and neck cancer. *Clin Cancer Res* 1999; 5:291–298.
121. Reigner B, Verweij J, Dirix L, et al. Effect of food on the pharmacokinetics of capecitabine and its metabolites following oral administration in cancer patients. *Clin Cancer Res* 1998; 4:941–948.
122. Schilsky RL, Hohneker J, Ratain MJ, et al. Phase I clinical and pharmacologic study of eniluracil plus fluorouracil in patients with advanced cancer. *J Clin Oncol* 1998; 16:1450–1457.
123. Hirata K, Horikoshi N, Okazaki M, et al. Pharmacokinetic study of S-1, a novel oral fluorouracil anti-tumor drug. *Clin Cancer Res* 1999; 5:2000–2005.
124. Van Groeningen CJ, Peters GJ, Schornagel JH, et al. Phase I clinical and pharmacokinetic study of oral S-1 in patients with advanced solid tumors. *J Clin Oncol* 2000; 18:2772–2779.
125. Peters GJ, Ackland SP. New antimetabolites in preclinical and clinical development. *Expert Opinion Invest Drugs* 1996; 5:637–679.
126. Porter DJT, Chestnut WG, Merrill BM, et al. Mechanism-based inactivation of dihydropyrimidine dehydrogenase by 5-ethynyluracil. *J Biol Chem* 1992; 267:5236–5242.

127. Spector T, Porter DJT, Nelson DJ. 5-Ethynyluracil (776C85), a modulator of the therapeutic activity of 5-fluorouracil. *Drugs Future* 1994; 19:565–571.
128. Baccanari DP, Davis ST, Knick VC et al. 5-Ethynyluracil: Effects on the pharmacokinetics and antitumor activity of 5-fluorouracil. *Proc Natl Acad Sci USA* 1993; 90:11064–11068.
129. Cao S, Rustum YM, Spector T. 5-Ethynyluracil (77C85): modulation of 5-fluorouracil efficacy and therapeutic index in rats bearing advanced colorectal carcinoma. *Cancer Res* 1994; 54:1507–1510.
130. Unemi N, Takeda S, Tajima K, et al. Studies on combination therapy with 1-(tetrahydro-2 furanyl)-5-fluorouracul plus uracil. I. Effect of coadministration of uracil on the antitumor activity of 1-(tetrahydro-2-furanyl)-5-fluorouracil and the level of 5-fluorouracil in AH 130 bearing rats. *Chemotherapy* 1981; 29:164–175.
131. Komatsu T, Yamazaki H, Shimada N, et al. Involvement of microsomal cytochrome P450 and cytosolic thymidine phosphorylase in 5-fluorouracil formation from tegafur in human liver. *Clin Cancer Res* 2001; 7:675–681.
132. Naguib FN, El Kouhni MH, Cha S. Structure-activity relationship of ligands of dihydrouracil dehydrogenase from mouse liver. *Biochem Pharmacol.* 1989; 38:1471–1480.
133. Ikenaka K, Shirasaka T, Kitano S, Fujii, S. Effect of uracil on metabolism of 5-fluorouracil in vitro. *Gann* 1979; 70:353–359.
134. Yamamoto J, Toide K, Haruno A, Yoshimura Y, Unemi N. General pharmacological properties of UFT, a new type of anti-cancer agent consisting of 1-(2-tetrahydrofuryl)-5-fluorouracil (FT) and uracil. I: Pharmacological analysis of the combined effect of FT and uracil. *Arzneimittelforschung* 1981; 31:1268–1278.
135. Taguchi T, Nakano Y, Fujii S, Shirasaka, T. Determination of 5-fluorouracil levels in tumors, blood, and other tissues. *Jpn J Cancer Chemother* 1978; 5:1167–1172.
136. Fujii S, Ikenada K, Fukushima M, Shirasaka, T. Effect of uracil and its derivatives on antitumor activity of 5-fluorouracil and 1-(2-tetrahydrofuryl)-5-fluorouracil. *Gann* 1978; 69:763–772.
137. Cao S, Frank C, Shirasaka, T, Rustum YM. 5-Fluorouracil Prodrug: Role of Anabolic and Catabolic Pathway Modulation in Therapy of Colorectal Cancer. *Clin Cancer Res* 1995; 1:839–845.
138. Takechi T, Nakano K, Uchida J, et al. Antitumor activity and low intestinal toxicity of S-1, a new formulation of oral tegafor, in experimental tumor models in rats. *Cancer Chemother Pharmacol* 1977; 39:205–211.
139. Tatsumi K, Fukushima M, Shirasaka T, et al. Inhibitory Effects of Pyrimidine, Barbituric Acid and Pyridine Derivatives on 5-Fluorouracil Degradation in Rat Liver Extracts. *Jpn J Cancer Res* (GANN) 1987; 78:748–755.
140. Yoshisue K, Masuda H, Matsushima E, et al. Tissue distribution and biotransformation of potassium oxonate after oral administration of a novel antitumor agent (drug combination of tegafur, 5-chloro-2,4-dihydroxypyridine, and potassium oxonate) to rats. *Drug Metab Dispos.* 2000; 28:1162–1167.
141. Shirasaka T, Shimamoto Y, Fukushima M. Inhibition by oxonic acid of gastrointestinal toxicity of 5-fluorouracil without loss of its antitumor activity in rats. *Cancer Res* 1993; 53:4004–4009.
142. Fukushima M, Shimamoto Y, Kato T, et al. Anticancer activity and toxicity of S-1, an oral combination of tegafur and two biochemical modulators, compared with continuous i.v. infusion of 5-fluorouracil. *Anticancer Drugs* 1998; 9:817–823.
143. Van der Wilt CL, Marinelli A, Pinedo HM, et al. The effect of different routes of administration of 5-fluorouracil on thymidylate synthase inhibition in the rat. *Eur J Cancer* 1995; 31A:754–760.
144. Van der Wilt CL, Van Groeningen CJ, Pinedo HM, et al. 5-Fluorouracil/leucovorin-induced inhibition of thymidylate synthase in normal tissues of mouse and man. *J Cancer Res Clin Oncol* 1999; 123:595–601.
145. Yoshisue K, Hironaga K, Yamaguchi S, Yamamoto A, Nagayama S, Kawaguchi Y. Reduction of 5-fluorouracil (5-FU) gastrointestinal (GI) toxicity resulting from the protection of thymidylate synthase (TS) in GI tissue by repeated simultaneous administration of potassium oxonate (Oxo) in rats. *Cancer Chemother Pharmacol* 2000; 46:51–56.
146. Fujita H, Okamoto M, Takao A, et al. Preclinical studies of S-1, a new oral tegafur, plus modulators: pharmacokinetics. *Recent Adv Chemother Proc Int Congr Chemotherapy* 1993; 928–929.
147. Tsunoda A, Shibusawa M, Tsunoda Y, et al. Antitumor effect of S-1 on DMH induced colon cancer in rats. *Anticancer Res.* 1998; 18:1137–1141.
148. Nishimura G, Yanoma S, Mizuno H, et al. Therapeutic effect of 1 M tegafur-0.4 M 5-chloro-2, 4-dihydroxypridine-1 M potassium oxonate (S-1) on head and neck squamous carcinoma cells. *Cancer Lett* 2000; 159:1–7.
149. Shirasaka T, Nakano K, Takechi T, et al. Antitumor activity of 1 M tegafur-0.4 M 5-chloro-2,4-dihydroxypyridine-1 M potassium oxonate (S-1) against human colon carcinoma orthotopically implanted into nude rats. *Cancer Res* 1996; 56:2602–2606.

150. Fukushima M, Satake H, Uchida J, et al. Preclinical antitumor efficacy of S-1: a new oral formulation of 5-fluorouracil on human tumor xenografts. *Int J Oncol* 1998; 13:693–698.
151. Kitamura M, Arai K, Iwasaki Y, et al. [Combined effect of S-1 and CDDP as a modulator for colon 26 liver metastasis]. *Gan To Kagaku Ryoho* 2000; 27:559–563.
152. Cao S, Lu K, Toth K, Slocum HK, Shirasaka T, Rustum YM. Persistent inducion of apoptosis and suppression of mitosis as the basis for curative therapy with S-1, an oral 5-fluorouracil prodrug in a colorectal tumor model. *Clin Cancer Res* 1999; 5:267–274.
153. Kindler HL, and Schilsky RL. Clinical trials of the Eniluracil/5-fluorouracil combination. In: Fluoropyrimidine in Cancer Therapy (Y.M. Rustum, ed.). Humana Press Inc., Totowa, 2002, pp. 235–247.
154. Peters GJ, Noordhuis P, Van der Born K, et al. Limited 5-Fluorouracil (5FU) Pharmacokinetics (PK) in EORTC/ECSG Phase II Clinical Trials of S-1; Disease-Dependent Relation with Toxicity. *Proc Am Assoc Cancer Res* 2001; 42:698 (Abstract 3753).
155. Vermorken JB, Schoffski P Schellens J, et al. S-1 in colorectal cancer (CRC): Interim results of an early phase II study. *Ann Oncol* 2000; 11:(Suppl 4), 60:(abstract 262P).
156. Chollet P, Schoffski P, Weigang K, et al. Phase II study with S-1 in patients with advanced gastric cancer. Proc 11th NCI-EORTC-AACR meeting, 2000. *Clin Cancer Res* 6(Supp), 2000; 129(#430).
157. Shimada T, Yamazaki H, Guengerich P. Ethnic-related differences in coumarin 7-hydroxylation activities catalyzed by cytochrome P4502A6 in liver microsomes of Japanese and Caucasian populations. *Xenobiotica* 1996; 26:395–405.
158. Noordhuis P, Peters GJ, Van Groeningen CJ, et al. The effect of food on the pharmacokinetcs (pk) of s-1 after single oral administration to patients with solid tumors. *Proc Am Assoc Cancer Res* 2000; 41:492. (Abstract 3137).
159. Sugimachi K, Maehara Y, Horikoshi N, et al. An early phase II study of oral S-1, a newly developed 5-fluorouracil derivative for advanced and recurrent gastrointestinal cancers. The S-1 *Gastrointestinal Cancer Study Group. Oncology* 1999; 57:202–210.
160. Koizumi W, Kurihara M, Nakano S, Hasegawa K. Phase II study of S-1, a novel oral derivative of 5-fluorouracil, in advanced gastric cancer. For the S-1 Cooperative *Gastric Cancer Study Group Oncology* 2000; 58:191–197.
161. Ohtsu A, Baba H, Sakata Y, et al. Phase II study of S-1, a novel oral fluorophyrimidine derivative, in patients with metastatic colorectal carcinoma. S-1 Cooperative Colorectal Carcinoma Study Group. *Br J Cancer* 2000; 83:141–145.
162. Sakata Y, Ohtsu A, Horikoshi N, Sugimachi K, Mitachi Y, Taguchi T. Late phase II study of novel oral fluoropyrimidine anticancer drug S-1 (1 M tegafur-0.4 M gimestat-1 M otastat potassium) in advanced gastric cancer patients. *Eur J Cancer* 1998; 34:1715–1720.
163. Taguchi T, Morimoto K, Horikoshi N, et al. [An early phase II clinical study of S-1 in patients with breast cancer. S-1 Cooperative Study Group (Breast Cancer Working Group)]. *Gan To Kagaku Ryoho* 1998; 25:1035–1043.
164. Inuyama Y, Kida A, Tsukuda M, Kohno N, Satake B. Early phase II study of S-1 in patients with advanced head and neck cancer. S-1 Cooperative Study Group (Head and Neck Working Group)] *Gan To Kagaku Ryoho* 1998; 25:1151–1158.
165. Martin DS. Biochemical modulation: perspectives and objectives. In: Harrap KR, Connors TA, (eds.) in Proc. 8th Bristol-Myers Symp. on Cancer Res. New Avenues in Developmental Cancer Chemother. Academic Press, London, 1987; 113–162.
166. Ardalan B, Singh G, Silberman H. A randomized Phase I and II study of Short-Term infusion of high-dose fluorouracil with or without N-(phosphonacetyl)-L-Aspartic acid in patients with advanced pancreatic colorectal cancers. *J Clin Oncol* 1988; 6:1053–1058.
167. O'Dwyer PJ, Paul AR, Walczak J, Weiner LM, S, Comis RL. Phase II study of biochemical modulation of fluorouracil by low dose PALA in patients with colorectal cancer. *J Clin Oncol* 1990; 8:1497–1503.
168. Kemeny N, Conti JA, Seiter K, et al, Biochemical modulation of bolus fluorouracil by PALA in patients with advanced colorectal cancer. *J Clin Oncol* 1992; 10:747–752.
169. Leichman CG, Fleming TR, Muggia FM, et al. Phase II study of fluorouracil and its modulation in advanced colorectal cancer: a Southwest Oncology Group study. *J Clin Oncol* 1995; 13:1303–1311.
170. Van der Wilt CL, Braakhuis BJM, Pinedo HM, De Jong M, Smid K, Peters GJ. Addition of leucovorin in modulation of 5-fluorouracil with methotrexate: potentiating or reversing effect? *Inter J Cancer* 1995; 61:672–678.
171. Jackson RC. Unresolved issues in the biochemical pharmacology of antifolates. *NCI Monographs* 1989; 5:9–15.
172. Westerhof GR, Schornagel JH, Kathmann I, et al. Carrier- and receptor-mediated transport of folate antagonists targeting folate-dependent enzymes: correlates of moleculare structure and biological activity. *Mol Pharmacol.* 1995; 48:659–671.

173. Romanini A, Li WW, Colofiore JR, Bertino JR. Leucovorin enhances cytotoxicity of trimetrexate/fluorouracil, but not methotrexate/fluorouracil, in CCRF-CEM cells. *J Nat Cancer Instit* 1992; 84:1033–1038.
174. Conti JA, Kemeny N, Seiter K, et al. Trial of sequential trimetrexate, fluorouracil, and high-dose leucovorin in previously treated patients with gastrointestinal carcinoma. *J Clin Oncol* 1994; 12:695–700.
175. Blanke CD, Kasimis B, Schein P, Capizzi R, Kurman M. Phase II study of trimetrexate, fluorouracil, and leucovorin for advanced colorectal cancer. *J Clin Oncol* 1997; 15:915–920.
176. Martin DS, Stolfi RL, Sawyer RC, et al. High-dose 5-fluorouracil with delayed uridine "rescue" in mice. *Cancer Res* 1982; 42:3964–3970.
177. Nord LD, Stolfi RL, Martin DS. Biochemical modulation of 5-fluorouracil with leucovorin or delayed uridine rescue – correlation of antitumor activity with dosage and FUra incorporation into RNA. *Biochem Pharmacol* 1992; 43:2543–2549.
178. Nadal JC, Van Groeningen CJ, Pinedo HM, Peters GJ. Schedule-dependency of in vivo modulation of 5-fluorouracil by leucovorin and uridine in murine colon carcinoma, *Investigational New Drugs* 1989; 7:163–172.
179. Colofiore JR, Sawyer RC, Balis ME, Martin DS. Effect of uridine diphosphoglucose on levels of 5-phosphoribosyl pyrophosphate and uridine triphosphate in murine tissues. *Pharm Res* 1989; 6:863–866.
180. Codacci-Pisanelli, G., Kralovansky, J., Van der Wilt, C.L., et al. Modulation of 5-fluorouracil in mice using uridine diphosphoglucose. *Clin Cancer Res* 1997; 3:309–315.
181. Leyva A, Van Groeningen CJ, Kraal I, et al. Phase I and pharmacokinetic studies of high-dose uridine intended for rescue from 5-fluorouracil toxicity. *Cancer Res* 1984; 44:5928–5933.
182. Peters GJ, Van Groeningen CJ, Laurensse E, Kraal I, Leyva A, Lankelma J, Pinedo HM. Effect of pyrimidine nucleosides on body temperature of man and rabbit in relation to pharmacokinetic data. *Pharmaceut Res* 1987; 4:113–119.
183. Van Groeningen CJ, Leyva A, Kraal I, Peters GJ & Pinedo HM. Clinical and pharmacokinetic study of prolonged administration of high-dose uridine intended for rescue from 5-fluorouracil toxicity. *Cancer Treatm Rep* 1986; 70:745–750.
184. Van Groeningen CJ, Peters GJ, Leyva A, Laurensse EJ, Pinedo HM. Reversal of 5-fluorouracil-induced myelosuppression by prolonged administration of high-dose uridine. *J Nat Cancer Instit* 1989; 81:157–162.
185. Seiter K, Kemeny N, Martin D, et al. Uridine Allows Dose Escalation of 5-Fluorouracil When Given with N-Phosphonacetyl-L-Aspartate, Methotrexate, and Leucovorin. *Cancer* 1993; 71:1875–1881.
186. Schwartz GK, Christman K, Saltz L, et al. A phase I trial of a modified, dose intensive FAMTX regimen (high dose 5-fluorouracil+doxorubicin+high dose methotrexate+leucovorin) with oral uridine rescue. *Cancer* 1996; 78:1988–1995.
187. Bagrij T, Kralovanszky J, Gyergyay F, Kiss E, Peters GJ. Influence of Uridine Treatment in Mice on the Protection of Gastrointestinal Toxicity Caused by 5-Fluorouracil. *Anticancer Res* 1993; 13:789–794.
188. Klubes P, Leyland-Jones B. Enhancement of the antitumor activity of 5-fluorouracil by uridine rescue. *Pharmacol Ther* 1989; 41:289–302.
189. Martin DS, Stolfi RL, Sawyer RC. Use of oral uridine as a substitute for parenteral uridine rescue of 5-fluorouracil therapy, with and without the uridine phosphorylase inhibitor 5-benzylacyclouridine. *Cancer Chemother Pharmacol* 1989; 24:9–14.
190. Van Groeningen CJ, Peters GJ, Nadal JC, Laurensse EJ, Pinedo HM. Clinical and pharmacologic study of orally administered uridine. *J Natl Cancer Inst* 1991; 83:437–441.
191. Van Groeningen CJ, Peters GJ, Pinedo HM. Reversal of 5-fluorouracil-induced toxicity by oral administration of uridine. *Annals of Oncol* 1993; 4:317–320.
192. Kelsen DP, Martin D, O'Neil J, et al. Phase I trial of PN401, an oral prodrug of uridine, to prevent toxicity from fluorouracil in patients with advanced cancer. *J Clin Oncol* 1997; 15:1511–1517.
193. Pritchard DM, Watson AJM, Potten CS, Jackman AL, Hickman JA. Inhibition of uridine but not thymidine of p53-dependent intestinal apoptosis initiated by 5-fluorouracil: evidence of the involvement of RNA perturbation. *Proc Nat Acad Sci USA* 1997; 94:1795–1799.
194. Van der Wilt CL, Peters GJ. New targets for pyrimidine antimetabolites for the treatment of solid tumors. Part 1, thymidylate synthase. *Pharmacy World and Science* 1994; 16:84–103.
195. Peters GJ, Van der Wilt CL, Van Groeningen CJ. Predictive value of thymidylate synthase and dihydropyrimidine dehydrogenase. *Eur J Cancer* 1994; 30A:1408–1411.
196. Spears CP, Shahinian AH, Moran RG, Heidelberg C, Corbett TH. In vivo kinetics of thymidylate synthethase inhibition in 5-fluorouracil-sensitive and -resistant murine colon adenocracinomas. *Cancer Res* 1982; 42:450–456.
197. Houghton HA, Houghton PJ. On the mechanism of cytotoxicity of fluorinated pyrimidines in four human colon adenocarcinoma xenografts maintained in immune-deprived mice. *Cancer* 1980; 45(Suppl):1159–1167.

198. Arbuck SG. Overview of clinical trials using 5-fluorouracil and leucovorin for the treatment of colorectal cancer. *Cancer* 1989; 63:1036–1044.
199. Piedbois P, Buyse M, Rustum Y, et al. Modulation of fluorouracil by leucovorin in patients with advanced colorectal cancer: Evidence in terms of response rate. *J Clin Oncol* 1992; 10:896–903.
200. Kohnewompner CH, Schmoll HJ, Harstrick A, Rustum YM. Chemotherapeutic Strategies in Metastatic Colorectal Cancer – An Overview of Current Clinical Trials. *Semin Oncol* 1992; 19:105–125.
201. Poon MA, O'Connell MJ, Wieand HS, et al. Biochemical modulation of fluorouracil with leucovorin: confirmatory evidence of improved therapeutic efficacy in advanced colorectal cancer. *J Clin Oncol* 1991; 9:1967–1972.
202. Machover D, Grison X, Goldschmidt E, et al. Fluorouracil combined with the pure (6S)-stereoisomer of folinic acid in high doses for treatment of patients with advanced colorectal carcinoma – a phase-I-II study. *J Nat Cancer Instit* 1992; 84:321–327.
203. Meta-Analysis Group in Cancer. Reappraisal of hepatic arterial infusion in the treatment of nonresectable liver metastasis from colorectal cancer. *J Nat Cancer Instit* 1996; 88:252–258.
204. Meta-Analysis Group in Cancer. Efficacy of intravenous continuous infusion of fluorouracil compared with bolus administration in advanced colorectal cancer. *J Clin Oncol* 1998; 16:301–308.
205. Köhne CH, Schöffski P, Wilke H, et al. Effective biomodulation by leucovorin of high dose infusional fluorouracil given as a weekly 24-hour infusion: Results of a randomized trial in patients with advanced colorectal cancer. *J Clin Oncol* 1998; 16:418–426.
206. Van der Wilt CL, Smid K, Peters GJ. Effects of antifolates on the binding of 5-fluoro-2′-deoxyuridine monophosphate to thymidylate synthase. *Biochem Pharmacol.* 2002; 64:669–675.
207. Weichsel A, Montfort WR, Ligand-induced distortion of an active site in thymidylate synthase upon binding anticancer drug 1843U89. *Nat Struct Biol* 1995; 2:1095–1101.
208. Van der Wilt CL, Kuiper CM, Peters GJ. Combination studies of antifolates with 5-fluorouracil in colon cancer cell lines. *Oncol Res* 1999; 11:383–391.
209. Longo GSA, Izzo J, Chang YM, et al. Pretreatment of colon carcinoma cells with Tomudex enhances 5-fluorouracil cytotoxicity. *Clin Cancer Res* 1998; 4:469–473.
210. Peters GJ, Van der Wilt CL, Van Moorsel CJA, Kroep JR, Bergman AM, Ackland SP. Basis for effective combination cancer chemotherapy with antimetabolites. *Pharmacol Ther* 2000; 87:227–253.

2 Dihydropyrimidine Dehydrogenase and Treatment by Fluoropyrimidines

Past and Future Directions

Gérard Milano, PhD

CONTENTS

1. INTRODUCTION

5-Fluorouracil (5-FU) is still one of the most commonly prescribed anticancer drugs, with activity against cancers of the gastrointestinal tract, head and neck, and breast. In addition, new oral 5-FU prodrugs like UFT, S_1, capecitabine are emerging in the arena of the new drugs in oncology *(1,2)*. Thus, treatment by fluoropyrimidines including 5-FU itself or its prodrugs represents a significant part of the chemotherapy agents currently in use or under investigation. The administration of oral fluoropyrimidines underscores the importance of the enzyme dihydropyrimidine dehydrogenase (DPD), which not only controls the catabolic route of 5-FU but also limits its oral absorption *(3)*. In addition, DPD inhibition represents a major objective for the development of oral fluoropyrimidines like UFT and S_1 *(4)*. DPD has highest activity in liver and mononuclear cells, but is also found in most human tissues. The aim of this chapter is to cover the role of DPD in treatment by fluoropyrimidines with considerations on the link between DPD and 5-FU pharmacokinetics, the importance of DPD deficiencies, the existence of DPD circadian rhythm with its clinical consequences, the comparison between DPD genotyping and DPD phenotyping, the role of DPD in 5-FU resistance in vitro and in vivo, and the role of DPD inhibition in the development of new oral fluoropyrimidines.

From: *Fluoropyrimidines in Cancer Therapy*
Edited by: Y. M. Rustum © Humana Press Inc., Totowa, NJ

2. DPD AND PHARMACOKINETICS OF 5-FU

More than 80% of an administered dose of 5-FU is eliminated by catabolism through DPD, the rate-limiting enzyme *(3)*. DPD activity is found in most tissues, exhibiting the highest activity in the liver *(5)*. However, peripheral blood mononuclear cells (PBMC) are used for clinical monitoring of DPD activity, as these cells are obviously more accessible than hepatic tissue. We reported on a significant, but weak ($r^2 = 0.32$), correlation between PBMC and liver DPD activity *(6)*. This observation validates the use of DPD determination in PBMC for estimating the individual capacity to clear 5-FU. It is however important to mention that marked discrepancies may exist between hepatic and PBMC-DPD activity particularly in the case of patients with altered liver function who can exhibit a low DPD activity and a normal PBMC-DPD activity *(7)*. The evidence of an association between DPD activity in PBMC and plasma 5-FU concentration was initially published a decade ago by the group of R. Diaso *(8)*. The relationship between PBMC-DPD activity and 5-FU systemic clearance was then evaluated by Fleming and associates *(9)*. A significant linear correlation was observed between PBMC-DPD activity and 5-FU clearance *(9,10)*. However, this relationship is very weak ($r^2 = 0.10$), and we feel that simply determining PBMC-DPD is not sufficient to accurately predict 5-FU clearance. The NONMEN population pharmacokinetic analysis that we conducted had the aim to identify patient covariables, which could influence interpatient variability in 5-FU clearance *(10)*. 5-FU clearance was significantly reduced by increased age, high serum alkaline phosphatase, length of infusion, and low PBMC-DPD. However, a relatively high error was found in the estimate between observed and predicted 5-FU clearance and thus this multifactorial approach including PBMC-DPD did not allow faithful 5-FU dose adaptation prior to treatment. In addition, DPD activity may vary from one cycle to the other without any evidence of a trend for an increase or decrease during the treatment course *(9)*. McLeod and coworkers conducted a clinical study and an experimental study on laboratory animals, aiming to examine the evolution of DPD activity under 5-FU treatment *(11)*. They found that PBMC-DPD decreased by a median of 39% following the administration of 5-FU ($p = 0.001$). In addition, 5-FU induced alterations in rat liver DPD were noted by these authors with the lowest activity occurring 48 h after drug administration *(11)*. In total, PBMC-DPD–based 5-FU dose adaptation strategy is not justified in our opinion. However, marked 5-FU dose reductions can be proposed for patients showing more or less marked DPD deficiency (*see* below).

3. DPD DEFICIENCIES

Lu and associates *(12)* were the first to provide population data on DPD activity and demonstrated a Gaussian distribution for PBMC-DPD in 124 healthy subjects. Prospective studies on 185 unselected cancer patients and 75 colorectal cancer patients were performed *(13,14)*. In these populations, DPD activity also showed an unimodal distribution and no subject with complete DPD deficiency was identified in these studies. Multifactorial analysis of variance showed that neither liver function tests (biological evaluation) nor age influenced DPD activity. It was also found that DPD activity was, on average, 15% lower in women as compared with men ($p = 0.03$) *(14)*. Interestingly, this 15% difference in DPD activity is the same order as the difference observed in 5-FU clearance between men and women *(15)*. However, in the study by Lu and colleagues, DPD activity was not influenced by sex *(12)*. The discrepancy in the effect of gender on DPD activity between these studies could be explained by the difference in the age range covered, with influences from the hormonal status: Premenopausal women were the majority in the Lu study *(12)* vs postmenopausal women in the majority studied by Etienne and colleagues *(14)*. However, this hypothesis could not be confirmed from the limited set of women studied (n = 33), since no difference in DPD activity was demonstrated between pre- and postmenopausal women. We recently reported PBMC-DPD data concerning a group of 53 patients (23 men, 30 women) *(16)* treated by 5-FU-based chemotherapy in different French institutions and who developed unanticipated 5-FU-related toxicity. Among the whole group of 53 patients, 19 had a significant DPD deficiency (DD; below 150 fmol/min/mg protein, i.e., less than 70% of the mean value observed from previous population study). There was a greater majority of women in the DD group (15 out of 19, 79%) compared with the remaining 34 patients (15 out of 34, 44%, $p < 0.014$). Toxicity was often severe, leading to patient death in two cases (both women). The toxicity score (sum of WHO grading, theoritical range 0–20) was twice as high in patients with marked DD (below 100 pmol/min/mg protein, n = 11, mean score = 13.2) compared with patients with moderate DD (between 150 and 100 pmol/min/mg protein, n = 8, mean score = 6.8), $p = 0.008$. In the DD group, there was a high frequency of neurotoxic syndromes (7 out of 19, 37%). The two deceased patients both had severe neurotoxicity. The occurrence of cardiac toxicity was relatively rare (1 out of 19, 5%). These data confirm that women are particularly prone to DPD deficiency. In total, from these above-discussed studies, it is clear that complete DPD deficiency is a very rare event. However, if we consider the PBMC-DPD value of 100 pmol/min/mg protein as the upper threshold indicative of an increased risk for developing 5-FU-related toxicity *(16)*, one can estimate that approx 3% of an unselected group of cancer patients are located below this threshold value *(14)*. DPD-associated morbidity, and in some cases mortality, among patients who often do not have detectable disease (adjuvant therapy) has great personal and economic implications. It follows that, in our opinion, the practical interest to determine DPD before 5-FU treatment must be carefully weighed in terms of cost–benefit balance. Current methods, requiring PBMC isolation and high performance chromatography analysis, are difficult to apply for general screening. In addition, Van Kuilenburg and colleagues have recently reported on a positive correlation they observed between DPD activity in PBMC and the percentage of monocytes *(17)*. The proportion of monocytes can vary during anticancer treatment, thus the variable proportion of monocytes in PBMC can introduce intra- and interpatient variability in DPD activity determination. An interesting alternative approach to identify DPD deficient patients could be to use surrogate markers like the dihydrouracil (UH_2)–uracil (U) ratio, easy to determine in plasma before treatment; Gamelin and coworkers recently reported on this ratio, which was determined in a group of 81 patients with advanced colorectal cancer receiving weekly infusions of 5-FU–folinic acid *(18)*. They found that the UH_2–U ratio was normally distributed and was correlated to 5-FU clearance (r = 0.64). Interestingly, toxic side effects were observed only in patients with initial UH_2–U ratio of less than 1.8.

4. CIRCADIAN RHYTHM OF DPD

The existence of a circadian rhythm for DPD activity has been suggested from both human and animal investigations *(19)*. Harris and associates *(8)* measured lymphocyte DPD activity and 5-FU plasma concentrations in cancer patients receiving 5-FU by protracted continuous infusion. A circadian rhythm was observed in 5-FU plasma concentrations with a peak observed at 11 AM and a trough at 11 PM on average. The inverse relationship observed between the circadian profile of 5-FU plasma concentration and PBMC-DP activity suggested a link between DPD activity and 5-FU pharmacokinetics. Our group performed a pharmacokinetic study of FU in patients treated by continuous venous infusion of a constant rate for 5 d *(20)*. All patients had stage C blader carcinoma and received *cis*-diamminedichloroplatinum (II) *(45–91)* mg/m^2) on d 1 as 30-min venous infusion at 5 PM. Continuous venous infusion of 5-FU (450–966 mg/m^2/day) was started on d 2 at 8:30 AM via a volumetric pump and lasted for 5 d (until d 6). Blood samples were obtained every 3 h on d 2, d 4, and d 6 on each patient (20 samples/patient). Data were analyzed by both multiple analysis of variance and cosinor. Mean lowest and highest 5-FU plasma concentrations ($\pm$ SEM) were, respectively, 254 $\pm$ 33 ng/mL at 1 PM and 584 $\pm$ 160 ng/mL at 1 AM ($p < 0.03$). Both analysis of variance and cosinor analysis further validated ($p < 0.0001$) a circadian rhythm with a double amplitude (total extent of variation) of 50% of the 24-h mean and an acrophase located at approx 1 AM (estimated time of peak). It was thus felt that circadian modulation of the infusion rate of 5-FU may further optimize the therapeutic index of such treatment modality. Besides continuous venous infusion, the impact of the time of drug administration was also studied for short venous infusions by Nowakowska-Dulawa *(21)*. 5-FU (15 mg/kg) was administered in over 15 min every 4 d for 12 d and this at various times during the day. The authors noted marked differences in pharmacokinetic parameters and clearance value was found to be 70% at 13.00 h as compared to 01.00 h. Several studies have described a wide interindividual variation in peaks and troughs in DPD activity *(22,23)*. More precisely, in the work recently reported Grem and coworkers *(23)* the authors wished to determine whether peak and trough in DPD activity occurred at uniform times in six subjects, whether individual patterns fit a discernible profile and whether such patterns were consistent and reproducible over time. In that purpose mononuclear cells were isolated from peripheral blood at 3-h intervals over a 24-h period on three different dates over a 6-mo period. When the data were averaged by study date for each subject, the median value for the average DPD activity was significantly different from both the median peak and median trough activities. Within the six subjects, the average DPD activity for the three study dates differed by a median of 2.4-fold. The time at which peak and trough DPD activities occurred varied between subjects: 8 of the 17 peaks (47%) occurred between 10:00 PM and 6:00 AM, 6 (35%) occurred between 8:00 AM and 3:00 PM, and 3 (18%) occurred between 5:00 PM and 8:15 PM. Thus, it could be concluded by the authors that the time of day when the peak occurred was essentially randomly distributed over the 24-h period of observation ($p = 0.68$). Sixty percent of the trough DPD activities occurred between 7:00 AM and 3:00 PM. The median interval between the peak and trough was 6.5 h. When the combined data for all cycles was considered, the trough occurred 6–9 h after the peak, and the DPD levels subsequent to the peak did not display merely random variation ($p = 0.0055$). The authors concluded that DPD activity levels and the times at which peak and trough DPD activities occurred varied both between and within subjects. A limitation from this latter study may be the fact that subjects were not synchronized.

5. DPD GENOTYPING VS DPD PHENOTYPING

Chromosome mapping of human *DPYD* gene was first described in 1994 *(24)*. *DPYD* gene is located on chromosome 1 (1p22). *DPYD* gene is a large gene (> 950 kb) containing 23 exons leading to 3 kb of coding region *(25,26)*. Seventeen *DPYD* mutations have been reported *(27)*; these mutations lead to single amino acid substitutions, nucleotide deletions, or a donor splice site mutation resulting in exon skipping (GA mutation in the exon 14 splice site, *27)*. This latter mutation results in the production of a truncated mRNA and has been consistently associated with low DPD activity and 5-FU toxicity. In addition, Van Kuilenburg reported that this mutation was found in 8 out of 11 patients suffering from a complete deficiency of DPD *(28)*. More recently, Johnson and coworkers identified this latter molecular defect as being responsible for a complete lack of DPD enzymatic activity having induced a life-threatening toxicity in a patient treated by topical 5-FU *(29)*. A molecular study was conducted in a cohort of cancer patients with reduced or normal DPD activity with the aim to analyze the 10 *DPYD* exons (exons 2, 4, 7, 10, 11, 13, 14, 18, 21, 23), where *DPYD* mutations were previously identified, *(27)*. From this study a patient with a heterozygous intron 14G1A mutation had normal DPD activity. Kouwaki and colleagues undertook an expression analysis for three mutant *DPYD* genes found in Japanese patients *(30)*. Only two mutations led to mutant DPD proteins with significant loss of enzymatic activity; the third one, however, resulted in no decrease in enzymatic activity compared with the wild-type. The conclusion from these studies is that *DPYD* mutations do not entirely explain polymorphic DPD activity and toxic response to 5-FU.

6. DPD IN TUMORS AND RESISTANCE TO 5-FU-BASED THERAPY

DPD activity can be considered as a potential factor for controlling 5-FU responsiveness at the tumoral level. The concept is simple: A high level of tumor DPD would metabolize 5-FU to inactive products before cytotoxic nucleotides can be formed. The potential role of DPD for influencing 5-FU activity also concerns new 5-FU prodrugs like UFT or capecitabine, where 5-FU is metabolically produced at the target site. Previous in vitro data revealed that DPD activity in tumor cells was significantly related to 5-FU sensitivity *(31)*; the lower the DPD enzymatic activity, the greater the cytotoxicity. Interestingly, from this experimental study it was shown that DPD activity and thymidylate synthase activity were independent variables significantly correleted with 5-FU cytotoxic activity. Recent studies in human cancer xenografts demonstrated that the efficacy of capecitabine correlated very well with the ratio of thymidine phosphorylase/DPD *(32)*. The role of tumoral DPD activity was then evaluated in the clinical setting. For head and neck cancer patients, DPD activity was detectable in all tumor samples (median tumoral DPD activity was 60, range 13–193 pmol/min/mg protein) *(33)*. Tumoral DPD activity was not influenced by tumor staging. The patients with a complete response to 5-FU-based induction chemotherapy, exhibited lower tumoral DPD activities as compared with partial or nonresponding patients *(33)*. In an attempt to reduce the variability due to confounding factors, including a possible circadian variability for DPD activity, we tested a normalized DPD value defined as the tumoral:adjacent nontumoral ratio of DPD activity. Interestingly, the distribution of normalized DPD revealed that complete responders exhibited a significantly lower normalized DPD than partial or nonresponding patients ($p = 0.03$) *(33)*. However, the tumor:normal tissue ratio is not the same for all tumor types. A recent study of 63 colorectal tumors found a median tumor:normal ratio of 0.76 *(34)*. Although a subset of patients did have up to three times higher tumor DPD, the majority of patients had highest DPD in adjacent normal tissue. Although resistance to 5-FU is multifactorial, it can be considered that tumoral DPD activity may be a determining factor for 5-FU responsiveness in a subset of cancer patients. These data provide further pharmacological rationale for the use of DPD-specific inhibitors.

7. DPD INHIBITORS

There were recently four agents under development that interacted with DPD activity (Table 1); 5 ethynyluracil was the only one that is a DPD inactivitor (irreversible inhibition)

Table 1
5-FU Oral Prodrugs Under Clinical Evaluation that Contain a DPD Inhibitor

Compound	*Chemical name*	*Effect on DPD*
Eniluracil (Glaxo-Wellcome)	5-Ethynyluracil	Inactivor
UFT (Orzel(R), Bristol-Myers Squibb, contains UFT plus leucovorin)	Uracil + tegafur	Inhibitor
S1 (Bristol-Myers Squibb)	5-Chloro-2, 4 dihydropyridine + tegafur + potassium oxonate	Inhibitor
BOF-A2 (Emitefur(R), Otsuka America Pharmaceutical)	1-Ethoxymethyl-5-fluorouracil + 3-cyano- 2,6-dihydropyrimidine	Inhibitor

while the three others act as DPD inhibitors (competitive inhibition). Details on the clinical development on these compounds will be given in other chapters in this book. We will insist on the main characteristics of these DPD inhibitors. With 5-ethynyluracil pretreatment, the biovailability of 5-FU becomes complete and thus renal clearance becomes the main source of drug elimination with significant correlations having been shown between 5-FU clearance and creatinine clearance *(35)*. A consequence could be that dosage reductions would need to be made in patients with reduced renal function who are candidates for 5-ethynyluracil and 5-FU combined treatment. Competitive inhibitors of DPD activity are also part of the new products UFT, S_1, and BOF-A_2. UFT contains uracil and tegafur in a 4:1 ratio and S_1 includes 5-chloro-2,4-dihydropyrimidine (CDHP) in combination with tegafur and potassium oxonate. BOF-A_2 is an oral prodrug of 5-FU and 3-cyano-2,6-dihydropyrimidine (CNDP). CNDP is a much stronger DPD inhibitor compared to uracil. When uracil, CDHP or CNDP compete with 5-FU for the uracil binding site on the DPD protein, more 5-FU can be activated through the anabolic pathway. The consequence of competive inhibition is that the effects of this inhibition are rapidly reversible; in comparison, a single dose of 5-ethynyluracil maintains a complete DPD inhibition for several days *(36)*. A striking feature of the DPD inhibitor clinical studies is the very low incidence of hand/foot syndrome. In comparison, capecitabine, another 5-FU oral prodrug that does not contain a DPD inhibitor, induces a relatively high frequence of more or less severe hand/foot toxicity *(37)*. It is thought that the presence of 5-FU related hand/foot syndrome can be due to the production of 5-FU catabolites that are absent when a DPD inhibitor is associated to the 5-FU oral prodrug. One of the major critical points for the clinical use of DPD inhibitors is to define the dose of DPD inhibitor so as to permit a significant inhibition of DPD activity to take place in the organism but to also keep a basal level of DPD activity in normal cells (intestinal, hematological) to maintain a minimal level of 5-FU detoxification through DPD activity.

REFERENCES

1. Lamont EB, Schilsky RL. The oral fluoropyrimidines in cancer chemotherapy. *Clin Cancer Res* 1999;5:2289–2296.
2. Sobrero A, Kerr D, Glimelius B, et al. New directions in the treatment of colorectal cancer: a look to the future. *Eur J Cancer* 2000;36:559–566.
3. Diasio RB, Harris BE. Clinical Pharmacology of 5-fluorouracil. *Clin Pharmacokin* 1989;16:215–237.
4. Milano G, Mc Leod HL. Can dihydropyrimidine dehydrogenase impact 5-fluorouracil-based treatment? *Eur J Cancer* 2000;36:37–42.
5. Naguib FNM, El Kouni MH, Cha S. Enzymes of uracil catabolism in normal and neoplastic human tissues. *Cancer Res* 1985;45:5402–5412.

6. Chazal M, Etienne MC, Renée N, Bourgeon A, Richelme H, Milano G. Link between dihydropyrimidine dehydrogenase activity in peripheral blood mononuclear cells and liver. *Clin Cancer Res* 1996;2:507–510.
7. Stephan F, Etienne MC, Wallays C, Milano G, Clergue F. Depressed hepatic dihydropyrimidine dehydrogenase activity and fluorouracil related toxicities. *J Med* 1995;99:685–688.
8. Harris BE, Song R, Soong SJ, Diasio RB. Relationship between dihydropyrimidine dehydrogenase activity and plasma 5-fluorouracil levels with evidence for circadian variation of enzyme activity and plasma drug levels in cancer patients receiving 5-fluorouracil by protracted continuous infusion. *Cancer Res* 1990;50:197–201.
9. Fleming R, Milano G, Thyss A, et al. Correlation between dihydropyrimidine dehydrogenase activity in peripheral mononuclear cells and systemic clearance of fluorouracil in cancer patients. *Cancer Res* 1992;52:2899–2902.
10. Etienne MC, Chatelut E, Pivot X, et al. Covariables influencing 5-fluorouracil clearance during continuous venous infusion. A NONMEM analysis. *Eur J Cancer* 1998;34:92–97.
11. McLeod HL, Sludden J, Hardy SC, Lock RE, Hawksworth GM, Cassidy J. Autoregulation of 5-fluorouracil metabolism. *Eur J Cancer* 1998;34:1623–1627.
12. Lu Z, Zhang R, Diasio RB. Dihydropyrimidine dehydrogenase activity in human peripheral blood mononuclear cells and liver: population characteristics, newly identified patients and clinical implication in 5-fluorouracil chemotherapy. *Cancer Res* 1993;53:5433–5438.
13. Ridge SA, Sludden J, Wei X, et al. Dihydropyrimidine dehydrogenase pharmacogenetics in patients with colorectal cancer. *Br J Cancer* 1998;77:497–500.
14. Etienne MC, Lagrange JL, Dassonville O, et al. Population study of dihydropyrimidine dehydrogenase in cancer patients. *J Clin Oncol* 1994;12:2248–2253.
15. Milano G, Etienne MC, Thyss A, et al. Influence of sex and age on fluorouracil clearance. *J Clin Oncol* 1992;10:1171–1175.
16. Milano G, Etienne MC, Pierrefite V, Barberi-Heyob M, Deporte-Fety R, Renée N. Dihydropyrimidine dehydrogenase deficiency and fluorouracil-related toxicity. *Br J Cancer* 1999;79:627–630.
17. Van Kuilenburg ABP, Van Lenthe H, Blom MJ, Mul EPJ, Van Gernip AH. Profound variation in dihydropyrimidine dehydrogenase activity in human blood cells: major implications for the detection of partly deficient patients. *Brit J Cancer* 1999;79:620–626.
18. Gamelin E, Boisdron-Celle M, Guerin-Meyer V, et al. Correlation between uracil and dihydrouracil plasma ratio, fluorouracil (5-FU) pharmacokinetic parameters, and tolerance in patients with advanced colorectal cancer: a potential interest for predicting 5-FU toxicity and determining optimal 5-FU dosage. *J Clin Oncol* 1999;17:1105–1110.
19. Harris BE, Song R, He YS, Soong SJ, Diasio RB. Circadian rhythm of rat liver dihydropyrimidine dehydrogenase. Possible relevance to fluoropyrimidine chemotherapy. *Biochem Pharmacol* 1988;37:4759–4762.
20. Petit E, Milano G, Levi F, Thyss A, Bailleul F, Schneider M. Circadian rhythm-varying plasma concentration of 5-fluourouracil during a five-day continuous venous infusion at a constant rate in cancer patients. *Cancer Res* 1988;48:1676–1679.
21. Nowakowska-Dulawa E. Circadian rhythm of 5-fluorouracil and pharmacokinetics and tolerance. *Chronobiologia* 1990;17:27–30.
22. Tuchman M, Von Roemeling R, Lanning RM, Sothern R, Hrushesky WJM. Sources of variability of dihydropyrimidine dehydrogenase activity in human blood mononuclear cells. (In Reinberg A., Smolensky M., Lebrecque G., eds.) 1998. Annual Review of Chronopharmacology. Oxford, Perganom Press, pp. 399–402.
23. Grem JL, Yee LK, Venzon DJ, Takimoto CH, Allegra CJ. Inter-and intraindividual variation in dihydropyrimidine dehydrogenase activity in peripheral blood mononuclear cells. *Cancer Chemother Pharmacol* 1997;40:117–125.
24. Yokota H, Fernandez-Salguero P, Furuya H, et al. cDNA cloning and chromosome mapping of human dihydropyrimidine dehydrogenase, an enzyme associated with 5-fluorouracil toxicity and congenital thymine uraciluria. *J Biol Chem* 1994;269:23192–23196.
25. Johnson MR, Wang K, Tillmanns S, Albin N, Diasio RB. Structural organization of the human *Dihydropyrimidine Dehydrogenase* gene. *Cancer Res* 1997;57:1660–1663.
26. Wei X, Elizondo G, Sapone A, et al. Characterization of the human dihydropyrimidine dehydrogenase gene: gene structure and genetic polymorphism. *Genomics* 1998;51:391–400.
27. Collie-Duguid ESR, Etienne MC, Milano G, Mc Leod HL. Known variant *DPYD* alleles do not explain DPD deficiency in cancer patients. *Pharmacogenetics* 2000;10:217–223.
28. Van Kuilenburg ABP, Vreken P, Beex LVAM, et al. Heterozygosity for a point mutation in a invariant splice donor site of dihydropyrimidine dehydrogenase and severe 5-fluorouracil related toxicity. *Eur J Cancer* 1997;33:2258–2264.

29. Johnson MR, Hageboutros A, Wang K, High L, Smith JB, Diasio RB. Life-threatening toxicity in a dihydropyrimidine dehydrogenase deficient patient after treatment with topical 5-fluorouracil. *Clin Cancer Res* 1999;5:2006–2011.
30. Kouwaki M, Hamafima N, Sumi S, et al. Identification of novel mutations in the dihydropyrimidine dehydrogenase gene in a Japanese patient with 5-fluorouracil toxicity. *Clin Cancer Res* 1998;4:2999–3004.
31. Beck A, Etienne MC, Cheradame S, et al. A role for dihydropyrimidine dehydrogenase and thymidylate synthase in tumor sensitivity to fluorouracil. *Eur J Cancer* 1994;30:1517–1522.
32. Ishikawa T, Sekiguchi F, Fukase Y, Sawada N, Ishitsuka H. Positive correlation between the efficacy of capecitabine and doxifluridine and the ratio of thymidine phosphorylase to dihydropyrimidine dehydrogenase activities in tumors in human cancer xenografts. *Cancer Res* 1998;58:685–690.
33. Etienne MC, Cheradame S, Fischel JL, Formento P, Dassonville O, Renée N, Schneider M, Thyss A, Demard F, Milano G. Response to fluorouracil therapy in cancer patients: the role of tumoral dihydropyrimidine dehydrogenase activity. *J Clin Oncol* 1995;13:1663–1670.
34. McLeod HL, Sludden J, Murray GI, et al. Characterization of dihydropyrimidine dehydrogenase in human colorectal tumors. *Brit J Cancer* 1998;77:461–465.
35. Baker SD, Khor SP, Adjei AA, et al. Pharmacokinetic, oral bioavailability, and safety study of fluorouracil in patients treated with 776C85, an inactivator of dihydroprimidine dehydrogenase. *J Clin Oncol* 1996;14:3085–3096.
36. Schilsky RL, Hohneker J, Ratain MJ, et al. Phase I clinical and pharmacologic study of eniluracil plus fluorouracil in patients with advanced cancer. *J Clin Oncol* 1998;16:1450–1457.
37. Van Custen E, Findlay M, Osterwalder B, et al. Capecitabine, an oral fluoropyrimidine carbamate with substantial activity in advanced colorectal cancer: results of a randomized phase II study. *J Clin Oncol* 2000;18:1337–1345.

3 Biochemical Bases of the 5-Fluorouracil–Folinic Acid Interaction and of its Limitations

A Retrospective Analysis

Richard G. Moran, PhD

CONTENTS

1. SUMMARY

The sensitivity of many, but not all, human carcinoma cell lines to 5-fluorouracil (5-FU) is substantially increased by exposure of cells to 0.3–10 μ*M* concentrations of reduced folates. The synergism is due to an enhanced kinetic trapping of thymidylate synthase (TS) in an inactive ternary complex, which, although covalent, is in dynamic equi-

From: *Fluoropyrimidines in Cancer Therapy*
Edited by: Y. M. Rustum © Humana Press Inc., Totowa, NJ

librium with unbound, active enzyme. Several factors interact to prevent or reverse complete inhibition of TS by fluoropyrimidines. Yet, cellular TS must be maintained completely inactive for a length of time equivalent to one cell generation before any appreciable cell kill ensues. Successful blockade for longer periods yields extensive commitment to cell death, and antitumor kill has been faithfully mirrored by the duration of complete inhibition of TS in those few studies that allow assessment of the time course of enzyme inhibition. In spite of the potency of 5-FU as an inhibitor of TS, maintenance of such a prolonged complete blockade of tumor TS is quite difficult under clinical conditions. These counterintuitive concepts are borne out by abundant preclinical information, and may lie behind the limited clinical activity of the drug. However, the current literature would support the conclusions that the therapeutic objective of fluoropyrimidine therapy is a sustained complete inhibition of TS for periods of 48 h or more, that such inhibition should permit substantial therapeutic effects against human colon carcinomas, and that this objective is probably seldom met.

2. THE FLUOROPYRIMIDINES

The initial discovery by Heidelberger and his colleagues *(1)* that pyrimidines substituted at the 5-position with fluorine had remarkable and broad spectrum activity against transplanted rodent tumors led to four decades of sustained effort to improve that activity and to apply it to human neoplastic diseases. Hundreds of structural analogs and blocked derivatives of the parent drugs were synthesized and tested as inhibitors of tumor cell growth and of the development of tumors in vivo from tumor inocula. The antitumor and toxic mechanisms of the three lead compounds, 5-fluorouracil (5-FU), 5-fluoro-2′-deoxyuridine (FUdR), and 5-fluorouridine (FUR) have been studied in substantial detail, and the therapeutic activity of the several hundred derivatives of 5-FU have been examined. Thousands of basic biochemical and molecular studies have been published that sought to explain the growth inhibitory and cytotoxic effects of these compounds. And, as the final step in this escalating series, several million patients with gastrointestinal (GI) cancers have been treated with 5-FU. For 40 yr, the clinical activity of 5-FU against carcinoma of the colon and rectum and carcinoma of the stomach has been the benchmark against which the activity of all compounds and combinations tested against these diseases has been measured.

All in all, the discovery of 5-FU and the systematic exploitation of the effects of this compound and its close relatives has been one of the most doggedly pursued areas within the field of cancer research. This experience represents the prototypical approach needed to break the barriers preventing the effective treatment of human carcinomas. And yet, 50 yr after the publication of the activity of 5-FU against experimental tumors, there is still debate over the events precipitated by the fluoropyrimidines. More disturbing is the fact that, after 40 yr of clinical use, 5-FU has not yet been displaced by another drug more active against GI cancers. 5-FU remains in use because of the lack of a better substitute. Hence, the onus is on the field to understand exactly what the limitations of 5-FU are due to under clinical circumstances and to minimize their effects on therapy as much as humanly possible.

The purposes of this chapter are to furnish a basic biochemical framework with which to place into perspective the other chapters in this volume. Along the way, it is the author's purpose to discuss the points of confusion and disagreement within this substantial literature in the hope that these will spark work that leads to a thorough understanding of this fascinating and important drug.

3. THE TS-DIRECTED AND RNA-DIRECTED EFFECTS OF THE FLUOROPYRIMIDINES

Early studies by Heidelberger and his students and colleagues unraveled the anabolism and catabolism of 5-FU, FUdR, and FUR; these studies have been summarized in several reviews (*see,* for instance, refs *2* and *3*). It became clear early on that these drugs followed the metabolic pathways that were in place to metabolize uracil and its nucleosides and nucleotides (reviewed in ref. *3*). Several points became evident from those earlier metabolic studies:

1. The incorporation of 5-FU into RNA was a striking aspect of the biochemistry of the drug, and several of the therapeutic strategems that enhanced the activity of 5-FU against animal tumors also increased incorporation of 5-FU into RNA. Thus, scheduling of a dose of methotrexate before 5-FU resulted in increased cellular phosphoribosyl pyriphosphate (PRPP), and hence, synthesis of FUMP *(4)*. Similar mechanisms occurred with coadministration of inhibitors of *de novo* pyrimidine synthesis *(5)*. Incorporation of 5-FU into various species of RNA is perhaps most remarkable in that it has broad, often nonspecific, but usually minor effects, although the net sum of these effects appears involved in the overall activity of 5-FU on mammalian tumor cells *(3)*.
2. The incorporation of 5-FU into DNA did not appear to contribute to the cytotoxicity of the drug. Incorporation of 5-FU into DNA was measurable, but barely so, and it was often confused with the more frequent event of metabolic dehalogenation of nucleotides of 5-FU followed by incorporation of these metabolites into DNA *(6,7)*. Destruction of FdUTP by cellular dUTPase and removal of any incorporated 5-FU from DNA by DNA-uracil glycosylase appear to be very efficient and redundant protective mechanisms *(8,9)*.
3. The potency of FdUMP as an inhibitor of TS was impressive (see below), but the cellular levels of FdUMP derived from 5-FU itself were always much lower than those of cellular FU ribonucleotides. In addition, any strategy which increased incorporation of 5-FU into RNA also increased the concentration of and residency of FdUMP.

Prior to the introduction of the combinations of 5-FU and reduced folates, the critical experiment was performed in which the mechanism of 5-FU and its derivatives was tested by challenging growth-inhibited cells with either thymidine, as a means of bypassing inhibition of *de novo* thymidylate synthesis, or uridine, as a means of competitively preventing 5-FU from being metabolized to ribonucleotides and, thence, incorporation into RNA. (The initial studies that used this experimental design are reported in refs. *10* and *11*, subsequent studies reviewed in ref. *3*.) In some cell lines, thymidine shifted the dose-response curve of 5-FU to a small degree but uridine was without effect; in other cell lines uridine shifted the curve some and thymidine was without effect. In no cell line ever studied did one of these end products prevent the cytotoxicity of 5-FU, but rather any protective effect of uridine or thymidine was manifested only by a shift in the dose-response curve. In contrast, thymidine dramatically altered the sensitivity of most cell lines to FUdR, but uridine was without effect. Although many investigators chose to ignore these experiments, the inescapable conclusion was that neither incorporation of 5-FU into RNA nor the inhibition of TS were sufficient, taken individually, to explain the growth inhibitory and cytotoxic effects of 5-FU; years of searching for yet a third mechanism underlying these results did not yield results. On the other hand, FUdR appeared to act as an almost pure inhibitor of TS in many cell lines. Perhaps one of the most inexplicable aspects of the pharmacology of the fluoropyrimidines is that FUdR is much more potent than 5-FU in cell culture, with typical IC_{50}s for the two compounds of 5×10^{-10} and 1×10^{-7} *M*, respectively, but 5-FU is substantially more potent than FUdR in vivo.

4. THE FLUOROPYRIMIDINE-REDUCED FOLATE SYNERGISM IN TISSUE CULTURE CELLS AND ITS RELATIONSHIP TO CLINICAL EFFECTIVENESS OF THE COMBINATION

In a classic paper published in *PNAS* in 1978 *(12)*, Ullman and his colleagues demonstrated that inclusion of higher levels of (6-R,S)5-formyltetrahydrofolate (leucovorin, citrovorin factor, CF, folinic acid) in tissue culture medium enhanced the growth inhibitory activity of FUdR against a line of mouse leukemia cells, the L1210 cell. The effect resulted in a threefold shift in the concentration of drug needed to half-maximally inhibit the growth of L1210 cells, a reasonably small effect, but one which ultimately resulted in clinical trials of the combination of 5-FU and folinic acid in several adult human epithelial tumors. Several other studies followed up on that seminal paper, and this result initially appeared to be general. Perhaps the most important of these studies were the very careful and insightful experiments of Hakala and her colleagues *(13,14)*. This group studied the mechanism of 5-FU by itself and in combination with reduced folates in a series of mouse tumor cell lines and in a battery of human carcinoma cell lines in culture. They drew the conclusion that the growth inhibitory effects of 5-FU on the mouse cell lines were primarily due to effects on TS, based on the ability of exogenous thymidine to prevent growth inhibition, a pivotal expectation for any drug active against TS. On the other hand, the effects of 5-FU on the human lines studied were not prevented by concurrent inclusion of thymidine, and appeared to best correlate with the incorporation of 5-FU into RNA. However, for any of the human cell lines studied, addition of folinic acid to the medium changed the site of action of 5-FU to inhibition of TS, again, as judged by reversibility of the growth inhibition by thymidine in the medium. Inclusion of high levels of folinic acid in the medium of the mouse tumor cells studied intensified the growth inhibition observed, and the site of the enhanced growth inhibitory activity of 5-FU for mouse tumor cells remained TS.

In retrospect, it is amazing that clinical trials of this combination resulted from the initial observation of a threefold shift in the growth-inhibitory potency of FUdR in L1210 cells, a model tumor cell of questionable relevance to human GI tumors, together with the related studies by Hakala and her colleagues at Roswell Park on established epithelial tumor cells in tissue culture. Nevertheless, clinical trials of the combination were initiated and the initial reports *(15–17)* on these trials were very encouraging; it appeared that a major change in the effectiveness of this old drug against human cancers had been realized. At first, it seemed hard to rationalize that enhanced clinical activity of 5-FU was attending a combination that only careful experimentation in vitro could demonstrate as superior to 5-FU itself.

The change in potency of FUdR originally reported by Ullman et al. was easily reproducible *(18)*, in spite of its modest magnitude (threefold). Interestingly, the potentiation of the growth-inhibitory potency of 5-FU against the L1210 cells was even more modest *(18)* (Fig. 1A). However, when the viability of L1210 cells treated with 5-FU or the combination of 5-FU and folinic acid was examined using the ability of treated cells to produce progeny in a clonigenic assay, as an index of true cytotoxicity, it appeared that the growth-inhibition assays performed underestimated the magnitude of the potentiation produced by the combination *(18)* (Fig. 1B,C). A concentration of 5-FU that was barely cytotoxic would result in several logs of tumor cell kill in the presence of folinic acid. Subsequent studies on the WIdR human colon carcinoma cell line confirmed this conclusion *(19)*, and suggested that

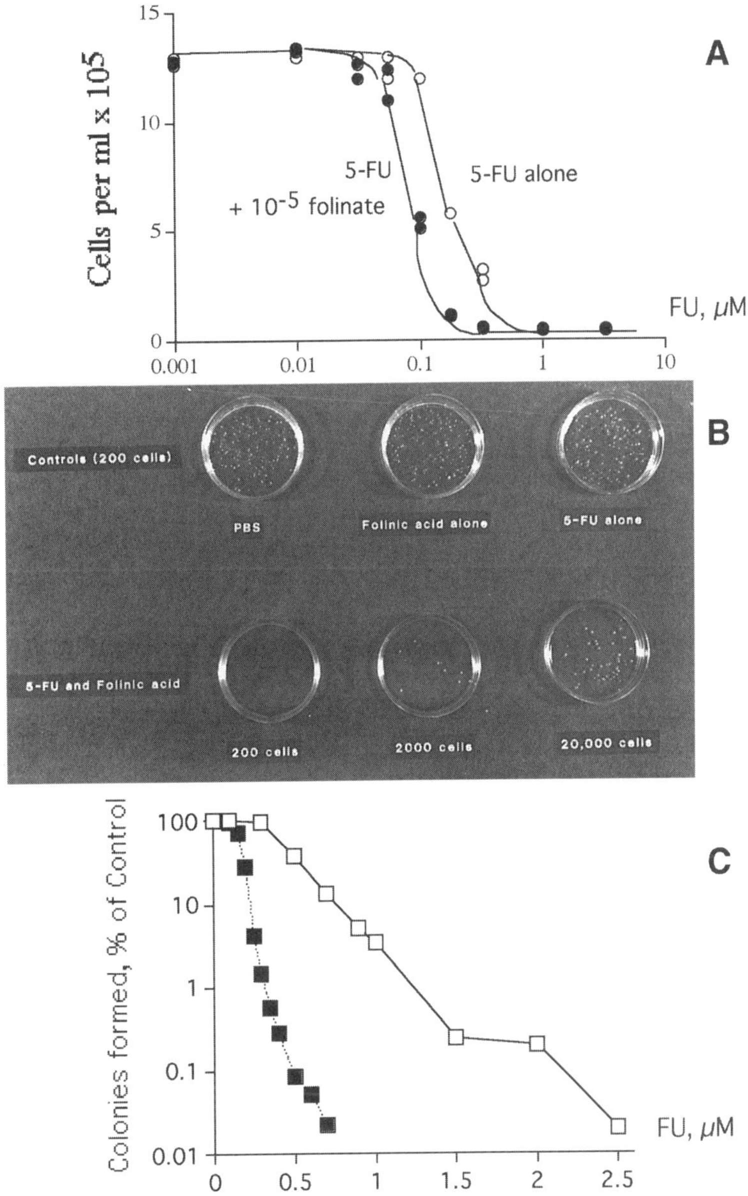

Fig. 1. *Enhancement of the growth inhibition and the cytotoxicity of 5-FU to mouse leukemic cells by folinic acid.* **(A)** The growth inhibition of 5-FU for mouse L1210 leukemic cells is increased in the presence of 10 μ*M* folinic acid. Cultures of L1210 cells were exposed to the indicated concentrations of 5-FU in the presence (filled circles) or absence (open circles) of folinic acid starting with an initial culture density of 2×10^4 cells/mL. After 72 h, the culture densities were determined. In other experiments, L1210 cells were exposed to 5-FU in the presence or absence of 10 μ*M* 5-FU for 72 h, then were plated into soft agarose in the absence of drugs, and the number of colonies formed after an additional 10 d incubation were determined. **(B)** Cells were incubated with 0.3 μ*M* 5-FU with or without folinic acid, and the viability of 200, 2000, or 20,000 cells was determined. It can be seen that the number of colonies formed from 200 cells treated with 5-FU alone was greater than the number of colonies formed from 20,000 cells treated with 5-FU plus folinic acid. **(C)** depicts the viability of cells treated with varying concentrations of 5-FU in the presence (filled squares) or absence (open squares) of 10 μ*M* folinic acid. (The data were adapted from ref *18* with the permission of *Cancer Research.*)

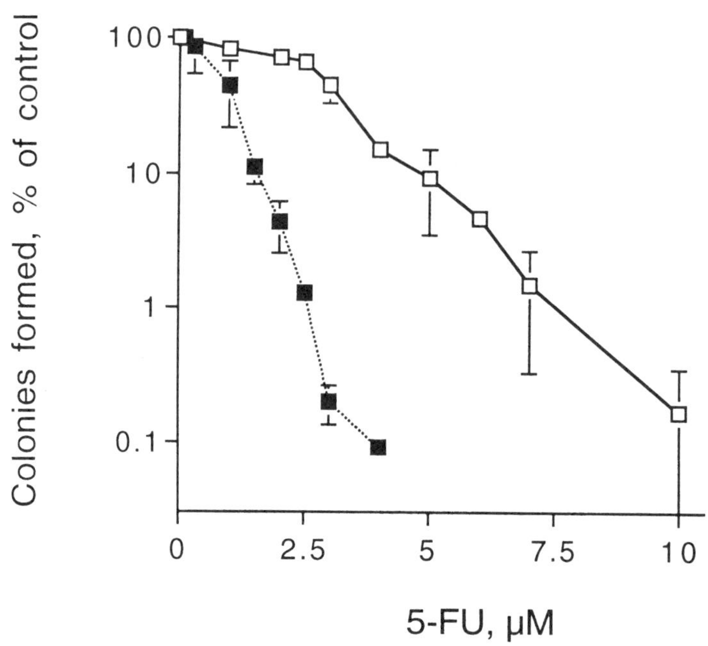

Fig. 2. *Enhancement of the cytotoxicity of 5-FU to human WiDr colon carcinoma cells by folinic acid.* WiDr cells were plated at 250–25,000 cells per 60 mm dish, and treated with 5-FU at the indicated concentrations starting 24 h after plating for a total of 72 h of drug exposure in the presence (filled squares) or absence (open squares) of 10 μ*M* folinic acid. Colonies formed were determined after fixing and staining the dishes 3–3.5 wk later. (The data were adapted from ref. *19* with permission of *Cancer Research.*)

the ability of 5-FU to kill tumor cells was substantially increased at the levels of drug that were clinically achievable (Fig. 2). However, it should be noted from the data of Figs. 1C and 2 that the synergy seen with the combination of 5-FU and folinic acid is only a shift in a dose-log cell kill curve, that is, if higher concentrations of 5-FU are clinically achievable, the same level of cell kill would be seen with 5-FU alone. So, the judgment of whether the combination of 5-FU and folinic acid made sense, clinically, would rely on a decision of what portion of the dose-response curve is in play during clinical use of 5-FU: if the achievable dose of drug is giving an insufficient exposure for efficient tumor cell kill, then an enhanced clinical response would be expected from the coadministration of folinic acid. If, on the other hand, one is currently working on the higher end of the fluoropyrimidine dose scale seen in Figs. 1C and 2, then one should not expect any therapeutic enhancement of the effects of 5-FU by coadministration of reduced folates.

The cell culture studies above raised several questions:

1. To what degree is the clinical activity of 5-FU enhanced by coadministration of folinic acid? This key question has been answered only by extensive large-scale clinical trials and is the subject of much continuing debate. It is safe to say, however, that the clinical effectiveness of the combination of 5-FU and folinic acid is not yet sufficient to provide major increases in mean survival time of populations of patients treated with the 5-FU/folinic acid combination compared to populations treated with 5-FU alone, although numerous cases of complete responses of colonic carcinoma have been documented with the combination which would not be expected with 5-FU alone. Most clinical studies have concluded that the combination offers better clinical results than 5-FU administered on intermittent schedules. This is discussed at length in chapters 13 and 14 of this volume.

2. Exactly what is folinic acid doing to enhance the effects of 5-FU against TS?
3. Would other folates offer the same potentiation as does folinic acid?
4. How much folinic acid is required for the effect?
5. Can the combination be further enhanced by manipulation of factors related to the mechanism of the synergy?
6. Is the extent of the 5-FU/folinic acid synergy dependent on the length of exposure to 5-FU or folinic acid?
7. How general is the antitumor synergy seen in cell culture? Is it safe to assume that the effects of 5-FU against all colonic carcinomas would be enhanced by folinic acid? If this is not the case, what factor or factors would determine the applicability of the combination, and could individual human tumors be tested in advance of therapy for effectiveness of 5-FU/folinic acid?
8. For tumors that are refractory to the combination, what is the mechanism of the resistance?

The literature that deals with these and related aspects of the treatment of human carcinomas with the combination of 5-FU and folinic acid represents an impressive body of biochemical, pharmacological, and clinical experimentation. With apologies to the investigators whose contributions I inadequately cover in this summary, I have attempted to mold the core of this literature into a coherent view of the biochemistry of the 5-FU–folinic acid combination. The review attempted here does not extend to the biochemical and molecular events downstream whereby inhibition of TS initiates apoptosis, but this central area is addressed by Dr. Houghton in Chapter 6.

5. PHARMACOLOGY OF THE 5-FU/CF COMBINATION

There has been a heavy reliance on cell culture experiments to understand the therapeutic and pharmacologic aspects of the 5-FU-reduced folate interaction as a result of an important species difference between man and mouse, which compromised the interpretation of mouse studies. The level of thymidine circulating in mouse serum (≈ 1.5–3 μ*M*) would easily prevent the effects of FUdR against cultured cells, whereas the thymidine concentration in human plasma (≈ 0.15 μ*M*) has been commonly thought to be too low to bypass the effect of inhibition of TS *(20–23)*. Hence, it was not surprising that a therapeutic effect of FU plus reduced folates has not been observed in some mouse studies in vivo, and has been observed to be rather weak in others. However, when human tumor cells deficient in thymidine kinase (which would, consequently, be incapable of salvage of circulating thymidine) were studied as xenografts in immune deficient mice, a strong synergy was seen with the 5-FU/folinic acid combination *(23)* (Fig. 3). The magnitude of this effect is of concern: If the common assumption that the level of thymidine in human serum is without effect on the cytotoxicity of 5-FU/folinic acid is incorrect, then the reason for the therapeutic failure of many patients treated with this regimen has been obvious for some time but has been ignored.

A very practical set of questions came to the fore related to how little or how much folate was necessary and sufficient to elicit the synergy seen between 5-FU and folinic acid. Initial studies *(13,14)* performed by Hakala's laboratory demonstrated that much higher levels of folinic acid (10 μ*M*) were required to promote the 5-FU/folinic acid synergism than to promote cell growth. This level set a target for the clinical trials, and promoted the development of the "high CF" or Roswell Park regimen, in which (6-R,S)-5-formyltetrahydrofolate is given at 400–550 mg/m^2 *(16)*. Subsequent studies on other cell lines in culture suggested that there were some cell line to cell line differences in how much extracellular reduced folate was required for optimal stimulation of the effects of 5-FU. Concentrations of 0.3 μ*M*

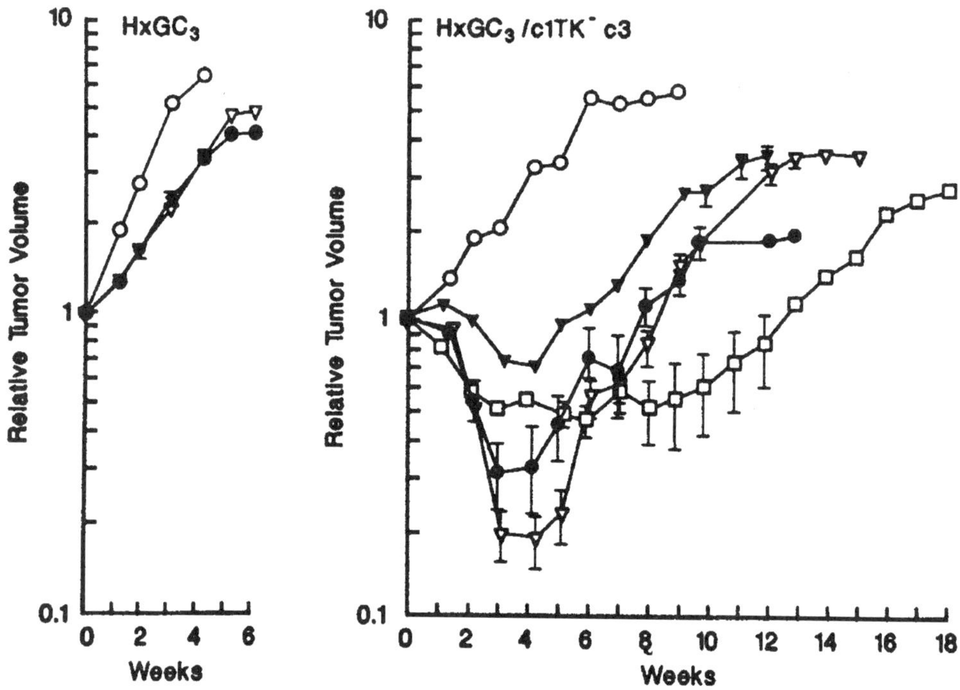

Fig. 3. *The chemotherapeutic effectiveness of 5-fluorouracil is enhanced by folinic acid in xenografts of human colon carcinoma which cannot salvage serum thymidine but not in xenografts capable of thymidine salvage.* Immune deficient mice were innoculated with the HxGC3 colon carcinoma (left panel) or a subline of HxGC3 selected in culture for deficiency of thymidine kinase (right panel). Groups of HxGC3 tumor-bearing mice were treated with control (open circles), three courses of 5-FU (filled circles); or FU plus 500 mg/m^2 folinic acid (triangles). Mice bearing the HxGC3/clTK-c3 tumor were treated with control (open circles), 5-FU (filled triangles), or 5-FU plus 50 (filled circles), 500 (open triangles), or 800 mg/m^2 folinic acid (open squares). (This figure was reproduced from Houghton et al. *(23)* with the permission of Dr. Houghton and *Cancer Chemotherapy and Pharmacology.* It clearly demonstrates that folinic acid substantially increases the activity of 5-FU against human colon carcinoma cells in vivo if plasma thymidine is not available for salvage.)

folinic acid were sufficient to maximally enhance the effects of 5-FU on either the growth inhibition or the cytotoxicity of 5-FU to L1210 cells *(18).* Optimal cytotoxicity of 5-FU was attained only with the use of 3–10 μ*M* folinic acid for the WIdR colonic carcinoma cell *(19)* or the Hep-2 carcinoma cell *(13,14).* In a very extensive French study of the response of multiple human carcinoma cell lines to the 5-FU/folinic acid combination, Beck et al. *(24)* reported that there was substantial variation in the concentration of folinic acid required to maximally enhance 5-FU. For 9 out of 17 cell lines, maximal synergy was observed at concentrations of folinic acid less than or equal to 5 μ*M,* whereas three other cell lines required 10–200 μ*M* folinic acid for optimal effect. In the remaining five cell lines, little or no synergy was observed at any reasonable concentration of folinic acid.

Faced with the substantial cost and availability problems caused by the perceived need to administer very high levels of folinic acid to patients, a large-scale clinical trial was performed by the Mayo group, which pitted high dose folinic acid against a much lower dose (20 mg/m^2). This trial *(25)* made the surprising observation that there was no detectable advantage to the high-dose folinate schedule, and this was confirmed in more extensive studies by this group *(26)*. This set the stage for further trials that compared the use of 20 mg/m^2 folinic acid with high dose leucovorin. Some large Phase III studies confirmed the superiority of high-dose leucovorin over the lower-dosage leucovorin introduced by the Mayo group *(27)*. On the other hand, a multifaceted SWOG study concluded that there was no difference in therapeutic effect of low- or high-dose folinic acid regimens in combination with 5-FU *(28)*. The extensive clinical literature on this combination and the effect of dosage regimens and schedules on clinical outcome and toxicities has been reviewed *(29)* and is discussed at length elsewhere in this volume.

6. SCHEDULING OF 5-FU AND FOLINIC ACID FOR OPTIMAL THERAPEUTIC SYNERGISM

In Chapter 8 of this monograph, Dr. Sobrero discusses the issue of how much of a change in thereapeutic synergism results from differences in the schedule of administration of either the 5-FU or the folinic acid components of the combination. Therapeutic synergism relates not only to the effects on tumor but also the interaction of the two agents in normal, toxicity-limiting stem cells, and hence, can only be definitively described in vivo. However, the effects of lengths of exposure to 5-FU or folinic acid on the cytotoxicity of the combination to tumor cells can and have been described on cells in culture *(19)*. The results were somewhat predictable, and somewhat surprising:

1. Short-term exposure to 5-FU, at any dose, resulted in minimal synergism with folinic acid, no matter how high the concentration of the latter, nor how long of an exposure to folinic acid.
2. The longer the exposure to 5-FU, the greater the degree of enhancement of cytotoxicity to 5-FU by folinic acid (Fig. 4).
3. At a constant length of exposure to 5-FU, the longer the exposure to folinic acid, the higher the cytotoxicity. This implies that extended continuous infusions of 5-FU plus folinic acid up to the limits of toxicity would yield a high therapeutic synergism. This may reflect the requirement for extended inhibition of thymidylate synthase for cell kill.

One of the most informative studies to date was performed by the Dutch group who studied the complete time course of TS after a maximally tolerated single dose of 5-FU and compared it with the effectiveness of equimolar and equitoxic doses of FUdR. In that study *(30)*, Van Laar and his colleagues found that maximally tolerated doses of intermittent FUdR were far superior to 5-FU in the treatment of the murine colon-26 transplanted tumor, and that the duration of TS inhibition explained this therapeutic superiority (see below).

7. BIOCHEMISTRY OF TS AND OF ENHANCEMENT OF THE INHIBITION OF TS IN MAMMALIAN CELLS BY REDUCED FOLATES

There are five aspects of the biochemistry of TS relevant to the enhancement of the effectiveness of 5-FU by high levels of exogenous reduced folates:

1. The characteristics of the active sites of TS.
2. The binding order of the TS reaction.
3. The mechanism of binding of FdUMP to TS.
4. The results of inhibition of TS on deoxypyrimidine pools.
5. The reversibility of the TS–FdUMP–methylenetetrahydrofolate binding reaction.

Each of these is discussed briefly.

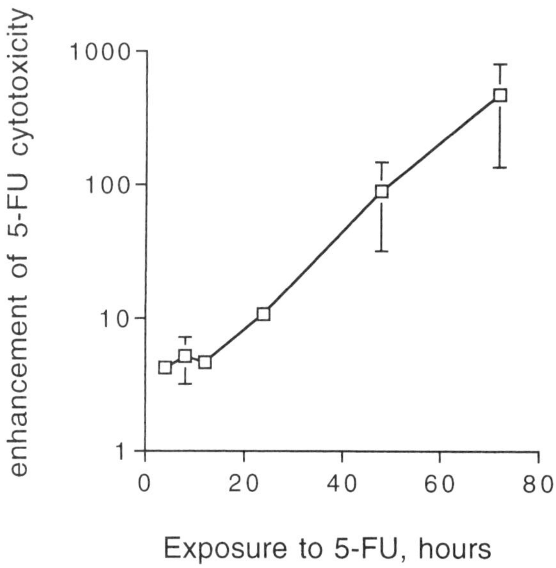

Fig. 4. *The 5-FU/folinic acid synergy becomes more exaggerated with longer exposures to 5-FU.* Cells were exposed to concentrations of 5-FU that killed 75–95% of exposed WiDr cells in the absence of folinic acid, and the survival of this cell line was compared to that observed with the same concentrations of 5-FU in the presence of 10 μ*M* folinic acid. The enhancement plotted is the ratio of the survival of cells treated with 5-FU divided by the survival of cells treated with the combination. (Reprinted from ref. 19 with permission of *Cancer Research.*)

Thymidylate synthase is a dimer of identical monomers each of which carries a catalytically active site. The monomeric molecular weight is 32–37,000 Daltons depending on species, but a comparison of mammalian enzymes reveals a very tightly conserved primary structure *(31)*. Each of the two subunits of mammalian TS donates a short peptide to the active site on the other monomer and two arginines on this peptide are involved in substrate binding sufficiently important to be conserved from bacteria to human *(32,33)*. Two very elegant studies have demonstrated that one subunit can be active on a dimer in which the other is inactivated either genetically *(34)* or chemically *(35)* but even then, the two monomers both contribute to the active site. Another aspect of the TS reaction that has complicated the field is the clear crosstalk between the two active sites *(36–38)*. In order to explain the beautiful complexities of this enzyme, it has been proposed that only one active site of mammalian TS can be active at any given time, but that the enzyme uses each active site in alternative catalytic cycles *(37,38)*. Although aspects of this proposal remain conjectural, the binding of FdUMP to the two active sites appears to be nonequivalent. An examination of the binding of FdUMP to pure human TS at low temperature (7°C) demonstrated that the first binding event to dimeric enzyme is rapid, but the rate of binding of FdUMP to the second active site of dimeric TS occurs much more slowly *(39)*. Although the rate of binding of FdUMP to the two sites differed 1000-fold, the rate of dissociation from the two sites were equivalent. These differences have not been observed at higher temperatures, and certainly not at physiological temperature, but it constitutes direct evidence for nonequivalence in FdUMP binding events at the two subunits. Several other studies have also indicated such a nonequivalence.

Mammalian TS follows an ordered sequential mechanism (Fig. 5) with deoxyuridylate binding to an active site first, followed by the folate cosubstrate *(3,37,40,41)*. An ordered

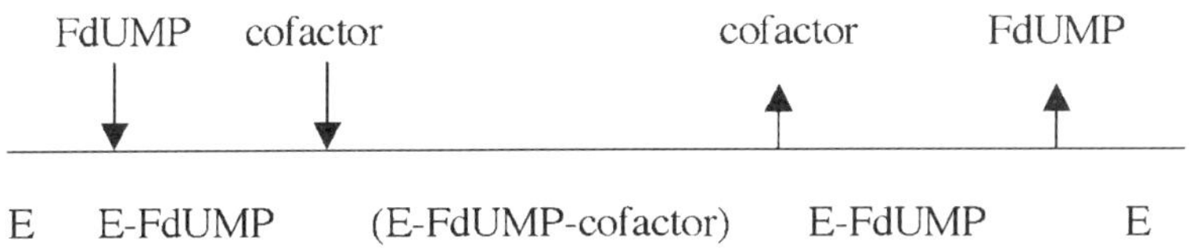

Fig. 5. *Mammalian thymidylate synthase follows an ordered sequential order of binding of substrates/ligands.*

sequential binding order is usually interpreted to mean either that the bound first substrate forms part of the binding surface for the second substrate or that the binding of the first substrate induces a conformational change in the protein that induces the formation of the binding site for the second substrate. Either mechanism has the effect that the second substrate (5, 10-methylene tetrahydrofolate) cannot bind to TS in a catalytically productive manner without prior binding of dUMP. Likewise, FdUMP binds to TS first, followed by binding of folate cosubstrate (Fig. 5), and the noncovalently bound ternary complex is thought to then rapidly proceed to a tightly bound complex followed by formation of covalent bonds between the active site cysteine and the 6-position of FdUMP, and the 5-position of FdUMP and the exocyclic methylene group of the folate cofactor. In the course of a detailed and careful analysis of the kinetics of these binding events, Danenberg and his colleagues *(3,37,42)* came to two crucial conclusions:

1. The observed rate of formation of a ternary complex among TS, folate, and FdUMP was a hyperbolic function of the concentration of folate cosubstrate, that is

$${}_k\text{on,obs} = {}_k1\{{}_k3(\text{folate})\}\{{}_k2 + {}_k3(\text{folate})\}{-1}$$

   where k_1, k_2 and k_3 were the kinetic constants determining the rate of formation of a enzyme–dUMP binary complex, the rate of addition of folate cofactor to the enzyme–dUMP binary complex, and the rate of dissociation of the enzyme–dUMP binary complex, respectively (Fig.5). In other words, the rate of formation of ternary complex was constant at high folate cofactor concentration, but was potentially quite a bit lower at low cofactor concentrations.
2. On the other hand, the observed rate of dissociation of the ternary complex was inversely related to the concentration of folate cofactor, and, at very high concentrations of folate cofactor, dissociation would be very slow indeed. This presumably did not reflect a slower dissociation of FdUMP from the enzyme–FdUMP binary complex, but rather the reformation of ternary complex in the presence of higher 5,10-methylenetetrahydrofolate after initial formation of binary complex from ternary complex.

Hence, the effective strength of binding of a noncovalent ternary complex was dramatically dependent on the concentration of 5,10-methylenetetrahydrofolate available at the surface of TS. The noncovalent ternary complex then rapidly formed covalent bonds, and the covalently bound ternary complex would have more opportunity for formation and less chance of productive dissociation at higher concentrations of folate cofactor. This, then, represents a kinetic trapping mechanism at the heart of the 5-FU–folinic acid combination.

The question comes up: Does the covalently bound ternary complex of TS, FdUMP, and 5,10-methylenetetrahydrofolate ever dissociate on a time scale of practical significance to 5-FU chemotherapy? The answer is rather astounding: TS trapped in a covalently bound ternary complex in intact mouse leukemic cells, in the presence of folate pools adequate for maximal cell growth rates, dissociated back to free enzyme with a half-time of two h (Fig. 6)

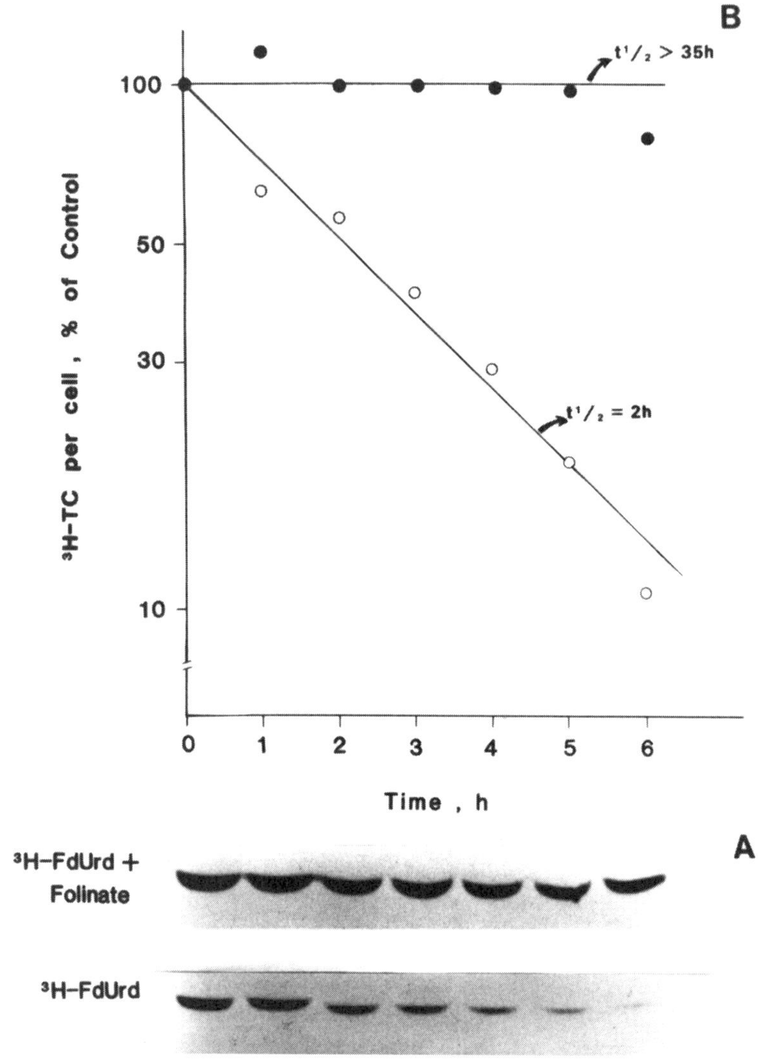

Fig. 6. *Stabilization of ternary complex by folinic acid in vivo.* Mouse L1210 leukemia cells were exposed to 0.7 n*M* FUdR in the presence (filled circles) or absence (open circles) of 10 μ*M* folinic acid for 12 h. The cells were washed and resuspended in 10 μ*M* unlabeled FUdR for the indicated times, the cells were harvested and sonicated, and cellular protein was subjected to electrophoresis on SDS-PAGE gels. The gel was impregnated with beta-ray enhancer, dried, and subjected to autoradiography. The only labeled band on the gels was at the position of the monomer of thymidylate synthase **(A).** The data of panel **A** were quantitated, corrected for the content of protein per cell, and plotted as a function of time in **B.** (Reprinted from ref. *43* with the permission of the *Journal of Biological Chemistry.*)

(43)! On the other hand, when these same cells were exposed to exogenous 5-formyltetrahydrofolate, at concentrations that optimally stimulated cell kill by 5-FU, the rate of dissociation of the covalent ternary complex was unmeasurable (> 35 h) *(43).* Hence, the addition of folinic acid to 5-FU converts 5-FU to what it originally was thought to be, namely, a pseudo-irreversible, titrating inhibitor of TS. How can one comprehend such a rapid reversal of covalent bonds in the ternary FdUMP–TS–methylenetetrahydrofolate complex that is ini-

tially formed in 5-FU exposed cells? The potency of the inhibition of TS by FdUMP is the result of the enzymatically catalyzed formation of covalent bonds by TS. By microscopic reversibility, it is clear that TS also catalyzes the breakage of the same covalent bonds that tie the complex together.

The remarkable decrease in the rate of turnover of the covalently bound ternary complex in cells in which the 5, 10-methylenetetrahydrofolate pools was expanded, as demonstrated in vivo in Fig. 6 appears to be somewhat at odds with prior data on pure human TS studied in vitro. Danenberg *(37,42)* had first demonstrated that the effective rate at which complexes of purified human TS, FdUMP, and 5,10-methylenetetrahydrofolate dissociate to native enzyme could be slowed substantially in the presence of 5,10-methylenetetrahydrofolate, and that the rate of dissociation became negligible at infinite free 5,10-methylenetetrahydrofolate. In both that study and the extensions of their work by Radparvar et al. *(44)*, concentrations of 5, 10-methylenetetrahydrofolate in excess of 1000 μ*M* were required to stabilize complex as much as is seen in Fig. 6. However, Radparvar et al. (44) demonstrated that long chain poly-γ-glutamate derivatives of 5, 10-methylenetetrahydrofolate were much more potent at trapping human TS in inhibited ternary complexes than was 5,10-methylenetetrahydrofolate monoglutamate, and that results *(43)* such as seen in Fig. 6 were compatible with intracellular concentrations of long-chain methylenetetrahydrofolate polyglutamate concentrations on the range of 5–10 μ*M*. The concentration of 5,10-methylenetetrahydrofolate polyglutamates in the experiment of Fig. 6 was on this range *(43)*. Hence, the data of Fig. 6 indicate that exposure of tumor cells to 5-formyltetrahydrofolate results in the kinetic trapping of TS by an expanded pool of long-chain 5,10-methylenetetrahydrofolate polyglutamates. The experiments of Milano and his colleagues (see below) draw attention to the cellular folate polyglutamate pool in primary human colon and head and neck tumors as a central variable determining the response of individual tumors to 5-FU.

8. METABOLIC ACCUMULATION OF dUMP IN TS-INHIBITED CELLS

The enzymatically catalyzed dissociation of the FdUMP–TS–cofactor ternary complex becomes even more significant because of the accumulation of dUMP in FU-treated cancer cells. Early studies demonstrated that dUMP is present in rather low concentrations, even in S-phase cells, and that these steady-state dUMP concentrations are in the range of the K_m for dUMP with human TS, 3 μ*M* (reviewed in ref. *3*). However, the binding constant for dUMP to human TS was determined to be about 0.36 μ*M (42)*, implying that dUMP would interfere with initial binding of FdUMP even at micromolar concentrations of dUMP. This is consistent with the fact that concentrations of dUMP as low as 1 μ*M* decreased the rate of binding of FdUMP to isolated human TS *(42)*. In some, but not all, tumor cells, blockage of TS results in the accumulation of dUMP often to millimolar concentrations, that is, to concentrations that are 3000 times the K_d for dUMP binding to TS *(45–47)*. In the face of such an expanded dUMP pool, any initially inhibited TS, upon dissociation of the ternary complex, would be protected from inactivation of FdUMP, due to competition of FdUMP and dUMP for binding to free TS; the binding constants for these two nucleotides for free TS for the initial formation of a binary complex appears to be equivalent. The effects of high dUMP and low 5,10-methylenetetrahydrofolate have been shown to have a multiplicative effect on the binding of FdUMP to TS *(42)*.

In vitro, the rate of inactivation of pure human TS by FdUMP is dramatically slowed in the presence of dUMP concentrations; for instance, 50 μ*M* dUMP slowed the binding of FdUMP to enzyme by 140-fold *(42)*. At the millimolar dUMP concentration seen to accu-

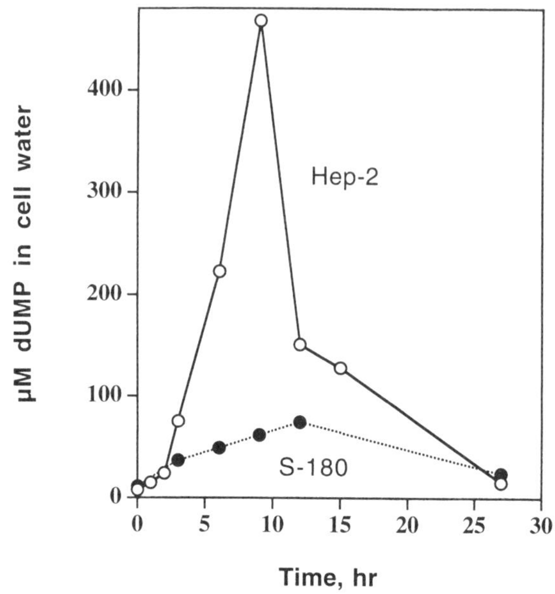

Fig. 7. *Expansion of the cellular dUMP pool in human Hep-2 hepatoma (open circles) and mouse S-180 sarcoma (filled circles) cells following treatment with 5-FU.* Cultures were treated with 5-FU for the first three hours of the period shown, and dUMP was measured with time thereafter. (Reproduced from Berger and Hakala (ref. *46*) with the permission of *Molecular Pharmacology* and Dr Berger.) The accumulation of dUMP is strikingly different in different cell types.

mulate in CEM cells after 5-FU *(45)*, any newly synthesized TS or active enzyme dissociating from ternary complex would be protected from all but extemely high concentrations of FdUMP. The technologies available for measurement of dUMP in small samples are a problem. One of the most widely used assays is one we developed based on the enzymatic conversion of dUMP to C^{14} thymidylate using 5,10-$^{14}CH_2$-tetrahydrofolate *(45)*. Although this technique is very cumbersome, it has been used quite extensively by Spears and his colleagues to estimate dUMP in biopsy material of primary human tumors and hepatic metastases *(48–50)*. In an exhaustive set of technically and tactically challenging clinical experiments *(49)*, this group analyzed biopsy specimens of more than 50 breast, colon, gastric, and pancreatic carcinomas and a moderate number of normal tissue samples at times ranging from 75 to 150 min after a single dose of 5-FU at 500 mg/m^2. The concentration of dUMP in the tumors ranged from 20 to 50 µ*M*. However, the level of dUMP in cellular elements of normal human bone marrow aspirates rose to > 1.5 m*M* 80 min after exposure to 5-FU *(49)*. Hence, the dUMP concentrations in tumor tissue in this study were at low to moderate levels, although certainly enough to slow the binding of FdUMP to TS, whereas the level of dUMP in bone marrow was high enough to preclude binding of FdUMP to TS. The timing of such biopsy samples is important and affects interpretation of these experiments. Thus, the level of dUMP in a human leukemia cell in culture did not rise until TS was substantially inhibited, which took about 4 h *(45)*. Likewise, studies by Berger and Hakala *(46)* demonstrated striking accumulation of dUMP in Hep-2 carcinoma cells after a 3-h treatment with either 5-FU alone or in combination with folinic acid. In the latter study by these investigators, dUMP pools accumulated progressively up to as much as 0.8 m*M* over several hours, then decreased progressively over 24 h back to control levels (Fig. 7). That is, the accumulation of dUMP is time dependent, even when marked, and probably will not occur until TS is substantially inhibited.

Perhaps one of the central questions in this area is why some mammalian cells respond to 5-FU treatment with a dramatic increase in dUMP and others do not *(46,47)*. The studies of Spears and his colleagues *(48–50)* suggested that dUMP does not accumulate at short times after 5-FU treatment in human tumors under clinical conditions, even though such an increase may or may not have occurred later in the time course after bolus drug. Yet, Spears et al. observed millimolar concentrations of dUMP in human bone marrow cells from individuals treated with 5-FU *(49)*. With the advantages of cell culture to work with, some studies have demonstrated dUMP accumulation behind a TS block *(45–47)*; there were orders of magnitude increases of dUMP in Hep-2 cells, but not in S-180 cells *(47)* (Fig.7). However, the distinct possibility exists that the reason why dUMP did not accumulate in primary human carcinomas studied under clinical circumstances is that the inhibition of TS was insufficient to cause buildup of substrate.

In other relevant studies, Calvert and his colleagues *(51)* noted that deoyxyuridine accumulated in the serum of patients treated with doses of folate-based TS inhibitors, indicating that inhibition of TS results in accumulation of dUMP with subsequent seepage of deoxyuridine into the general circulation. The tissue of origin of the deoxyuridine in these clinical study is not known, but the effect is striking.

9. ACCUMULATION OF TS IN FLUOROPYRIMIDINE-INHIBITED TUMOR CELLS

It has been known for decades that, following inhibition of the growth of mammalian cells by any inhibitor of TS, cells undergo the process of "unbalanced growth" whereby the cellular content of RNA and protein expands, but, since DNA synthesis is blocked, division does not occur *(52,53)*. This also occurs after treatment of tumor cells with fluoropyrimidines and is somewhat more pronounced in the presence of folinic acid *(43)* (Fig. 8). Interestingly, the total cellular content of TS increases to an extent which substantially surpasses the accumulation of bulk protein after inhibition of TS by fluoropyrimidines (Fig. 8). The interpretation of this accumulation of enzyme is controversial. Early studies by Washtien *(54)*, which have been somewhat ignored in favor of more molecular explanations, clearly demonstrated that the stability to proteolysis of TS bound in a ternary complex is greatly increased and, as a result, total cellular TS would be expected to accumulate. This has been more recently confirmed in an elegant series of experiments *(55)* which concluded that stabilization against proteolysis was sufficient to explain the accumulation of enzyme in fluoropyrimidine-inhibited tumor cells. However, the interpretation of this effect may be more complex. Chu and his colleagues *(56)* have offered an alternative explanation based on their finding that recombinant TS can bind to its own cognate mRNA, and that this binding is disrupted by binding of either FdUMP or folate-based inhibitors to the active site of TS. This group has mapped the binding site for mRNA to the protein and that of protein to TS mRNA *(56–58)*. The binding of enzyme to its mRNA is a very attractive mechanism, which has been termed "translational detainment" and has been widely accepted as the mechanism explaining the accumulation of TS in 5-FU-inhibited tumor cells. This area has been discussed in detail by Chu in Chapter 4 of this book. There is evidence that this binding of TS to its cognate mRNA is the mechanism reponsible for the cell cycle oscillations in the level of TS *(59)*. This accumulation of enzyme, whether it is in a protease-stabilized inactive state or as a result of an increased rate of translation from preexisting mRNA, is an important factor in the recovery

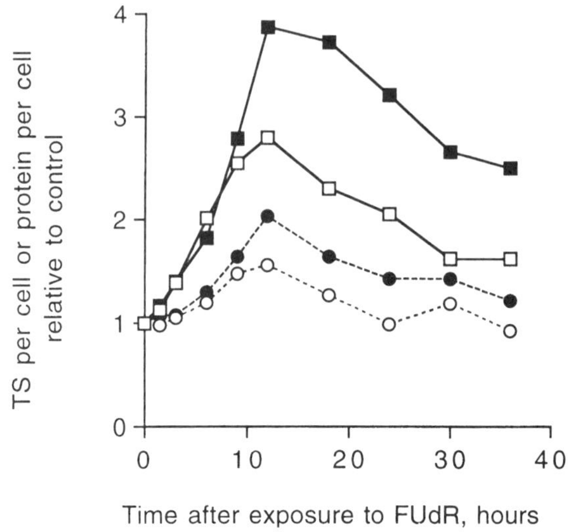

Fig. 8. *Accumulation of TS in L1210 cells treated with FudR with or without folinic acid.* Cultures of mouse L1210 cells were treated with 0.7 n*M* FUdR with (filled symbols) or without (open symbols) 10 μM folinic acid. With time after initiation of drug exposure, total levels of TS per cell (FdUMP-bound plus unbound) (squares) was measured, as was total cellular protein (circles). The total cellular content of TS per cell increased more than the protein content per cell, but the latter also increased after inhibition of cell growth with FudR. (Adapted from ref *43*.)

of active TS following 5-FU treatment, given that such inhibition is reversible (see above) and marginal under human therapeutic conditions (*see* below).

The literature on levels of TS in tumors in vivo supports the concept that TS accumulates under clinically relevant circumstances and this accumulation may confound therapy. The treatment of murine tumors in vivo with fluoropyrimidines resulted in higher levels of total TS (free plus FdUMP bound) and, as FdUMP decreased in the tumors, free enzyme was present in excess over that originally present in the tumors *(60)*. Likewise, a few studies that have addressed this factor in clinical specimens have reported higher TS levels after treatment than before *(60)*.

10. FOLATE POLYGLUTAMATES IN TUMORS AND OPTIMAL LEVELS OF REDUCED FOLATES FOR 5-FU ENHANCEMENT

Virtually all of the intracellular pool of folate cofactors exist as poly-γ-glutamate derivatives, and the normal endogenous substrate used by TS in mammalian tumor cells and normal stem cells is 5,10-methylenetetrahydropteroyl-pentaglutamate and -hexaglutamates. The chain length of the polyglutamate side chain of the folate cosubstrate available to intracellular TS will change depending on the level of folates available in the mileau in which the tumor cell or normal stem cell finds itself, and the level of folylpolyglutamate synthetase. There appears to be some hysteresis in this system, that is, the chain length of available folate cofactors in the cell depends on the concentration of exogenous folates at the moment and the level to which it has been exposed over the most recent period of perhaps 10–200 h, depending on the mitotic activity of the cell.

Folylpolyglutamate synthetase (FPGS) is present both in the mitochondrial compartment and in the cytosol in all tissues that express this enzyme *(63,64)*. The ratio of enzyme content in these two compartments is usually between 2:1 and 1:2. In human tissues, the same species of FPGS is expressed in liver and all dividing tissues, including those tumors that have been studied to date *(65)*. The same enzyme adds each of the glutamic acid residues to substrates, although some substrates are only promoted to diglutamates, and others rapidly progress to long chain polyglutamates without accumulation of diglutamates *(66)*. In mouse, a different enzyme is made in liver and kidney than in normal or malignant dividing tissues *(67,68)*.

Early studies emphasized that FPGS was present at very low levels in even enzyme-rich tissues *(69)*, and FPGS is certainly present at much lower catalytic capacities than TS or methenyltetrahydrofolate synthetase in any tumor studied to date *(70)*. However, reasonable amounts of FPGS protein are, in fact, present in almost all tumor cells, but the human enzyme has a very low turnover number (approx 0.5 s^{-1}) *(65,71)*. It is very interesting to note that cells in culture can survive and, in fact, grow at optimal rates, on levels of FPGS that are only 2–3% of those found in continuous cell lines *(72–74)*. In order for any effects to be seen on the intracellular folate pool or cell growth, FPGS levels must be less than 1–2% of normal levels *(72–74)*. At low cellular levels of FPGS, the distribution of folates favors higher polyglutamate chain length. The folate polyglutamate chain length is a biphasic function of extracellular folate concentration. As extracellular folate concentration increases, the total folate pool increases but the intracellular folate polyglutamate chain length shifts to shorter lengths. This appears to be a characteristic of FPGS itself, given that the phenomenon can be replicated with isolated pure FPGS. Hence, if too high a level of 5-formyltetrahydrofolate is used in combination with 5-FU, the cellular content of 5,10-methylenetetrahydrofolate will shift to shorter polyglutamate chain length *(75)*. One could reason that this effect might result in less effective trapping of FdUMP in ternary complex, but there is little reason to be concerned: The effectiveness of polyglutamate forms of 5,10-methelenetetrahydrofolate of chain lengths from 3–6 have been shown to be almost equivalent *(44)*.

Most of the preclinical and clinical studies on the 5-FU–folinic acid combination have utilized the mixture of diastereomers of 5-formyltetrahydrofolate about carbon 6 that results from the chemical synthesis of folinic acid. When administered to animals, the naturally occurring diastereomer of 5-formyltetrahydrofolate [(6-S)-5-formyltetrahydrofolate] is more rapidly cleared from the plasma than is (6-R)-5-formyltetrahydrofolate, so that the unnatural isomer can reach a substantial molar excess in plasma *(76,77)*. Although it is commonly thought that only the natural diastereomer has biological activity, there have been concerns that the (6-R) diastereomer could interfere with the biological effects of the (6-S)-diastereomer at high concentrations. However, studies by Zhang and Rustum *(78)* have carefully shown that (6-S)-5-formyltetrahydrofolate enhances the activity of 5-FU at exactly twice the potency of (6-R,S)-5-formyltetrahydrofolate in cell culture assays, and that (6-R)-5-formyltetrahydrofolate does not interfere with the enhancement of 5-FU caused by (6-S)-5-formyltetrahydrofolate even at a 100-fold molar excess. Several other studies support this conclusion. Hence, although both diastereomers have been shown to bind to the carrier responsible for transport of reduced folates through the plasma membrane of mammalian cells *(79)*, it would appear that the 6-R-diastereomer of folinic acid is, by and large, an inert material. In spite of these facts, it remains the case that some of the best clinical results reported with the 5-FU–reduced folate combination were obtained in trials which administer the pure (6-S) diastereomer of 5-formyltetrahydrofolate *(80,81)*, so the question of superiority of the single diastereomer in combination with 5-FU viv-a-vis the mixture of diastereomers in humans may ultimately need to be resolved by large randomized clinical trials.

However, later perspective randomized clinical trials have not shown a therapeutic advantage of FU combined with single diastereomer 5-formyltetrahydrofolate compared with FU plus the mixture of diastereomers *(82)*.

Preclinical studies demonstrated that 5-methyltetrahydrofolate was as effective as 5-formyltetrahydrofolate at enhancing the growth inhibitory activity of limiting doses of 5-FU *(83,84)*. This was a very important observation, for (6-S)-5-formyltetrahydrofolate administered to man is rapidly converted to (6-S)-5-methyltetrahydrofolate *(76,77)*, which is present at micromolar concentrations in human serum for extended periods after bolus dosage or continuous infusions of folinic acid. The chemical lability of 5-methyltetrahydrofolate is well known, and the decomposition of this compound has been shown to be much faster in oxygenated solutions, such as cell culture medium *(85)*. In addition, mammalian cells require the activity of the B_{12}-dependent 5-methyltetrahydrofolate homocysteine methyltransferase (methionine synthase) to convert 5-methyltetrahydrofolate to the cofactor for TS *(84)*. The need for transcobalamin II to allow transport of B_{12} into cells has caused some confusion in the literature on the utility of 5-methyltetrahydrofolate to enhance the activity of 5-FU. Of course, these problems are artifacts of cell culture and do not apply to in vivo use of such combinations. Presumably, the lability of 5-methyltetrahydrofolate to oxidation is circumvented by protein binding in human plasma.

As a result of demand for large amounts of folinic acid for clinical studies, methods for the large-scale preparation of individual diastereomers of 5-formyltetrahydrofolate were improved dramatically by the Swiss pharmaceutical group SAPEC, and very high purity 5,10-methylenetetrahydrofolate also became available as an offshoot of this substantial chemical effort. This compound is a Shiff base adduct of tetrahydrofolate and formaldehyde and had never been widely available as a stable chemical entity before SAPEC's considerable accomplishments in this area. Subsequent studies made it clear that single isomer (6-S)5-formyltetrahydrofolate can act as an effective substitute for the mixture of (6-R,S)diastereomers, that is, for folinic acid. Indeed, 5,10-methylenetetrahydrofolate itself could serve as an exogenous source of an expanded intracellular pool of 5,10-methylenetetrahydrofolate polyglutamates *(86)*, although the sensitivity of 5,10-methylenetetrahydrofolate to dissociation into formaldehyde and tetrahydrofolate and the chemical instability of the latter made 5,10-methylenetetrahydrofolate a source of an expanded pool of intracellular cofactor of questionable value. Other studies *(87)* used the stable form folic acid to expand the pools of 5,10-methylenetetrahydrofolate derivatives available to TS. The use of folic acid as a exogenous source of folates would require the activity of hepatic and cellular dihydrofolate reductase for production of tetrahydrofolate available to tumor cells, and older literature had shown *(88)* that systemic dihydrofolate reductase can be saturated by pharmacological doses of folic acid, potentially resulting in inefficient production of reduced folates at high doses.

11. RELATIONSHIP BETWEEN FOLINIC ACID-INDUCED ENHANCEMENT OF 5-FU AND INTRACELLULAR POOLS OF TETRAHYDROFOLATES

Early studies by Hougthon et al. *(89)* found that the intracellular pool of methylenetetrahydrofolate in a series of human colon carcinoma xenographs was suboptimal for maximal formation and stabilization of the ternary complex in these tumors. This group subsequently measured the content of tetrahydrofolate and 5,10-methylenetetrahydrofolate in these tumors after the administration of increasing doses of folinic acid to the mice *(90,91)*. In these studies, there were large differences among the tumors in how much the pool could be expanded with administered folinic acid, and also the pool size of these

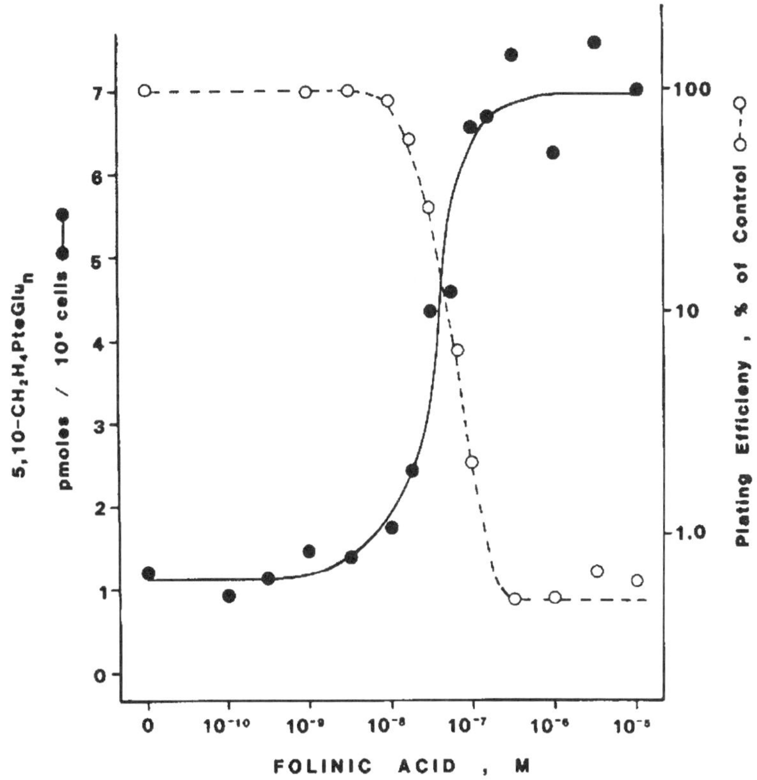

Fig. 9. *Relationship of 5-FU enhancement by folinic acid and intracellular folate cofactor pools.* Mouse L1210 cells were exposed to the indicated concentrations of folinic acid in the presence of 0.32 µ*M* 5-FU for 72 h, and the cells were harvested and assayed for 5,10-methylenetetrahydrofolate (polyglutamate) pools. Another aliquot of each culture was plated in soft agarose to determine cell viability by colony formation. (Taken from ref. *43* with the permission of the *Journal of Biological Chemistry.*)

tetrahydrofolates in tumors from animals not administered exogenous folinic acid varied from 0.5 to 3 µ*M.* However, in animals treated with 100–300 mg/m^2 folinic acid, the pool of these reduced folates was from 2.2 to 10 µ*M (89–91).* Treatment of tumor-bearing mice with increasing doses of folinic acid caused a decrease in the mean chain length of the side chain of the tetrahydrofolates, similarly to that seen in cell culture. The authors did not see any relationship between the size or expansion of the tetrahydrofolate pool and the level of tumor cell FPGS; however, the level of FPGS in these tumors ranged from high to very high.

An early study from our laboratory *(43)* demonstrated that the dependence of the 5-FU/folinic acid combination on folinic acid concentration was directly related to the ability of each concentration of folinic acid to expand the pool of 5,10-methylenetetrahydrofolate and tetrahydrofolate available as substrate for TS (Fig. 9). Thus, exactly the same range of folinic acid concentrations that expanded the intracellular pool of 5,10-methylenetetrahydrofolate, presumably present as polyglutamates, enhanced the cytotoxic effects of exposure to 5-FU. A critical set of studies by Milano and his colleagues *(92,93)* found that the concentration of intracellular cofactors for TS needed to enhance the efficacy of 5-FU in a series of cell lines was in the range of 8–40 pmol/mg protein, a range of only five-fold. whereas the extracellular range of folinic acid concentrations to stimulate 5-FU activity in this same group of cell lines was much wider (0.7–108 µ*M,* a 150-fold range). This is a very important observation, and it suggests that the concentration dependence for stimulation of 5-FU by folinic acid reflects differences among cell types in the metabolism of extracellular 5-formyltetrahydrofolate to 5,10-methylenetetrahydrofolate or the ability of cells to accumulate folates in this form in the steady state. Making reasonable assumptions from the method of preparation of cell extracts in these papers *(92)*, it appears that the concentrations required to stimulate binding to FdUMP to TS in these cells were about 0.8 to 4 pmol/mg tissue or 1–5 μ*M* in cell water. The data for L1210 cells (Fig. 9) suggest an intracellular concentration of tetrahydrofolate and 5,10-methylenetetrahydrofolate polyglutamates of about 5–10 μ*M* would maximally enhance 5-FU cytotoxicity *(43)*. Interestingly, the experiments of Cheradame et al. *(92)* demonstrated that the enhancement of 5-FU by folinic acid was maximal under conditions that expanded the tetrahydrofolate plus 5,10-methylelene tetrahydrolfolate pool to 3–6 μ*M*, yet expansion of these pools to equivalent or higher levels in the CAL51 cell was without effect on the growth-inhibitory efficacy of 5-FU. This potentially central observation has yet to be explained.

Cheradame et al. *(93,94)* also measured the level of tetrahydrofolate plus 5,10-methylelene tetrahydrofolate in a series of 50 primary head and neck tumors, 16 colon carcinomas, and 30 biopsies of colon cancer metastatic to the liver. The levels of these critical cofactors were below those that enhance binding to FdUMP to TS in most of the head and neck and colon carcinomas (calculated from their data to have mean values of (approx 0.5–0.6 pmol/mg tissue), but were higher in liver metastases (approx 1.8 pmol/mg tissue). Preclinical studies had demonstrated that extreme deficiency of FPGS results in frank resistance to 5-FU with or without folinic acid *(95,96)*. As a result, the French group *(93,94)* studied the link between sensitivity to 5-FU, tumor tetrahydrofolate pool size and FPGS level in a series of human colon and head and neck carcinoma biopsies. Their results suggested that head and neck tumors with a low tetrahydrofolate pools were not likely to respond to regimens containing 5-FU (without folinic acid), while those patients that responded tended to have higher tetrahydrofolate pools in tumor tissue. The FPGS levels in liver metastasis samples from individuals with colon cancer that responded to 5-FU plus folinic acid were significantly higher than in patients who did not respond to this treatment. This agrees with the prior experiments from this group *(92)* that showed a direct relationship between the level of FPGS and the sensitivity to 5-FU plus folinic acid in a series of eighteen human carcinoma cell lines. Overall, the data emerging from these critical clinical and preclinical studies *(92–96)* support the concept that the level of 5,10-methylenetetrahydrofolate (polyglutamates) available in human carcinomas is too low to allow maximal stabilization of the inhibited TS complex without supplementation by folinic acid treatment, and that the level of FPGS in a tumor is a factor in the ability of that tumor to respond to 5-FU/folinic acid.

12. LENGTH OF TIME THAT TS MUST BE INHIBITED TO YIELD EFFICIENT CELL KILL

The question has been debated with little solution as to how long TS must be inhibited in order to irreversibly initiate cell kill. Given the multiple mechanisms possible for 5-FU, the timing of inhibition of TS by this agent needed for induction of cytotoxicity could always be debated, with little hope of a definitive answer. However, two test systems have yielded the answer: Cell lines genetically modified to be deficient in TS *(97,98)* and cell lines inhibited by the pure TS inhibitor tomudex (D-1694, ralitrexid) *(99)*. For both of these model systems, tumor cells will grow quite normally with genetically or pharmacologically deleted TS in the presence of exogenous thymidine, but thymine-less conditions will be induced rapidly after

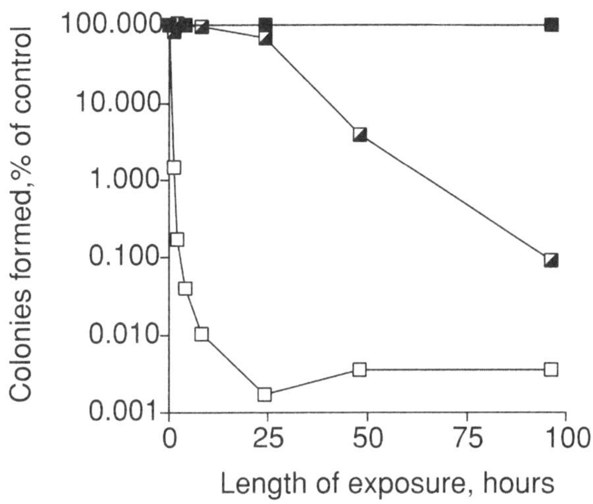

Fig. 10. *Length of inhibition of thymidylate synthase required for efficient cell kill of WiDr cells.* Human WiDr colon carcinoma cells were plated out at 300–250,000 cells per dish and treated with 1 μ*M* tomudex (D-1694), a folate antimetabolite specifically inhibitory to TS. After the indicated time periods, the drug was removed and fresh medium added every 3 d for 3.5 wk on some of the cultures (open squares). For other cultures (filled squares), thymidine (5.6 μ*M*) was added to the cultures during drug exposure, and in all culture medium changes after drug removal. For the third group of cultures (half-filled squares), thymidine was added to the medium after drug exposure but not during drug exposure. Thus, the open symbols show the time course of drug toxicity, including accumulation of drug polyglutamates in the cells. The filled symbols show the complete reversibility of tomudex effects by thymidine, direct evidence of the specificity of this drug only for TS. The half-filled symbols demonstrate the time course with which blockage of thymidylate synthase leads to irreversible commitment to cell death. (This figure was adapted from ref. *99* with the permission of *Cancer Research.*)

removal of thymidine from the medium. Given that the cellular pool of thymidine nucleotides in cells grown on thymidine is not higher than 10 μ*M,* a cell will consume the preexisting pool of thymidine nucleotides during the first 0.5% of S-phase, or in about 3 min. By maintaining cells in the continuous presence of drug under clonogenic conditions, then removing the culture medium and changing to medium containing thymidine but no drug, one can determine how long TS must be inhibited to induce irreversible commitment to cell death *(99).* As shown in Fig. 10, complete inhibition of TS can be maintained in the human WiDr colon carcinoma cell (a p53 null cell line), for 24 h (equivalent to one cell generation time for the WiDr cell) without cytotoxicity; with longer inhibition of this pathway, commitment to cell death proceeds exponentially and with a very steep slope. The cell cycle traverse time for the WiDr cell is about 24 h. Hence, we conclude that the therapeutic objective of treatment of tumors with TS inhibitors should be to maintain complete inhibition for >> 24 h. If tumor TS is completely inhibited after treatment of patients with 5-FU ± folinic acid for periods of one cell generation time (for *stem cells* of many human tumors, one could take 24 h as an estimate of the fastest reasonable cell cycle time) or less, it is to be expected that no cell kill would result. Longer periods of complete suppression of TS would be very effective in inducing irreversible commitment to cell death *(99).* Very similar conclusions could be drawn from prior literature on the survival of cell lines deficient in TS when thymidine is withdrawn from the medium *(97,98,100).*

This is a somewhat surprising conclusion. Clearly, lesser degrees of inhibition of TS would be met with much lower success in forcing cells to commit to death. Hence, we are faced with the question: How often does therapy with 5-FU with or without folinic acid result in complete enzyme inhibition, and how often is that inhibition maintained for extended periods of time in human colon carcinomas?

13. INHIBITION OF TS BY THE COMBINATION OF 5-FU AND FOLINIC ACID

The net effect of exposure of tumors to fluoropyrimidines on the availability of enzymatically active TS has been studied in cells in culture, in mice, and in humans being treated with 5-FU. Several assays are available which measure either true catalytic rates in tumor extracts *(101),* or the number of open TS active sites in extracts (by titration with ^{3}H-FdUMP) *(45)* or that estimate catalytic rates in intact cells *(102).* The first two of these assays are sensitive enough for and appropriate for assays in patient biopsies or experimental animals and have been modified in the process of application to tissues. The ^{3}H-FdUMP binding assay has been modified to allow estimation of both free TS active sites and FdUMP-bound active sites *(60,103).* However, the inhibition of TS by fluoropyrimidines with or without reduced folates under therapeutic conditions has remained a challenging exercise, and a surprisingly small amount of information is available. Much of the difficulty is based on the characteristics of the assay procedures and on the ethical and practical considerations in estimating TS in primary human tumor tissue. Thus, catalytic assays sufficiently sensitive for such experiments rely on conversion of ^{3}H-dUMP to ^{3}H-H_2O and are, hence, susceptible to isotope dilution by tissue dUMP. FdUMP titration experiments must also deal with dilution of isotope by tissue FdUMP and with the surprisingly rapid release of FdUMP bound to TS during assay and subsequent exchange with ^{3}H-FdUMP during labeling incubations *(60).* This latter effect can and has caused difficulty in accurately estimating the therapeutically critical level of uninhibited TS in the presence of enzyme bound to FdUMP, namely the difference between zero and 20% residual enzyme activity. Finally, the level of TS in clinical samples of colon carcinoma is quite low, reducing signal to the levels comparable to a few times background in many if not most tumor biopsies. Thus, compared with the experimental tumor and tumor cells studied which have TS levels of 20–150 pmol of FdUMP binding sites per gram wet weight *(60),* a series of 123 advanced human colon, stomach, and pancreatic tumor biopsies were reported to have a range clustering about 2–6 pmol enzyme per gram wet weight and 13 breast carcinoma biopsies has TS levels on the same range *(103,104).* Comparing these numbers with the level of TS shown to allow rapid recovery of L1210 cells (Fig. 11) after FUdR treatment (approx 4 pmol/g of FdUMP binding sites; see below), one sees that TS in these tumors is, in fact, quite low and can be viewed as close to limiting to GI tumor cell growth. Of course, the interpretation of biochemical assays on tissue biopsies is plagued with concerns about heterogeneity, so that all of this active enzyme might be in 10% of the cells in a specimen, which would put the level of TS to be as high in a subset of expressing cells in a tumor as in the most rapidly growing experimental tumor. Tumor immunohistochemistry would not agree with this concept, and would suggest that the large fraction of cells in a GI tumor express the TS found by bulk enzyme assays.

Spears and his colleagues followed the level of free TS in a series of colon tumors of the mouse that differed in sensitivity to 5-FU as a function of time after a bolus dose of drug *(60).* Only one of the four tumors responded to 5-FU, and that response was somewhat limited (a 58% increase in life span after four doses of 5-FU). That tumor showed complete

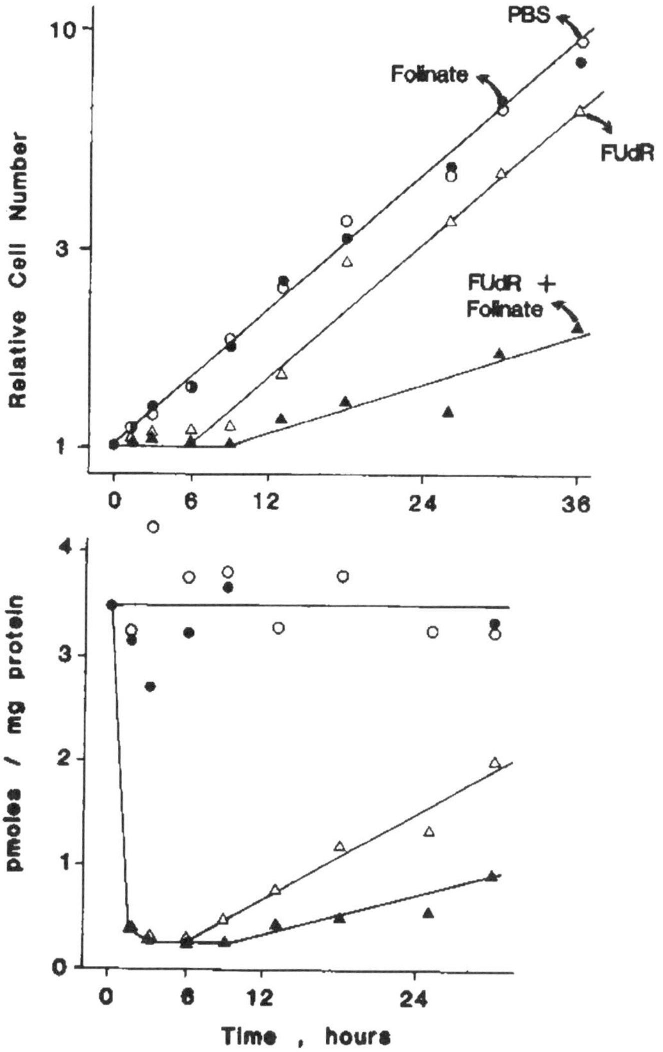

Fig. 11. *Rapid recovery of TS in L1210 cells treated continuously with FudR.* Cultures of mouse L1210 cells were exposed to 0.7 n*M* FudR alone (open triangles) or combined with 10 μ*M* folinic acid for the indicated periods of time, culture density was measured using a Coulter counter, and cellular TS activity was quantitated using a catalytic assay that measured the release of tritium from the 5-position of dUMP. Control cultures were exposed to folinic acid (filled circles) or an equivalent amount of phosphate-buffered saline. Note that cell growth resumed in FudR-treated cells after 3–5% of the enzyme activity had reappeared in the cells, in spite of the continued presence of FudR. The presence of folinic acid suppressed the reappearance of active enzyme and proportionally extended the period of cell growth inhibition. (Modified from ref. *43* with the permission of the *Journal of Biological Chemistry.*)

inhibition of TS after a single test dose of drug, which was maintained for 6 h, followed by recovery of free enzyme. The three insensitive colon tumors showed inhibition of TS, but inhibition was not complete nor was it sustained. This in vivo experiment, then, reinforces the concept that a complete and sustained depletion of TS activity is required for therapeutic effect. Some aspects of the augmentation of inhibition of cellular TS by folinic acid in human *(95)* or mouse *(43)* leukemia cells in culture after exposure to FudR bear directly on this point. At high concentrations of FUdR, enzyme was completely inhibited whether or not folinic acid was present. At lower concentrations, a very interesting pattern emerged (Fig 11). Cells exposed to FUdR alone were initially prevented from further growth, but rapid growth resumed after 6 h *(43,95)*. In contrast, for the same concentration of FUdR, in the presence of folinic acid, growth inhibition was maintained longer, and when growth resumed, the rate of growth was stunted. TS levels mirrored the tumor cell growth: In FUdR alone *(43)*, enzyme was completely inhibited for about 6 h, then progressively recovered, while in cells treated with FUdR and folinic acid, enzyme levels were held at zero for 10–12 h, and recovered only slowly thereafter. Perhaps the most important aspect of this study, however, was the observation that cell growth recovered to control rates in FUdR-treated cells at a time when only about 5% of control enzyme was uninhibited. Although this fraction will clearly depend upon how much enzyme is present in a tumor cell population to begin with, it suggests that measurement of tumor enzyme levels must be carefully interpreted, since tumors do not care about percentages but rather grow or die depending only on whether sufficient enzyme is active to allow TMP synthesis. Thus, the only pertinent parameter for assessing the biochemical effect of 5-FU against TMP synthesis is the absolute amount of active enzyme left in dividing tumor stem cells after 5-FU therapy.

A related study from Peters' group *(105)* nicely explained the therapeutic activity of maximally tolerated doses of 5-FU and FUdR in terms of the time course of inhibition of TS. In that study, treatment with either 5-FU or FUdR at high bolus doses depressed tumor TS and held it depressed for extended periods of time, but the antitumor effect of FUdR was far superior to that of 5-FU. There were several other quite striking effects demonstrated by this very complete study:

1. Residual TS was found by both a catalytic assay, run over 30 min, and an FdUMP binding assay, run over 60 min; the residual activity was 10% and 20–30% of control in these two assays, which were performed on the same extracts. Viewed for the perspective of the characteristics of these assays, this technique-dependent, residual, apparently uninhibited, TS is almost certainly artifact due to dissociation of ternary complex during experimental procedures. Unfortunately, this serves to underscore the fact that reliable determination of complete enzyme inhibition is still technically challenging in vivo under even well-controlled and executed preclinical conditions. The judicious interpretation of these results is that TS was, in fact, completely inhibited for extended periods in these tumors.
2. The difference between a good therapeutic fluoropyrimidine exposure and one of marginal therapeutic effect was complete and prolonged TS inhibition: 5-FU treatment completely suppressed TS at early times as well as FUdR, but allowed recovery of TS after 3 d, whereas FUdR completely suppressed enzyme for 7 d.
3. The level of FdUMP in the tumors was only slightly more than stoichiometric with the level of TS active sites after 5-FU, yet TS was either completely inhibited after treatment or was very close to completely inhibited. The level of FdUMP immediately after FUdR was in 2.5 molar excess over the level of TS active sites, yet the level of inhibition of TS was not meaningfully more than after 5-FU, where FdUMP was only slightly more than stoichiometric with binding sites. Hence, FdUMP was a very effective enzyme inhibitor in this tumor.
4. FdUMP rapidly disappeared from tumor cytosols in both cases. The peak levels of FdUMP in tumor in these and other studies suggests that the binding of this metabolite to newly synthesized TS is probably involved in the rate of dissapearance of free FdUMP from the tumor.

Hence, the reason that TS remained suppressed in FUdR-treated tumors longer than in 5-FU-treated tumors was not apparent in this study, which applied current biochemical techniques available for TS and FdUMP in the meticulous manner consistent with preclinical experiments. Perhaps dUMP and methylene tetrahydrofolate determinations might have allowed an understanding of the mechanism of recovery of enzyme activity, perhaps it would not have.

Although such studies are much more difficult to design and execute on clinical samples, the results of a few studies are available. Spears, Gustavsson, and Frosing biopsied multiple individual hepatic and peritoneal metastases of a colon carcinoma as a function of time during a 2 h surgical procedure *(106)*. A single dose of 5-FU at 500 mg/m^2 reduced the level of FdUMP-titratable TS in these biopsies from 2–3.5 pmol/g to levels below 0.5 pmol/g within 1 h in the face of excess FdUMP in some of the metastases, but there was evidence that inhibition was not maintained following loss of adequate FdUMP in the tumors. In a one-of-a-kind study *(49)*, Spears et al. measured the parameters of FdUMP inhibition of TS in biopsies of more than 20 human tumors, chiefly GI malignancies, 1–3 h after a single dose of 500 mg/m^2 5-FU. Single biopsies were taken from each patient, but composite time courses of tumor levels of FdUMP, dUMP, and free and inhibited TS were deduced. As had been seen in animal tumors, substantial levels of FdUMP formed very quickly, peaking before 30 min after 5-FU treatment, but FdUMP was rapidly lost, reaching levels near or equivalent to enzyme levels within about 3 h. Free TS dropped after drug dosage, reaching a nadir of about 25% of uninhibited levels after 1.5–2 h. dUMP levels hovered around 25 μ*M* for several hours after drug. At face value, the results of this study *(49,104)* said that free TS coexisted with excess FdUMP for the length of the observation time possible, and the level of active enzyme remaining might not be consistent with cytotoxic effects of the 5-FU dose. From preclinical experience, it appears that the key to interpretation of these critical clinical experiments is whether the residual enzyme levels found were real or artifacts, and, in either case, why they are found.

Hence, the conclusion that appears to be correct is that FdUMP in tumor cells rises to a peak within about 0.5–4 h after exposure to 5-FU, but was usually not maintained long after bolus administration of drug to animals or patients, and the level of residual active TS following dosage and the difficulty supressing enzyme activity may not be consistent with a therapeutic effect. However, assessment of the absolute levels of residual active enzyme in colon carcinoma biopsies certainly pushes the limit of existing technique, and the approx 25% of pretreatment enzyme seeen in the clinical experiments in the face of adequate FdUMP might represent either analytical artifact or intrinsic limitations of therapy with 5-FU.

14. ASSESSMENT OF TUMOR LEVELS OF MRNA ENCODING TS

In view of the substantial difficulties of following the biochemical pharmacology of inhibition of TS in human carcinomas under clinical conditions, alternative parameters predictive of the responsiveness of individual tumors have been widely sought. A very informative parameters that is of current interest is the relative level of mRNA encoding TS. Although a surrogate measure for TS itself, reverse transcription-polymerase chain reaction (RT-PCR) analysis of TS mRNA has proven to be a technically approachable, robust, and useful technique *(107)*. Following the initial suggestion from Spears and his colleagues that individuals with low TS were more likely to have a therapeutic response to tolerated doses of 5-FU than individuals with high TS content, TS expression studies demonstrated this correlation quite convincingly for metastatic colon carcinoma and for carcinoma of the stomach *(108,109)*. The technique has now been widely applied *(110–113)*, and the details of correlations of RT-PCR data to clinical response is described in detail by Danenberg, by Leichman, and by Lenz and their colleagues.

REFERENCES

1. Heidelberger C, Chaudhuri NK, Danneberg P, et al. Fluorinated pyrimidines, a new class of tumor inhibitory agents. *Nature* 1957; 179:663–666.
2. Heidelberger C. "Fluorinated Pyrimidines and their Nucleosides." In Antineoplastic and Immunosuppressive Agents II (A.C. Sartorelli and D.G. Johns, eds.) Springer-Verlag, New York, NY pp 193–231.
3. Heidelberger C, Danenberg PV, Moran RG. Fluorinated Pyrimidines and Their Nucleosides. *Adv Enzymol* 1983; 54:57–119.
4. Cadman E, Heimer R, Davis L. Enhanced 5-fluorouracil nucleotide formation after methotrexate administration: explanation for drug synergy. *Science* 1979; 205:1135–1137.
5. Martin DS, Stolfi RL, Sawyer RC, Spiegelman S, Casper ES, Young CW. Therapeutic utility of utilizing low doses of N-(phosphonacetyl)-L-aspartic acid in combination with 5-fluorouracil: a murine study with clinical relevance. *Cancer Res* 1983; 43:2317–2321.
6. Danenberg PV, Heidelberger C, Mulkins MA, Peterson AR. The incorporation of 5-fluoro-2′-deoxyuridine into DNA of mammalian tumor cells. *Biochem Biophys Res Commun* 1981; 102:654–658.
7. Major PP, Egan E, Herrick D, Kufe DW. 5-Fluorouracil incorporation in DNA of human breast carcinoma cells. *Cancer Res* 1982; 42:3005–3009.
8. Ingraham HA, Tseng BY, Goulian M. Mechanism for exclusion of 5-fluorouracil from DNA. *Cancer Res* 1980; 40:998–1001.
9. Caradonna SJ, and Cheng YC. Uracil DNA-glycosylase. Purification and properties of this enzyme isolated from blast cells of acute myelocytic leukemia patients. *J Biol Chem* 1980; 255:2293–2300.
10. Umeda M, Heidelberger C. Comparative studies of fluorinated pyrimidines with various cell lines. *Cancer Res* 1968; 28:2529–2538.
11. Rich MA, Bolaffi JL, Knoll JE, Cheong L, Eidinoff ML. Growth inhibition of a human cell strain by 5-fluorouracil, 5-fluorouridine, and 5-fluoro-2-deoxyuridine-reversal studies. *Cancer Res* 1958; 18:730–735.
12. Ullman B, Lee M, Martin DW Jr, Santi DV. Cytotoxicity of 5-fluoro-2′-deoxyuridine: requirement for reduced folate cofactors and antagonism by methotrexate. *Proc Natl Acad Sci USA* 1978; 75:980–983.
13. Evans RM, Laskin JD, Hakala MT. Assessment of growth-limiting events caused by 5-fluorouracil in mouse cells and in human cells. *Cancer Res* 1980; 40:4113–22.
14. Evans RM, Laskin JD, Hakala MT. Effect of excess folates and deoxyinosine on the activity and site of action of 5-fluorouracil. *Cancer Res* 1981; 41:3288–3295.
15. Machover D, Goldschmidt E, Chollet P, et al. Treatment of advanced colorectal and gastric adenocarcinomas with 5-fluorouracil and high-dose folinic acid. *J Clin Oncol* 1986; 4:685–696.
16. Petrelli N, Herrera L, Rustum Y, et al. A prospective randomized trial of 5-fluorouracil versus 5-fluorouracil and high-dose leucovorin versus 5-fluorouracil and methotrexate in previously untreated patients with advanced colorectal carcinoma. *J Clin Oncol* 1987; 5:1559–1565.
17. Erlichman C, Fine S, Wong A, Elhakim T. A randomized trial of fluorouracil and folinic acid in patients with metastatic colorectal carcinoma. *J Clin Oncol* 1988; 6:469–475.
18. Keyomarsi K, Moran RG. Folinic acid augmentation of the effects of fluoropyrimidines on murine and human leukemic cells. *Cancer Res* 1986; 46:5229–5235.
19. Moran RG, Scanlon KL. Schedule-dependent enhancement of the cytotoxicity of fluoropyrimidines to human carcinoma cells in the presence of folinic acid. *Cancer Res* 1991; 51:4618–4623.
20. Howell SB, Mansfield SJ, Taetle R. Significance of variation in serum thymidine concentration for the marrow toxicity of methotrexate. *Cancer Chemother Pharmacol* 1981; 5:221–226.
21. JH Semon and GB Grindey Potentiation of the antitumor activity of methotrexate by concurrent infusion of thymidine *Cancer Res* 1978; 38:2905–2911.
22. Jackman AL, Taylor GA, Calvert AH, Harrap KR Modulation of anti-metabolite effects. Effects of thymidine on the efficacy of the quinazoline-based thymidylate synthetase inhibitor, CB3717. *Biochem Pharmacol* 1984; 33:3269–3275.
23. Houghton JA, Williams LG, Loftin SK, et al. Factors that influence the therapeutic activity of 5-fluorouracil [6RS]leucovorin combinations in colon adenocarcinoma xenografts. *Cancer Chemother Pharmacol* 1992; 30:423–432.
24. Beck A, Etienne MC, Cheradame S, Fischel JL, Formento P, Guillot T, Milano G. Wide range for optimal concentration of folinic acid in fluorouracil modulation—experimental data on human tumour cell lines. *Eur J Cancer* 1994; 30A:1522–1526.
25. O'Connell MJ. A phase III trial of 5-fluorouracil and leucovorin in the treatment of advanced colorectal cancer. A Mayo Clinic/North Central Cancer Treatment Group study. *Cancer* 1989; 63:1026–1030.

26. Poon MA, O'Connell MJ, Wieand HS, et al. Biochemical modulation of fluorouracil with leucovorin: confirmatory evidence of improved therapeutic efficacy advanced colorectal cancer. *J Clin Oncol* 1991; 9:1967–1972.
27. Petrelli N, Douglass HO Jr, Herrera L, et al. The modulation of fluorouracil with leucovorin in metastatic colorectal carcinoma: a prospective randomized phase III trial. Gastrointestinal Tumor Study Group. *J Clin Oncol* 1989; 7:1419–1426.
28. Leichman CG, Fleming TR, Muggia FM, et al. Phase II study of fluorouracil and its modulation in advanced colorectal cancer: a Southwest Oncology Group study. *J Clin Oncol* 1995; 13:1303–1311.
29. Machover D. A comprehensive review of 5-fluorouracil and leucovorin in patients with metastatic colorectal carcinoma. *Cancer* 1997; 80(7):1179–1187.
30. van Laar JA, van der Wilt CL, Rustum YM, et al. Therapeutic efficacy of fluoropyrimidines depends on the duration of thymidylate synthase inhibition in the murine colon 26-B carcinoma tumor model. *Clin Cancer Res* 1996; 2:1327–1333.
31. Perry KM, Fauman EB, Finer-Moore JS, et al. Plastic adaptation toward mutations in proteins: structural comparison of thymidylate synthases. *Proteins* 1990; 8:315–33.
32. Hardy LW, Finer-Moore JS, Montfort WR, Jones MO, Santi DV, Stroud RM. Atomic structure of thymidylate synthase: target for rational drug design. *Science* 1987; 235:448–455.
33. Sayre PH, Finer-Moore JS, Fritz TA, et al. Multi-targeted Antifolates Aimed at Avoiding Drug Resistance Form Covalent Closed Inhibitory Complexes with Human and Escherichia coli Thymidylate Synthases. *J Mol Biol* 2001; 313(4):813–829.
34. Pookanjanatavip M, Yuthavong Y, Greene PJ, Santi DV. Subunit complementation of thymidylate synthase. *Biochemistry* 1992; 31:10303–10309.
35. Bradshaw TP, Dunlap RB. Characterization of a novel form of thymidylate synthase: a heterodimer isolated after specific chemical modification of the immobilized native enzyme. *Biochemistry* 1993; 19932:12774–12781.
36. Finer-Moore JS, Montfort WR, Stroud RM. Pairwise specificity and sequential binding in enzyme catalysis: thymidylate synthase. *Biochemistry* 1990; 29:6977–6986.
37. Danenberg KD, Danenberg PV. Evidence for a sequential interaction of the subunits of thymidylate synthetase. *J Biol Chem* 1979; 254:4345–4348.
38. Maley F, Pedersen-Lane J, Changchien L. Complete restoration of activity to inactive mutants of *Escherichia coli* thymidylate synthase: evidence that *E. coli* thymidylate synthase is a half-the-sites activity enzyme. *Biochemistry* 1995; 34:469–1474.
39. Reilly RT, Barbour KW, Dunlap RB, Berger FG. Biphasic binding of 5-fluoro-2′-deoxyuridylate to human thymidylate synthase. *Mol Pharmacol* 1995; 48:72–79.
40. Lorenson MY, Maley GF, Maley F. The purification and properties of thymidylate synthetase from chick embryo extracts. *J Biol Chem* 1967; 242:3332–3344.
41. Daron HH, Aull JL. A kinetic study of thymidylate synthase from Lactobacillus casei. *J Biol Chem* 1978; 253:940–945.
42. Lockshin A, Danenberg PV. Biochemical factors affecting the tightness of 5-fluorodeoxyuridylate binding to human thymidylate synthetase. *Biochem Pharmacol* 1981; 30(3):247–257.
43. Keyomarsi K, Moran RG. Mechanism of the cytotoxic synergism of fluoropyrimidines and folinic acid in mouse leukemic cells. *J Biol Chem* 1988; 263:14402–14409.
44. Radparvar S, Houghton PJ, Houghton JA. Effect of polyglutamylation of 5,10-methylenetetrahydrofolate on the binding of 5-fluoro-2′-deoxyuridylate to thymidylate synthase purified from a human colon adenocarcinoma xenograft. *Biochem Pharmacol* 1989; 38:335–342.
45. Moran RG, Spears CP, Heidelberger C. Biochemical determinants of tumor sensitivity to 5-fluorouracil: ultrasensitive methods for the determination of 5-fluoro-2′-deoxyuridylate, 2'-deoxyuridylate, and thymidylate synthetase. *Proc Natl Acad Sci USA* 76:1456–1460.
46. Berger SH, Hakala MT. Relationship of dUMP and free FdUMP pools to inhibition of thymidylate synthase by 5-fluorouracil. *Mol Pharmacol* 1984; 25:303–309.
47. Webley SD, Welsh SJ, Jackman AL, Aherne GW. The ability to accumulate deoxyuridine triphosphate and cellular response to thymidylate synthase (TS) inhibition. *Br J Cancer* 2001; 85:446–452.
48. Spears CP, Gustavsson BG, Mitchell MS, et al. Thymidylate synthetase inhibition in malignant tumors and normal liver of patients given intravenous 5-fluorouracil. *Cancer Res* 1984; 44:4144–4150.
49. Spears CP, Gustavsson BG, Berne M, Frosing R, Bernstein L, Hayes AA. Mechanisms of innate resistance to thymidylate synthase inhibition after 5-fluorouracil. *Cancer Res* 1988; 48:5894–5900.
50. Spears CP, Gustavsson BG, Frosing R. Folinic acid modulation of fluorouracil: tissue kinetics of bolus administration. *Invest New Drugs* 1989; 7:27–36.

51. Rafi I, Taylor GA, Calvete JA, et al. Clinical pharmacokinetic and pharmacodynamic studies with the antifolate thymidylate synthase inhibitor 3, 4-dihydro-2-amino-6-methyl-4-oxo-5-(4-pyridylthio)-quinazolone dihydrochloride (AG337) given by 24-hour continuous intravenous infusion. *Clin Cancer Res* 1995; 1:1275–1284.
52. Cohen LS, Studzinski GP. Correlation between cell enlargement and nucleic acid and protein content of HeLa cells in unbalanced growth produced by inhibitors of DNA synthesis. *J Cell Physiol* 1967; 69:331–339.
53. Cohen SS. On the nature of thymineless death. *Ann N Y Acad Sci* 1971; 186:292–301.
54. Washtien WL. Increased levels of thymidylate synthetase in cells exposed to 5-fluorouracil. *Mol Pharmacol* 1984; 25:171–177.
55. Kitchens ME, Forsthoefel AM, Barbour KW, et al. Mechanisms of acquired resistance to thymidylate synthase inhibitors: the role of enzyme stability. *Mol Pharmacol* 1999; 56:1063–1070.
56. Chu E, Voeller D, Koeller DM, et al. Identification of an RNA binding site for human thymidylate synthase. Proc Natl Acad Sci U S A. 1993; 90:517–521.
57. Chu E, Copur SM, Ju J, et al. Thymidylate *Mol Cell Biol* 1999; 19:1582–1594.
58. Lin X, Parsels LA, Voeller DM, et al. Characterization of a cis-acting regulatory element in the protein coding region of thymidylate synthase mRNA. *Nucleic Acids Res* 2000; 28:1381–1389.
59. Keyomarsi K, Samet J, Molnar G, Pardee AB. The thymidylate synthase inhibitor, ICI D1694, overcomes translational detainment of the enzyme. *J Biol Chem* 1993; 268:15142–15149.
60. Spears CP, Shahinian AH, Moran RG, et. al. In vivo kinetics of thymidylate synthetase inhibition of 5-fluorouracil-sensitive and -resistant murine colon adenocarcinomas. *Cancer Res* 1982; 42:450–456.
61. Swain SM, Lippman ME, Egan EF, et. al. Fluorouracil and high-dose leucovorin in previously treated patients with metastatic breast cancer. *J Clin Oncol* 1989; 7:890–899.
62. Lin BF, Huang RF, Shane B. Regulation of folate and one-carbon metabolism in mammalian cells. III. Role of mitochondrial folylpoly-gamma-glutamate synthetase. *J Biol Chem* 1993; 268:21674–21679.
63. Freemantle SJ, Taylor SM, Krystal G, et.al. Upstream organization of and multiple transcripts from the human folypoly-gamma-glutamate synthetase gene. *J Biol Chem* 1995; 270:9579–9584.
64. Turner FB, Taylor SM, Moran RG. Expression patterns of the multiple transcripts from the folypolyglutamate synthetase gene in human leukemias and normal differentiated tissues. *J Biol Chem* 2000; 275:35960–35968.
65. Sanghani PC, Moran RG. Purification and characteristics of recombinant human folypoly-gamma-glutamate synthetase expressed at high levels in insect cells. *Protein Expr Purif* 2000; 18:36–45.
66. Moran RG, Colman PD. Measurement of folypolyglutamate synthetase in mammalian tissues. *Anal Biochem* 1984; 140:326–342.
67. Turner FB, Andreassi 2nd JL, Ferguson J, et al. Tissue-specific expression of functional isoforms of mouse folypoly-gamma-glutamate synthetase: a basis for targeting folate antimetabolites. *Cancer Res* 1999; 59:6074–6079.
68. Roy K, Mitsugi K, Sirotnak FM. Additional organizational features of the murine folypolyglutamate synthetase gene. Two remotely situated exons encoding an alternate 5′ end and proximal open reading frame under the control of a second promoter. *J Biol Chem* 1997; 272:5587–5593.
69. Barredo J, Moran RG. Determinants of antifolate cytotoxicity: folypolyglutamate synthetase activity during cellular proliferation and development. *Mol Pharmacol* 1992; 42:687–694.
70. van der Wilt CL, Cloos J, de Jong M, et.al. Screening of colon tumor cells and tissues for folypolyglutamate synthetase activity. *Oncol. Res* 1995; 317–321.
71. Chen L, Qi H, Korenberg J, et.al. Purification and properties of human cytosolic folypoly-gamma-glutamate synthetase and organization, localization, and differential splicing of its gene. *J Biol Chem* 1996; 271:13077–13087.
72. Lowe KE, Osborne CB, Lin BF, Kim JS, Hsu JC, Shane B. Regulation of folate and one-carbon metabolism in mammalian cells. II. Effect of folylpoly-gamma-glutamate synthetase substrate specificity and level on folate metabolism and folypoly-gamma-glutamate specificity of metabolic cycles of one-carbon metabolism. *J Biol Chem* 1993; 268:21665–21673.
73. McCloskey DE, McGuire JJ, Russell CA, et al. Decreased folypolyglutamate synthetase activity as a mechanism of methotrexate resistance in CCRF-CEM human leukemia. *J Biol Chem* 1991; 266(10): 6181–6187.
74. Zhao R, Titus S, Gao F, et al. Molecular analysis of murine leukemia cell lines resistant to 5, 10-dideazatetrahydrofolate identifies several amino acids critical to the function of folylpolyglutamate synthetase. *J Biol Chem* 2000; 275:26599–25606.
75. Houghton JA, Williams LG, de Graaf SS, et al. Relationship between dose rate of [6RS]Leucovorin administration, plasma concentrations of folates, and pools of 5, 10-methylenetetra-hydrofolates and tetrahydrofolates in human colon adenocarcinoma xenografts. *Cancer Res* 1990; 50:3493–3502.

76. Newman EM, Straw JA, Doroshow JH. Pharmacokinetics of diastereoisomers of (6R,S)-folinic acid (leucovorin) in humans during constant high-dose intravenous infusion. *Cancer Res* 1989; 49:5755–5760.
77. Straw JA, Szapary D, Wynn WT. Pharmacokinetics of the diastereoisomers of leucovorin after intravenous and oral administration to normal subjects. *Cancer Res* 1984; 44:3114–3119.
78. Zhang ZG, Rustum YM. Effects of diastereoisomers of 5-formyltetrahydrofolate on cellular growth, sensitivity to 5-fluoro-2′-deoxyuridine, and methylenetetrahydrofolate polyglutamate levels in HCT-8 cells. *Cancer Res* 1991; 51:3476–3481.
79. Sirotnak FM, Chello PL, Moccio DM, Kisliuk RL, Combepine G, Gaumont Y, Montgomery JA. Stereospecificity at carbon 6 of formyltetrahydrofolate as a competitive inhibitor of transport and cytotoxicity of methotrexate in vitro. *Biochem Pharmacol* 1979; 28:2993–2997.
80. Machover D, Grison X, Goldschmidt E, et al. Fluorouracil combined with thc pure (6S)-stereoisomer of folinic acid in high doses for treatment of patients with advanced colorectal carcinoma: a phase I-II study. *J Natl Cancer Inst* 1992; 84:321–327.
81. Rosso R, Mazzei T, Sobrero A, et al. Phase II trial of 5-fluorouracil and the natural 1 isomer of folinic acid in the treatment of advanced colorectal carcinoma. *Eur J Cancer* 1994; 30A:338–343.
82. Goldberg RM, Hatfield AK, Kahn M, et al. Prospectively randomized North Central Cancer Treatment Group trial of intensive-course fluorouracil combined with the 1-isomer of intravenous leucovorin, oral leucovorin, or intravenous leucovorin for the treatment of advanced colorectal cancer. *J Clin Oncol* 1997; 15:3320–3329.
83. Mini E, Mazzei T, Coronnello M, et al. Effects of 5-methyltetrahydrofolate on the activity of fluoropyrimidines against human leukemia (CCRF-CEM) cells. *Biochem Pharmacol* 1987; 36:2905–2911.
84. Chello PL, Bertino JR. Dependence of 5-methyltetrahydrofolate utilization by L5178Y murine leukemia cells in vitro on thepresence of hydroxycobalamin and transcobalamin II. *Cancer Res* 1973; 33:1898–1904.
85. Etienne MC, Fischel JL, Formento P, et al. Combination of reduced folates with methotrexate or 5-fluorouracil. Comparison between 5-formyltetrahydrofolate (folinic acid) and 5-methyltertrahydrofolate in vitro activities. *Biochem Pharmacol* 1993; 46:1767–1774.
86. Carlsson G, Hafstrom LO, Spears CP, et.al. 5-fluorouracil (5-FU) and 5,10-methylene tetrahydrofolate (5,10-CH2FH4) as adjuvant therapy in an experimental rodent colon carcinoma model. *Anticancer Res* 1997; 17:3671–3674.
87. Raghunathan K, Priest. Modulation of fluorouracil antitumor activity by folic acid in a murine model system. *Biochem Pharmacol* 1999; 58:835–839.
88. Olinger EJ, Bertino JR, Binder HJ. Intestinal folate absorption. II. Conversion and retention of pteroylmonoglutamate by jejunum. *J Clin Invest* 1973; 52:2138–2145.
89. Houghton JA, Williams LG, Radparvar S, et al. Characterization of the pools of 5,10-methylenetetrahydrofolates and tetrahydrofolates in xenografts of human colon adenocarcinoma. *Cancer Res* 1988; 48:3062–3069.
90. Houghton JA, Williams LG, Cheshire PJ, et.al. Influence of dose of [6RS]leucovorin on reduced folate pools and 5-fluorouracil-mediated thymidylate synthase inhibition in human colon adenocarcinoma xenografts. *Cancer Res* 1990; 50:3940–3946.
91. Houghton JA, Williams LG, de Graaf SS, et al. Relationship between dose rate of [6RS]Leucovorin administration, plasma concentrations of reduced folates, and pools of 5,10-methylenetetrahydrofolates and tetrahydrofolates in human colon adenocarcinoma xenografts. *Cancer Res* 1990; 50:3493–3502.
92. Cheradame S, Etienne MC, Chazal M, et al. Relevance of tumoral folypolyglutamate synthetase and reduced folates for optimal 5-fluorouracil efficacy: experimental data. *Eur J Cancer* 1997; 33:950–959.
93. Cheradame S, Etienne MC, Formento P, et al. Tumoral-reduced folates and clinical resistance to fluorouracil-based treatment in head and neck cancer patients. *J Clin Oncol* 1997; 15:2604–2610.
94. Chazal M, Cheradame S, Formento JL, et al. Decreased folylpolyglutamate synthetase activity in tumors resistant to fluorouracil-folinic acid treatment clinical data *Clin Cancer Res* 1997; 3:553–557.
95. Romanini A, Lin JT, Niedzwiecki D, Bunni M, Priest DG, Bertino JR. Role of folylpolyglutamates in biochemical modulation of fluoropyrimidines by leucovorin. *Cancer Res* 1991; 51:789–793.
96. Wang FS, Aschele C, Sobrero A, Chang YM, Bertino JR. Decreased folypolyglutamate synthetase expression: a novel mechanism of fluorouracil *Cancer Res* 1993; 53:3677–3680.
97. Ayusawa D, Koyama H, and Seno T. Resistance to methotrexate in thymidylate synthetase-deficient mutants of cultured mouse mammary tumor FM3A cells. *Cancer Res* 1981; 41:1497–1501.
98. Houghton PJ, Germain GS, Hazelton BJ, Pennington JW, Houghton JA. Mutants of human colon adenocarcinoma selected for thymidylate synthase deficiency. *Proc Natl Acad Sci USA* 1989; 86:1377–1381.
99. Smith SG, Lehman NL, Moran RG. Cytotoxicity of antifolate inhibitors of thymidylate and purine synthesis to WiDr colonic carcinoma cells. *Cancer Res* 1993; 53:5697–5706.

100. Houghton JA, Harwood FG, Tillman DM. Thymineless death in colon carcinoma cells is mediated via fas signaling. *Proc Natl Acad Sci USA* 1997; 94:8144–8149.
101. Roberts D. An isotopic assay for thymidylate synthetase. *Biochemistry* 1966; 5:3546–3548.
102. Yalowich JC, Kalman TI. Rapid determination of thymidylate synthase activity and its inhibition in intact L1210 leukemia cells in vitro. *Biochem Pharmacol* 1985; 34:2319–2324.
103. Spears CP, Gustavsson BG. Methods for thymidylate synthase pharmacodynamics: serial biopsy, free and total TS, FdUMP and dUMP and H4PteGlu and CH2-H4PteGlu assays. *Adv Exp Med Biol* 1988; 244:97–106.
104. Larsson PA, Carlsson G, Gustavasson B et.al. Thymidylate synthase in advanced gastrointestinal and breast cancers. *Acta Oncol* 1996; 35:469–472.
105. van Laar JA, van der Wilt CL, Rustum YM, et al. Therapeutic efficacy of fluoropyrimidines depends on the duration of thymidylate synthase inhibition in the murine colon 26-B carcinoma tumor model. *Clin Cancer Res* 1996; 2:1327–1333.
106. Spears CP, Gustavasson BG, Frosing R. Folinic acid modulation of fluorouracil: tissue kinetics of bolus administration. *Invest New Drugs* 1989; 7:27–36.
107. Horikoshi T, Danenberg KD, Stadlbauer TH, et al. Quantitation of thymidylate synthase, dihydrofolate reductase, and DT-diaphorase gene expression in human tumors using the polymerase chain reaction. *Cancer Res* 1992; 52:108–116.
108. Johnston PG, Lenz HJ, Leichman CG, et al. Thymidylate synthase gene and protein expression correlate and are associated with response to 5-fluorouracil in human colorectal and gastric tumors. *Cancer Res* 1995; 55:1407–1412.
109. Lenz HJ, Leichman CG, Danenberg KD, et al. Thymidylate synthase mRNA level in adenocarcinoma of the stomach: a predictor for primary tumor response and overall survival. *J Clin Oncol* 1996; 14:176–182.
110. Lenz HJ, Danenberg KD, Leichman CG, et al. p53 and thymidylate synthase expression in untreated stage II colon cancer: associations with recurrence, survival, and site. *Clin Cancer Res* 1998; 4:1227–1234.
111. Lenz HJ, Hayashi K, Salonga D, et al. p53 point mutations and thymidylate synthase messenger RNA levels in disseminated colorectal cancer: an analysis of response and survival. *Clin Cancer Res* 1998; 4: 1243–1250.
112. Gorlick R, Metzger R, Danenberg KD, et al. Higher levels of thymidylate synthase gene expression are observed in pulmonary as compared with hepatic metastases of colorectal adenocarcinoma. *J Clin Oncol* 1998; 16: 1465–1469.
113. Salonga D, Danenberg KD, Johnson M, et al. Colorectal tumors responding to 5-fluorouracil have low gene expression levels of dihydropyrimidine dehydrogenase, thymidylate synthase, and thymidine phosphorylase. *Clin Cancer Res* 2000; 6:1322–1327.

4 Molecular Mechanisms Regulating the Expression of Thymidylate Synthase

John C. Schmitz, PhD, *Ashwin Gollerkeri,* MD,
Xiukun Lin, MD, PhD, *Jun Liu,* MD, PhD,
and Edward Chu, MD

CONTENTS

1. INTRODUCTION

Thymidylate synthase (TS) is a folate-dependent enzyme that catalyzes the reductive methylation of 2′-deoxyuridine-5′-monophosphate (dUMP) by the reduced folate 5,10-methylenetetrahydrofolate (CH_2THF) to thymidylate (dTMP) and dihydrofolate (Fig. 1) *(1,2)*. Once synthesized, dTMP is then further metabolized intracellularly to the dTTP triphosphate form, an essential precursor for DNA synthesis. Although dTMP can be formed through the salvage pathway catalyzed by thymidine kinase, the TS-catalyzed reaction provides for the sole intracellular *de novo* source of dTMP. Given its central role in DNA biosynthesis, and given that inhibition of this reaction results in immediate cessation of cellular proliferation and growth, TS represents an important target for cancer chemotherapy *(3,4)*.

There are several lines of evidence that provide additional support to the view that TS is an important chemotherapeutic target. The first comes from in vitro, in vivo, and clinical studies that show a strong association between the level of expression of TS enzyme activity and TS protein and fluoropyrimidine sensitivity *(5–7)*. It is well established that neoplastic cell lines and tumors expressing higher levels of TS are relatively more resistant to the cytotoxic and antitumor effects of the fluoropyrimidines and antifolate analogs targeting TS. Second, there is a strong correlation between the level of inhibition of TS enzyme activity

From: *Fluoropyrimidines in Cancer Therapy*
Edited by: Y. M. Rustum © Humana Press Inc., Totowa, NJ

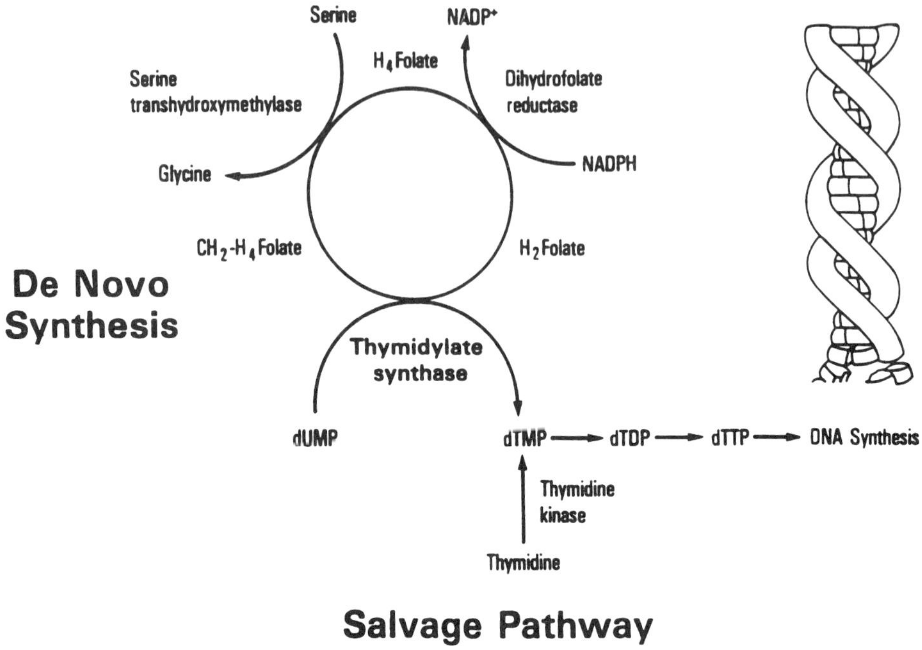

Fig. 1. The TS-catalyzed reaction.

within patient tumor specimens following treatment with 5-FU and eventual clinical response to 5-FU-based chemotherapy *(8,9)*. Third, the improved response rates observed when 5-FU is combined with the reduced folate leucovorin (LV) as compared to single-agent 5-FU provide support to the cell-free studies which showed that TS enzyme inhibition was optimally maintained in the presence of increasing concentrations of the reduced folate CH_2THF (10–15). Finally, clinical trials with the antifolate analog ZD1694, a specific inhibitor of TS, have shown good activity against advanced colorectal cancer with response rates in the range of 25–30%. These responses are comparable to those observed with the combination of 5-FU and LV, and, for this reason, ZD1694 has been approved for use as first-line therapy for metastatic colorectal cancer in several countries in Europe, Asia, Australia, and Canada *(16–18)*.

2. GENE AMPLIFICATION

Gene amplification is a well-characterized mechanism for increased gene expression, and its role in mediating drug resistance has been well established. Schimke et al. were the first to identify amplification of the dihydrofolate reductase (DHFR) gene in Chinese hamster ovary cells made resistant to the antifolate analog methotrexate (MTX) *(19)*. There is now growing evidence that the process of DHFR gene amplification with resultant overexpression of the DHFR protein may have clinical relevance *(20–22)*. With regard to TS, amplification of the TS gene has been observed in various experimental model systems including human cancer cell lines such as hepatoma HEp-2, colon cancer H630, and breast cancer MCF-7, and murine cancer cell lines, including breast FM3A, and leukemic L1210 after treatment with the fluoropyrimidines 5-fluorouracil (5-FU) and 5-fluoro-2′-deoxyuridine (FdUrd) or with the TS inhibitor antifolate compounds CB3717 and ZD1694 *(23–26)*. In each of these preclinical studies, a strong association between the level of TS expression and relative fluoropyrimidine and/or antifolate sensitivity was observed. Thus, malignant cell lines and tumors expressing higher levels of TS protein are more resistant to the cytotoxic effects of these agents.

Although TS gene amplification is well documented in various in vitro and in vivo model systems, to date there remains little direct evidence to link this process with the development of clinical drug resistance. Clark et al. *(27)* reported a 4- to 6-fold increased level in the TS gene copy number in a tumor sample obtained from a patient with progressive colon cancer relative to other tumor specimens following treatment with 5-FU and LV chemotherapy. However, a pretreatment biopsy sample was not obtained to determine the baseline tumor TS gene copy number. Gorlick et al. *(28)* observed low-level amplification of TS gene copy number (two to three copies) in 4 of 7 pulmonary metastases and 2 of 12 hepatic metastases. This level of amplification was detected in tumor samples from patients who had received prior 5-FU treatment as well as from patients who had received no prior therapy. Since treatment outcome was not included in this study, a correlation between TS gene amplification and response rate could not be made. Moreover, TS gene amplification was determined by comparing the TS gene copy number in the tumor tissue relative to that expressed in the peripheral blood of healthy volunteers. Thus, a comparison of the TS gene copy number expressed in either the original tumor tissue prior to therapy or to that in corresponding normal lung and/or liver tissue was not performed. For this reason, the determined TS gene copy number may not accurately reflect the effect of drug treatment on the final expression of TS. Taken together, these clinical studies provide, at best, only suggestive evidence that the process of TS gene amplification may play a role in the development of clinical resistance following fluoropyrimidine therapy.

3. TRANSCRIPTIONAL REGULATION

The majority of the initial studies on the regulation of expression of TS focused on cell-cycle-directed events. TS enzyme activity increases maximally at the G1/S-phase boundary of the cell cycle in eukaryotic cells *(29)*. In quiescent cells, the levels of TS mRNA and TS protein are present at relatively low levels. However, when resting cells are stimulated to proliferate upon addition of serum, both TS mRNA and TS protein levels increase by more than 10- to 20-fold as cells progress from the G1- to S-phase *(30,31)*. These initial findings suggested that the expression of TS as it relates to growth stimulation and the cell cycle may be regulated, in part, at the transcriptional level.

The essential *cis*-acting regulatory elements that control expression of TS at the transcriptional level have been characterized for both the murine and human TS gene. The promoters are G-C rich with bidirectional activity but both lack a TATA box as well as a transcriptional initiator element. A sequence located between –104 and –75 relative to the AUG start codon within the 5′-flanking region of the mouse gene is sufficient for promoter activity *(32)*. Extensive analysis of this region identified several elements that were critical for promoter activity: an Sp1 binding site and two potential binding sites for members of the Ets family of transcription factors *(33)*. With regard to the human gene, the essential promoter region (EPR) is located between –161 to –141 relative to the AUG start codon *(34)*. Analysis of this region, which has high homology to the mouse sequence, revealed similar promoter elements: an Sp1 binding site and an Ets element. However, an additional Sp1 binding site was identified 15 nt upstream of the human EPR *(35)*. Of interest, this site acts as a negative regulatory sequence (NRS). Mutation of this sequence resulted in a 70% increase in TS promoter activity. A second NRS has been identified and is located between nts –212 to –202 in the human TS gene. Using a standard CAT assay, Takeishi et al. *(35)* reported a 2.5-fold increase in promoter activity following mutation of four bases in this sequence. The role of these NRS elements in determining the expression of human TS at the transcriptional level remains to be more fully elucidated. These negative regulatory sequences have yet to be identified in the mouse gene.

The CACCC motif, located at –228 to –221 in the 5′ flanking region of the human TS gene and upstream of the NRS, is another important regulatory element *(31)*. This motif appears to have a positive effect on TS promoter activity since mutation of nucleotides within this element reduced promoter activity to 65% of that of the wild-type sequence *(35)*. Although the murine TS genes contain a CACCC box 160 nt upstream of the Spl binding element, its effect on TS expression remains to be characterized.

Several other binding elements have recently been identified that are critical for S-phase expression of TS. Putative E2F binding sites are present upstream of the EPR in the mouse TS gene and downstream of the human EPR *(34)*. The E2F consensus sequence has been implicated as playing an important role in regulating the expression of several essential S-phase-specific genes such as thymidine kinase, ribonucleotide reductase, dihydrofolate reductase, and DNA polymerase-α *(36)*. However, deletion of the E2F element did not affect mouse TS promoter activity nor did it inhibit growth-regulated expression of mouse TS *(37)*. Furthermore, cotransfection experiments revealed that overexpression of the mouse E2F1 gene was not sufficient to increase transcription from the TS promoter *(38)*. These findings suggest that the expression of mouse TS may not be directly controlled by E2F transcription factors. With regard to the human gene, inactivation of the E2F motif (TTCCC) at position –125 resulted in a 50–75% increase in promoter activity. In contrast, inactivation of a weaker E2F motif (TTCCG) at position –115 resulted in a slight decrease in promoter activity. Mutations in both E2F sites resulted in only a slight increase in promoter activity compared to the wild-type sequence, suggesting that the E2F motif represents a relatively weak negative sequence for S-phase regulation of TS in human cells. There is recent evidence to suggest a different role for E2F in TS expression. Overexpression of E2F-1 in human fibrosarcoma HT-1080 cells resulted in high levels of TS protein *(39)*. Moreover, analysis of clinical tumor samples revealed a close correlation between levels of mRNA expression of E2F-1 and TS suggesting a possible role for E2F-1 in the upregulation of TS *(40,41)*. However, additional studies are required to further characterize the specific effect of the E2F transcription factor on the expression of human TS.

In addition to E2F, the LSF transcription factor plays a key role in S-phase regulation of both the mouse and human TS gene *(42)*. The ability of LSF to stimulate gene expression from the SV40 major late promoter suggested a potential role for LSF in cell growth control *(43)*. One of the binding motifs for LSF in the TS gene overlaps with the essential promoter region containing the Ets and Sp1 binding elements. Other LSF sites are located within introns 1 and 5 and upstream of the mouse EPR (–160 to –142). Powell et al. *(42)* determined that mutation of the mouse LSF binding sites inhibits G1/S phase induction of TS mRNA derived from a transfected TS minigene. They also showed that expression of a dominant-negative LSF, which bound to and inactivated endogenous LSF, prevented an increase in levels of TS protein during serum stimulation resulting in programmed cell death in both mouse and human cell lines. The process of programmed cell death was prevented upon addition of thymidine to the growth medium or by cotransfection of the TS gene driven by a heterologous promoter. Thus, LSF appears to be critical for progression of cells through S-phase by controlling the expression of the TS gene.

While the 5′ flanking region of the TS gene contains sequences that are important for S-phase-specific expression, these elements, alone, do not appear to be sufficient for regulation of the TS gene during the cell cycle *(33)*. Constructs consisting of the 5' flanking region of TS linked to reporter genes were expressed at a constant level throughout the cell cycle. Thus, regions downstream of the AUG start site must be critical for S-phase regulation. Johnson and coworkers confirmed that S-phase expression of the mouse TS gene was not dependent on a single intron as introns 1, 2, 5, or 6 were capable of inducing growth-regulated expression from TS minigene constructs *(44)*. Deletion of nearly all of the interior of the intron did not effect S-phase expression. However, mutation of the splice donor and acceptor sites resulted in constant TS expression during growth stimulation. These results suggest that S-phase expression of mouse TS requires some form of communication between the 5′ flanking promoter region and the exon/intron splicing machinery. Since, the transcription rate of TS does not change significantly during growth stimulation *(31,45)*, effective expression of TS during S-phase might be because of some unknown S-phase specific regulatory factor that binds to the promoter region of the unspliced transcript and stimulates splicing. In contrast, the inclusion of intron 1, but not intron 2, was necessary for growth-stimulated expression of the human TS gene *(46)*. Deletion analysis revealed that the 5′ end of intron 1 contains two positive and one negative regulatory sequences *(47)*. Further studies are needed to investigate the potential role of the donor/acceptor splice sites of the introns in regulating the expression of human TS.

In addition to cell-cycle-related events, chronic exposure of malignant cells to various anticancer agents can result in increased expression of TS that is controlled at the transcriptional level. Work by Scanlon et al. *(48)* demonstrated that selection of human ovarian cancer cells in cisplatin led to the development of cross-resistance to 5-FU. They found that cisplatin-resistant cells expressed 3- to 4-fold higher levels of TS when compared to wild-type parental cells. Moreover, the increased level of expression of TS was not associated with TS gene amplification but rather was the direct result of an increased transcriptional rate. A series of adriamycin-resistant human breast cancer MCF-7 and human colon cancer DLD-1 cells were established by Chu et al. *(49)* to investigate the process of multidrug resistance, and characterization of these cell lines revealed that they were cross-resistant to the fluoropyrimidines, 5-FU and FdUrd. Of note, these resistant cell lines had not previously been exposed to either of these compounds. Further evaluation revealed that the development of fluoropyrimidine resistance was associated with an increased expression of TS protein. The increased expression of TS was not the result of gene amplification but was caused by enhanced transcription of the TS gene. Although the precise molecular mechanism(s) by which this process occurs remains to be characterized, these two studies suggest that the ability to increase the expression of TS in response to chronic exposure to cytotoxic agents other than fluoropyrimidine may serve as an important adaptive response mechanism for malignant cells to circumvent the effects of various cytotoxic stress and, thereby, maintain cellular synthetic function.

4. TRANSLATIONAL REGULATION

The potential for translational regulation of TS was first proposed by Belfort et al. *(50)* upon cloning and characterization of the structural features of the *Escherichia coli* TS *thy*A gene. Kisliuk and colleagues *(51,52)* then made the interesting observation that the TS protein isolated from a MTX-resistant *Streptococcus faecium* species was bound to a poly-G tetraribonucleotide sequence. Although the precise nature of this RNA–protein interaction was not further characterized, this finding suggested that the short RNA sequence might, in some way, alter TS enzyme activity. An alternative possibility was that this sequence might be part of a longer RNA sequence with an intrinsic regulatory function. In their initial characterization of the human TS cDNA sequence, Takeishi et al. *(53)* also suggested the potential for translational control. They identified three tandem repeat sequences in the 5′-untranslated region, and secondary structure analysis predicted for three interconvertible stem-loop structures. Kaneda et al. *(54)* extended this work to show that deletion of any one of these tandem repeat sequences significantly altered the translational efficiency of TS mRNA in vivo. These findings suggested that these tandem repeat sequences regulate the translation of TS mRNA, perhaps through their interaction with other cellular proteins and/or cofactors.

Several groups have described rapid increases in TS enzyme levels in various in vitro, in vivo, and clinical experimental model systems following short-term exposure to the fluoropyrimidines *(8,9,55,56)*. Although the underlying mechanism(s) for the enhanced expression of TS in response to 5-FU was not well characterized in these initial studies, several possibilities were proposed including increased transcription of TS-specific sequences, enhanced stability of TS mRNA, increased efficiency of TS mRNA translation, and enhanced stability of TS protein. Because this observation represented a potentially important mechanism for the rapid development of resistance to 5-FU chemotherapy in the clinical setting, significant research efforts have focused on elucidating the critical biochemical and molecular events that control the 5-FU-mediated acute induction of TS. Studies by Keyomarsi and Pardee *(57)* showed that treatment of human breast cancer MCF-7 cells with the folate-based quinazoline analog ZD1694 (Tomudex, raltitrexed) resulted in a 10- to 40-fold increase in TS enzyme levels with no associated change in TS mRNA levels. The presence of cycloheximide, a protein synthesis inhibitor, blocked the elevation in TS enzyme levels following exposure to ZD1694, providing suggestive evidence that a translational regulatory event was involved. Using a human colon cancer H630 cell line as a model system, studies from our own lab have shown that the increase in both TS enzyme activity and TS protein expression that arises in response to exposure to 5-FU was not associated with a corresponding change in the level of TS mRNA expression *(58,59)*. Although the majority of the increased level of TS was in the form of protein complexed with the 5-FU metabolite FdUMP, there was also an approx 30–45% increase in free levels of TS protein *(23)*. Thus, the induction of TS protein in response to 5-FU exposure allowed free TS to remain at levels 40% above baseline, so that thymidylate and DNA biosynthesis could be maintained in the face of a cytotoxic stress such as 5-FU. Further work revealed that the increase in TS protein expression was the direct result of new synthesis of TS protein as opposed to alterations in protein stability. In addition, repression of the 5-FU-mediated induction of TS by γ-IFN, at nongrowth inhibitory drug concentrations, was associated with a nearly 20-fold increase in the cytotoxic effects of 5-FU. Of note, the negative effect of γ-IFN on TS expression was controlled at the translational level. Thus, this study provided the first direct evidence for the role of translational regulation in an intact biological system and suggested that this regulatory process has biological relevance. Taken together, these findings suggested that the ability to regulate the expression of TS at the translational level may represent:

1. An important mechanism by which normal cellular synthetic function can be tightly regulated.
2. A critical protective mechanism for the rapid development of cellular resistance is response to exposure to a cytotoxic stress such as 5-FU or ZD1694 so as to maintain cellular synthetic function.

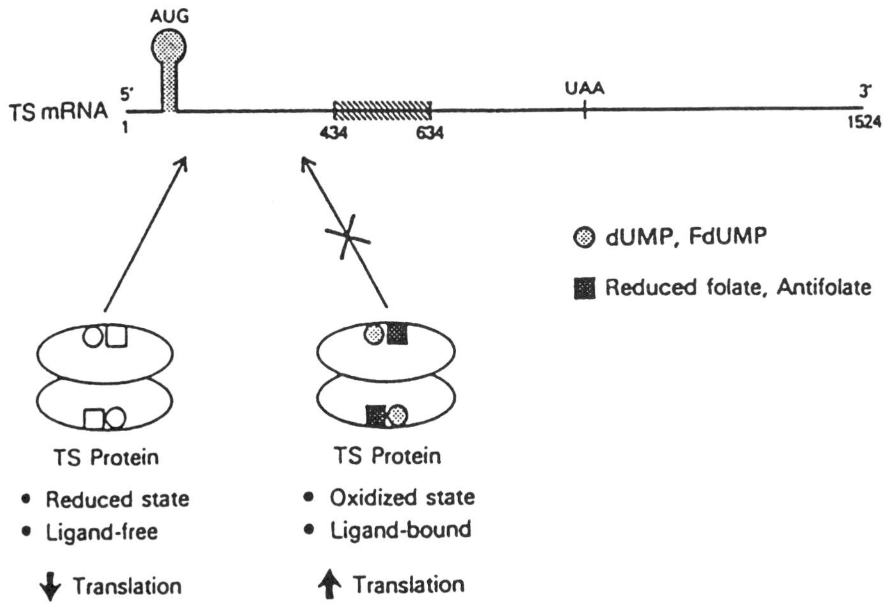

Fig. 2. Model of TS translational autoregulation.

5. TRANSLATIONAL AUTOREGULATION

Because the expression of TS during the cell cycle and in response to exposure to cytotoxic agents is controlled, in part, by a translational regulatory event, an extensive series of studies were performed to more carefully elucidate the regulation of TS mRNA translation. The current working model for the translational autoregulatory control of TS and the interaction between TS protein and its own TS mRNA is presented in Fig. 2. Two different sequences have been identified on TS mRNA that bind with high affinity, on the order of 1–2 n*M*, to TS *(60–62)*. The first site is located within the first 188 nucleotides and includes the translational start site. Because many of the earlier studies identified the 5′-untranslated region (5′-UTR) as playing a key role in mediating the repression of translation initiation of a number of other genes *(63–65)*, significant efforts were initially placed on defining the 5′-upstream binding site on TS mRNA. A Zuker RNA fold analysis predicted that this particular sequence could adopt a stable stem-loop secondary structure with the translational AUG start site contained within the loop aspect. A series of mutant and deletion RNA sequences subsequently confirmed that such a structure was indeed important for RNA binding and that the hexanucleotide GCCAUG sequence contained within the loop aspect of this putative stem-loop structure was critical for RNA recognition *(61,62)*.

The second site is contained within a 200-nt sequence corresponding to nts 434 to 634 in the protein-coding region of TS mRNA. This *cis*-acting element is sufficient to confer the property of translational regulation onto a heterologous luciferase reporter gene and requires the presence of an intact TS protein for its biological effect. Further studies using a series of in vitro RNA gel mobility shift and in vivo transfection experiments have localized this element to a 70 nt sequence corresponding to nts 480 and 550 of TS mRNA *(66)*. Although this sequence can function independently of the 5′-upstream *cis*-acting element in vivo, the presence of both this RNA sequence and the 5′-upstream element is required in order for human TS protein to exhibit its full range of translational autoregulatory activity.

One issue raised by these findings relates to how binding of TS to a *cis*-acting element in the protein-coding region of TS mRNA results in translational repression. In order for such events to occur, some type of interaction between the 5′ end of the mRNA and the protein-coding region must take place. Several groups have identified sequences within the protein-coding region and the 3′-UTR as being critical for the translational control of various genes *(67–70)*. Although the specific molecular mechanism(s) by which the process of translational repression occurs remains to be determined, there is growing evidence to suggest that sequences in both the protein-coding region and in the 3'-UTR play a key role in controlling the process of translational initiation. Sophisticated molecular modeling studies will be required, however, to more precisely characterize the molecular events mediating this complex process.

Careful sequence analysis has yet to reveal a consensus nucleotide sequence within the 5'-upstream and the protein-coding region binding sites. However, one potential drawback to such a "consensus" approach is that many of the RNA binding proteins characterized, to date, seem to recognize a combination of sequence and structure *(71,72)*. Thus, identification of a consensus RNA binding site by simple sequence analysis may be inadequate. A preliminary analysis using the Zuker RNA fold algorithm predicts for the existence of stable secondary structures in the TS434-634 and TS480-550 sequences. However, these structures appear to be somewhat different from the one predicted for the *cis*-acting element located within the 5′-upstream binding site. Studies are now in progress to perform a more-detailed analysis of the sequence and/or structural determinants required for binding of TS protein to its respective *cis*-acting elements. This work should provide critical insight into the essential elements required for RNA recognition by TS protein and enhance our understanding of the specific molecular events mediating the translational regulation of TS.

Significant efforts have been placed on defining the essential molecular factors that determine RNA–protein interactions. The R17 bacteriophage coat protein *(73–75)* and aminoacyl-tRNA synthetase *(76,77)* represent two particularly well-studied examples of RNA binding proteins. In an elegant series of experiments, Starzyk et al. *(77)* conclusively demonstrated that the C-6 position of uridine 8 in aminoacyl-tRNA was subject to direct nucleophilic attack by a cysteine sulfhydryl group within the aminoacyl-tRNA synthase protein. This interaction resulted in formation of a transient covalent bond, referred to as the Michael adduct. Subsequent studies revealed that the interaction between the R17 replicase protein and its target mRNA was also mediated by a cysteine sulfhydryl group *(75)*.

Both TS catalytic activity and TS enzyme–ternary complex formation with FdUMP and 5, 10-methylenetetrahydrofolate require the highly conserved cysteine sulfhydryl positioned in the nucleotide active site of TS to be in a fully reduced state *(2,3,78,79)*. During the catalytic reaction, the C-6 on the uracil ring of dUMP undergoes nucleophilic attack by the active site cysteine to form a Michael adduct. Since Michael addition of a protein nucleophile represents the critical step in the TS enzyme-catalyzed reaction and since this process appears to be essential in mediating RNA–protein interactions, the potential role of the redox state in determining the interaction between TS protein and its target TS mRNA was examined. Studies from our laboratory have shown that the RNA binding activity of human recombinant TS is markedly sensitive to the presence of reducing agents and requires the presence of at least one free sulfhydryl group *(80)*. In the presence of either 2-mercaptoethanol (2-ME) or dithiothreitol, the RNA binding activity of TS was significantly enhanced. In contrast, treatment of TS with an oxidizing agent such as diamide inhibited RNA binding in a dose-dependent manner. This inhibitory effect was readily reversible in that the simultaneous presence of a reducing agent such as 2-ME fully restored RNA binding activity. In addition, the catalytic activity of this human TS protein was significantly enhanced in the presence of 2-ME, a finding that initially suggested the potential for a single common redox site on TS to simultaneously control RNA binding and catalysis by switching TS from inactive to active forms. A detailed mathematical analysis revealed that the reduced form of TS involved in the processes of RNA binding and enzyme catalysis was not mediated by a single common redox site. This model suggested that the process of RNA binding was complex, potentially involving multiple redox sites on the protein. Although the precise mechanism(s) by which the cysteine sulfhydryl group(s) on TS mediates RNA binding remains to be more precisely defined, several possibilities exist to explain its central role. They include:

1. Direct formation of a covalent Michael adduct between the active site sulfhydryl and the C-6 position of a uracil ring on TS mRNA.
2. Occupation of the active site cysteine alters RNA binding via a steric hindrance mechanism.
3. The cysteine sulfhydryl groups in their maximally reduced state maintain TS protein in a certain conformation that allows for optimal RNA binding elsewhere on the protein.

In addition to the redox state of TS, the state of occupancy of the protein appears to play an important role as a determinant of RNA binding. Specifically, when TS is ligand-free, maximal RNA binding activity is maintained, thereby resulting in complete translational repression of TS mRNA. In contrast, when TS is bound by either of its physiologic substrates dUMP or 5,10-methylenetetrahydrofolate or bound by the 5-FU nucleotide metabolite FdUMP, TS is no longer able to bind to its target mRNA. The end result of this decreased RNA binding activity is to relieve translational repression, a process that leads to increased synthesis of new TS protein *(80)*. Such a condition would exist in cells exposed to direct inhibitor compounds of TS, whether it be nucleotide analogs such as 5-FU or to antifolate analogs such as ZD1694. Thus, this model can be used to explain the acute induction of TS that arises in response to exposure to 5-FU and antifolate analogs. Moreover, it offers a novel mechanism for the development of acute drug resistance to compounds that specifically target TS.

To begin to define the domain(s) on TS involved in RNA binding, the ability of various mutant TS proteins to form an RNP complex with human TS mRNA was investigated. For this initial series of experiments, mutant *E. coli* TS proteins were used given their ready availability, the relative difficulty in expressing and purifying mutant human recombinant TS proteins, and the fact that TS is one of the most highly conserved proteins identified to date. Binding studies have shown that proteins with point mutations in the nucleotide-binding region retained RNA binding activity with the sole exception of the C146S mutant *(81)*. In contrast, proteins with point mutations in the folate-binding region were completely devoid of RNA binding activity *(81)*. These initial experiments suggest that the active site cysteine sulfhydryl and the folate-binding site may represent domains on TS required for RNA binding. It is noteworthy that each of the nucleotide site mutant TS proteins expressed little to no enzymatic activity. This observation confirms that the functions of RNA binding and enzyme catalysis are not controlled by a single common site on TS. At this time, the specific mechanism(s) by which the cysteine sulfhydryl and the folate-binding region mediate RNA binding remains to be determined. It is possible that these regions either form a direct covalent bond with their target RNA or that they maintain the protein in a particular conformation that then allows for optimal RNA binding. Although definitive analysis of the specific RNA binding domain(s) on TS awaits the results of molecular modeling studies such as X-ray crystallography and/or NMR spectroscopy of the TS RNA–TS protein complex, studies are now in progress to identify the critical amino acid residues on TS that are directly involved in RNA binding.

TS represents the first eukaryotic gene whose expression is governed by a translational autoregulatory process. However, such a mechanism has been shown to play an important role in the regulation of various bacteriophage *(82–85)* and *E. coli* proteins *(86–88)*. Since TS is a highly conserved protein, one issue to address was whether the process of translational autoregulation observed in the human system was, in fact, conserved in evolution. Given the ready availability of both wild-type and mutant *E. coli* recombinant TS proteins, the bacterial *E. coli* TS system was selected for further study. Using the RNA gel mobility shift assay, a specific interaction between recombinant *E. coli* TS protein and its own *E. coli* TS mRNA was observed *(81)*. A series of RNA gel shift competition experiments identified at least three different binding sites in the protein-coding region of *E. coli* TS mRNA with the affinity of *E. coli* TS for each of these sites being approximately the same as that observed for the full-length *E. coli* TS mRNA (relative binding affinity, 1 n*M*) *(81)*. Preliminary analysis of these binding sites has, thus far, failed to identify a consensus sequence and/or secondary structure. In addition, no apparent consensus has been detected upon comparison of the binding sites on *E. coli* TS mRNA with those identified on human TS mRNA. However, definitive studies including direct RNA sequencing experiments are required before definitive conclusions can be made regarding the presence of a consensus nucleotide sequence and/or secondary structure.

An extensive analysis has shown that the interaction between *E. coli* TS protein and its own TS mRNA results in translational repression. This observation suggests that the synthesis of *E. coli* TS is indeed controlled by a translational autoregulatory event identical to that described for human TS. At the present time, it remains unclear as to how binding of *E. coli* TS to RNA sequences in the protein-coding region actually leads to translational repression. Of note, a *cis*-acting element was also identified in the coding region of the human TS mRNA. As in the case of the human system, it is conceivable that formation of this RNA–protein complex might interfere with either binding of the translational initiation machinery or with ribosomal scanning. For such an event to occur, this would suggest that some type of interaction between the 5′-end and the RNA sequences within the protein-coding region must take place. Further studies are needed to more fully characterize the underlying molecular events for this process. Nonetheless, the fact that TS translational autoregulation is conserved in evolution provides strong evidence that this mechanism represents a fundamental regulatory process underlying the expression of TS.

6. POSTTRANSLATIONAL REGULATION

There is now growing evidence to suggest that posttranslational mechanisms are involved in controlling the expression of TS. Maley et al. were the first to investigate the induction of TS, along with several other enzymes involved in DNA synthesis including deoxycytidylate deaminase and thymidine kinase, in regenerating rat liver cells. They observed that the induction of TS was not inhibited by the addition of either actinomycin-D or puromycin, agents that disrupt the processes of transcription and translation, respectively. These findings suggested that a posttranslational mechanism was mediating the expression of TS in these cells *(89)*. Subsequent studies in rats following partial hepatectomy demonstrated that intraperitoneal injections of methotrexate (MTX) gave rise to the rapid induction of TS enzyme activity *(90)*. In follow-up studies, Maley et al. *(91)* investigated the effect of MTX on TS expression in cultured parenchymal cells isolated from regenerating rat liver cells as well as from rats who were treated intraperitoneally with MTX. In both cases, they observed that exposure to MTX resulted in an approx 5-fold higher level of TS enzyme activity than in control untreated cells. They subsequently measured TS enzyme activity at various time points following exposure to MTX. In both rat hepatic parenchymal cells as well as in the remaining hepatic tissue in rats following partial hepatectomy, TS enzyme activity was maintained for up to 48 h with prior exposure to MTX in marked contrast to untreated controls in which TS activity decreased by more than 50% within 18–24 h. This dramatic effect of MTX on TS enzyme activity was not affected by the presence of transcriptional or translational inhibitors, a finding that implicated the process of enzyme stabilization as a mechanism for the increased levels of TS enzyme activity.

Using the human colon cancer HCT-15 cell line as their model system, Berger et al. *(92)* observed a 2- to 3-fold increase in TS enzyme levels following treatment with the fluoropyrimidine analog FdUrd for 24 h. RNase protection assay revealed the levels of TS mRNA to be unchanged with drug treatment. A polysome analysis was subsequently performed and showed that the polysome profiles in drug-treated and control, untreated, cells were identical with nearly all of the TS mRNA sedimenting with the higher-molecular-weight polysomes. This finding suggested that the translational efficiency of TS mRNA was not altered with FdUrd treatment. To provide further support to these findings, they then went on to use a FdUrd-resistant subline HCT-15/200, which was established by chronic exposure of the parent HCT-15 cells to FdUrd. Treatment of HCT-15/200 cells with 200 n*M* FdUrd for 24 h resulted in a 10- to 15-fold induction of TS enzyme activity with no change in TS mRNA levels. Polysome analysis revealed that the TS mRNA in drug-treated cells was primarily associated with higher-molecular-weight polysomes, on the order of 4–7 ribosomes/mRNA. The polysome distribution pattern was identical in both treated and control cells. These findings suggested that the expression of TS in both parent HCT-15 and TS-overexpressing, HCT-15/200 cells in response to treatment with FdUrd was controlled at the posttranslational level. In support of the role of enzyme stabilization as a possible mechanism for the induction of TS, protein half-life studies were performed which revealed that the half-life of TS protein in HCT-15 parent cells was 7.3 h in the absence of drug treatment and 25 h in the presence of FdUrd treatment. In HCT-15/200 cells, the half-life of TS protein was 2.3 h in untreated cells and increased by nearly 9-fold to 18 h following treatment with FdUrd. Thus, stabilization of protein appeared to be the primary mechanism underlying the induction of TS in both HCT15 and HCT15/200 cells following treatment with FdUrd *(92)*.

Further evidence for posttranslational regulation of TS comes from the work of Keyomarsi and Pardee *(11)*, who investigated the differential expression of TS protein and TS mRNA levels in human breast cancer MCF-7 cells in response to lovastatin treatment. Lovastatin synchronized the cells in the G_1 phase of the cell cycle, and synchrony was followed for several cycles. During the first three cell cycles, the levels of TS protein were induced by up to 10-fold during the S phase and returned to baseline during the subsequent G_1 phases. During the first G_1 phase, the levels of TS mRNA were barely detectable. However, they increased markedly by 10-fold upon entry into the S-phase and remained at relatively high levels during the next few cycles. Thus, although TS protein expression varied with the cell cycle, TS mRNA expression remained at a constant level following the initial lag in the first G_1 phase. Given the differential levels of expression of TS protein and TS mRNA, it was initially concluded that the regulation of TS during the cell cycle was mainly due to a translational mechanism. However, the dramatic decrease, by nearly 10-fold, in the levels of TS protein, as determined by the radioenzymatic FdUMP binding assay, also suggested the possibility of altered stability of the enzyme as a relevant regulatory mechanism. Since the half-life of TS protein in normal mammary epithelial cells was determined to be on the order of 12 h, the fact that the level of TS protein was reduced by 50% in a time frame of

5–6 h suggests that enhanced degradation of the protein may also play a role in the discordant expression of TS protein and TS mRNA in MCF-7 cells during the cell cycle.

Jackman et al. *(93)* recently investigated the effect of the third generation antifolate TS inhibitor compound ZD9331 on TS expression. Using the human lymphoblastoid W1L2 cell line, they observed that levels of TS protein were maximally induced 10-fold following treatment with 1 μM ZD9331 for 24 h. To determine the duration of induction following drug removal, cells were treated with 1 μM ZD9331 for 24 h and then resuspended in drug-free media. The levels of TS protein were then determined at various time points thereafter. Although the expression of TS was induced 10-fold following exposure to ZD9331, these levels decreased approx 25% within 4 h of drug removal. By 12 h after removal of ZD9331, TS expression decreased to a level, approx 4-fold less, than that present in control, untreated, cells and remained at this reduced level for up to 24 h. While the half-life of TS protein was not specifically measured in this series of experiments, the fact that the levels of TS were reduced to below pretreatment values within a period of 12 h suggests a process of enhanced degradation of the protein.

Finally, recent findings by Schmitz et al. *(94)* provide further evidence that the expression of TS is regulated, at least in part, at the posttranslational level. They investigated the effect of an antisense RNA oligoribonucleotide (ORN) targeted to the 5′ upstream *cis*-acting element on TS mRNA, on expression of TS protein in the human colon cancer RKO cell line. The antisense ORN repressed TS protein expression in a dose- and time- dependent fashion. In order to determine the effect of the antisense ORN on protein stability, half-life experiments were performed by treating the RKO cells with the antisense ORN for 6 h prior to incubation with ^{35}S methionine. Although the labeling studies following the antisense treatment did not suggest an effect of the antisense RNA on the half-life of TS protein, the Western blot analysis revealed a marked 60% decrease in levels of TS protein during the 6-h antisense treatment. Based on the calculated half-life of the protein (14 h), the decrease in TS protein levels during this time frame should be, at most, only 20–25%. Thus, the observed reduction in TS expression was significantly greater than predicted, suggesting that an effect of the antisense ORN on stability of the TS protein could not be ruled out. The effect on protein stability appears to occur during antisense treatment, since decreased expression of TS protein at later time points does not appear to be due to enhanced protein degradation based on the determined half-life of TS. Since TS is an RNA binding protein, it is conceivable that TS binds directly to the antisense ORN itself or to the TS mRNA:ORN complex resulting in activation of a protein degradation pathway. Taken together, these experiments suggest that the antisense ORN controls the expression of TS at the posttranscriptional level, most likely through a combination of translational arrest of TS mRNA and posttranslational processes that may involve enhanced degradation of TS protein.

7. CONCLUSIONS

TS plays an essential role in the biosynthesis of key precursors required for DNA biosynthesis. The ability to increase the expression of TS in response to growth stimuli and/or exposure to cytotoxic stresses either on an acute or chronic basis serves as an important adaptive response mechanism that allows for normal synthetic function to be maintained. It is now well established that regulation at the level of gene amplification, transcription, translation, and posttranslation are all involved in regulating the expression of TS with regard to cell-cycle-directed events, growth proliferation, and in response to exposure to cytotoxic agents. Moreover, there is growing evidence that the regulatory events involved in the expression of TS are complex and may not be restricted to only one specific control mechanism. It is quite possible that the precise control of TS expression requires multiple levels of regulation acting in close concert with one another. The specific cellular and/or cytotoxic stress, the timing of exposure to a particular cytotoxic agent, as well as the dose of a given cytotoxic compound may be especially relevant issues that must be taken into account. Certainly, an enhanced understanding of each of these basic control mechanisms should offer new insights as to how the expression of TS is regulated. Moreover, these molecular-based studies may provide rationale for the design and development of novel therapeutic approaches that are directly targeted against TS.

ACKNOWLEDGMENTS

The authors wish to thank the members of our laboratory, both past and present, for the dedicated research efforts and contributions to this work. This work was supported by grants from the National Cancer Institute (CA16359 and CA75712 to E.C.) and from the Department of Veterans Affairs (VA Merit Review Award to E.C.).

REFERENCES

1. Santi DV, Danenberg PV. Folates in pyrimidine nucleotide biosynthesis. In Folate and Pteridines. (Blakely, R.L., Benkovic, S.J., eds.) Wiley, New York, 1984; 345–398.
2. Carreras C, Santi DV. The catalytic mechanism and structure of thymidylate synthase. *Annu Rev Biochem* 1995; 64:721–762.
3. Danenberg PV. Thymidylate synthase: a target enzyme in cancer chemotherapy. *Biochem Biophys Acta* 1977; 473:73–79.
4. Hardy LW, Finer-Moore JS, Montfort WR, Jones MO, Santi DV. Stroud RM. Atomic structure of thymidylate synthase: target for rational drug design. *Science* 1987; 235:448–455.
5. Johnston PG, Liang CM, Henry S, Chabner BA, Allegra CJ. Production and characterization of monoclonal antibodies that localize thymidylate synthase in the cytoplasm of human cells and tissu. *Cancer Res* 1991; 51:6668–6676.
6. Leichman L, Danenberg K, Baranda J, et al. Quantitation of intratumoral thymidylate synthase expression predicts for disseminated colorectal cancer response and resistance to protracted-infusion fluorouracil and weekly leucovorin. *J Clin Oncol* 1997; 10:3223–3230.
7. Lenz HJ, Hayashi K, Salonga D, et al. p53 mutations and thymidylate synthase messenger RNA levels in disseminated colorectal cancer: an analysis of response and survival. *Clin Cancer Res* 1998; 4:1243–1250.
8. Swain SM, Lippman MC, Egan EF, Drake JC, Steinberg SM, Allegra CJ. 5-Fluorouracil and high-dose leucovorin in prevsiouly treated patients with metastatic breast cancer. *J Clin Oncol* 1989; 7:890–899.
9. Van der Wilt CL, Pinedo HM, Smit K, Peters GJ. Elevation of thymidylate synthase following 5-fluorouracil treatment is prevented by the addition of leucovorin in murin colon tumors. *J Clin Oncol* 1994; 12:2035–2042.
10. Santi DV, McHenry CS, Sommer H. Mechanism of interaction of thymidylate synthetase with 5-fluorodeoxyuridylate. *Biochemistry* 1974; 13:471–480.
11. Keyomarsi K, Moran RG. Folinic acid augmentation of the effects of fluoropyrimidines on murine and human leukemic cells. *Cancer Res* 1988; 46:5229–5235.
12. Erlichman C, Fine S, Wong A, Elhakim T. A randomized trial of fluorouracil and folinic acid in patients with metastatic colorectal carcinoma. *J Clin Oncol* 1988; 6:469–475.
13. Poon MA, O'Conell MJ, Moertel CG, et al. Biochemical modulation of fluorouracil: evidence of a significant improvement of survival and quality of life in patients with advanced colorectal carcinoma. *J Clin Oncol* 1989; 10:1407–1418.
14. Advanced colorectal cancer meta-analysis project. Modulation of fluororuacil by leucovorin in patients with advanced colorectal cancer: evidence in terms of response rate. *J Clin Oncol* 1992; 10:896–903.
15. Rustum YM, Harstrick A, Cao S, et al. Thymidylate synthase inhibitors in cancer therapy: direct and indirect inhibitors. *J Clin Oncol* 1997; 15:389–400.
16. Cunningham D, Zalcberg JR, Rath U, et al. Tomudex Colorectal Cancer Study Group. Tomudex (ZD1694): results of a randomized trial in advanced colorectal cancer demonstrate efficacy and reduced mucositis and leucopenia. *Eur J Cancer* 1995; 12:1945–1954.

17. Zalcberg JR, Cunningham D, van Cutsem E, et al. ZD1694: a novel thymidylate synthase inhibitor with substantial activity in the treatment of patients with advanced colorectal cancer. *J Clin Oncol* 1996; 14:716–721.
18. Cocconi G, Cunninghman D, van Cutsem E, et al. Open, randomized, multicenter trial of raltitrexed versus fluorouracil plus high-dose leucovorin in patients with advanced colorectal cancer. *J Clin Oncol* 1998; 16:2943–2952.
19. Alt FW, Kellems RE, Bertino JR, Schimke RT. Selective multiplication of dihydrofolate reductase genes in methotrexate-resistant variants of cultured mouse cells. *J Biol Chem* 1998; 253:1357–1370.
20. Trent JM, Buick RN, Olson S, et al. Cytologic evidence for gene amplification in methotrexate-resistant cells obtained from a patient with ovarian adenocarcinoma. *J Clin Oncol* 1984; 2:8–16.
21. Horns RC, Jr Dower WJ, Schimke RT. Gene amplification in a leukemic patient treated with methotrexate. *J Clin Oncol* 1984; 2:2–7.
22. Carman MD, Schornagel JH, Rivest RS, et al. Resistance to methotrexate due to gene amplification in a patient with acute leukemia. *J Clin Oncol* 1984; 2:16–23.
23. Danenberg, KD Danenberg, PV. Activity of thymidylate synthetase and its inhibition by 5-fluorouracil in highly enzyme-overproducing cells resistant to 10-propargyl-5,8-dideazafolate. *Mol Pharmacol* 1989; 36:219–223.
24. Berger SH, Jenh CH, Johnson LF, Berger FG. Thymidylate synthase overproduction and gene amplification in fluorodeoxyuridine-resistant human cells. *Mol Pharmacol* 1985; 28:461–467.
25. Copur MS, Aiba K, Drake JC, Allegra CJ, Chu E. Thymidylate synthase gene amplification in human colon cancer cells resistant to 5-fluorouracil. *Biochem Pharm* 1995; 49:1419–1426.
26. Drake JC, Allegra CJ, Moran RG, Johnston PG. Resistance to Tomudex (ZD1694) is multifactorial in human breast and colon carcinoma cell lines. *Biochem Pharm* 1996; 51:1349–1355.
27. Clark JL, Berger SH, Mittleman A, Berger F. Thymidylate synthase gene amplification in a colon tumor resistant to fluoropyrimidine chemotherapy. *Cancer Treat Rep* 1987; 71:261–265.
28. Gorlick R, Metzger R, Danenberg KD, et al. Higher levels of thymidylate synthase gene expression are observed in pulmonary as compared with hepatic metastases of colorectal adenocarcinoma. *J. Clin Oncol* 1998; 16:1465–1469.
29. Conrad AH. TS activity in cultured mammalian cells. *J Biol Chem* 1971; 246:1318–1323.
30. Navalgund LG, Rossana C, Muench AL, Johnson LF. Cell cycle regulation of thymidylate synthetase gene expression in cultured mouse fibroblasts. *J Biol Chem* 1980; 255:7386–7390.
31. Ayusawa D, Shimizu K, Koyama H, Kaneda S, Takeishi K, Seno T. Cell-cycle-directed regulation of thymidylate synthase messenger RNA in human diploid fibrolbasts stimulated to proliferate. *J Mol Biol* 1986; 190:559–567.
32. Geng Y Johnson LF. Lack of an initiator element is responsible for multiple transcriptional initiation sites of the TATA-less mouse thymidylate synthase promoter. *Mol Cell Biol* 1993; 13:4894–4903.
33. Li D, Osborn K, Johnson LF. The 5′-flanking region of the mouse TS gene is necessary but no sufficient for normal regulation in growth stimulated cells. *Mol Cell Biol* 1991; 11:1023–1029.
34. Dong S, Lester L, Johnson LF. Transcriptional control elements and complex initiation pattern of the TATA-less bidirectional human thymidylate synthase promoter. *J Cell Biochem* 2000; 77:50–64.
35. Horie N, Takeishi K. Identification of functional elements in the promoter region of the human gene for thymidylate synthase and nuclear factors that regulate the expression of the gene. *J Biol Chem* 1997; 272:18375–18361.
36. Farnham PJ, Slansky JE, Kollmar, R. The role of E2F in the mammalian cell cycle. *Biochem Biophys Acta Rev Cancer* 1993; 1155:125–131.
37. Ash J, Ke Y, Korb M, Johnson LF. Regulation of mouse thymidylate synthase gene expression in growth-stimulated cells: upstream S phase control elements are indistinguishable from the essential promoter elements. *Nucleic Acids Res* 1995; 23:4649–4656.
38. Li Y, Slansky JE, Myers DJ, Drinkwater NR, Kaelin WG, Farnhan PJ. Cloning, chromosomal location, and characterization of mouse E2F1. *Mol Cell Biol* 1994; 14:1861–1869.
39. Banerjee D, Schnieders B, Fu JZ, Adhikari D, Zhao SC, Bertino JR. Role of E2F-1 in chemosensitivity. *Cancer Res* 1998; 58:4292–4296.
40. Banerjee D, Gorlick R, Liefshitz A, et al. Levels of E2F1 expression are higher in lung metastasis of colon cancer as compared with hepatic metastasis and correlate with levels of thymidylate synthase. *Cancer Res* 2000; 60:2365–2367.
41. Kasahara M, Takahashi Y, Nagata T, et al. Thymidylate synthase expression correlates closely with E2F1 expression in colon cancer. *Clin Cancer Res* 2000; 6:2707–2711.
42. Powell C, Rudge TL, Zhu Q, Johnson LF, Hansen U. Inhibition of the mammalian transcription factor LSF induces S-phase-dependent apoptosis by downregulating thymidylate synthase expression. *EMBO J* 2000; 19:4664–4675.

43. Kim CH Heath C, Bertuch A, Hansen U. Specific stimulation of simian virus 40 late transcription in vitro by a cellular factor binding the simian virus 40 21-base-pair repeat promoter element. *Proc Natl Acad Sci USA* 1987; 84:6025–6029.
44. Ke Y, Ash J, Johnson LF. Splicing signals are required for S-phase regulation of the mouse thymidylate synthase gene. *Mol Cell Biol* 1996; 16:376–383.
45. Jenh CH Geyer PK, Johnson LF, Control of thymidylate synthase mRNA content and gene transcription in on overproducing mouse cell line. *Mol Cell Biol* 1985; 5:2527–2532.
46. Kaneda S, Horie N, Takeishi K, Takayanagi A, Seno T, Ayusawa D. Regulatory sequences clustered at the 5′ end of the first intron of the human thymidylate synthase gene function in cooperation with the promoter region. Somat. *Cell Mol Genet* 1992; 18:409–415.
47. Takayanagi A, Kaneda S, Ayusawa D, Seno T. Intron 1 and the 5′-flanking region of the human thymidylate synthase gene as a regulatory determinant of growth-dependent expression. *Nucleic Acids Res* 1992; 20:4021–4025.
48. Scanlon KJ, Kashani-Sabet M. Elevated expression of thymidylate synthase cycle genes in cisplatin-resistant human ovarian carcinoma A2780 cells. *Proc Natl Acad Sci USA* 1988; 85:650–653.
49. Chu E, Drake JC, Koeller DM, et al. Induction of thymidylate synthase associated with multidrug resistance in human breast and colon cancer cell lines. *Mol Pharmacol* 1991; 39:136–143.
50. Belfort M, Maley G, Pedersen-Lane J. Maley F. Primary structure of the *Escherichia coli* thyA gene and its thymidylate synthase product. *Proc Natl Acad Sci USA* 1983; 80:4914–4918.
51. Rao KN, Kisliuk RL. Association of RNA with thymidylate synthase from methotrexate-resistant Streptococcus faecium. *Proc Natl Acad Sci USA* 1983; 80:916–920.
52. Thorndike J, Kisliuk RL. Identification of poly G bound to thymidylate snythase. *Biochem Biophys Res Commun* 1986; 139:461–465.
53. Takeishi K, Kaneda S, Ayusawa D, Shimizu K, Gotoh O, Seno T. Nucleotide sequence of a functional cDNA for human thymidylate synthase. *Nucleic Acids Res* 1985; 13:2035–2043.
54. Kaneda S, Takeishi K, Ayusawa D, Shimuzu K, Seno T. Altman S. Role in translation of a triple tandemly repeated sequence in the 5' untranslated region of human thymidylate synthase mRNA. *Nucleic Acids Res* 1987; 15:1259–1270.
55. Spears CP, Shahinian AH, Moran RG, et al. In vivo kinetics of thymidylate synthase inhibition in 5-fluoruracil-sensitive and-resistant murine colon adenocarcinoma. *Cancer Res* 1982; 42:450–456.
56. Washtein WL. Increased levels of thymidylate synthetase in cells exposed to 5-fluorouracil. *Mol Pharmacol* 1984; 25:171–177.
57. Keyomarsi K, Samet J, Molnar G. Pardee AB. The thymidylate synthase inhibitor, ICI D1694, overcomes translational detainment of the enzyme. *J Biol Chem* 1993; 268:15142–15149.
58. Chu E, Zinn S, Boarman D. Allegra CJ. Interaction of gamma interferon and 5-fluorouracil in the H630 human colon carcinoma cell line. *Cancer Res* 1990; 50:5834–5840.
59. Chu E, Koeller DM, Johnson PG, Zinn S, Allegra CJ. Regulation of thymidylate synthase in human colon cancer cells treated with 5-fluorouracil and interferon-gamma. *Mol Pharmacol* 1993; 43:527–533.
60. Chu E, Koeller DM, Casey JL, et al. Autoregulation of human thymidylate synthase messenger RNA translation by thymidylate synthase. *Proc. Natl. Acad. Sci. USA* 1991; 88:8977–8981.
61. Chu E, Voeller DM, Koeller DM, et al. Identification of an RNA binding site for human thymidylate synthase. *Proc Natl Acad Sci USA* 1993; 90:517–521.
62. Chu E, Allegra CJ. The role of thymidylate synthase as an RNA binding protein. *Bioessays* 1996; 18:191–198.
63. Klausner RD, Harford JB. Cis-trans models for post-transcriptional gene regulation. *Science* 1989; 246:870–872.
64. Kozak M. Structural features in eukaryotic mRNAs that modulate the initiation of translation. *J Biol Chem* 1991; 266:19867–19870.
65. McCarthy JEG, Kollmus H. Cytoplasmic mRNA-protein interactions in eukaryotic gene expression. *Trends Biochem Sci* 1995; 20:191–197.
66. Lin X, Parsels LA, Voller DM, et al. Characterization of a cis-acting regulatory element in the protein coding region of thymidylate synthase mRNA. *Nucleic Acids Res* 2000; 28:1381–1389.
67. Jackson RJ, Standard N. Do the poly (A) tail and 3′ untranslated region control mRNA translation? *Cell* 1990; 62:15–24.
68. Gallie DR. The cap and poly (A) tail function synergistically to regulate mRNA translational efficiency. *Genes Dev* 1991; 5:2108–2116.
69. Jackson RJ, Cytoplasmic regulation of MRNA function: the importance of the 3′ untranslated region. *Cell* 1993; 74:9–14.

70. Ostareck-Lederer AD, Ostareck DH, Standard N, Thiele BJ. Translation of 15-lipoxygenase mRNA is inhibited by a protein that binds to a repeated sequence in the 3′ untranslated region. *EMBO J* 1994; 13:1476–1481.
71. Uhlenbeck OC, Wu H-N, Sampson JR. Recognition of RNA by proteins. In Molecular Biology of RNA, 1987; pp. 285–294. Academic Press, New York.
72. Henderson BR, Menotti E, Bonnard C, Kühn, LC. Optimal sequence and structure of iron-responsive elements. *J Biol Chem* 1994; 269:17481–17489.
73. Carey J. Uhlenbeck IC. Kinetic and thermodynamic characterization of the R17 coat protein-ribonucleic acid interaction. *Biochemistry* 1983; 22:2610–2615.
74. Carey J, Cameron V, de Haseth PL, Uhlenbeck OC. Sequence-specific interaction of R17 coat protein with its ribonucleic acid binding site. *Biochemistry* 1983; 22:2601–2610.
75. Romaniuk PJ, Uhlenbeck OC. Nucleoside and nucleotide inactivation of the R-17 coat protein: evidence for the transient covalent RNA-protein bond. *Biochemistry* 1985; 24:4239–4244.
76. Koontz SW, Schimmel PR. Aminoacyl-tRNA synthetase-catalyzed cleavage of the glycosidic bond of 5-halogenated uridines. *J Biol Chem* 1979; 254:12277–12280.
77. Starzyk RM, Koontz SW, Schimmel P. A covalent adduct between the uracil ring and the active site of an aminoacyl tRNA synthetase. *Nature* 1982; 298:136–140.
78. Leary RP, Beaudette N, Kisliuk RL. Interaction of deoxyuridylate with thymidylate synthetase. *J Biol Chem* 1975; 250:4864–4968.
79. Plese PC, Dunlap RB. Sulfhydryl group modification of thymidylate synthetase and its effect on activity and ternary complex formation. *J Biol Chem* 1977; 252:6139–6144.
80. Chu E, Voeller DM, Morrison PF, et al. The effect of reducing reagents on binding of thymidylate synthase protein to thymidylate synthase messenger RNA. *J Biol Chem* 1994; 69:20289–20293.
81. Voeller DM, Changchein, L-M, Maley GF, et al. Characterization of a specific interaction between Escherichia coli thymidylate synthase and Escherichia coli thymidylate synthase mRNA. *Nucleic Acids Res* 1995; 23:869–875.
82. Bernardi A, Spahr P-F. Nucleotide sequence at the binding site for coat protein on RNA of bacteriophage R17. *Proc Natl Acad Sci USA* 1972; 69:3033–3037.
83. Trimble RB, Maley F. Level of specific prereplicative mRNA's during bacteriophage T4 regA-, 43- and T4 43- infection of Escherichia coli B1. *Virology* 1976; 17:538–549.
84. Winter RB, Morrissey L, Gauss P, Godl L, Hsu T, Karam J. Bacteriophage T4 regA protein binds to mRNAs and prevents translation initiation. *Proc Natl Acad Sci USA* 1987; 94:7822–7826.
85. Andrake M, Guild N, Hsu T, Gold L, Tuerk C, Karam J. DNA polymerase of bacteriophage T4 is an autogenous translational repressor. *Proc Natl Acad Sci USA* 1988; 85:7942–7946.
86. Gold L. Posttranscriptional regulatory mechanisms in Escherichia coli. *Ann Rev Biochem* 1988; 57:199–233.
87. Wu H, Wower I, Zimmermann RA. Mutagenesis of ribosomal protein S8 from Escherichia coli: expression, stability, and RNA-binding properties of S8 mutants. *Biochemistry* 1993; 32:4761–4768.
88. Spedding G, Draper DE. Allosteric mechanism for translational repression in the Escherichia coli alpha operon. *Proc Natl Acad Sci USA* 1993; 90:4399–4403.
89. Maley GF, Lorenson MG, Maley F. Inhibitors of protein synthesis: effect on the levels of deoxycytidylate deaminase, thymidylate synthetase, and thymidine kinase in regenerating rat liver. *Biochem Biophys Res Comm* 1965; 18:364–370.
90. Labow R Maley GF, Maley F. The effect of methotrexate on enzyme induced following partial hepatectomy. *Cancer Res* 1969; 29:366–372.
91. Bonney RJ, Maley F. Effect of methotrexate on thymidylate synthetase in cultured parenchymal cells isolated from regenerating rat liver. *Cancer Res* 1975; 35:1950–1956.
92. Kitchens ME, Forshoefel AM, Rafique Z, Spencer HT, Berger FG. Ligand-mediated induction of thymidylate synthase occurs by enzyme stabilization. *J. Biol. Chem.* 1999; 274:12544–12547.
93. Welsh SJ, Titley J, Brunton L, et al. Comparison of thymidylate synthase (TS) protein up-regulation after exposure to TS inhibitors in normal and tumor cell lines and tissues. *Clin. Cancer Res.* 2000; 6:2538–2546.
94. Schmitz JC, Yu D, Agrawal S, Chu E. Effect of 2′-O-methyl antisense ORNs on expression of thymidylate synthase in human colon cancer RKO cells. *Nucleic Acids Res.* 2001; 29:415–422.

5

Regulation of Thymidylate Synthase Gene Expression and Drug Response

Posttranscriptional Regulation and Cell Population Density

Bruce J. Dolnick, PhD

CONTENTS

1. INTRODUCTION

Thymidylate synthase (TS) is a major target for anticancer drug action. Understanding of the mode of regulating TS expression is of great importance to developing strategies to reducing TS levels and activity, and inhibiting the enzyme with paramount efficacy. Over the years investigations of TS levels have alternatively produced evidence supporting the contributions of transcriptional or posttranscriptional regulation, as well as evidence for cell cycle phase-specific or phase-independent mechanisms in regulating TS levels. Most of the literature in this area concludes that TS is a cell cycle, S-phase-specific enzyme. However, as will be discussed, the data frequently rely on biological models that utilize questionable, although widely accepted, assumptions of biological validity. These models may not always be appropriate for generating generalized conclusions of the mechanism for regulationg TS levels. This chapter presents and overview of the key data concerning the regulation of TS gene expression with the perspective that much of the prevailing view that TS is an S-phase enzyme is incorrect. The iconoclastic view of the regulation of TS discussed in this chapter has its origins in the investigations of the rTS gene, a gene that overlaps the 3′-end of the TS gene and codes for an RNA that is partially complementary (antisense) to the TS

From: *Fluoropyrimidines in Cancer Therapy*
Edited by: Y. M. Rustum © Humana Press Inc., Totowa, NJ

mRNA and pre-mRNA and two proteins that may be responsible for controlling a large fraction of TS gene expression at the posttranscriptional through effects on TS pre-mRNA and protein stability.

2. TS AS AN ENZYME OF CELL PROLIFERATION:S-PHASE OR GROWTH SPECIFIC?

TS function is required for the *de novo* synthesis of thymidine, a precursor for DNA biosynthesis. Because of this fact, it is expected that TS would be associated with cell proliferation, as proliferating cells need to synthesize DNA and require DNA precursors (deoxyribonucleoside triphosphates). All investigations involving the characterization of TS activity in cells, both in vivo and in cell culture, have found increased TS levels and TS enzyme activity in actively dividing cell, compared with cells in stasis *(1,2)*. A discrepancy arises when cultured cells are studied. This discrepancy is the cell cycle dependence or independence of TS expression depending on whether cells are arrested for growth prior to examination.

When cells are growth arrested by serum starvation, by nutrient depletion or by exposure to cytotoxic and cytostatic agents and then allowed to reenter the proliferating state, elevations in TS protein and enzyme activity are invariably associated with the onset of S-phase *(2–6)*. However, in stark contrast to these results, when TS levels or activity are assayed in cells from different phases of the cell cycle when cells have not been subjected to various means of cell cycle arrest followed by release, TS or TS mRNA levels do not vary with S-phase *(7–10)*. The results obtained with each model are at strict odds mechanistically and have fairly wide ranging implications. To conclude that the studies performed with growth-arrested cells are an accurate reflection of the regulation of TS requires that and assumption be made that the arrest of cells has no meaningful effect upon the cell cycle and pattern of expression of TS. On the other hand, to conclude that the studies performed with cells that have not been perturbed are an accurate reflection of how TS is regulated requires no assumptions. Despite the requirement that fundamental assumptions be made that the means to achieve cell cycle arrest do not impinge upon the behavior of gene expression in cells following release from a cell cycle block, the cell cycle S-phase-specific model predominates overwhelmingly in the literature view of TS regulation.

Since quiescent cells in vivo can reenter the cell cycle (as in the case of wound healing recruitment of tumor cells following debulking, or even organ regeneration), it is clear that models that employ nutrient deprivation or other means to impose synchronization are likely to be an accurate representation of many in vivo situations for simulating TS regulation. In the case of cells that are growing and are not recovering from some form of imposed growth arrest, however (as in the case of unperturbed tumor growth or normal cell replicative events), it is likely that the proliferation-dependent S-phase-independent model is likely to be more applicable. A combination of the two models may be most appropriate when considering the behavior of TS in the tumors of patients undergoing therapy, where the growth fraction of the tumor and number of cells in the quiescent phase (G_0) may change in response to therapy. Based upon the difference in the cell culture models, the proliferation-dependent, S-phase-independent mechanism is more likely to be an accurate reflection of how TS is regulated the majority of the time in tumor cells when the cell cycle composition of a cell population is in a relatively steady-state distribution, with the S-phase-dependent behavior likely to be restricted to circumstances shortly after quiescent cells have reentered the cell cycle.

3. EXPRESSION OF THE TS GENE: CONSTITUTIVE OR REGULATED?

Studies of TS expression in cells synchronized by arrest methods where TS is an S-phase enzyme imply TS is regulated by control mechanisms associated with S-phase. The mammalian TS genes sequenced to date show that for the most part the 5′-flanking regions are highly conserved and contain binding sites for Ets, Sp1, E2F, and LSF transcription factors. It has been shown that enhanced E2F expression can upregulate TS gene expression, leading to interpretations that the gene is regulated by E2F *(11,12)*. Despite these reports, the involvement of E2F in the transcription of the TS gene was never verified by direct transcriptional analyses. One of the most significant observations is that made by Ayusawa et al., who investigated the expression of the human TS gene in diploid fibroblasts *(8)*. The results of these studies demonstrated that the rate of TS gene transcription was constant during the cell cycle transition, although TS and TS mRNA levels increased with S-phase, leading to the conclusion that regulation of the human TS gene is posttranscriptional. Recent studies using transient transfection assays demonstrate that deletion of the E2F motifs have no effect upon TS promoter activity, casting doubt on the role of E2F in the cell cycle regulation of TS *(13)*. The association between E2F and TS gene expression may be more closely related to the role of E2F in the transition of cells from quiescence to a proliferative state, which would correlate with an increase in S-phase cells but suggests the relationship is one that is circumstantial and not controlled by transcription *(14)*. On the other hand, the connection between cell cycle regulation and TS gene expression is affected by the presence or absence of introns in TS minigenes, with the presence of spliceable introns being a requisite to demonstrate cell cycle regulation *(15–17)*. The requirement for spliceable introns to enact some form of regulation on the expression of the TS gene is intriguing and indicates that a portion (if not most) of the regulation of TS gene expression is posttranscriptional. These data, taken together, provide evidence that the TS gene is likely to be transcriptionally turned on most of the time and that fluctuations in the levels of TS mRNA and TS protein are controlled by other cell growth related mechanisms *(vide infra)*. These mechanisms are also likely to be cell cycle independent to a degree, but depending on how cell cycle related studies are performed may lead to the interpretation that regulation of TS is cell cycle related when it is not.

4. POSTTRANSCRIPTIONAL REGULATION OF TS

The evidence that the TS gene is regulated posttranscriptionally comes from transcriptional studies that demonstrated alterations in the rates of transcription are insufficient to explain changes in the levels of TS mRNA and protein, the need for spliceable introns for S-modulation of the translation of TS mRNA by TS protein. There are three major sites for the posttranscriptional regulation of TS levels. These are TS RNA (pre-mRNA and mRNA) processing and stability, protein stability, and TS mRNA translation. Regulation of TS protein levels by autoregulation of TS mRNA translation has been discussed in detail by E. Chu. The role of pre-mRNA processing and stability and TS mRNA stability in regulating TS protein levels have not been extensively described, but are affected by the rTS gene through the production of a naturally occurring antisense RNA to TS pre-mRNA *(18–20)*. The rTS gene is colocalized with the TS gene on chromosome 18 and is transcribed convergently with the TS gene such that one of the rTS gene transcripts (rTSα RNA) forms an extensive complementary (antisense) RNA to TS pre-mRNA *(21–24)*. This naturally occurring antisense RNA is responsible for regulating the levels of TS pre-mRNA, and consequently, TS mRNA in cells through an novel RNA editing mechanism. The rTS gene also encodes proteins that appear to play a role in the regulation of TS protein levels. Although both of these mechanisms for the regulation of TS mRNA and TS protein levels. are related by the role of the rTS gene in providing active antisense RNA and protein components that function in both distinct and complementary pathways, the regulation of the rTS gene itself appears to be controlled not by cell cycle, but by cell population density.

5. THE rTS GENE AND REGULATION OF TS

The relation of rTS to TS in manifested by both rTSα RNA and the two rTS proteins (rTSα and rTSβ). Evidence for the effects of rTS upon TS is experimental but the effects may be easier to understand in light of what is known of the organization and expression of the rTS gene. The rTS gene is comprised of 17 exons and 16 introns *(24)*. Transcription of the gene leads to the generation of RNA transcripts of which are alternatively spliced to generate either rTSα RNAs (mRNA and other nuclear species) as well as rTSβ mRNA. Both rTSα and β mRNAs utilize 16 of the 17 exons present in the rTS gene, with the α transcripts lacking exon 3 and the β transcripts lacking exon 17. The rTSα RNAs are antisense to TS RNAs because they incorporate exon 17 at the 3′-ends. In addition, most of the rTSα RNA is not spliced to mRNA but remains as higher-molecular-weight species retained by the nucleus, in great excess to TS pre-mRNA. The rTSβ RNAs do not contain exon 17 and as a result do not have an antisense RNA component, but do code for most of the rTS protein produced in vivo. Exon 17 of the rTS gene is complementary to 521 bases of the TS pre-mRNA, and this comprises the extent of complementarity between rTSα mRNA and TS pre-mRNA. However, since most of rTSα RNA is nuclear, the rTSα pre-mRNA is also likely to provide for a source of TS pre-mRNA:rTSα RNA duplexes. In this case the extent of complementarity consists of 973 bases due to the additional contribution of rTS intron 16 that is spliced out during the maturation of rTS pre-mRNA.

Amplification of the region of TS pre-mRNA (by RT-PCR using gene specific primers) from exon 7 that is complementary to rTSα mRNA and sequencing of this region demonstrates that editing (adenosine to inosine) occurs at five sites (Fig. 1). We have developed a method to quantitate TS pre-mRNA and editing of TS pre-mRNA using DNA dendrimer probes complementary to the region of TS pre-mRNA with the 5′-most editing site *(25)*. Examination of the levels of TS pre-mRNA and the extent of TS pre-mRNA editing as function of cell population density demonstrate that the amount of editing (for H630 cells) correlates with the decrease in TS pre-mRNA levels and TS mRNA levels (Fig. 2). As demonstrated in Fig. 2, the level of unedited TS pre-mRNA decreases approx 90% by the time the cells have reached a population density of 10^5 cells/cm^2, 24 h after plating. Under these conditions, changes in the fraction of the cells in S-phase are not observed until the cell population density increases above 2×10^5 cells/cm^2 (unpublished results). In the experiment shown, TS mRNA also declines, subsequent to the decrease in TS pre-mRNA, although in other experiments the decline in TS mRNA was found not to be quite as extensive over this 24-h period. It has also been demonstrated by Chu that rTSα RNA levels correlate inversely with TS mRNA levels in Hep2 cells during asynchronous cells growth and that transient transfection of Hep2 cells with inducible rTSα mRNA can effect downregulation of TS mRNA and protein *(18,19)*. Taken together the data suggest that rTSα RNA interacts with TS pre-mRNA, or possibly TS mRNA, in transfected cells and causes the degradation of TS RNA species, subsequent to editing of the TS pre-mRNA. Since rTSα RNA is always present in excess to TS pre-mRNA in the nucleus, rTSα RNA:TS pre-mRNA duplex formation, presumed to be an essential step to trigger TS pre-mRNA degradation is either a regulated process, or the enzymes that recognize these duplexes must be regulated

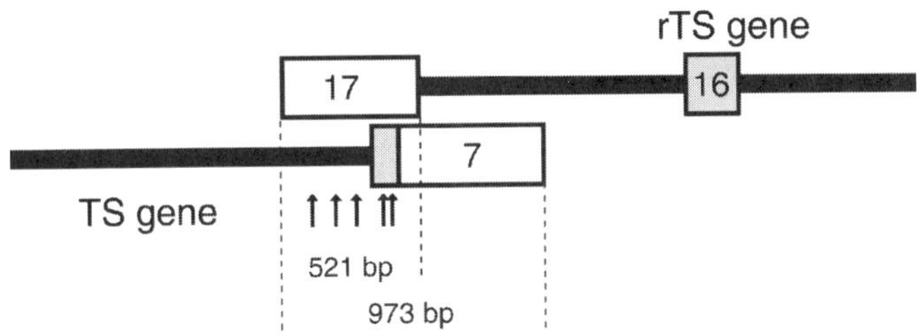

Fig. 1. Overlap of the rTS and TS genes and sites of RNA editing. The cartoon shows the relation of the rTS and TS genes in the region of overlap. The degrees of overlap with the TS mRNA (521 bp) and the TS pre-mRNA (973 bp) are shown. The overlapping lengths are based upon the sequence data obtained for the rTS gene, and differ from that published elsewhere *(24,37)*. TS pre-mRNA editing sites are indicated by arrows. Exons are indicated by boxes, with protein coding regions shaded.

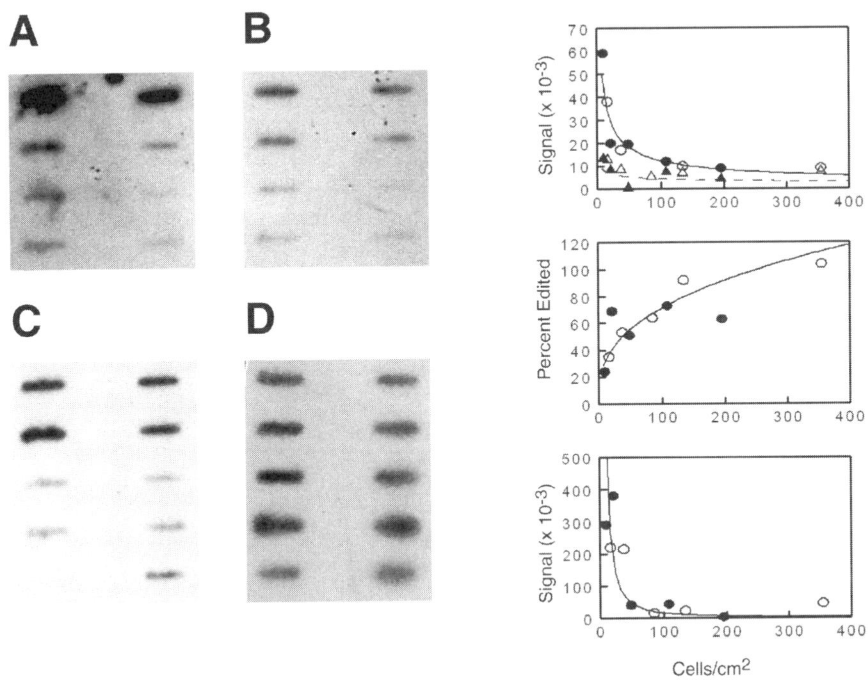

Fig. 2. Cell-population-dependent editing and downregulation of TS RNAs. H630 cells were seeded at different population densities and extracted for RNA after 24 h. TS pre-mRNAs (edited and unedited) were detected by ^{32}P-DNA dendrimer probes and quantitated by comparison with standard RNAs. TS mRNA and GAPDH mRNA were detected using antisense ^{32}P-RNA probes. Signal strength was determined using a phosphor imager. Panels: **A**, TS pre-mRNA; **B**, Edited TS pre-mRNA; **C**, TS mRNA; **D**, GAPDH mRNA. Panels **A–D** show results for 10 µg RNA from two experiments (left- and right-hand columns) where H630 cells were plated at different population densities and extracted for RNA after 24 h. Cell population densities increase from the top to bottom in each panel. A graphic presentation of the data is shown in the three graphs on the right. Top graph, TS pre-mRNA (circles) and edited TS pre-mRNA (triangles). Center graph, percent edited TS pre-mRNA. Bottom graph, TS mRNA. GAPDH is not shown but was blotted as a control for mRNA loading. The closed and open symbols represent experiments 1 and 2, respectively.

themselves. It is known that at least some of the ADAR (adenosine deaminases that act on RNA) that are responsible for editing of double-stranded RNA are regulated by factors such as interferon *(26,27)*. The activation of the processes responsible for the degradation of TS pre-mRNA as a function of cell population density suggests there may be either a cell-to-cell contact function responsible for the phenomenon or that the accumulation of a signal molecule or molecules in the cell culture medium is responsible for activating the degradation of TS pre-mRNA.

Expression of the rTS proteins increases with cell population density (going from mid-log to late-log/plateau phase), as TS protein levels drop, suggesting an inverse relationship between rTS protein expression and TS protein levels during asynchronous cell growth *(23)*. As previously reported, the only exception to this observation was found in KB cells, where rTSβ protein levels did not change as cells progressed from mid-log to plateau phase and TS protein levels were also found not to change *(23)*. Thus, there is a good correlation between growth-related expression of rTS and regulation of TS levels, downregulation of TS observed with growth to high cell population densities when rTSβ is upregulated, and no downregulation of TS when rTSβ is not upregulated. Although the two rTS mRNAs differ at their 3′-ends such that rTSα is antisense to TS RNA but rTSβ mRNA is not, they also differ in their protein coding regions, owing to the inclusion of exon 3 in the rTSβ mRNA but not in rTSα mRNA. This alternative splicing leads to the production of two proteins that are identical for most of their carboxy region but differ in their amino region sequences.

The rTS proteins are members of the enolase superfamily of proteins *(28,29)*. Members of this family catalyze the abstraction of protons from the α-carbons of carboxylic acids, and catalyze a wide variety of reactions. Examples of members of this family include lactonizing enzymes and racemases. One member, RspA, is an *Escherichia coli* protein that has a pattern of expression in bacteria similar to that of rTS in cultured human cells, showing elevated levels of expression as cultures reach high population densities *(30)*. This protein has been found to interfere with quorum sensing functions in other bacterial cells. The significance of this is related to the quorum sensing phenomenon, a widespread mechanism of regulating biological function in Gram negative bacterial cells as a function of cell population density *(31,32)*. In quorum sensing, bacteria continually synthesize and release into the bacterial milieu signaling molecules that regulate a wide variety of biological functions. As the bacterial population increases, so does the concentration of signaling molecules. Once the population reaches a significant density, the concentration of the signaling molecules reaches the level where specific receptors become activated, triggering quorum sensing responses. The activation of a quorum sensing pathway depends on the amount of signaling molecule in the environment relative to the binding affinity for its cognate receptor. Different bacterial species utilize different signaling molecules and one species may also use multiple variants of the same type of signaling molecule to regulate multiple genes. In bacteria the biologic responses are varied and include synthesis of virulence factors, bioluminescence, and ion transport.

Cultured cell lines that overproduce rTS proteins (e.g., H630-1, K562 B1A) grow slower than their cognate cell lines (i.e., H630, K562) that do not overproduce rTS and reach the plateau phase at lower cell population densities. These cell lines are also altered in their ability to regulate TS with cell growth *(33,34)*. These studies suggest that rTS protein expression is related to alternations in TS activity and altered cell growth rates. This conclusion is tempered by the nature of the biological system in which these results were obtained. In the drug-resistant cell lines studied, other genetic changes aside from increased rTS have been shown to occur *(35,36)*. Transfection experiments have not been overly helpful in resolving this issue because of the extreme growth suppressive nature of transfected rTS gene products observed in mammalian cells, yeast, and even bacteria. However, recent results support a hypothesis that rTS proteins serve as the equivalent of quorum sensing enzymes in human cells. Cell culture medium from cells that overproduce rTS can effect the downregulation of TS protein in other cells, compared with medium obtained from cells that do not overproduce rTS. In addition, cell culture media from cells that overproduce rTS can elicit a response using a recombinant quorum sensing bioassay (Dolnick, unpublished results), suggesting that rTS overproduction is associated with the production of a signaling molecule or molecules present in cell culture medium similar to the molecules produced by Gram negative bacteria. Current ongoing studies to define the pathway for the synthesis of these signaling molecules and to examine analogs of these molecules as bioactive reagents further support the role of rTS proteins as the enzymes responsible for their synthesis. If this turns out to be the case, one possible reason for the cell cycle dependency of TS in synchronized cells (synchronized by nutritional or inhibitor mediated methods) vs cell cycle independency in asynchronously growing cells may be related to the technical requirement to change cell culture media after cell synchronization. Adding fresh medium would reduce the amount of the rTS-generated signal molecules from the cellular milieu (although not eliminate them entirely), downregulating their negative effects on TS pre-mRNA stability, and allowing for new TS synthesis to coincide with proliferation. This would have the effect of TS appearing to be an S-phase enzyme as cells are recruited back into the proliferative state and enter S-phase. The same effect would then occur subsequent to each change of cell culture medium.

6. REGULATION OF TS (BY rTS) AND DRUG RESPONSE

The best evidence that rTS may play a role in drug response involving TS comes from the demonstration that rTS protein expression is elevated in a cell line that was made resistant to methotrexate, not a specific TS inhibitor *(33,35)*. The significance of this is that the elevation of rTSβ in this cell line occurred independently of amplification of the TS gene and coincided with the downregulation of TS *(35)*. Although developed to be resistant to methotrexate, this cell line, has twofold decreased levels of TS *(33,35)*. Although the K562 B1A cell line has increased sensitivity to the TS inhibitor fluorodeoxyuridine (IC_{50}s: 2.7×10^{-8} *M* for K562, 6.7×10^{-9} *M* for K562 B1A after 120 h), it has greatly increased resistance to some other specific TS inhibitors such as Tomudex® (IC_{50}s: 2.4×10^{-9} *M* for K562, 2.4×10^{-6} *M* for K562 B1A after 120 h). Thus, a cell line that is resistant to methotrexate due to elevations in the level of dihydrofolate reductase, but also has elevated levels of rTSβ has altered sensitivity to TS inhibitors as well. These changes in drug sensitivity cannot be explained by the levels of TS and suggest that other changes, such as the elevated levels of rTS are involved.

As has been stated previously, cell lines that overproduce rTSβ have an altered ability to regulate TS activity with cell growth *(23,33)*. In addition, transfection of cells that can induce rTSα, and the antisense RNA portion of rTSα exhibit downregulation of TS mRNA and protein *(19)*. It is clear that altering expression of the rTS gene products will alter the level and activity of TS and therefore cellular sensitivity to TS inhibitors. The importance of rTS to tumor response in vivo and the detailed mechanisms by which the rTS proteins and antisense RNA affect TS levels and functions are currently the topic of ongoing and future investigations.

REFERENCES

1. Maley F, Maley GF. Nucleotide interconversion II. Elevation of deoxycytidylate deaminase and thymidylate synthetase in regenerating rat liver. *J Biol Chem* 1960;235:2968–22970.
2. Conrad AH. Thymidylate synthetase activity in cultured mammalian cells. *J Biol Chem* 1971;246:1318–1323.

3. Conrad AH, Ruddle F, H. Regulation of thymidylate synthetase activity in cultured mammalian cells. *J Cell Sci* 1972;10:471–486.
4. Navalgund LG, Rossana C, Muench AJ, Johnson LF. Cell cycle regulation of thymidylate synthetase gene expression in cultured mouse fibroblasts. *J Biol Chem* 1980;255:7386–7390.
5. Rode W, Scanlon KJ, Moroson BA, Bertino JR. Regulation of thymidylate synthetase in mouse leukemia cells (L1210). *J Biol Chem* 1980;255:1305–1311.
6. Keyomarsi K, Samet J, Molnar G, Pardee AB. The thymidylate synthase inhibitor, ICI D1694, overcomes translational detainment of the enzyme. *J Biol Chem* 1993;268:15142–15149.
7. Cadman E, Heimer R. Levels of thymidylate synthetase during normal culture growth of L1210 cells. *Cancer Res* 1986;46:1195–1198.
8. Ayusawa D, Shimizu K, Koyama H, Kaneda S, Takeishi K, Seno T. Cell-cycle-directed regulation of thymidylate synthase messenger RNA in human diploid fibroblasts stimulated to proliferate. *J Mol Biol* 1986;190:559–567.
9. Ali Imam AM, Crossley PH, Jackman AL, Little PFR. Analysis of thymidylate synthase gene amplification and of mRNA levels in the cell cycle. *J Biol Chem* 1987;262:7368–7373.
10. Pestalozzi BC, McGinn CJ, Kinsella TJ, et al. Increased thymidylate synthase protein levels are principally associated with proliferation but not cell cycle phase in asynchronous human cancer cells. *Brit J Cancer* 1995;71:1151–1157.
11. DeGregori J, Kowalik T, Nevins JR. Cellular targets for activation by the E2F1 transcription factor include DNA synthesis- and G1/S-regulatory genes *Mol Cell Biol* 1995;15:4215–4224.
12. Li WW, Fan J, Hochhauser D, Bertino JR. Overexpression of p21waf1 leads to increased inhibition of E2F-1 phosphorylation and sensitivity to anticancer drugs in retinoblastoma-negative human sarcoma cells. *Cancer Res* 1997;57:2193–2199.
13. Lee Y, Johnson LF. Transcriptional control elements of the rat thymidylate synthase promoter:evolutionary conservation of regulatory features. *Exp Cell Res* 2000;258:53–64.
14. Johnson DG, Schwarz JK, Cress WD, Nevins JR. Expression of transcription factor E2F1 induces quiescent cells to enter S phase. *Nature* 1993;365:349–52.
15. Li Y, Li D, Osborn K, Johnson LF. The 5′-flanking region of the mouse thymidylate synthase gene is necessary but not sufficient for normal regulation in growth-stimulated cells. *Mol Cell Biol* 1911;11:1023–1029.
16. Takayanagi A, Kaneda S, Ayusawa D, Seno T. Intron 1 and the 5′-flanking region of the human thymidylate synthase gene as a regulatory determinant of growth-dependent expression. *Nucleic Acids Res* 1992;20:4021–4025.
17. Ke Y, Ash J, Johnson LF. Splicing signals are required for S-phase regulation of the mouse thymidylate synthase gene. *Mol Cell Biol* 1996;16:376–383.
18. Chu J, Dolnick BJ. Effects of transfected rTSa expression on thymidylate synthase and cell growth. *Proceedings of the American Association for Cancer Research* 1998;39:257.
19. Chu J. Natural antisense (rTSalpha) RNA mediated down-regulation of thymidylate synthase gene expression. *Mol Pharmacol Cancer Ther* Buffalo, NY: SUNY at Buffalo, 1999.
20. Dolnick BJ. Regulation of Thymidylate Synthase mRNA Levels by RNA Editing. Proceedings AACR 2000;40:945.
21. Dolnick BJ. Cloning and characterization of a naturally occurring antisense RNA to human thymidylate synthase mRNA. *Nucleic Acids Res* 1993;21:1747–1752.
22. Dolnick BJ. Naturally occurring antisense RNA. *Pharmacol Ther* 1997;75:179–184.
23. Dolnick BJ, Lu K, Yin MB, Rustum YM. Recent advances in the study of rTS proteins. rTS expression during growth and in response to thymidylate synthase inhibitors in human tumor cells. *Adv Enzyme Regul* 1997;37:95–109.
24. Dolnick B, Su J. Homo sapiens RTS (RTS) gene, complete cds, alternatively spliced. GenBank, 2000;AF305057.
25. Nilsen T, Grayzel J, Prensky W. Dendritic nucleic acid structures. *J Theor Biol* 1997;187:273–284.
26. Patterson JB, Samuel CE. Expression and regulation by interferon of a double-stranded-RNA- specific adenosine deaminase from human cells: evidence for two forms of the deaminase. *Mol Cell Biol* 1995;15:5376–5388.
27. Liu Y, Samuel C. Editing of glutamate receptor subunit B pre-mRNA by splice-site variants of interferon-inducible double-stranded RNA-specific adenosine deaminase ADAR1. *J Biol Chem* 1999;274:5070–5077.
28. Babbitt P, Mrachko G, Hasson M, et al. A functionally diverse enzyme superfamily that abstracts the alpha protons of carboxylic acids. *Science* 1995;267:1159–1161.
29. Babbitt PC, Hasson MS, Wedekind JE, et al. The enolase superfamily: a general strategy for enzyme-catalyzed abstraction of the alpha-protons of carboxylic acids. *Biochemistry* 1996;35:16489–16501.

30. Huisman G, Kolter R. Sensing starvation: a homoserine lactone—dependent signaling pathway in Escherichia coli. *Science* 1994;265:537–539.
31. Parsek M, Greenberg E. Acyl-homoserine lactone quorum sensing in gram-negative bacteria: A signaling mechanism involved in associations with higher organisms. *Proc Nat Acad Sci USA* 2000;97:8789–8793.
32. Swift S, Bainton NJ, Winson MK. Gram-negative bacterial communication by N-acyl homoserine lactones: a universal language? *Trends Microbiol* 1994;2:193–198.
33. Black AR, Dolnick BJ. Expression of rTS correlates with altered growth regulation of thymidylate synthase. *Cancer Res* 1996;56:700–705.
34. Dolnick BJ, Black AR. Alternate splicing of the rTS gene product and its overexpression in a 5-fluorouracil-resistant cell line. *Cancer Res* 1996;56:3207–3210.
35. Srimatkandada S, Medina WD, Cashmore AR, et al. Amplification and organization of dihydrofolate reductase genes in a human leukemic cell line, K-562, resistant to methotrexate. *Biochemistry* 1983;22:5774–5781.
36. Chu E, Drake JC, Koeller DM, et al. Induction of thymidylate synthase associated with multidrug resistance in human breast and colon cancer cell lines. *Mol Pharmacol* 1991;39:136–143.
37. Kaneda S, Nalbantoglu J, Takeishi K, et al. Structural and functional analysis of the human thymidylate synthase gene. *J Biol Chem* 1990;265:20277–20284.

6 Death Receptor Signaling in the Mechanism of 5-Fluorouracil Action

Janet A. Houghton, PhD

CONTENTS

1. INTRODUCTION

5-Fluorouracil (5-FU) was the first fluoropyrimidine to be synthesized in 1957 by Heidelberger and colleagues, by replacement of a fluorine atom in the place of hydrogen at the C-5 position of the pyrimidine ring *(1)*. Since then, compounds of this class have received extensive preclinical and clinical development. Fluoropyrimidines currently remain some of the most widely employed antineoplastic agents with activity against breast, gastrointestinal, and head and neck cancers. Their use in cancer therapy continues to progress with the identification of new modulators that enhance their cytotoxic activity (interferon-γ [IFN]-γ; *2*), with the exploration of new orally active compounds that are currently in clinical trial (tegafur, capecitabine, S1; reviewed in refs. *3–5*), and with new antifolate inhibitors of thymidylate synthase (TS; ZD1694 [Ralitrexed, Tomudex], ZD9331, LY231514, AG337 [Thymitaq], GW1843U89, reviewed in refs. *6 and 7*). The antineoplastic activity of 5-FU has been enhanced by biochemical modulation that increases the metabolism of the agent. These modulators include L-phosphonacety-L-aspartate (PALA;*8*), inhibitors of dihydrofolate reductase (methotrexate [MTX]; *9,10;* trimetrexate [TMQ]; *11*), and inhibitors of the 5-FU degradative enzyme dihydropyrimidine dehydrogenase (5-chlorodihydropyridine [tegafur],

From: *Fluoropyrimidines in Cancer Therapy*
Edited by: Y. M. Rustum © Humana Press Inc., Totowa, NJ

5-ethynyluracil; reviewed in refs. *3–5*). Interferon-α has also increased the cytotoxic activity of 5-FU by influencing thymidine kinase activity *(12)*, and, in particular, by enhancing 5-FU-induced DNA damage *(13)*. 5-FU continues to be the standard agent and mainstay in the treatment of advanced colorectal cancer in combination with the reduced folate, leucovorin (LV), which has proven the most effective modulator in enhancing the therapeutic selectivity of 5-FU *(14,15)*. Thus advancing therapeutic strategies for the treatment of colorectal cancer will build upon the activity obtained with 5-FU/LV combinations.

More recently it has been demonstrated that genes downstream of thymineless stress-induced or 5-FU-induced DNA damage can determine the sensitivity of cancer cells to this agent, including E2F-1 *(16,17)*, Bcl-2 family members *(18–21)*, and oncogenic K-Ras *(22,23)*. However, more extensive studies have demonstrated that thymineless stress-induced apoptosis may be induced by signaling via the Fas (CD95/APO-1) death receptor *(2,24)*, and 5-FU cytotoxicity may also be influenced by the status of the p53 tumor suppressor gene *(25–27)*. This chapter discusses how, in addition to biochemical modulation, the cytotoxic action of 5-FU may be enhanced in malignant cells by modulation of gene expression. Furthermore, the review will focus on how modulation of the Fas death receptor and the functional status of p53 may impact the therapeutic application of 5-FU in the treatment of human malignancies with an emphasis on colorectal cancer.

2. MECHANISM OF 5-FU ACTION

Following entry within the cell, 5-FU is extensively metabolized. The active metabolite 5-fluorodeoxyuridylate (FdUMP) binds to the enzyme TS in a covalent ternary complex with the reduced folate cofator 5,10-methylenetetrahydrofolate (CH_2-H_4PteGlu) thereby inhibiting enzyme function and the synthesis of deoxythymidine triphosphate (dTTP) *de novo* (Fig. 1). The stability of the ternary complex, degree and duration of TS inhibition, and the cytotoxic action of 5-FU are enhanced when the folate is polyglutamylated, and when 5-FU is combined with LV to elevate the pool of CH_2-H_4PteGlu and its polyglutamylated derivatives (reviewed in refs. *3,4 and 28*). Thymineless stress or 5-FU/LV treatment induces an imbalance in the pools of dTTP and deoxyadenosine triphosphate (dATP) where dTTP is depleted and dATP is significantly elevated, a process which precedes inhibition of DNA synthesis, DNA damage, and the induction of apoptosis in human colon carcinoma cells *(29)*. In other systems, the misincorporation of FdUTP or dUTP into DNA may also contribute to the induction of DNA damage *(28)*. In TS^- colon carcinoma cells apoptosis is signaled via the Fas death receptor after dThd deprivation *(24)*, and in other colon carcinoma cell lines *(2)* or in other cell types *(30,31)*, a Fas-dependent component has been demonstrated following 5-FU treatment both in vitro *(2,30)* and in vivo *(31)*. The Fas dependency of FUra-induced cytotoxicity depends upon the induction of DNA damage but is independent of the status of p53 *(2)*. However, the induction of apoptosis by 5-FU is acute in the presence of wtp53, or delayed if p53 is mutated *(25)*. 5-FU treatment also upregulates Fas expression in the presence of wtp53 *(25)*. The improved response rates observed clinically when 5-FU is combined with LV *(14,15)* and the relationship between high TS expression and resistance to 5-FU-based therapy *(32–34)*, strongly suggest that this mechanism of 5-FU-induced cytotoxicity is critical in clinical therapy with 5-FU.

Alternatively following metabolism to ribonucleotides, fluoridine triphosphate (FUTP) is incorporated into both nuclear and cytoplasmic RNA species, resulting in alterations in the secondary structure of RNA and in protein synthesis. The effect of 5-FU incorporation

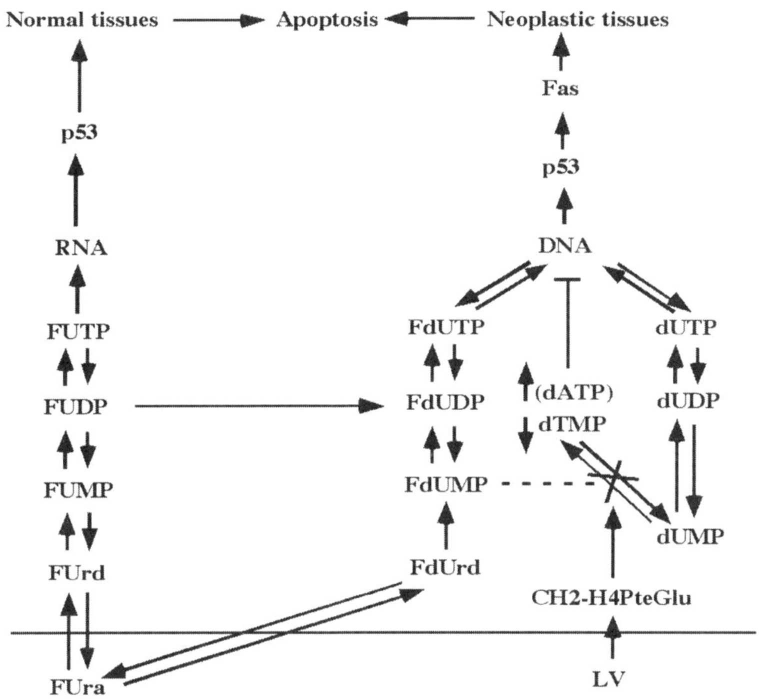

Fig. 1. Metabolism and mechanism of 5-FU action.

may be related to pre-RNA processing resulting in aberrant transcriptional and posttranscriptional processing, which may lead to the cytotoxic effect of 5-FU (reviewed in ref. *28*). RNA-directed 5-FU cytotoxicity has been demonstrated in cultured cells including some colon carcinoma cell lines *(2,35)*. Furthermore, evidence suggests that this is the mechanism by which 5-FU toxicity is induced in normal gastrointestinal tissues *(27,36)*, where the toxic action of 5-FU is reversible in mice following administration of uridine (Urd) but not dThd, and is also p53-dependent *(27)*. The importance of the anti-TS effects of 5-FU in the therapeutic response of human cancers, and the RNA-directed mechanism of 5-FU-induced toxicity in normal gastrointestinal tissues thus provides a rationale for the selective action of 5-FU/LV in the treatment of human cancers, in particular those of epithelial origin.

3. Fas SIGNALING IN THYMINELESS DEATH

Fas, a type I integral membrane protein, belongs to the tumor necrosis factor receptor (TNFR) superfamily and expresses an intracellular death domain (DD) required for rapid signaling from the receptor. Following ligation of the natural ligand, Fas ligand (FasL), or agonistic anti-Fas antibodies to Fas, an apoptotic signal is induced *(37)*. Fas and FasL are known regulators of apoptosis in cells of the immune system including activation-induced cell death *(38)* and apoptosis induced by cytotoxic T cells *(39)*. Fas is expressed in tissues that posses a high rate of cell turnover including epithelial tissues *(40)*, and has demonstrated functional activity in cell lines derived from a variety of different histiotypes

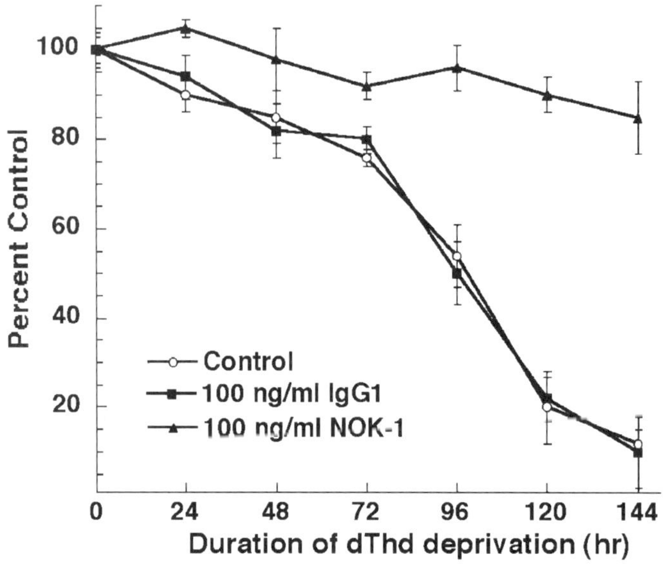

Fig. 2. Fas-dependent cytotoxicity following thymineless stress in TS⁻ colon carcinoma cells.

(reviewed in ref. *41*) including colon carcinomas *(2,42,43)* and breast carcinomas *(45)*. Studies conducted in normal human colonic epithelium *(42)* demonstrated constitutive expression of Fas in every cell, suggesting that the Fas system may be involved in the regulation of normal cell turnover, in colonic tissue homeostasis, and in the regulation of apoptosis. The first study to demonstrate that the Fas death receptor was involved in regulating apoptosis following the induction of thymineless stress was conducted in thymidylate synthase-deficient (TS^-) colon carcinoma cells with high Fas expression (*24;* Fig. 2). The TS^- clone of wt GC_3/c1 cells deficient in TS mRNA and protein committed to cell death following dThd deprivation thereby allowing examination of events downstream of dTTP depletion in an unambiguous manner. Following dThd deprivation in TS^- cells clonogenic survival was reduced to 50% in 3 d, and to 5% by 5 d, with the onset of apoptosis occurring at 24 h (Fig. 2; *29*). However complete protection from thymineless death was obtained following exposure to the NOK-1 MoAb that binds FasL and inhibits Fas/FasL interactions, even at 5 d, when survival would be anticipated to be minimal. The kinetics of loss in clonogenic survival following dThd deprivation correlated with the upregulated expression of FasL *(24)*, and a close correlation existed between loss in clonogenic survival, expression of FasL, and the induction of apoptosis *(45)*. In contrast TS^- clones selected for resistance to the cytolytic anti-Fas MoAb CH-11 and hence to Fas-mediated apoptosis, were cross resistant to apoptosis induced by thymineless stress where clonogenic survival was maintained *(45)*, providing further confirmation of the involvement of Fas in this mechanism of cell death. The requirement of Fas in thymineless stress-induced apoptosis in TS^- cells appeared unique to this form of cell death. A similar Fas dependency for the induction of apoptosis by topotecan, VP-16, or doxorubicin could not be demonstrated in these cells. In this study drug-induced loss in clonogenic survival could not be blocked in the presence of NOK-1, and did not correlate with FasL expression. Furthermore, the Fas-resistant TS^- clones were not cross resistant to these DNA damaging agents in contrast to the effects of dThd deprivation.

4. DETERMINANTS OF FAS-MEDIATED APOPTOSIS IN HUMAN COLON CARCINOMA CELL LINES

For Fas-dependent apoptosis to occur, all components of the Fas signaling pathway must be present. Following ligation and subsequent trimerization of the receptor, several proteins bind to the intracellular death domain of Fas to form the death-inducing signaling complex (DISC). The adaptor protein FADD is recruited to Fas via the DD *(46,47)*, followed by recruitment of procaspase-8 (a FADD-homologous ICE/CED-3-like protease) via the respective death effector domains (DED; 48–60). Following release of active caspase-8 from the DISC, downstream effector caspases are activated. Recently small accelerator for death signaling (SADS) has been identified, is involved in accelerating FADD-dependent cell death, and may be downregulated in certain colon carcinomas *(51)*.

Modification of any one component of the Fas signaling pathway by mutation or reduced expression, or elevated expression of proteins that are inhibitory at various steps in the pathway, may reduce or eliminate Fas-mediated apoptosis. Mutations in the death domain of Fas *(52)*, expression of soluble Fas (sFas; *53*), or reduced receptor expression, may prevent Fas-induced apoptosis, and reduced expression of Fas has been identified in certain colon carcinomas *(42)*. Cells must also express sufficient levels of all components of the DISC to induce apoptosis. Inhibitory factors that may be expressed include:

1. FAP-1 (A Fas-associated phosphatase, which associates with the negative regulatory domain of Fas; *54,55*).
2. DcR3, a soluble Fas decoy receptor, which binds FasL but cannot transmit an apoptotic signal *(56)*.
3. c-FLIP (long [$cFLIP_L$] and short [$cFLIP_S$] forms), which is recruited to the DISC and inhibits caspase-8 activation *(57,58)*.
4. High Bcl-2 expression which can inhibit Fas signaling, and has correlated with decreased anti-Fas sensitivity in colorectal carcinomas *(59)* and their derived cell lines *(24,60)*.

In a series of 10 human colon carcinoma cell lines, four were sensitive to the anti-Fas Ab CH-11, and six were resistant *(61)*. In nine lines expressing Fas PCR-sequencing indicated the death domains to be of wt sequence. Downstream of Fas, expression of FADD, procaspase-8, sFas, FAP-1, Bcl-2 *(61)*, and DcR3, c-FLIP, and SADS (unpublished) demonstrated no correlation between levels of expression and sensitivity to anti-Fas. However, levels of the Fas antigen varied by > 1,000-fold, and correlated with the sensitivity of the lines to CH-11. Fas expression is relatively high in TS^- cells *(29)*, whereas Fas-mediated apoptosis may be limited in other colon carcinoma cell lines because of reduced expression of Fas, but may be elevated following treatment with the cytokine recombinant human IFN-γ *(29,43,61)*. In HT29 cells, four-fold elevation in Fas expression in the presence of IFN-γ (100 IU/mL noncytotoxic) caused a synergistic effect when combined with CH-11 (50–200 ng/mL noncytotoxic) in a clonogenic assay ($\leq$ 10% survival; *2*). These studies demonstrated the significance of Fas expression in colon carcinomas, that this could be modulated to sensitize these cells to apoptotic mechanisms, and that this may be an important target to explore in the modulation of Fas-dependent and chemotherapy-induced apoptosis.

5. FAS SIGNALING AS A DETERMINANT OF THE MECHANISM OF 5-FU ACTION

There are now several published studies that demonstrate the importance of the Fas signaling pathway in the induction of apoptosis and cytotoxicity in the mechanism of 5-FU action. Tillman et al. *(2)* investigated whether a Fas-dependent component existed in 5-FU/LV-induced cytotoxicity of human colon carcinoma cells, and whether this may be potentiated by IFN-γ-induced elevation in Fas expression. In HT29 the cytotoxic action of 5-FU/LV was inhibited by dThd and also in part by NOK-1 + NOK-2 MoAbs that prevent Fas/FasL interactions. 5-FU/LV-induced cytotoxicity was significantly potentiated by IFN-γ (which was reversed by dThd), reversed by exposure to NOK-1 + NOK-2 Abs, and correlated with a fourfold induction of Fas expression in the presence of IFN-γ and significant elevation in expression of FasL. Using six additional human colon carcinoma cell lines, 5-FU/LV-induced cytotoxicity was dThd-dependent in GC_3/c1, VRC_5/c1, RKO, and Caco2, but not in HCT8 or HCT116 (Fig. 3; *2*). Like HT29 cells, this cytotoxicity was potentiated by IFN-γ in GC_3/c1, VRC_5/c1, and RKO, but not in Caco2 that failed to express Fas, nor in HCT8 and HCT116, where no dThd-dependent 5-FU-induced cytotoxicity was demonstrated. This study demonstrated a Fas-dependent component, potentiated by IFN-γ, existed in 5-FU/LV-induced cytotoxicity, but required 5-FU/LV-induced DNA damage for IFN-γ-induced potentiation to occur (Fig. 3). The Fas dependency of 5-FU/LV-induced cytotoxicity was independent of p53 since HT29 and VRC_5/c1 expressed mp53.

Subsequently, Eichhorst et al. *(30)* demonstrated the importance of Fas in the mechanism of 5-FU-induced apoptosis of HepG2 hepatocellular carcinoma cells. In this study 5-FU treatment led to a significant increase in apoptosis determined 12–24 h after 5-FU administration in HepG2 cells in culture, that could be inhibited substantially by NOK-1 or the Fas–Fc chimeric fusion protein that also blocks Fas/FasL interactions. Apoptosis correlated temporally with upregulated expression of FasL, similar to the studies conducted in thymineless death of TS^- colon carcinoma cells. In a second study conducted in vivo, Eichhorst et al. *(31)* demonstrated that 5-FU induced apoptosis in mouse thymocytes via activation of the Fas system. Mice received an intraperitoneal injection of 5-FU, and 18 h later apoptotic cell death peaked in thymocytes, where total organ weight and cell number decreased by 40%, correlating with upregulated expression of FasL. Apoptosis was partially inhibited using neutralizing anti-Fas antibodies, not obtained in lpr mice with impaired Fas signaling due to a mutation in Fas. Therefore 5-FU-induced, Fas-dependent apoptosis can occur in diverse cell types, and under both in vitro and in vivo conditions.

6. TRANSCRIPTIONAL REGULATION OF FASL IN THYMINELESS DEATH

The response of cells to cytotoxic stress and DNA damage depend on the cell type, and the type and extent of DNA damage. In addition to the activation of p53, there have been reports in a variety of different systems that activation of other transcription factors including NF-κB *(62,63)* and AP-1 *(62,64)* are involved in the induction of apoptosis following drug-induced DNA damage. KB elements are found in promoter regions of genes that are crucial for acute or immune phase responses, including FasL *(62)*. AP-1 is a sequence-specific transcriptional activator composed of members of the Jun and Fos families (reviewed in *65*), and is activated via the JNK/SAPK signaling pathway. An AP-1 binding domain has also been identified in the promoter region of FasL *(62)*.

The importance of the transcriptional regulation of FasL in thymineless death of TS^- colon carcinoma cells and in 5-FU/LV-treated cells were initially reported by Harwood et al. *(66)*. In transient transfection assays with reporter constructs, both NF-κB and AP-1 were activated in TS^- colon cells deprived of dThd (Fig. 4), with confirmation by EMSA analysis. A human FasL reporter construct, hFasLPR, was also activated following dThd deprivation that was not obtained when mutations were introduced into the binding sites for either

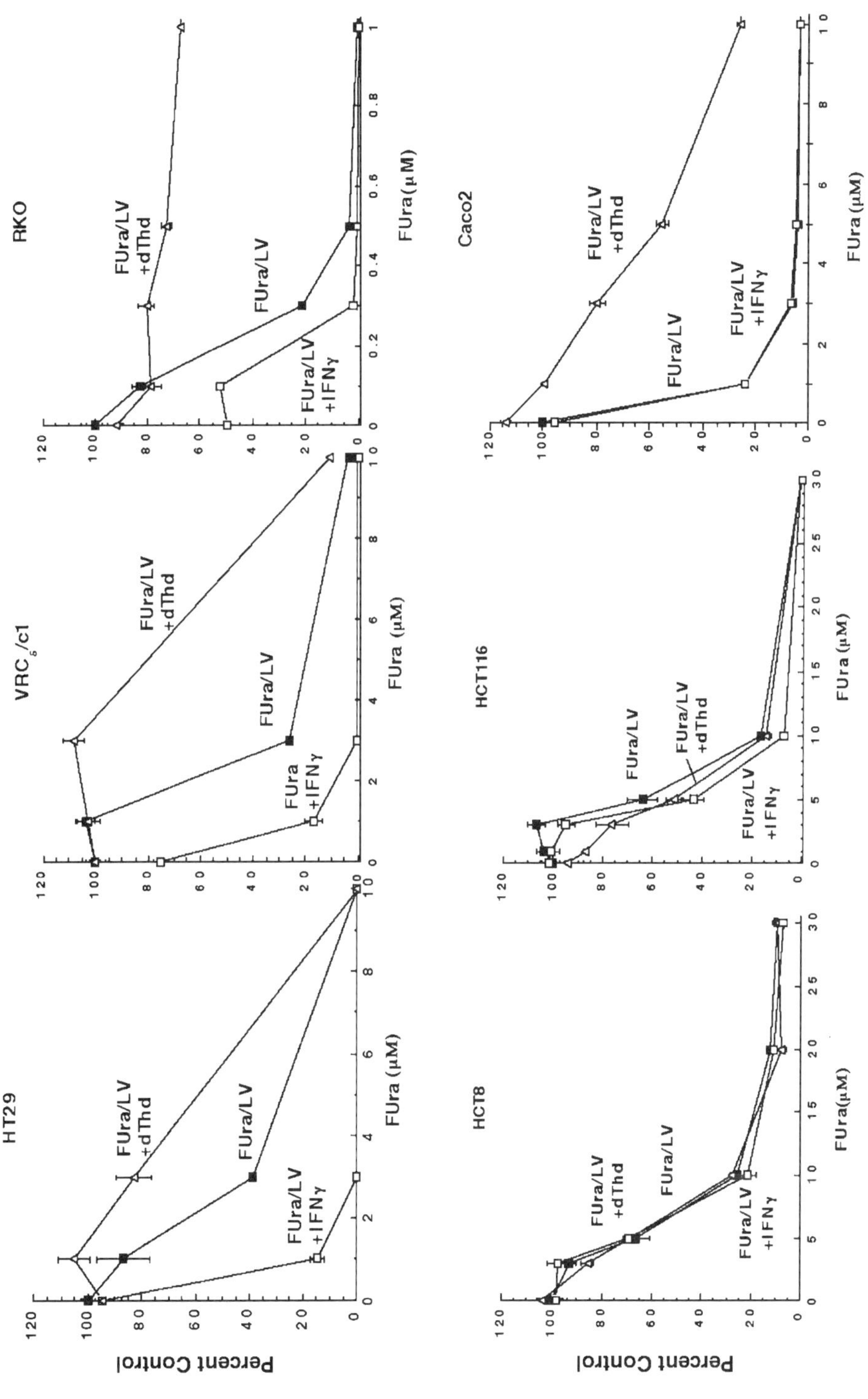

Fig. 3. Enhancement of 5-FU/LV cytotoxicity by modulation of Fas.

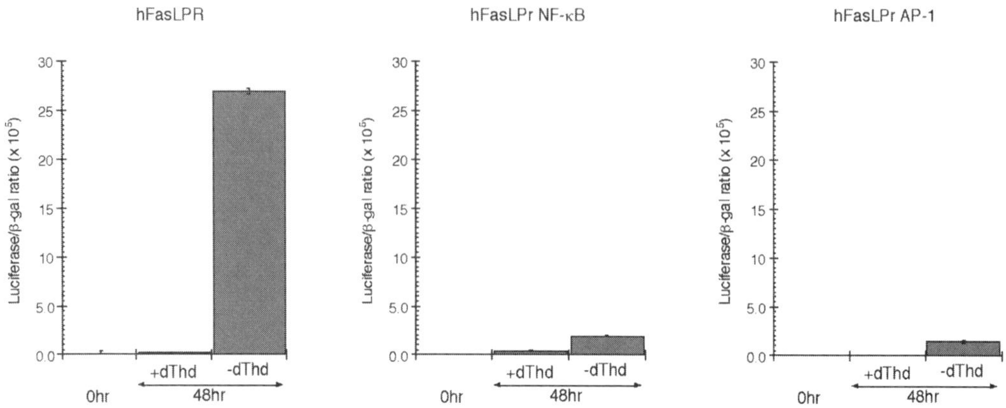

Fig. 4. Transcriptional regulation of FasL by NF-KB and AP-1 in TS$^-$ colon carcinoma cells.

NF-κB or AP-1 in the FasL promoter. Transient transfection of IκBαM or DN-MEKK that block the activation of NF-κB and AP-1, respectively, inhibited the activation of hFasLPR, and in stable transformants expressing IκBαM or DN-MEKK, enhanced clonogenic survival and delayed appearance of FasL following dThd deprivation. Furthermore, both NF-κB and AP-1 were activated following treatment of colon carcinoma cells with 5-FU/LV, which correlated with upregulated expression of FasL in these cells. Subsequently, the MEKK1/JNKK pathway and an AP-1 element in the FasL promoter were found to be required for 5-FU-induced upregulation of FasL in hepatoma cells *(30)*, thereby establishing this transcription factor as more generally applicable in the regulation of FasL in response to 5-FU.

7. ROLE OF P53 IN THE MECHANISM OF 5-FU ACTION

The relationship between apoptosis, p53, and the sensitivity of cancer cells to chemotherapeutic agents has been the subject of considerable debate (reviewed in ref. *67*). The relationship between wtp53 and induction of apoptosis following DNA damage has been well established, particularly in oncogenically transformed normal cells, which appear to have a lower threshold for apoptosis induction following drug treatment, as well as in tissues of lymphoid origin *(68)*. Loss of wtp53 function is considered the most common genetic abnormality in human cancers, and a major predictor of failure to respond to chemotherapy. However, for nonhematologic malignancies, this relationship is not clear *(67)*. Furthermore, increasing evidence indicates that p53 status may determine the threshold and kinetics of drug-induced apoptosis but not overall survival in a treated-cell population *(67)*. For 5-FU there is evidence that the presence of a functional wtp53 gene enhances the sensitivity of cultured cell lines to this agent *(25,69)*, that sensitization occurs following both DNA-directed *(25)* and RNA-directed *(25,69)* 5-FU cytotoxicity, that the status of the p53 gene determines the kinetics of 5-FU-induced apoptosis but not the overall survival of the population *(25)*, and that RNA-directed 5-FU toxicity in mice is also p53 dependent *(27)*.

In both mouse embryonic and NIH-3T3 fibroblasts with a wtp53 gene, 5-FU induced DNA strand breaks resulting in increased p53 levels by activation of p53–DNA binding *(70,71)*. Enhanced 5-FU cytotoxicity in the presence of a wtp53 gene has been demonstrated in human colon carcinoma cell lines *(25,69)* and in HL-60 cells *(72)*. However, there are few studies conducted in vitro in which cell lines have been cultured in the presence of dialyzed serum under dThd-free conditions, such that the anti-TS and hence DNA damaging effects of 5-FU may be analyzed. In the study by Petak et al. *(25)* under dThd-free conditions, acute apoptosis was induced in human colon carcinoma cell lines expressing wtp53 (RKO, HCT8, HCT116), independent of the mechanism of 5-FU action (RKO, DNA-directed; HCT8, HCT116, RNA-directed; Fig. 3), whereas in HT29 and VRC_5/cl that expressed mp53, apoptosis was delayed. Of the cell lines that underwent 5-FU/LV-induced DNA damage, RKO was the most sensitive to 5-FU with an IC_{50} for loss in clonogenic survival 10-fold lower than for HT29 or VRC_5/cl. Transduction of HT29 cells with Ad-wtp53 sensitized the cells to 5-FU/LV-induced and DNA damage-induced apoptosis.

Yang et al. *(69)* transfected an exogenous wtp53 allele under the control of the regulateable lac repressor into SW480 cells (mp53), which were cultured in nondialyzed serum-containing medium. Under these conditions of RNA-directed 5-FU cytotoxicity, SW480 cells were also sensitized to 5-FU when wtp53 was induced by isopropyl-B-thiogalactopyraniside. Furthermore, reduced apoptosis was observed following RNA-directed 5-FU cytotoxicity in p53 null (–/–) human colon carcinoma cells *(73)*. In vivo studies have also demonstrated the importance of wtp53 in 5-FU-induced toxicity of murine gastrointestinal tissues *(27)*. Administration of 5-FU to mice induced an acute p53-dependent apoptosis in the crypts of both the small intestine and midcolon, which was significantly reduced in tissues from p53 null mice. Therefore acute apoptosis induced by both DNA- and RNA-directed 5-FU cytotoxicity is dependent on wtp53, the presence of mp53 delayed the onset of apoptosis but did not change the outcome of 5-FU treatment, acute apoptosis could be induced by 5-FU in cells expressing mp53 alleles following transfection of wtp53, and p53-dependent effects can be demonstrated in vivo.

There have been several reports demonstrating that transfection of a wtp53 gene into mammalian cells elevates the expression of the Fas death receptor *(74–77)*, and sensitizes the cells to Fas-mediated apoptosis *(75,77)*. P53-mediated cytotoxicity has correlated with p53-mediated Fas induction *(75)*. Furthermore, adenoviral transfer of Fas to MCF-7 cells that were resistant to the transduction of Ad-wtp53 was not toxic alone, but sensitized cells to p53-mediated apoptosis *(75)*. Additional data demonstrate that in human vascular smooth muscle cells, p53 activation increased Fas expression at the cell surface by transport from the Golgi complex, and that disruption of this complex blocked both p53-induced surface Fas expression and apoptosis *(78)*. These findings suggest that Fas induction may be a rate-limiting step in p53-mediated apoptosis. Data derived in HT29 demonstrated that transduction of Ad-wtp53, which elevated Fas expression, was not cytotoxic when administered alone. However, when combined with 5-FU/LV that induced DNA damage, apoptosis increased significantly as the moi of Ad-wtp53 was increased *(25)*. Since > 75% of colon carcinomas have deleted or mutated p53 alleles *(79)* and ≈ 50% demonstrate reduced Fas expression *(42)*, this supports a model of tumor progression whereby tumors lose either p53 or Fas functional activity in the reduction of apoptosis-inducing mechanisms.

Clinically there are limited data available regarding the relationship between the status of the p53 tumor suppressor gene and response to 5-FU-containing regimens. A correlation was found between p53 gene status as a predictor of response to 5-FU-based therapy in treatment of squamous cell carcinomas of the head and neck *(80,81)* and in gastric carcinomas *(82)*. In colon cancer p53 status has correlated with Dukes' staging and therefore prognosis *(83)*. In patients with advanced hepatic metastases, p53 overexpression appears to be a dominant predictor of survival *(84)*. One study suggested that in stage III colorectal cancer patients, p53 overexpression predicted for lack of benefit from adjuvant 5-FU plus levamisole *(25)*, although results from other studies in advanced colorectal cancer have suggested that p53 status may not be a good predictor of response to 5-FU *(86,87)*, and hence this relationship remains unclear.

8. CONCLUSIONS

It is evident that 5-FU/LV-containing regimens must be built upon for the improvement of response rates and survival in the treatment of epithelial cancers, in particular colon cancer. As an alternative strategy to biochemical modulation, a promising approach is to effectively modulate the expression of specific genes that determine the degree of apoptosis and cytotoxicity induced by 5-FU/LV. In colon cancer cells the available evidence suggests that signaling of apoptosis and cell death via the Fas death receptor may be unique to the mechanism of action of 5-FU/LV and may not be a pathway utilized by other cytotoxic agents. Fas is reduced in expression in ≈ 50% of colon cancers and IFN-γ induces the expression of Fas in human colon carcinoma cell lines. This effect of IFN-γ is dependent on 5-FU/LV-induced DNA damage, independent of the status of the p53 tumor suppressor gene (mutated in high frequency in colon cancers), and sensitizes the cells to Fas-mediated, 5-FU/LV-induced cytotoxicity. Because IFN-γ does not sensitize cells demonstrating RNA-mediated 5-FU cytotoxicity (which occurs in normal gastrointestinal tissues), IFN-γ has the potential to yield a selective therapeutic approach in combination with 5-FU/LV for the treatment of colon carcinomas. In those colon carcinomas that express wtp53, the approach to sensitize tumors to Fas-mediated apoptosis by upregulating the expression of Fas, may be further enhanced from the effect of 5-FU/LV in elevating Fas expression in a p53-dependent manner. To test this therapeutic strategy a Phase I trial is nearing completion *(88)*, and given the poor prognosis of patients with unresectable colon cancer, it will be of importance to determine whether the 5-FU/LV/IFN-γ approach will translate into improved therapy for this disease.

ACKNOWLEDGMENTS

Supported by NIH Awards RO1 CA 32613, the Cancer Center Support (CORE) Grant CA 21765, and by the American Lebanese Syrian Associated Charities.

REFERENCES

1. Heidelberger C, Chaudhuri NK, Danenberg P, Mooreh D, Griesbach L, Duschinsky K, Schnitzer RJ, Pleven L. Fluorinated pyrimidines. A new class of tumor inhibitory compounds. *Nature* 1957;179:663–666.
2. Tillman DM, Petak I, Houghton JA. A Fas-dependent component in 5-fluorouracil/leucovorin-induced cytotoxicity in colon carcinoma cells. *Clin Cancer Res* 1999;5:425–430.
3. Rustum YM, Cao S. New drugs in colorectal cancer: preclinical studies. *Sem Oncol* 1999;26:612–620.
4. Sobrero A, Guglielmi A, Grossi F, Puglisi F, Aschele C. Mechanism of action of fluoropyrimidines: elevance to the new developments in colorectal cancer chemotherapy. *Sem in Oncol* 2000;27(5 Suppl 10):72–77.
5. Kohne CH, Peters GJ. UFT: mechanism of drug action. *Oncology* 2000;14(10 Suppl 9):13–18.
6. Van Triest B, Peters GJ. Thymidylate synthase: a target for combination therapy and deterninant chemotherapeutic response in colorectal cancer. *Oncology* 1999;57:179–194.
7. Danenberg PV, Malli H, Swenson S. Thymidylate synthase inhibitors. *Sem in Oncol* 1999;26:621–631.
8. O'Dwyer P. The role of low-dose PALA in biochemical modulation. *Pharmacol Ther* 1990;48:371–380.
9. Cadman E, Heimer R, Davis L. Enhanced 5-fluorouracil nucleotide formation after methotrexate administration; explanation for drug synergism. *Science* 1979;205:1135–1137.
10. Houghton JA, Tice AJ, Houghton PJ. The selectivity of action of methotrexate in combination with 5-fluorouracil in xenografts of human colon adenocarcinomas. *Mol Pharmacol* 1982;22:771–778.
11. Blanke CD, Messenger M, and Taplin SC. Trimetrexate: review and current clinical experience in advanced colorectal cancer. *Sem Oncol* 1997;24 (Suppl. 18):57–63.

12. Wadler S, Schwartz EL. Antineoplastic activity of the combination of interferon and cytotoxic agents against experimental and human malignancies. A review. *Cancer Res* 1990;50:3473–3486.
13. Houghton JA, Morton CL, Adkins DA, Rahman A. Locus of the interaction between 5-fluorouracil leucovorin and interferon-a2a in colon carcinoma cells. *Cancer Res* 1993;53:4243–4250.
14. Erlichman C, Fine S, Wong A, Tahani E. A randomized trial of fluorouracil and folinic acid in patients with metastatic colorectal carcinoma. *J Clin Oncol* 1988;6:469–475.
15. Doroshow JH, Multhauf P, Margolin K, et al. Prospective randomized comparison of fluorouracil versus fluorouracil and high-dose continuous infusion leucovorin calcium for the treatment of advanced measurable colorectal cancer in patients previously unexposed to chemotherapy. *J Clin Oncol* 1990;8:491–501.
16. Banerjee D, Schneiders B, Fu JZ, Adhikari D, Zhao SC, Bertino JR. Role of E2F-1 in chemosensitivity. *Cancer Res* 1998;58:4292–4296.
17. Hsueh CT, Kelsen D, Schwartz GK. UCN-01 suppresses thymidylate synthase gene expression and enhances 5-fluorouracil-induced apoptosis in a sequence-dependent manner. *Clin Cancer Res* 1998;4:2201–2206.
18. Sawa H, Kobayashi T, Mukai K, Zhang W, Shiku H. Bax overexpression enhances cytochrome c release from mitochondria and sensitizes KATOIII gastric cancer cells to chemotherapeutic agent-induced apoptosis. *Int J Oncol* 2000;16:745–749.
19. Nita ME, Ono-Nita SK, Tsuno N, et al. Bcl-X(L) antisense sensitizes human colon cancer cell line to 5-fluorouracil. *Jpn J Cancer Res* 2000;91:825–832.
20. Mirjolet JF, Barberi-Heyob M, Didelot C, et al. Bacl-2/Bax protein ratio predicts 5-fluorouracil sensitivity independently of p53 status. *Br J Cancer* 2000;83:1380–1386.
21. Agarwal B, Bhendwal S, Halmos B, Moss SF, Ramey WG, Holt PR. Lovastatin augments apoptosis induced by chemotherapeutic agents in colon cancer cells. *Clin Cancer Res* 1999;5:2223–2229.
22. Houghton JA, Ebanks R, Harwood FG, Tillman DM. Inhibition of apoptosis after thymineless stress is conferred by oncogenic K-Ras in colon carcinoma cells. *Clin Cancer Res* 1998;4:2841–2848.
23. Funato T, Ishii T, Kambe M, Scanlon KJ, Sasaki T. Anti-K-ras ribozyme induces growth inhibition and increased chemosensitivity in human colon cancer cells. *Cancer Gene Ther* 2000;7:495–500.
24. Houghton JA, Harwood FG, Tillman DM. Thymineless death in colon carcinoma cells is mediated via Fas signalling. *Proc Natl Acad Sci USA* 1997;94:8144–8149.
25. Petak I, Tillman DM, Houghton JA. P53-dependence of Fas induction amd acute apoptosis in response to 5-fluorouracil-leucovorin in human colon carcinoma cell lines. *Clin Cancer Res* 2000;6:4432–4441.
26. Yang B, Eshleman JR, Berger N, Markowitz SD. Wild-type p53 protein potentiates cytotoxicity of therapeutic agebts in human colon cancer cells. *Clin Cancer Res* 1996;2:1649–1657.
27. Pritchard DM, Watson AJM, Potten CS, Jackman AL, Hickman JA. Inhibition by uridine but not thymidine of p53-dependent intestinal apoptosis initiated by 5-fluorouracil: evidence for the involvement of RNA perturbation. *Proc Natl Acad Sci USA* 1997;94:1795–1799.
28. Grem JL. 5-Fluorouracil: forty plus and still ticking. A review of its preclinical and clinical development. *Invest New Drugs* 2000;18:299–313.
29. Houghton JA, Tillman DM, Harwood FG. Ratio of 2′-deoxyadenosine-5′-triphosphate/thymidine-5′-triphosphate influences the commitment of human colon carcinoma cells to thymineless death. *Clin Cancer Res* 1995;1:723–730.
30. Eichhorst ST, Muller M, Li-Weber M, Schulze-Bergkamen H, Angel P, Krammer PH. A novel AP-1 element in the CD95 ligand promoter is required for induction of apoptosis in hepatocellular carcinoma cells upon treatment with anticancer drugs. *Mol Cell Biol* 2000;20:7826–7837.
31. Eichhorst ST, Muerkoster S, Weigand MA, Krammer PH. The chemotherapeutic drug 5-fluorouracil induces apoptosis in mouse thymocytes in vivo via activation of the CD95 (APO-1/Fas) system. *Cancer Res* 2001;61:243–248.
32. Johnston PG, Lanz HJ, Leichman CG, Danenberg KD, Allegra CJ, Danenberg PV, Leichman L. Thymidylate synthase gene and protein expression correlate and are associated with response to 5-fluorouracil in human colorectal and gastric tumors. *Cancer Res* 1995;55:1407–1412.
33. Lenz HJ, Leichman CG, Danenberg KD, et al. Thymidylate synthase mRNA level in adenocarcinoma of the stomach: a predictor for primary tumor response and overall survival. *J Clin Oncol* 1995;14:176–182.
34. Leichman CG, Lenz HJ, Leichman L, et al. Quantitation of intratumoral thymidylate synthase expression predicts for disseminated colorectal cancer response and resistance to protracted infusion fluorouracil and weekly leucovorin. *J Clin Oncol* 1997;15:3223–3229.
35. Glazer RI, LLoyd LS. Association of cell lethality with incorporation of 5-fluorouracil and 5-fluorouridine into nuclear RNA in human colon carcinoma cells. *Mol Pharmacol* 1982;21:468–473.
36. Houghton JA, Houghton PJ, Wooten RS. Mechanism of induction of gastrointestinal toxicity in the mouse by 5-fluorouracil, 5-fluorouridine and 5-fluoro-2′-deoxyuridine. *Cancer Res* 1979;39:2406–2413.

37. Itoh N, Yonehara S, Ishii A, et al. The polypeptide encoded by the cDNA for human cell surface antigen Fas can mediate apoptosis. *Cell* 1991;66:233–243.
38. Brunner T, Mogil RJ, LaFace D, et al. Cell-autonomous Fas (CD95)/Fas-ligand interaction mediates activation-induced apoptosis in T-cell hybridomas. *Nature* 1995;373:441–444.
39. Rouvier E, Luciani ML, Golstein P. Fas invovvement in Ca(2+)-independent T-cell-mediated cytotoxicity. *J Exp Med* 1993;177:195–200.
40. French LE, Hahne M, Viard I, et al. Fas and Fas ligand in embryos and adult mice: ligand expression in several immune-privileged tissues and coexpression in adult tissues characterized by apoptotic cell turnover. *J Cell Biol* 1996;133:335–343.
41. Houghton JA. Apoptotis and drug response. *Curr Opinion Oncol* 1999;11:475–481.
42. Moller P, Koretz K, Leithauser F, et al. Expression of Apo-1 (CD95), a member of the NGF/TNF receptor superfamily, in normal and neoplastic colon epithelium. *Int J Cancer* 1994;57:371–377.
43. von Reyher V, Strater J, Kittstein W, Gschwendt M, Krammer PH, Moller P. Colon carcinoma cells use different mechanisms to escape CD95-induced apoptosis. *Cancer Res* 1998;58:526–534.
44. Ruiz-Ruiz M del C, Lopez-Rivas A: P53-mediated up-regulation of CD95 is not involved in genotoxic drug-induced apoptosis of human breast tumor cells. *Cell Death Diff* 1999;6:271–280.
45. Petak I, Tillman DM, Harwood FG, Mihalik R, Houghton JA. Fas-dependent and – independent mechanisms of cell death following DNA damage in human colon carcinoma cells. *Cancer Res* 2000;60:2643–2650.
46. Boldin MP, Varfolomeev EE, Pancer Z, Mett IL, Camonis JH, Wallach D. A novel protein that interacts with the death domain of Fas/APO1 contains a sequence motif related to the death domain. *J Biol Chem* 1995;270:7795–7798.
47. Chinnaiyan AM, O'Rourke K, Tewari M, Dixit VM. FADD, a novel death domain-containing protein, interacts with the death domain of Fas and initiates apoptosis. *Cell* 1995;81:505–512.
48. Boldin MP, Goncharov TM, Goltsev YV, Wallach D. Involvement of MACH, a novel MORT1/FADD-interacting protease, in Fas/APO-1-and TNF receptor-induced cell death. *Cell* 1996;85:803–815.
49. Medema JP, Scaffidi C, Kischkel FC, et al. FLICE is activated by association with the CD95 death-inducing signaling complex (DISC) *EMBO J* 1997;16:2794–2804.
50. Muzio M, Chinnaiyan AM, Kischkel FC, et al. FLICE, a novel FADD-homologous ICE/CED-3-like protease, is recruited to the CD95 (Fas/APO-1) death-inducing signaling complex. *Cell* 1996;85:817–827.
51. Suzuki A, Obata S, Hayashida M, Kawano H, Nakano T, Shiraki K. SADS: a new componenbt of Fas-DISC is the accelerator for cell death signaling and is downregulated in patients with colon carcinoma. *Nature Med* 2001;7:88–93.
52. Itoh N, Nagata S. A novel protein domain required for apoptosis. *J Biol Chem* 1993;268:10932–10937.
53. Cheng J, Zhou T, Liu C, et al. Protection from Fas-mediated apoptosis by a soluble form of the Fas molecule. *Science* 1994;263:1759–1762.
54. Sato T, Irie S, Kitada S, Reed JC. FAP-1: A protein tyrosine phosphatase that associates with Fas. *Science* 1995;268:411–415.
55. Yanagisawa J, Takahashi M, Kanki H, et al. The molecular interaction of Fas and FAP-1. *J Biol Chem* 1997;272:8539–8545.
56. Pitti RM, Marsters SA, Lawrence DA, et al. Genomic amplification of a decoy receptor for Fas ligand in lung and colon cancer. *Nature* 1998;396:699–703.
57. Irmler M, Thome M, Hahne M, et al. Inhibition of death receptor signals by cellular FLIP. *Nature* 1997;388:190–195.
58. Scaffidi C, Schmitz I, Krammer PH, Peter ME. The role of c-FLIP in modulation of CD95-induced apoptosis. *J Biol Chem* 1999;274:1541–1548.
59. Meterissian S, Kontogiannea M. Fas antigen expression and function in human colorectal carcinoma. Correlation with Bcl-2 expression. *Proc Am Assoc Cancer Res* 1996;37:15.
60. Houghton JA, Harwood FG, Gibson AA, Tillman DM. The Fas signalling pathway is functional in colon carcinoma cells and induces apoptosis. *Clin Cancer Res* 1997;2205–2209.
61. Tillman DM, Harwood FG, Gibson AA, Houghton JA. Expression of genes that regulate Fas signalling and Fas-mediated apoptosis in colon carcinoma cells. *Cell Death Diff* 1998;5:450–457.
62. Kasibhatla S, Brunner T, Genestier L, Echeverri F, Mahboubi A, Green DR. DNA damaging agents induce expression of Fas ligand and subsequent apoptosis in T lymphocytes via the activation of NF-kappa B and AP-1. *Mol Cell* 1998;1:543–551.
63. Piret B, Piette J. Topoisomerase poisons activate the transcription factor NF-kappaB in ACH-2 and CEM cells. *Nucl Acids Res* 1996;24:4242–4248.
64. Brach MA, Herrmann F, Kufe DW. Activation of the AP-1 transcription factor by arabinofuranosylcytosine in myeloid leukemia cells. *Blood* 1992;79:728–734.

65. Karin M. The regulation of AP-1 activity by mitogen-activated protein kinases. *J Biol Chem* 1995;270:16483–16486.66.
66. Harwood FG, Kasibhatla S, Petak I, Vernes R, Green DR, Houghton JA. Regulation of FasL by NF-KB and AP-1 in Fas-dependent thymineless death of human colon carcinoma cells. *J Biol Clin* 2000;275:10023–10029.
67. Brown JM, Wouters BG. Apoptosis, p53, and tumor cell sensitivity to anticancer agents. *Cancer Res* 1998;59:1391–1399.
68. Aldridge DR, Radford IR. Explaining differences in sensitivity to killing by ionizing radiation between human lymphoid cell lines. *Cancer Res* 1998;58:2817–2824.
69. Yang B, Eshleman R, Berger NA, Markowitz SD. Wild-type p53 protein potentiates cytotoxicity of therapeutic agents in human colon cancer cells. *Clin Cancer Res* 1996;2:1649–1657.
70. Lowe SW, Ruley HE, Jacks T, Housman DE. P53-dependent apoptosis modulates the cytotoxicity of anticancer agents. *Cell* 1993;74:957–967.
71. Tishler RB, Calderwood SK, Coleman CN, Price BD. Increases in sequence specific DNA binding by p53 following treatment with chemotherapeutic and DNA damaging agents. *Cancer Res* 1993;53(10 Suppl):2212–2216.
72. Ju J-F, Banerjee D, Lenz HJ, et al. Restoration of wild-type p53 activity in p53-null HL-60 cells confers multidrug sensitivity. *Clin Cancer Res* 1998;4:1315–1322.
73. Bunz F, Hwang PM, Torrance C, et al. Disruption of p53 in human cancer cells alters the responses to therapeutic agents. *J Clin Invest* 1999;104:263–269.
74. Owen-Schaub LB, Zhang W, Cusack JC, et al. Wild-type human p53 and a temperature-sensitive mutant induce Fas/APO-1 expression. *Mol Cell Biol* 1995;15:3032–3040.
75. Rakkar ANS, Katayose Y, Kim M, et al. A novel adenoviral vector expressing human Fas/CD95/APO-1 enhances p53-mediated apoptosis. *Cell Death Diff* 1999;6:326–333.
76. Fukazawa T, Fujiwara T, Morimoto Y, et al. Differential involvement of the CD95 (Fas/APO-1) receptor/ligand system on apoptosis induced by the wild-type p53 gene transfer in human cancer cells. *Oncogene* 1999;18:2189–2199.
77. Tamura T, Aoyama N, Saya H, et al. Induction of Fas-mediated apoptosis in p53-transfected human colon carcinoma cells. *Oncogene* 1995;11:1939–1946.
78. Bennett M, Macdonald K, Chan S-W, Luzio JP, Simari R, Weissberg P. Cell surface trafficking of Fas: a rapid mechanism of p53-mediated apoptosis. *Science* 1998;282:290–293.
79. Fearon ER, Vogelstein BA. A genetic model for colorectal tumorigenesis. *Cell* 1990;61:759–767.
80. Temam S, Flahault A, Perie S, et al. P53 gene status as a predictor of tumor response to induction chemotherapy of patients with locoregionally advanced squamous cell carcinomas of the head and neck. *J Clin Oncol* 2000;18:385–394.
81. Cabelguenne A, Blons H, de Waziers I, et al. P53 alterations predict tumor response to neoadjuvant chemotherapy in head and neck squamous cell carcinomas: a prospective series. *J Clin Oncol* 2000;18:1465–1473.
82. Kimura H, Konishi K, Kaji M, et al. Apoptosis, cell proliferation and expression of oncogenes in gastric carcinomas induced by preoperative administration of 5-fluorouracil. *Oncol Rep* 2000;7:971–976.
83. Flamini G, Curigliano G, Ratto C. Prognostic significance of cytoplasmic p53 overexpression in colorectal cancer. An immunohistochemical analysis. *Eur J Cancer* 1996;32A:802–806.
84. Nitti D, Belluco C, Montesco MC, et al. Nuclear p53 protein expression in resected hepatic metastases from colorectal cancer: an independent prognostic factor of survival. *Eur J Cancer* 1998;34:851–855.
85. Ahnen DJ, Feigl P, Quan G, et al. Ki-ras mutation and p53 overexpression predict the clinical behavior of colorectal cancer: a Southwest Oncology Group study. *Cancer Res* 1998;58:1149–1158.
86. Brett MC, Pickard M, Green B, et al. P53 protein overexpression and response to biomodulated 5-fluorouracil chemotherapy in patients with advanced colorectal cancer. *Eur J Surg Oncol* 1996;22182–22185.
87. Cascinu S, Catalano V, Aschele C, et al. Immunohistochemical determination of p53 protein does not predict clinical response in advanced colorectal cancer with low thymidylate synthase expression receiving a bolus 5-fluorouracil-leucovorin combination. *Ann Oncol* 2000;11:1053–1056.
88. Petak I, Tillman DM, Stewart C, et al. Phase I Trial of 5-Fluorouracil (FUra), Leucovorin (LV) and Interferon-γ (IFN-γ) based upon modulation of Fas (CD95/APO-1) signaling. *Proc Am Assoc Cancer Res* 2001;42:621.

7 Circadian Rhythms in 5-Fluorouracil Pharmacology and Therapeutic Applications

Francis Lévi, MD, PhD

CONTENTS

1. INTRODUCTION

5-Fluorouracil (5-FU) has been subjected to many delivery schedules and combined with many other drugs over its 40 yr of use against gastrointestinal, breast, and several other malignancies. Many studies have shown that the toxicologic and pharmacologic properties of this drug are modulated with circadian rhythms. These findings have led to chronomodulate the infusion rate of 5-FU along the 24-h time scale in order to improve its therapeutic index. 5-FU-based chronotherapy has been administered to over 2000 patients with gastrointestinal, breast, lung or other malignancy within prospective clinical trials. Specific methods, including study design, time series analyses, and drug delivery systems are required to demonstrate the rhythms in fluoropyrimidine pharmacology or their alterations and to take advantage of them for therapeutic purposes. This chapter summarizes our rapidly growing knowledge on mammalian circadian rhythms, the consequences of this circadian organization for 5-FU metabolism and cytotoxicity, and the main results from the clinical chronotherapy trials involving this drug.

2. CIRCADIAN RHYTHMS

Circadian rhythms have similar properties in all living beings: These about 24-h cycles persist in constant environmental conditions, hence they are not the mere reflection of the

From: *Fluoropyrimidines in Cancer Therapy*
Edited by: Y. M. Rustum © Humana Press Inc., Totowa, NJ

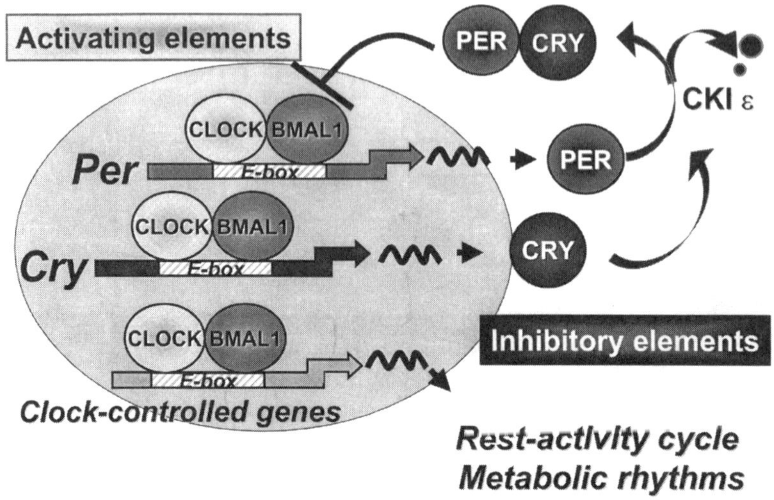

Fig. 1. Schematic representation of the mammalian cellular circadian clock. Activating elements consist of CLOCK and BMAL-1 and inhibiting elements consist of PER and CRY. These four proteins belong to the helix-loop-helix protein family (hlh) and share a common PAS domain that allows them to dimerize or to heterodimerize. The CLOCK–BMAL-1 heterodimer binds to an E-box on the *per* and *cry* genes and stimulate their transcription. PER and CRY proteins, in turn heterodimerize and inhibit CLOCK–BMAL-1 activation of their own transcription. Casein kinase Iε is involved into the degradation of PER and CRY thus exert a posttranscriptional control on these interacting feedback loops, which constitute the circadian oscillator. The CLOCK–BMAL-1 heterodimer also activates the transcription of several so-called clock-controlled genes, thereby generating circadian rhythms in cellular metabolism as well as the rest–activity circadian cycle.

regular alternation of light and darkness or other external cycles. The molecular mechanisms of mammalian circadian rhythms has been unraveled over the past few years. Interacting loops involving up to nine specific genes (*per1, per2, per3, cry1, cry2, tim, clock, bmal1,* and *ckIε*) generate the intracellular circadian oscillation. This cellular circadian clock modulates transcription and posttranscriptional processes of several other genes, thereby creating periodic 24-h changes in cell physiology *(1–4)* (Fig. 1).

The cellular clocks are coordinated by the suprachiasmatic nucleus (SCN), a central clock, located at the floor of the hypothalamus, through mechanisms yet to be determined *(5–6)*. The SCN generates the circadian rest–activity cycle and coordinates the "peripheral" oscillators. It is also essential for the adaptation of the whole circadian time structure to the environmental cycles, so-called synchronizers. The regular alternation of light and darkness over 24 h is the main synchronizer of the circadian system, with lights on representing a powerful signal, which resets the circadian system via activation of *per1* among several other "early response" genes *(fos, jun) (1–4)* (Fig. 2). For this reason, circadian time is usually expressed as *H*ours *A*fter *L*ight *O*nset (HALO), rather than as clock hours, in the experiments involving rodents. Melatonin, a hormone mostly secreted by the pineal gland during darkness, contributes to the calibration of the endogenous period to precisely 24 h *(7)*.

Under such synchronization, mammals with normal circadian function display 24-h rhythms in cellular metabolism and proliferation with predictable amplitude and times of

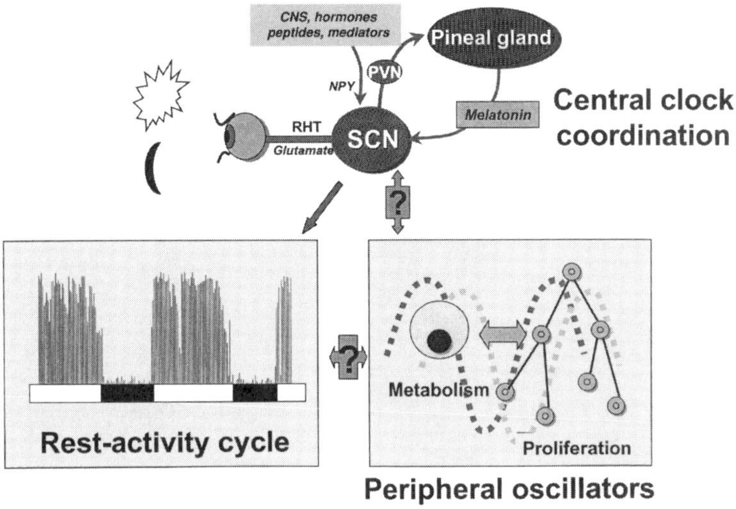

Fig. 2. Schematic view of the human circadian system. The mammalian SCN is a biological clock located at the floor of the hypothalamus. It displays an approx 24-h cycle in the expression of several genes and biochemical functions. Its period (cycle duration) is calibrated by the alternation of light (directly) and darkness (through melatonin secretion by the pineal gland). The SCN generates the rest–activity cycle *(left)* and coordinates many circadian rhythms in the body, and possibly those that modulate cellular metabolism and proliferation *(right)*. RHT, retinohypothalamic tract; PVN, paraventricular nucleus; NPY, neuropeptide Y.

peak and trough. These rhythms modulate anticancer drug pharmacology and ultimately tolerability and/or antitumor efficacy of cancer treatments *(8–11)*.

3. EXPERIMENTAL CHRONOPHARMACOLOGY OF 5-FU

3.1. Rhythms in 5-FU Cytoxicity Determinants

Circadian changes in cellular enzymatic activities by two- to eightfold appear to contribute to the chronopharmacology of antimetabolites (Fig. 3) *(10,11)*. Dehydropyrimidine dehydrogenase (DPD) activity, the rate-limiting catabolic enzyme of fluoropyrimidines, peaks in the early light span (early rest) in mouse or rat tissues *(12–14)*. Conversely, uridine phosphorylase (URDP), orotate phosphoribosyltransferase (OPRT), and deoxythymidine kinase (TK) activities—all three involved in the anabolism of the cytotoxic forms of fluoropyrimidines, FdUMP and FUMP—peak near the middle of darkness (mid-activity) in mouse or rat tissues *(12,13,15,16)*. Dihydrofolate reductase, a target enzyme for methotrexate cytotoxicity, which is also involved into fluoropyrimidine cytotoxicity, peaks at 18 HALO (middle of the activity span) in the liver of mice *(17)*. More recently, thymidylate synthase (TS) activity, a cellular target for fluoropyrimidine toxicity, was found to peak in the late activity span in mouse small intestine, tongue, and bone marrow. A second peak was also found in the late rest span in both latter organs *(18)*. The cellular rhythm in TS activity as well as that in DPD activity seem to be controlled by the circadian oscillator at both transcriptional and posttranscriptional levels *(14,18)*. All the data concur to support a better tolerability of 5-FU in the first half of the light span in mice or rats, i.e., during the early rest phase of their rest–activity cycle.

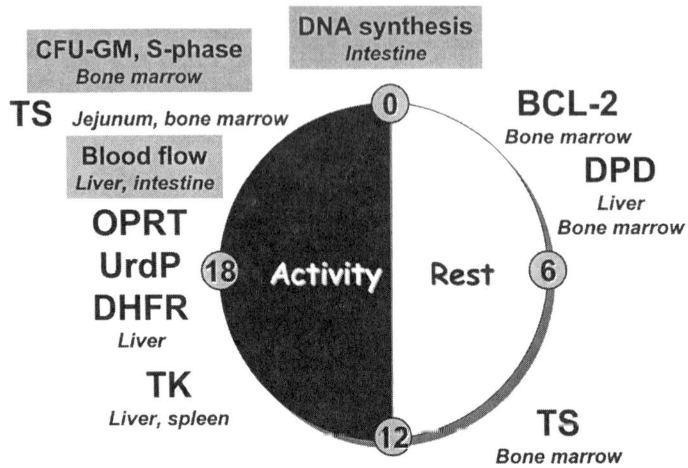

Fig. 3. Distribution of peak times of several biological functions relevant for 5-FU metabolism or cytotoxicity in mice or rats. Time is expresed in HALO. Mice or rats rest during the 12-h light span and are active during the 12-h dark span. Enzymatic activities are TS, thymidilate synthase; DPD, dehydropyrimidine dehydrogenase; TK, deoxythymidine kinase; DHFR, dehydrofolate reductase; UrdP, uridine phosphorylase; OPRT, orotate phosphoribosyltransferase. After data from Kouni et al. *(15),* Naguib et al. *(12),* Zhang et al. *(13),* Malmary-Nebot et al. *(17),* Lincoln et al. *(18),* Labrecque et al. *(19),* Scheving et al. *(20),* Haus et al. *(21),* Waldrop et al. *(23),* and Tampellini et al; *(29).*

Twenty-four hour changes in liver and intestinal blood flow also alter cellular exposure to 5-FU and can influence its metabolism and its cytotoxicity. The distribution of labeled microspheres to these organs following intracarotid injection was investigated in rats at four different times of day or night. The estimated blood flow in both organs was 50% larger near the middle of the activity span of the animal *(19).*

Target tissues such as bone marrow or intestinal mucosa exhibit circadian changes in metabolic and cell division activity. Several studies have reported that DNA synthetic activity in murine jejunal or colon mucosa was higher at the end of the nocturnal (activity) span or at the beginning of the diurnal (rest) span in mice or rats *(20–24).* Large and predictable changes in the proportion of myeloid progenitors of murine bone marrow (CFUs, CFU_{GM}, F-CFU) were found along the 24-h time scale, with the highest values usually occurring in the second half of the activity span, or at the beginning of the rest span of mice *(25–28).* Similar rhythms were found for the proportion of S-phase cells in total murine bone marrow *(27,29,30).* Figure 3 briefly summarizes these data.

3.2. Rhythm in 5-FU Toxicity

Three different teams have tested the relevance of 5-FU dosing time with regard to drug lethal toxicity in mice. Survival rate was 2–8 times as high if the same dose of 5-FU was injected near the middle of the rest span as compared to darkness in mice from different strains or sex (Fig. 4) *(31–33).* The extent of leukopenia and that of diarrhea were also significantly less during the light span, as compared to those given the drug during darkness *(34–35).* Nonetheless, toxicity to the intestinal mucosa of rats, as gauged by impairment of water absorption, was reduced following 5-FU injection at night in rats, indicating the complexity of the 5-FU toxicokinetics *(36).*

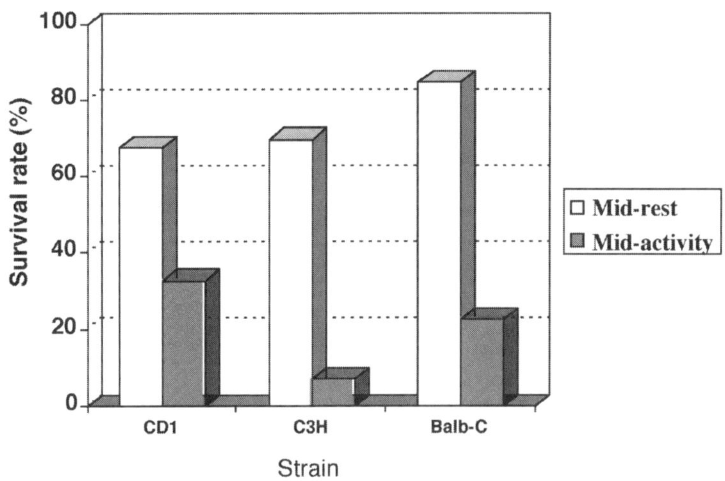

Fig. 4. Relevance of dosing time for the tolerability of 5-FU, as assessed with survival following a single administration of a toxic dose. Results from three independent studies, referred to the rest–activity circadian cycle. After Popovic et al. *(31)*, Burns et al. *(32)*, and Gonzalez et al. *(33)*.

3.3. Rhythm in 5-FU Efficacy

Subgroups of mice bearing the murine colon 38 or colon 26 carcinomas were treated with 5-FU once a week in the early rest span (at 2.30 HALO) or in the early activity span (12.30 HALO), respectively *(34)*. Treatment at 2.30 HALO was significantly most active against both tumors. Toxic effects (leukopenia) were observed only in the 12.30 HALO treatment group. Thus, a good correlation was observed between time of optimal effectiveness and that of least hematologic toxicity. These results were confirmed in a separate study using colon 26-bearing Balb/C mice *(35)*. In another study, 5-FU was given in the early rest or early activity span in nude mice bearing human squamous cell carcinoma xenograft *(37)*. Despite these xenografts, mice retained a circadian rhythm in rest–activity, and minimal differences in tumor growth inhibition were found between the two time points that were compared and that, respectively, corresponded to a high and to a low point in the proportion of tumor S-phase cell *(37)*. They emphasize that this parameter is not a *single* critical determinant for optimizing 5-FU anticancer activity through circadian timing.

3.4. Infusional Fluoropyrimidines and Circadian Rhythms

Prolonged infusion of 5-FU at a constant rate was performed in mice using 5-FU-containing pellets of various dosages that were implanted subcutaneously *(38)*. Plasma 5-FU concentration was measured at various circadian times on the tenth infusional day. A peak value was consistently found at 6 HALO, near the middle of the rest span, with nearly undetectable plasma levels at 12 HALO, despite continuous drug release. This prominent rhythm in the exposure of target tissues to 5-FU was associated with reduced hematological toxicity and greater antitumor activity against colon 26 and colon 38, as compared to bolus 5-FU injection *(38)*. Constant rate venous infusion of 5-FU was performed for 3 d in Yoshida sarcoma-bearing rats. The average plasma concentration of 5-FU nearly doubled between 16 HALO (trough) and 6 HALO (peak). 5-FU plasma level was highest at 6 HALO in each of the 10 rats that were studied *(39)*.

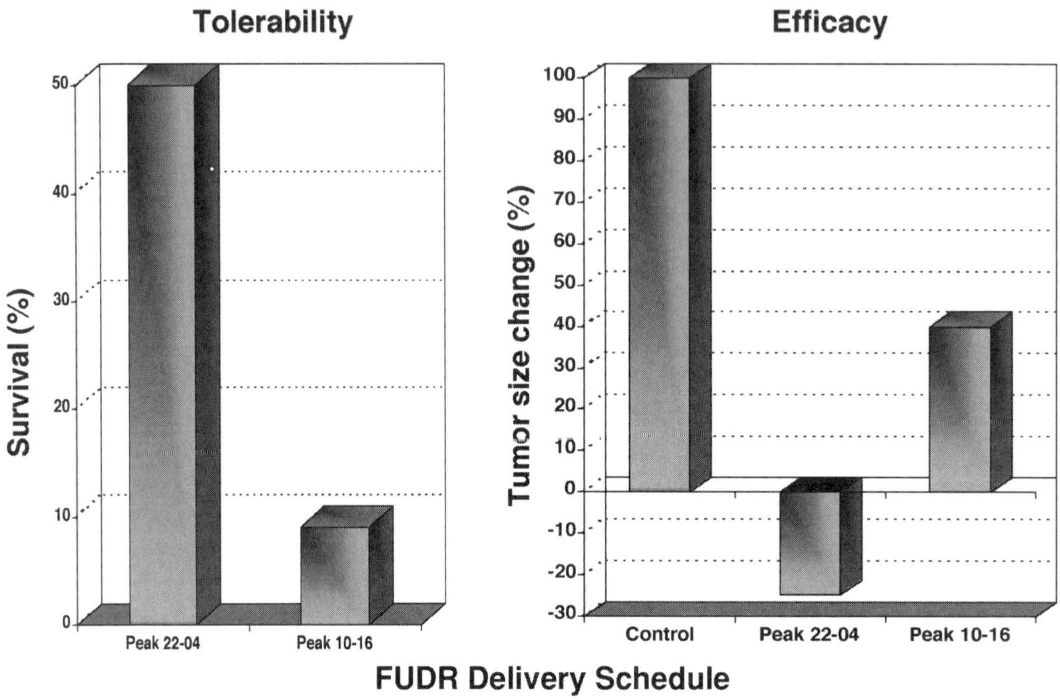

Fig. 5. Role of floxuridine (FUDR) scheduling upon tolerability and antitumor activity in rats. The drug was infused intravenously for 48 h to nontumor-bearing or to 13762 mammary carcinoma-bearing rats using one of several schedules. Left panel: Tolerability with best or worst schedule (1000 mg/kg), with peak delivery rate respectively set at 22 to 4 HALO and at 10 to 16 HALO. Right panel: Antitumor activity with same "best" and "worst" schedules (700 mg/kg); controls received saline infusion. After Roemeling et al. *(40)*.

The ability of chronomodulated fluoropyrimidine infusion to improve therapeutic index as compared to constant rate infusion was investigated using floxuridine (FUdR) in rats *(40)*. These animals received a 48-h infusion of this drug at a constant rate or according to one of four quasisinusoidal delivery patterns, with maximum delivery rate from 22 to 04 HALO or from 04 to 10 HALO or from 10 to 16 HALO or from 16 to 22 HALO.

While infusions at a constant rate or at a chronomodulated rate with a high rate at 22–04 HALO were equally well tolerated, the toxicity of the three other variable rate schedules was significantly worse. Furthermore, the antitumor activity of the five schedules was assessed in rats with transplanted mammary adenocarcinoma. The chronomodulated schedule with high FUdR delivery rate from 22 to 04 HALO was the only one to induce tumor shrinkage, while the other variable-rate schedules and the constant rate infusion only retarded tumor growth relative to controls.

Thus chronomodulated FUdR with maximum delivery rate from 22 to 04 HALO offered the best therapeutic index as compared to constant rate infusion or other variable rate infusion schedules (Fig. 5). This study also demonstrated that appropriate circadian chronomodulation rather than quasi-intermittency of FUdR administration was responsable for pharmacodynamic differences between infusional schedules *(40)*.

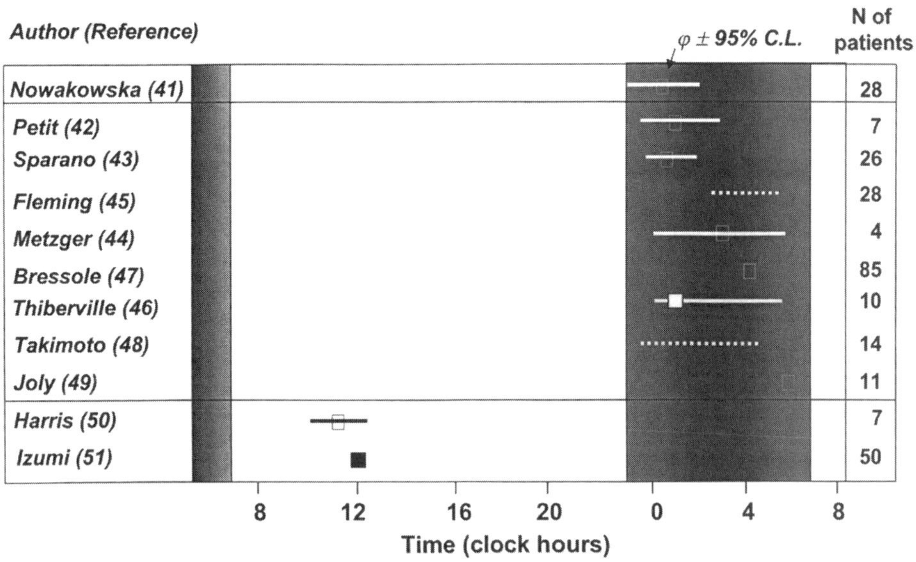

Fig. 6. Circadian changes in plasma 5-FU disposition in cancer patients related to day–night cycle in 10 separate studies (references in left panel). For each study, the time of maximum as estimated by the acrophase (filled circle) is shown with its 95% confidence limits, whenever they are reported. Otherwise, the time of reported average peak (filled square) or the range of individual peak times (dotted line) are shown. The time of lowest 5-FU clearance following bolus administration at different times is shown on the top lane. The times of maximum concentration of 5-FU are shown in the intermediate lane panel for 2–5 d constant rate infusions and in the lower lane for 14-d constant rate infusions.

4. CLINICAL CHRONOPHARMACOLOGY

4.1. Rhythm in 5-FU Pharmacokinetics

4.1.1. Bolus Injection

5-FU (15 mg/kg, e.g., approx 600 mg/m^2 was injected intravenously (bolus) at 01:00, 07:00, 13:00 or 19:00 h to 28 patients with metastatic gastrointestinal cancer in a randomized sequence, each injection being separated by 96 h from the next one. Both plasma pharmacokinetics and hematologic toxicity were assessed. 5-FU dosing at 01:00 h resulted in the longest half-life, in the largest VdSS and AUC, and in the lowest clearance (CI_B), as well as in the least depression of leukocyte count. All these differences were statistically validated and confirmed the predictions based upon the experimental model *(41)*.

4.1.2. Constant Rate Infusion

The lowest plasma clearance of 5-FU at night resulted in an accumulation of this drug between midnight and 6:00 h during continuous infusion at a constant rate. This finding has been reported in 8 of 10 studies, with various designs involving patients with bladder, gastrointestinal, lung, or head-and-neck cancer (Fig. 6) *(42–51)*. 5-FU was infused at a constant rate for durations ranging from 1 to 5 d as a single agent or combined with leucovorin and/or cisplatin, oxaliplatin, interferon-α, vinorelbine or *N*-(phosphonaletyl)-L-aspartate (PALA) *(42–49)*. In a study where a lower dose of 5-FU (300 mg/m^2/d) was continuously infused for 14 d, a significant circadian rhythm was also documented, yet the highest mean plasma level was found near 12:00 h and the lowest one near midnight *(50)*. A similar trend was found in a separate study in patients treated with this protracted continuous infusion schedule *(51)*. The main difference between both of these studies and the other eight was the daily dose level. Thus, all the 1–5 d schedules involved the administration of daily doses that were 1.5 to 3 times as high as those given in the 14-d schedule. As a result, the mean 24-h plasma levels ranged from 340 to 470 ng/mL in the 4- or 5-d schedules *(42,44)* as compared to 16 ng/mL in the 14-d schedule *(50)*, possibly as a result of the nonlinear pharmacokinetic disposition of the drug *(52)*.

The interpatient variability in 24-h mean level of 5-FU usually required to express each concentration relative to the 24-h mean in the same patient, in order to demonstrate synchronized circadian rhythmicity at a group level *(42,44,48)*. Furthermore, differences in individual circadian time structure, including the prominence of ultradian rhythms, with periods of one to several hours, could not be caught up by sampling times staggered every 4 h for 24 h, as was usually the case. Indeed, approx 30% of the patients with metastatic colorectal or breast cancer displayed a marked damping of their 24-h rhythms in rest–activity or cortisol *(53–55)*. These alterations might influence 5-FU disposition and ablate its rhythmicity especially in patients with extensive tumor burden or poor performance status *(49)*. Interestingly circadian function alteration predicted for poor outcome in advanced cancer patients independently of the known prognostic factors *(54–55)*, and exogenous glucocorticoids synchronized the circadian rhythm in 5-FU disposition *(49)*.

4.1.3. Chronomodulated Infusion

The patients on constant rate infusion who had a marked rhythm in 5-FU plasma concentration and a spontaneous peak near 4:00 displayed less toxicity than those who had not. This led us to chronomodulate the infusion rate of this drug and to assign peak delivery rate at 4:00 at night *(44)*. Circadian changes in 5-FU plasma levels matched rather well the sinusoidal delivery waveform over 3, 4, or 5 infusional days, irrespective of prior or concurrent administration of PALA, LV, or oxaliplatin *(44,48,56)*. Chronomodulated delivery of 5-FU and l-LV with respective peak flow rates at 4:00 h was associated with markedly reduced interpatient variability in the plasma levels of both 5-FU and l-LV as compared to constant rate infusions or to chronomodulated administrations with peak flow rates at 13:00 h or at 19:00 h (Fig. 7) *(57)*. These three latter schedules displayed increased toxicity as compared to the former one. Despite, the average time course of plasma 5-FU and l-LV concentrations closely matched chronomodulated delivery of 5-FU-LV with a peak at 04:00 h, this was not the case for plasma methyltetrahydrofolate (mTHF), a metabolite that reflects the intracellular active form of l-LV. The circadian maximum of mTHF was found approx 2 h after l-FA peak delivery *(58)*.

Chronomodulated 5-FU-LV was given near maximum tolerated dose to 22 patients with metastatic colorectal cancer (5-FU, 900 to 1100 mg/m^2/d × 4 d q 2 wk; dl-LV, 300 mg/m^2/d × 4 d). 5-FU plasma levels were measured every 2 h for 24 h on first and fourth infusional nights. The patients with altered 5-FU circadian disposition pattern displayed significantly worse toxicity and poorer antitumor activity, suggesting the need for specific chronotherapy schedules in the patients with disorganized circadian time structure *(56)*.

These pharmacokinetic studies ensured that an appropriate target rhythm in tissue exposure was produced by the chosen chronomodulated schedule for 5-FU for most patients. They suggest that some patients with altered circadian time structure could benefit from further optimization of the delivery patterns of 5-FU and LV.

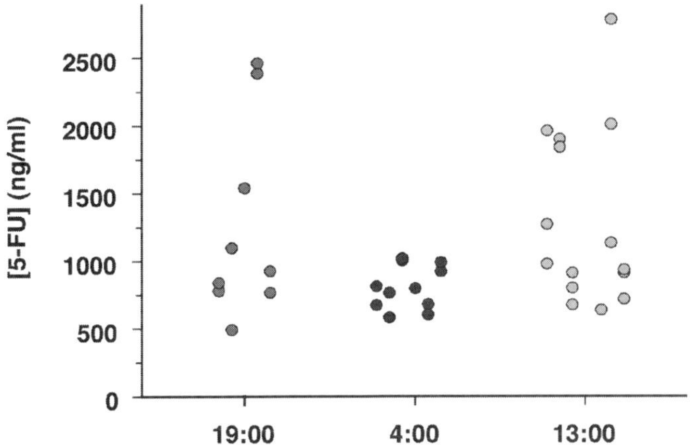

Fig. 7. Role of peak time of 5-FU chronomodulated delivery on (5-FU) C_{max} in patients with metastatic colorectal cancer. Eighteen patients received chronomodulated 5-FU/LV/1-OHP, with peak rate of 5-FU/LV infusion scheduled at 19:00, 4:00, or 13:00. Blood was sampled at time of peak delivery on first and fourth infusional day. Inter- and intra-patient variability were significantly least in the patients receiving chronomodulated 5-FU with peak delivery at 4:00 (after ref. *57*).

4.2. Rhythms in Cellular Determinants of Toxicity

The activity of DPD was measured every 4 h for 24 h in human mononuclear cells. Similar results were found in five healthy subjects *(59)* and in seven patients receiving continuous venous infusion of 5-FU at a constant rate *(50)*. In both studies, DPD varied two- to sixfold, with the highest activity occurring near 01:00 or 03:00 h at night. In 12 patients with colorectal cancer metastases, we also found a higher DPD activity in circulating mononuclear cells at midnight as compared to 10:00 h (Fig. 8) *(57)*. Quite interestingly, peak 5-FU concentration and peak DPD activity occurred 12 h apart, in the study where patients were receiving low dose 5-FU for 14 d *(50)*. This indeed suggested a prominent role for DPD rhythms as a mechanism in 5-FU rhythm. Nonetheless, DPD activity is saturable *(52)*, and other mechanisms also influence 5-FU disposition. Among these factors, liver blood flow, as estimated by indocyanine green plasma clearance, exhibited a 50% increase in the second half of the night and in the early morning in 10 healthy supine subjects. Lowest values were found at 13:00 h *(60)*. Quite strikingly, 5-FU clearance reportedly had a similar value as liver blood flow *(60)*. This suggests that the main mechanism of the circadian rhythm in 5-FU plasma levels is the rhythm in DPD activity when low doses of 5-FU are infused, whereas the rhythm in liver blood flow may be a more relevant mechanism when high daily doses of 5-FU are delivered.

The primary target organs of 5-FU toxicity also display large amplitude rhythms in healthy human subjects. Thus, an increased incidence of mitoses occurred at 01:00 h in the skin *(61)*, whereas a trough in DNA synthetic activity, as gaged by ex vivo ^{3}H-TdR incorporation or flow cytometric studies was found between 04:00 h and 09:00 h in this tissue *(62)*.

Mitotic activity in human bone marrow was higher at midnight. Peak DNA synthetic activity, as gaged by ex vivo ^{3}H-TdR synthesis or by cytometry-assessed proportion of S-phase cells occurred between 12:00 h and 18:00 h *(63–66)*.

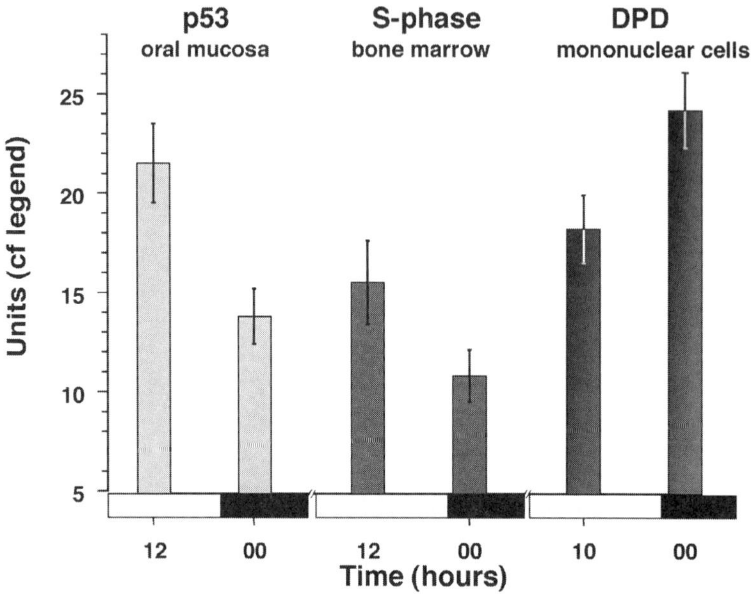

Fig. 8. Circadian changes in cellular functions relevant for 5-FU cytotoxicity in humans. P53 expression in oral mucosa of healthy human subjects (after ref. *70*), proportion of S-phase cells in the bone marrow of cancer patients (after ref. *66*) and DPD activity in circulating mononuclear cells of patients with colorectal cancer metastases (after ref. *57*).

DNA synthetic activity (ex vivo ^{3}H-TdR incorporation) was the highest near 08:00 h and remained elevated during daytime in the normal rectal mucosa of 16 normally fed or fasting healthy subjects *(67)*. Several enzymatic activities of the brush border of human jejunum also displayed prominent circadian rhythmicity *(68)*. This was also the case for several enzymatic activities in the superficial cells of the human oral mucosa *(69)*.

The circadian time structure of oral mucosa has recently been well documented with regard to both the expression of circadian genes *(per, clock, tim, bmall, cry)* and that of cell cycle-related proteins (cyclins, p53) and thymidilate synthase activity, a target enzyme for 5-FU cytotoxicity (Fig. 9) *(70–71)*.

Mitotic index and/or DNA synthesis have been used to evaluate the proliferative activity of many experimental and human breast, ovarian or lymphomatous tumors. Data suggest that well-differentiated, slow-growing tumors retain a circadian time structure, whereas poorly differentiated, fast-growing tumors tend to lose it *(72–75)*.

5. CLINICAL CHRONOTHERAPY WITH 5-FU BASED REGIMENS

5.1. Chronotherapy Tolerability and Efficacy (Phase I–II studies)

5.1.1. Hypotheses and Overall Strategy

A dose-response relationship characterized the antitumor efficacy of 5-FU against colorectal cancer *(76)*. The chronotherapy hypothesis has thus considered that high doses of this drug and proper circadian scheduling of drug delivery were needed to concurrently achieve maximum anticancer efficacy and good treatment tolerability and compliance. 5-FU has been the model drug to test these hypotheses, using sinusoidally-varying delivery schedules

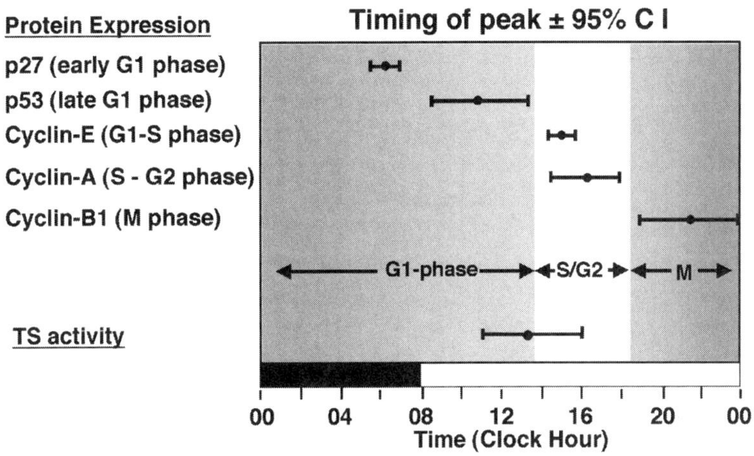

Fig. 9. Circadian time structure of human oral mucosa. The maxima in the expression of several cell cycle related proteins and TS activity are shown along the 24-h cycle, with their respective 95% confidence limits. After Bjarnason et al. *(70)*.

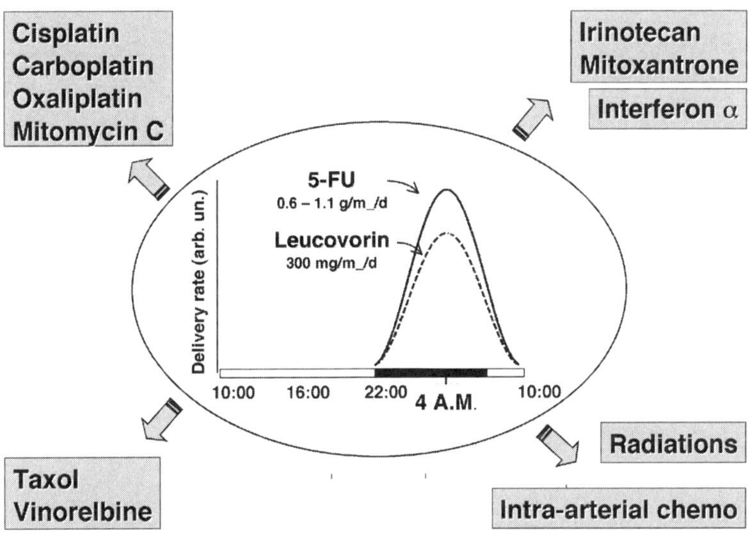

Fig. 10. Chronomodulated scheduling of 5-FU ± leucovorin, as automatically delivered with a programmable pump, without hospitalization. This schedule has been the basis for subsequent combination chronotherapy regimens involving chronomodulated or standard administrations of platinum complexes, antimitotic drugs or other agents, including radiation therapy.

(Fig. 10), based upon results from murine experiments and chronopharmacokinetic studies (see above).

The main results of phase I, II, and III clinical trials will be briefly reviewed in order to define the role of 5-FU-based chronotherapy in the medicosurgical management of patients with metastatic colorectal cancer. More limited data are available for breast and lung cancer chronotherapy.

5.1.2. Maximum Tolerated Dose and Antitumor Activity (Phase I–II) in Gastrointestinal Cancer

5.1.2.1. Chronomodulated 5-fluorouracil. The infusion rate of 5-FU alone was chronomodulated along the 24-h time scale for five consecutive days (every 3 wk), with peak delivery at 04:00 h and no infusion from 16:00 h to 22:00 h. Thirty-five patients with metastatic colorectal cancer participated to this Phase I–II trial with intrapatient dose escalation according to defined toxicity criteria. As a result of good tolerability (< 8% courses with severe—WHO grade 3—toxic symptoms), recommended dose could be escalated up to 1400 mg/m^2/d or more for 5 d in 80% of the assessable patients *(77)*. Similar results were found in a study involving 16 patients with advanced metastatic pancreatic cancer. The dose intensity of chronomodulated 5-FU was significantly correlated with progression-free survival *(78)*. This dose level represents a 40 to 100% increase in dose or dose intensity as compared to 5-d flat infusion, for which the recommended dose is 800–1000 mg/m^{2}d for 5 d every 3–4 wk.

5.1.2.2. Chronomodulated 5-FU/LV. In a Canadian study, 5-FU was infused for 14 d, with low-dose LV. Both drugs were delivered according to a quasisinusoidal 24-h rhythmic chronomodulated pattern with peak flow rate near 04:00 h at night. Maximum tolerated dose (MTD) was 250 mg/m^{2}d of 5-FU (3500 mg/m^2/course) with 20 mg/m^2/d of LV. The authors further suggested that peak delivery at early night (22:00 h) could improve tolerance in some patients *(79)*.

A phase I study established the MTD of the combination of 5-FU and l-LV given as a 5 d chronomodulated infusion every 3 wk to ambulatory patients with metastatic colorectal cancer. Thirty-four patients were included. Dose limiting toxicities were stomatitis and diarrhea. The recommended doses were 900 mg/m^2/d for 5-FU combined with 150 mg/m^2 for l-LV. Objective responses were achieved in 8 of 20 untreated patients and in 1 of 13 previously treated ones *(80)*.

The low toxicity profile and the apparently dose-related antitumor activity led us to further intensify this regimen. Both drugs were delivered near MTD as chronomodulated infusions for 4 d instead of 5 and every 2 wk rather than every 3 wk. The antitumor efficacy and tolerability of such intensified 5-FU-LV schedule was investigated in a multicenter European Phase II trial, which registered 100 patients with previously untreated metastatic colorectal cancer. While LV dose remains fixed (150 mg/m^2/d of l-LV or 300 mg/m^2/d of dl-LV), the 5-FU dose was escalated in the absence of grade 2 or greater toxicity from 900 mg/m^2/d at first course to 1000 mg/m^2/d at second course and 1100 mg/m^2/d at third course. The dose-limiting toxicity of this regimen was grade 3 hand–foot syndrome, which was encountered in 38% of the patients (8% of the courses). The median 5-FU dose intensity was 1800 mg/m^2/wk and the objective response rate, as assessed from computed tomography scans reviewed by an independent panel, was 41% (95% C.L., 31.5 to 50.5). Median survival was 17 mo, with 18.6% of the patients alive at 3 yr *(81)*. A 45% objective response rate was obtained by two Canadian teams using this same schedule *(82)*.

The good tolerability of chronomodulated 5-FU ± LV has allowed its combination with other drugs, eventually given as chronomodulated infusions, or with radiation therapy (Fig. 10).

5.1.2.3. Chronomodulated 5-Fluorouracil, Leucovorin, and Oxaliplatin Combination. Since chronomodulated oxaliplatin (l-OHP) was shown to be better tolerated than constant rate infusion *(83)*, this schedule was combined with chronomodulated 5-FU/LV. A phase II study of a 5-d schedule of chronomodulated chemotherapy with 5 FU, LV, and l-OHP (chronoFFL) was performed in 93 patients with unresectable colorectal metastases. Forty-six of these patients had received previous chemotherapy. Courses were repeated every

21 d. A 58% objective response rate was obtained. Moreover, all treatments were administered on an outpatient basis and less than 10% of the 784 courses given were associated with severe toxicity. Median overall survival was 16 mo irrespective of prior chemotherapy, with a 17% survival rate at 3 yr in chemotherapy-naive patients. We related the high antitumor efficacy of chronoFFL both to l-OHP and to chronomodulation, which allowed safe delivery of high drug doses *(84)*.

The role of l-OHP addition to chronomodulated 5-FU/LV was investigated in a multicenter, open randomized phase II–III study *(85)*. Two hundred patients from 15 centers with previously untreated measurable metastases from colorectal cancer were randomly assigned to receive chronomodulated 5-FU and LV (700 and 300 mg/m^2/d, respectively; peak delivery rate at 04:00) with or without l-OHP. Oxaliplatin (125 mg/m^2) was given as a 6-h flat infusion from 10:00 h to 16:00 h on the first day of each course every 3 wk. This infusion schedule was devised to remain close to the least toxic time of l-OHP. Response, the main judgment criteria was assessed with extramural review of computed tomography scans. Severe gastrointestinal toxicity (grade 3–4) occurred in 5% of the patients given chronomodulated 5-FU/LV as compared to 43% of those receiving additional l-OHP. An objective response was obtained in 16% of the patients on 5-FU/LV (CI: 9–24%) as compared to 53% of those receiving additional l-OHP (CI: 42–63%) ($p < 0.001$). Median progression-free survival time was 6.1 mo with 5-FU/LV (4.1 to 7.4) and 8.7 mo (7.4 to 9.2) with l-OHP and 5-FU/LV ($p = 0.048$). Median survival times were similar in both treatment groups (19.9 vs 19.4 mo respectively). A possible explanation was that 57% of the patients from the 5-FU/LV arm received second line therapy with the three-drug regimen, which was mostly given as an intensified chronomodulated schedule. Thus l-OHP added significant activity to chronomodulated 5-FU/LV as first line chemotherapy for metastatic colorectal cancer *(85)*.

5.1.2.4. Chronomodulated 5-Fluorouracil, Leucovorin, and Carboplatin Combination. Oxaliplatin was replaced by carboplatin in a single institution Phase II study of chronomodulated 5-FU, LV, and carboplatin. The trial accrued 60 patients with metastatic colorectal cancer, 50% of whom had failed up to three chemotherapy regimens. The chronomodulated delivery pattern of carboplatin (40 mg/m^2/d) was similar to that of oxaliplatin, based on the similar toxicity rhythms of both compounds in the experimental model. The daily doses of 5-FU and LV were 700 and 300 mg/m^2/d, respectively. Courses lasted 4 d and were repeated every 2 wk. Grade 3–4 granulocytopenia was encountered in 29% of the patients and was the main dose-limiting toxicity. An objective response was achieved in 47% of the patients, being 69% in 13 chemotherapy-naive patients. The median survival of the 60 patients was 14.6 mo *(86)*. The good therapeutic index of this regimen warrants further evaluation.

5.1.2.5. Chronomodulated 5-Fluorouracil, Leucovorin Combined with Irinotecan. A Phase I study was undertaken in order to define the tolerability of CPT11 (d 1) with 5-d chronomodulated 5-FU/LV infusion. Twenty-six patients with previously treated metastatic colorectal cancer were registered in this study. The recommended dose was 325 mg/m^2 as a 30 min infusion on d 1 for CPT11, 700 mg/m^2/d × 5 d for 5-FU and 150 mg/m^2/d > 5d for l-LV. An objective response was achieved in 23% of the patients. Quality of life, as assessed with the EORTC QLQ-C30+3 questionnaire, remained stable during the entire course of treatment.

The study demonstrated that the combination of CPT11 with chronomodulated 5-FU/LV did not require any reduction in CPT11 dose intensity as compared with single-agent CPT11 *(87)*. Ongoing studies currently assess the relevance of chronomodulated CPT11/5-FU/LV with or without oxaliplatin *(88,89)*.

5.1.2.6. Chronomodulated 5-FU with Concurrent Radiation Therapy. The maximum tolerated dose of a chronomodulated infusion of 5-FU combined with concurrent radiation

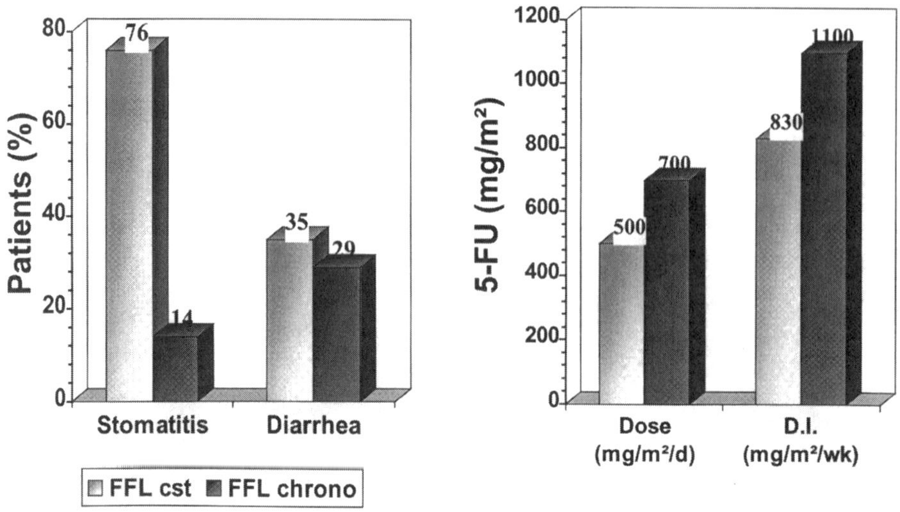

Fig. 11. Relevance of 5-FU/leucovorin/oxaliplatin infusional schedule for mucosal and intestinal tolerability (left panel) and for actually delivered 5-FU dose and dose intensity (left panel) in 186 patients with metastatic colorectal cancer. Constant rate infusion of the three drugs (FFL cst) was compared to chronomodulated infusion FFL chrono, peak delivery at 4:00 for 5-FU-LV and at 16:00 for I-OHP (After 93).

therapy for 5 wk was investigated in 18 patients with primary locally advanced or unoperable rectal cancer *(90)*. All the patients completed the whole treatment course and were subsequently resectable, so that the activity of the regimen was fully assessable. The MTD of 5-FU was 275 mg/m^2/d. Seven patients had a sphincter-sparing procedure and 10 had an abdominoperineal resection. Five complete pathologic resections were obtained (28%). The authors recommended a further evaluation of combined chronomodulated infusion of 5-FU and radiation therapy as a neoadjuvant treatment of rectal cancer. The feasibility of combining chronotherapy and radiotherapy has been independently confirmed *(91)*. An international trial testing the clinical relevance of this approach is being activated in biliary cancer (EORTC 05991) and is being discussed for rectal cancer.

5.2. Chronotherapy for Metastatic Colorectal Cancer

5.2.1. Role of Chronomodulated Delivery

Two consecutive European multicenter Phase III studies compared flat vs chronomodulated infusion of the same three-drug combination (5-FU/LV/l-OHP) in patients with previously untreated metastatic colorectal cancer.

A first randomized trial was undertaken in 92 patients. Grade 3 or 4 stomatitis, the main toxicity, was fivefold higher with constant rate infusion as compared to chronotherapy (89% vs 18%). Chronotherapy allowed a 22% increase in 5-FU dose intensity as compared to flat infusion. Response rate, the main judgment criterion, was significantly increased from 32% with flat infusion up to 53% with chronotherapy. Median progression-free survival and survival of all patients were 8 and 14.9 mo in the flat arm, and 11 and 19 mo in the chronotherapy schedule *(92)*.

A second multicenter trial registered 186 patients. Severe stomatitis was incurred by 76% on the flat infusion regimen as compared to 14% of those on chronotherapy, despite the 5-FU dose intensity was significantly larger in the chronotherapy schedule (Fig. 11). Cumulative peripheral sensory neuropathy with functional impairment was reported in 31% patients on constant delivery and in 16% patients on chronotherapy. This latter schedule allowed the administration of a higher dose of 5-FU (700 mg/m^2/d) than flat infusion (500 mg/m^2/d) and a 22% larger dose intensity. Objective response rate was 51% on chronotherapy and 29% on constant rate delivery. Median survival was 16 mo in both modalities, possibly because 24% of the patients crossed over from the flat schedule to chronotherapy. In these European multicenter randomized trials, the chronomodulated schedule was both the most active one and the least toxic one *(93)*.

5.2.2. Relation between Dose Intensity, Response Rate, Survival

The results from both of these latter studies led us to further densify and intensify the chronotherapy schedule. This involved its administration for 4 d every 2 wk (10 d interval) rather than for 5 d every 3 wk (16 d interval).

An intrapatient 5-FU dose escalation scheme was performed in 50 patients with metastatic colorectal cancer (37 previously treated and 13 chemotherapy naive). Courses were repeated every 14 d, 5-FU being escalated by 100 mg/m^2/d in each patient when toxicity was < grade 2. Median 5-FU and 1-OHP dose intensities were increased by 32% and 18%, respectively, as compared to the previous 5-d on–16-d off Phase II protocol. Objective response rate was 40% (95% C.L., 24% to 57%) in previously treated patients and 69% (48% to 90%) in chemotherapy-naive ones. Median progression-free survival was 9.3 mo (95% C.L.: 6.6 to 11.2) Median survival was 16.9 mo in previously treated patients and 20.7 mo in chemotherapy-naive patients *(94)*. This highly effective fully ambulatory outpatient regimen was subsequently confirmed in a multicenter European Phase II trial involving 90 patients. The main acute toxicities were WHO grade 3 or 4 diarrhea (41% of patients, 8.2% of courses), stomatitis (30% of patients, 5.1% of courses). The overall objective response rate was 66% (56% to 76%). The median progression-free survival and survival durations were 8.4 mo (5.9 to 10) and 18.5 mo (13.2 to 23.8) *(95)*.

Figure 12 summarizes the relationship between 5-FU dose intensity, treatment schedule, and objective response rate in those multicenter trials which involved chemotherapy-naive patients.

5.2.3. New medico-surgical strategy with curative intent

The achievement of a 50% or greater objective response rate with the three-drug chronomodulated regimen, allowed for a surgical resection of metastases in a substantial proportion of patients *(96)*. We examined the outcome of patients with initially unresectable colorectal metastases who underwent infusional chemotherapy with 5-FU, LV, and 1-OHP, followed by surgery at Paul Brousse hospital *(97)*. The cohort involves 389 patients with a median follow-up of 5.5 yr and a minimum follow-up of 3.5 yr. Out of 389 patients, 151 had unresectable liver-only metastases and have been analyzed. Seventy-seven patients (51%) underwent liver surgery with curative intent, 58 patients had a complete resection. A complete histologic response was documented in four patients. Median overall survival of the 151 patients with liver-only disease was 24 mo (19–28 mo) with 28% surviving at 5 yr (95% CI: 20 to 35). The 77 operated patients had a median overall survival of 48 mo (95% CI: 25 to 71). The estimated 5-yr survival rates of the operated patients was 50% (38 to 61). Median overall survival of the 58 patients in complete resection has not been reached. For comparison, the median overall survival of the 74 nonoperated patients was 15.5 mo (95% CI: 13.5 to 17.5) *(97)*. Surgery-related morbidity was < 10% and was comparable to that observed in patients with primary hepatic resection *(96–97)*.

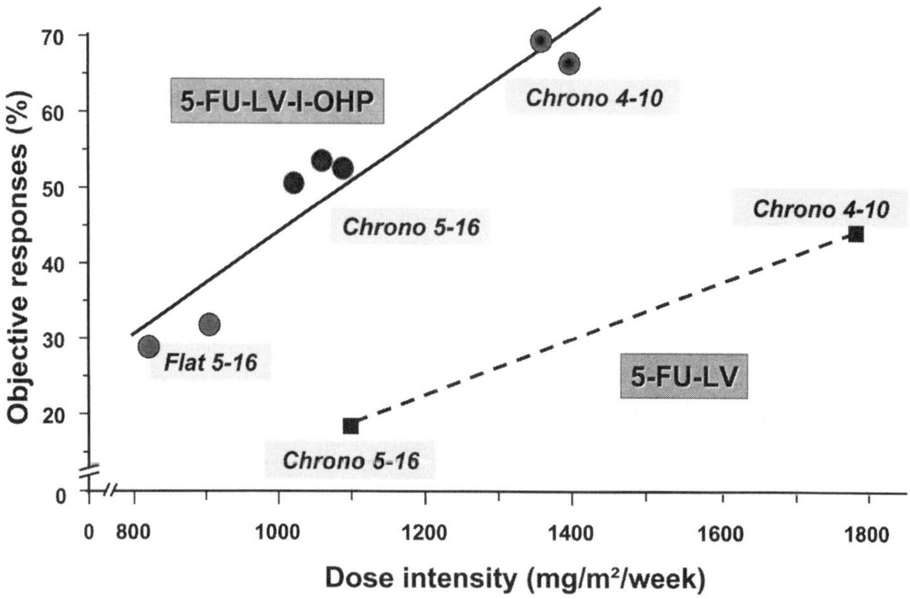

Fig. 12. Role of 5-FU dose intensity, constant rate (flat) or chronomodulated delivery schedule (chrono) and oxaliplatin (I-OHP) upon objective response rate in patients with metastatic colorectal cancer. Results from first line chemotherapy in multicenter European trials involving a total of 682 patients (After 81, 85, 87, 92–95). "5–16" and "4–10", respectively, mean that the chemotherapy infusion was given for 5 d on, 16 d off or for 4 d on, 10 d off.

Thus, combining effective and safe chemotherapy and surgery altered the natural history of unresectable colorectal cancer metastases. This study further emphasized the need for an active collaboration between surgeons and oncologists.

Figure 13 summarizes the relationship between the objective response rate produced by infusional 5-FU/LV/1-OHP and the rate of patients who could subsequently undergo a complete surgical resection of metastases within the multicenter setting of our group.

6. PERSPECTIVES AND CONCLUSIONS

Circadian rhythms in normal cell function and proliferation account for predictable changes in 5-FU tolerability and efficacy. The extrapolation of the least toxic time from mice to human beings has been validated in patients with metastatic colorectal cancer in Phase III clinical trials. The application of the chronotherapy concept has improved tolerability and activity of 5-FU-based combination involving new drugs such as oxaliplatin or irinotecan or radiation therapy. 5-FU-based chronotherapy has further given rise to a new medicosurgical strategy with curative potential in patients with metastatic colorectal cancer. Thus, the median survival of patients with colorectal cancer metastases receiving chronotherapy has consistently ranged from 16 to 21 mo, i.e., the longest figures reported for this disease in multicenter trials.

Most patients who participated to the control arm of chronotherapy trials did receive chronotherapy along the course of their disease however, once the main endpoint, i.e., tumor response, had been reached. This illustrates that the selection of survival as the main endpoint may be unrealistic for metastatic disease, because these patients can hardly be denied the benefit of proven active therapeutic modalities. Nevertheless, ongoing multicenter trials

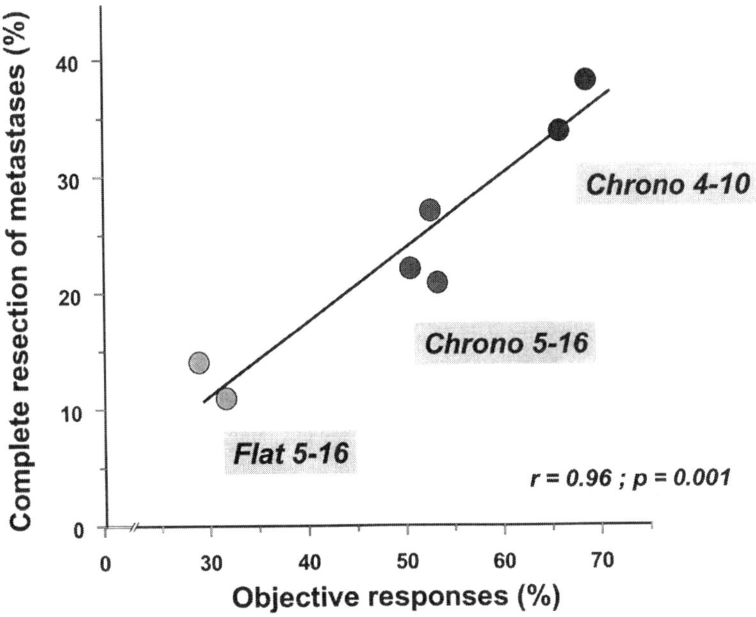

Fig. 13. Relation between objective response rate, delivery schedule and rate of patients with macroscopic complete surgical resection of metastases following chemotherapy. Data from multicenter European trials involving the administration of 5-FU/LV and I-OHP as first line chemotherapy for metastatic colorectal cancer (After 85, 92–95).

by the Chronotherapy Group of the European Organization for Research and Treatment of Cancer (EORTC) currently investigate the relevance of chronotherapy for prolonging the survival of patients with colorectal or pancreatic cancer (EORTC 05962 and 05963). Meta-analyses will possibly be required to demonstrate survival differences between chronotherapy and conventional treatment schedules in patients with metastatic disease, as survival was only weakly correlated with response rate in this setting *(98)*. Taken together, the findings warrant investigations of chronotherapy for prolonging survival in adjuvant situations. This possibility is supported by the fact that survival was largely improved with evening rather than morning administration of maintenance chemotherapy in children with acute lymphoblastic leukemia *(99,100)*.

The role of this treatment concept for improving the tolerability of other chemotherapeutic drugs combined with chronomodulated 5-FU is being further explored in breast cancer with taxol *(101)* or vinorelbine (EORTC 05971 trial), in lung cancer with cisplatin and vinorelbine, in pancreatic cancer with cisplatin (EORTC 05962 trial), and in colorectal cancer with irinotecan (EORTC 05011 trial). Infusional chronochemo-radiation also undergoes clinical Phase II evaluation in patients with primary biliary cancer (EORTC 05991 trial).

The results obtained in colorectal cancer further warrant the assessment of 5-FU-based chronochemotherapy in patients with breast, lung, or other gastrointestinal malignancies and in adjuvant situations. Yet circadian rhythms also modulate cell cycle proteins, growth factors, coagulation factors, immune functions, and the expression of many genes. Combination of 5-FU-based chronotherapy with chronomodulated delivery of cytokines, regulators of cell growth or angiogenesis or COX-2 inhibitors may improve therapeutic index in several malignancies. Finally, the circadian rhythms in fluoropyrimidine metabolism together with those which modulate drug absorption warrant to test the role of circadian timing for oral fluoropyrimidines and their inhibitors. Indeed several pharmacokinetic parameters are markedly dependent upon the circadian time of ingestion *(102)*. Circadian timing may well become a simple measure for decreasing toxicity and improving compliance for these oral compounds.

Thus, circadian scheduling of 5-FU is based upon extensive preclinical and clinical data and provides better tolerability, higher dose intensity, and greater antitumor activity as compared to constant rate infusion regimens. The principle likely also applies to other fluoropyrimidines, irrespective of their route of administration.

REFERENCES

1. Dunlap JC. Molecular bases for circadian clocks. *Cell* 1999;96(2):271–290.
2. Shearman LP, Sriram S, Weaver DR, et al. Interacting molecular loops in the mammalian circadian clock. *Science* 2000;288:1013–1019.
3. Cermakian N, Sassone-Corsi P. Multilevel regulation of the circadian clock. *Nature Rev Mol Cell Biol* 2000;1:59–67.
4. Lowrey PL, Takahashi JS. Genetics of the mammalian circadian system:photic entrainment, circadian pacemaker mechanisms and posttranslational regulation. *Ann Rev Genetics* 2000;34:533–562.
5. Klein DC, Moore RY, Reppert SM. *Suprachiasmatic Nucleus, the Mind's Clock.* Oxford University Press, Oxford, 1991;p.467.
6. Moore RY. Entrainment pathways and the functional organization of the circadian system. *Prog Brain Res* 1996;111:103–119.
7. Cassone VM. Melatonin's role in vertebrate circadian rhythms. *Chronobiol Int* 1998;15:457–473.
8. Hrushesky WJM, Bjarnason GA. Circadian cancer therapy. *J Clin Oncol* 1993;11:1403–1417.
9. Focan C. Circadian rhythms and cancer chemotherapy. *Pharmacol Ther* 1995;67:1–52.
10. Lévi F. Chronopharmacology of anticancer agents. In: *Handbook of Experimental Pharmacology.* Vol.: Physiology and Pharmacology of Biological Rhythms. (P.H. Redfern and B. Lemmer, eds.) Springer-Verlag, Berlin, pp. 299–331, 1997.
11. Lévi F. Circadian Chronotherapy for human cancers. *Lancet Oncology* 2001;2:307–315.
12. Naguib FNM, Soong SJ, El Kouni MH. Circadian rhythm of orotate phosphoribosyltransferase, pyrimidine nucleoside phosphorylases and dihydrouracil dehydrogenase in mouse liver. *Biochem Pharmacol* 1993;45:667–673.
13. Zhang R, Lu Z, Liu T, Soong SJ, Diasio RB. Relationship between circadian-dependent toxicity of 5-fluorodeoxyuridine and circadian rhythms of pyrimidine enzymes: possible relevance to fluoropyrimidine chemotherapy. *Cancer Res* 1993;53:2816–2822.
14. Porsin B, Formento JL, Filipski E, et al. Dihydropyrimidine dehydrogenase circadian rhythm in both enzyme activity and gene expression from mouse liver. Submitted.
15. El Kouni MH, Naguib FNM, Park KS, Cha S, Darnowski JW, Soong SJ. Circadian rhythm of hepatic uridine phosphorylase activity and plasma concentration of uridine in mice. *Biochem Pharmacol* 1990;40:2479–2485.
16. Daher G, Zhang R, Soon SJ, Diasio R. Circadian variation of fluoropyrimidine catabolic enzymes in rat liver: possible relevance to 5-fluorodeoxyuridine chemotherapy. *Drug Metab Disp* 1991;19:285–287.
17. Malmary-Nebot M, Labat C, Casanovas AM, Oustrin J. Aspect chronobiologique de I'action du methotréxate sur la dihydrofolate réductase. *Ann Pharm Fr* 1985;43:337–343.
18. Lincoln DW. 2nd, Hrushesky WJ, Wood PA. Circadian organization of thymidylate synthase activity in normal tissues: a possible basis for 5-fluorouracil chronotherapeutic advantage. *Int J Cancer* 2000;88:479–485.
19. Labrecque G, Bélanger PM, Doré F, et al. 24-hour variations in the distribution of labeled microspheres to the intestine, liver and kidneys. *Ann Rev Chronopharmacol* 1989;5:445–448.
20. Scheving LE, Burns ER, Pauly JE, et al. Circadian variation in cell division of the mouse alimentary tract, bone marrow and corneal epithelium. *Anat Rec* 1978;191:479–486.
21. Haus E, Lakatua D, Sackett-Lundeen L, White M. Circannual variation of intestinal cell proliferation in BDF1 male mice on three lighting regimens. *Chronobiol Intern* 1984;1:185–194.
22. Kennedy M, Tutton P, Barkla D. Comparison of the circadian variation in cell proliferation in normal and neoplastic colonic epithelial cells. *Cancer* 1985;28:169–175.
23. Waldrop R, Saydjari R, Rubin N, Rayford P, Townsend C Jr, Thompson J. DNA synthetic activity in tumor bearing mice. *Chronobiol Intern* 1989;6:237–243.
24. Scheving LA. Biological clocks and the digestive system. *Gastroenterology* 2000;119:536–549.

25. Stoney P, Halberg F, Simpson H. Circadian variation of colony-forming ability of presumably intact murine bone marrow cells. *Chronobiologia* 1975;2:319–327.
26. Perpoint B, Le Bousse-Kerdiles C, Clay D, Smadja-Joffe F, Deprés-Brummer P, Jasmin C, Lévi F. In vitro chronopharmacology of recombinant mouse IL-3, mouse GM-CSF and human G-CSF on murine myeloid progenitor cells. *Exp Hematol* 1995;23:362–368.
27. Laerum OD. Hematopoiesis occurs in rhythms. *Exp Hematol* 1995;23:1145–1147.
28. Li XM, Ezan E, Bindoula G, et al. Chronopharmacologic aspects of continuous AcSDKP infusion in mice. *Exp Hematol* 1999;27:19–27.
29. Tampellini M, Filipski E, Liu X-H, et al. Docetaxel chronopharmacology in mice. *Cancer Res* 1998;58:3896–3904.
30. Ohdo S, Makinosumi T, Ishizaki T, et al. Cell cycle-dependent chronotoxicity of irinotecan hydrochloride in mice. *J Pharmacol Exp Ther* 1997;283:1383–1388.
31. Popovic P, Popovic V, Baughman J. Circadian rhythm and 5-fluorouracil toxicity in C3H mice. *Biomed Thermol* (Gautherie M. and~ Albert E, (eds), Alan Liss, New York (U.S.A.), 1982;25:185–187.
32. Burns ER, Beland SS. Effect of biological time on the determination of the LD50 of 5-fluorouracil in mice. *Pharmacology* 1984;28:296–300.
33. Gonzalez RB, Sothern RB, Thatcher G, et al. Substantial difference in timing of murine circadian susceptibility to 5-fluorouracil and FUdR. *Proc Am Ass Cancer Res* 1989;30:A2452 (abstr.).
34. Peters GJ, Van Dijk J, Nadal JC, Van Groeningen CS, Lankelma J, Pinedo HM. Diurnal variation in the therapeutic efficacy of 5-fluorouracil against murine colon cancer. *In Vivo* 1987;1:113–118.
35. Kojima H, Sakamoto J, Yasue M. Circadian-rhythm modulated chemotherapy with high dose 5-fluorouracil against gastrointestinal cancers: evaluation and case report. *Nagoya J Med Sci* 1999;62:29–38.
36. Gardner ML, Plumb JA. Diurnal variation in the intestinal toxicity of 5-fluorouracil in the rat. *Clin Sci* 1981;61(6):717–722.
37. Rydell R, Wennerberg J, Willen R. Circadian variations in cell cycle phase distribution in a squamous cell-carcinoma xenograft; effects of cisplatin and fluorouracil treatment. *In Vivo* 1990;4(6):385–389.
38. Codacci-Pisanelli G, van der Wilt CL, Pinedo HM, et al. Antitumor activity, toxicity and inhibition of thymidylate synthase of prolonged administration of 5-fluorouracil in mice. *Eur J Cancer* 1995;31A(9):1517–1525.
39. Fujii S, Shimamoto Y, Ohshimo H, et al. Effects of the plasma concentration of 5-fluorouracil and the duration of continuous venous infusion of 5-fluorouracil with an inhibitor of 5-fluorouracil degradation on Yoshida sarcomas in rats. *Jpn J Cancer Res* 1989;80:167–172.
40. von Roemeling R, Hrushesky WJM. Determination of the therapeutic index of floxuridine by its circadian infusion pattern. *J Natl Cancer Inst* 1990;82:386–393.
41. Nowakowska-Dulawa E. Circadian rhythm in 5-fluorouracil (FU) pharmacokinetics and tolerance. *Chronobiologia* 1990;17:27–35.
42. Petit E, Milano G, Levi F, Thyss A, Bailleul F, Schneider M. Circadian varying plasma concentration of 5-FU during 5-day continuous venous infusion at constant rate in cancer patients. *Cancer Res* 1988;48:1676–1679.
43. Sparano JA, Wadler S, Diasio RB, et al. Phase I trial of low-dose, prolonged continuous infusion fluorouracil plus interferon-alfa: evidence for enhanced fluorouracil toxicity without pharmacokinetic perturbation. *J Clin Oncol* 1993;11(8):1609–1617.
44. Metzger G, Massari C, Etienne MC, et al. Spontaneous or imposed circadian changes in plasma concentrations of 5-fluorouracil coadministered with folinic acid and oxaliplatin: relationship with mucosal toxicity in cancer patients. *Clin Pharm Ther* 1994;56:190–201.
45. Fleming GF, Schilsky RL, Mick R, et al. Circadian variation of 5-fluorouracil (5-FU) and cortisol plasma levels during continuous-infusion 5-FU and leucovorin (LV) in patients with hepatic or renal dysfunction. *Proc Amer Soc Clin Oncol* 1994;13:abstr. 352.
46. Thiberville L, Compagnon C, Moore N, et al. Plasma 5-fluorouracil and alpha-fluorobeta-alanin accumulation in lung cancer patients treated with continuous infusion of cisplatin and 5-fluorouracil. *Cancer Chemother Pharmacol* 1994;35:64–70.
47. Bressolle F, Joulia JM, Pinguet F, et al. Circadian rhythm of 5-fluorouracil population pharmacokinetics in patients with metastatic colorectal cancer. *Cancer Chemother Pharmacol* 1999;44:295–302.
48. Takimoto CH, Yee LK, Venzon DJ, et al. High inter- and intrapatient variation in 5-fluorouracil plasma concentrations during a prolonged drug infusion. *Clin Cancer Res* 1999;5(6):1347–1352.
49. Joly AC. Perfusion continue de 5-FU et cancers bronchiques non à petites cellules: rythmes circadien et influence d'une corticothérapie. *Thèse* de DES (Diplôme d'Etudes Spécialisées) de Pharmacie Spécialisée, Octobre 1998, Université Paris XI, Faculté de Chatenay-Malabry.

50. Harris B, Song R, Soong S, et al. Relationship between dihydropyrimidine dehydrogenase activity and plasma 5-fluorouracil levels: evidence for circadian variation of plasma drug levels in cancer patients receiving 5-fluorouracil by protracted continuous infusion. *Cancer Res* 1990;50:197–201.
51. Izumi M, Ohwada S, Morishita Y. Evaluation of intravenous infusion with 5-fluorouracil for advanced or recurrent gastric or colorectal cancer. *J Jpn Soc Cancer Ther* 1995;30:24–29.
52. Diasio RB, Harris BE. Clinical pharmacology of 5-fluorouracil. *Clin Pharmacokinet* 1989;16:215–237.
53. Touitou Y, Bogdan A, Lévi F, Benavides M, Auzéby A. Disruption of the circadian patterns of serum cortisol in breast and ovarian cancer patients. Relationships with tumor marker antigens. *Brit J Cancer* 1996;74:1248–1252.
54. Mormont MC, Waterhouse J, Bleuzen P, et al. Marked 24-h rest-activity rhythms are associated with better quality of life, better response and longer survival in patients with metastatic colorectal cancer and good performance status. *Clin Cancer Res* 2000;6:3038–3045.
55. Sephton SE, Sapolsky RM, Kraemer HC, Spiegel D. Diurnal cortisol rhythm as a predictor of breast cancer survival. *J Natl Cancer Inst* 2000;92:994–1000.
56. Kwaitkowski F, Chevrier R, De Renzis JP, et al. Chronopharmacocinétique du 5-FU dans le traitement du cancer colorectal métastatique et indicateurs de réponse métabolique. *J Pharm Clin* 1999;18:138–143.
57. Langouët AM, Metzger G, Comisso M, et al. Plasma drug concentration control through time-programmed administration. *Proc 87th meeting Am Ass Cancer Res* Washington DC, U.S.A., March 20–24 1996, vol. 37, abstr. 1253.
58. Assier I, Léger-Enreille A, Kwiatowski F, et al. Relationship of dose-limiting toxicity (DLT) with plasma 5-fluorouracil (5-FU) accumulation in high-dose chronomodulated (CM) infusion of 5-FU and L-folinic acid (L-FA). *Proc 33rd Annual Meeting Am Soc Clin Oncol* May 17–20, 1997, Denver, CO, U.S.A., abstr. # 808.
59. Tuchman M, Roemeling Rv, Lanning RM, Sothern RB, Hrushesky WJM. Sources of variability of dihydropyrimidine dehydrogenase activity in human blood mononuclear cells. *Ann Rev Chronopharmacol* 1989;5:399–402.
60. Lemmer B, Nold G. Circadian changes in estimated hepatic blood flow in healthy subjects. *Brit J Clin Pharm* 1991;32:627–629.
61. Scheving LE, Burns ER, Pauly JE, et al. Circadian variation in cell division of the mouse alimentary tract, bone marrow and corneal epithelium. *Anat Rec* 1978;191:479–486.
62. Brown WR. A review and mathematical analysis of circadian rhythms in cell proliferation in mouse, rat and human epidermis. *J Invest Dermatol* 1991;97(2):273–280.
63. Killman SA, Cronkite ZEP, Fliedner TM, et al. Mitotic indices of human bone marrow cells. 1. Number and cytologic distribution of mitoses. *Blood* 1962;19:743–750.
64. Mauer AM. Diurnal variation of proliferative activity in the human bone marrow. *Blood* 1965;26:1–7.
65. Smaaland R, Laerum OD, Lote K, Sletvold O, Sothern RB, Bjerknes R. DNA synthesis in human bonne marrow is circadian stage dependent. *Blood* 1991;77:2603–2611.
66. Smaaland R, Abrahamsen JF, Svardal AM, Lote K, Ueland PM. DNA cell cycle distribution and glutathione (GSH) content according to circadian stage in bone marrow of cancer patients. *Brit J Cancer* 1992;66:39–45.
67. Buchi KN, Moore JG, Hrushesky WJM, Sothern RB, Rubin NH. Circadian rhythm of cellular proliferation in the human rectal mucosa. *Gastroenterology* 1991;101:410–415.
68. Markiewick A, Lelek A, Panz B, et al. Chronomorphology of jejunum in man. Proc. XVIII Intern. Conf. on Chronobiol, (Leiden, July 12–17th, 1987), *Chronobiologia* 1987;14:abstra. 131.
69. Rietweld W, Boon M. Variation in size and glycogen content of exfoliating epithelial cells at different times of day. In *Chronobiology*, 1982–1983, H. Kabat ed, S. Karger (Basel), 22–24.
70. Bjarnason GA, Jordan RCK, Sothern RB. Circadian variation in the expression of cell-cycle proteins in human oral epithelium. *Am J Pathol* 1999;154(2):613–622.
71. Bjarnason GA, Jordan RCK, Wood PA, et al. Circadian expression of clock genes in human oral epithelium and skin: association with cell cycle progression. *Am J Pathol* 2001;158:1793–1801.
72. Garcia-Sainz M, Halberg F. Mitotic rhythms in human cancer reevaluated by electronic computer programs. Evidence for chronopathology. *J Natl Cancer Inst* 1966;37:279–292.
73. Klevecz R, Shymko R, Braly P. Circadian gating of S phase in human ovarian cancer. *Cancer Res* 1987;47:6267–6271.
74. Smaaland R, Lote K, Sothern RB, et al. DNA synthesis and ploidy in non-Hodgkin's lymphomas demonstrate variation depending on circadian stage of cell sampling. *Cancer Res* 1993;53:3129–3138.
75. Mormont MC, Lévi F. Circadian system alterations during cancer processes: a review. *Int J Cancer* 1997;70:241–247.

76. Hryniuk WM, Figueredo A, Goodyear M. Applications of dose-intensity to problems in chemotherapy of breast and colorectal cancer. *Semin Oncol* 1987;14:3–11.
77. Lévi F, Soussan A, Adam R, et al. A Phase I-II trial of five-day continuous intravenous infusion of 5-fluorouracil delivered at circadian rhythm modulated rate in patients with metastatic colorectal cancer. *J Infus Chemother* 1995;5(3):153–158.
78. Bertheault-Cvitkovic F, Lévi F, Soussan S, et al. Circadian-rhythm modulated chemotherapy with high-dose 5-fluorouracil: a pilot study in patients with pancreatic adenocarcinoma. *Eur J Cancer* 1993;29A(13):1851–1854.
79. Bjarnason GA, Kerr IG, Doyle N, Macdonald M, Sone M. Phase I study of 5-fluorouracil and leucovorin by a 14-day circadian infusion in metastatic adenocarcinoma patients. *Cancer Chemother Pharmacol* 1993;33:221–228.
80. Garufi C, Lévi F, Aschelter AM, et al. A Phase I trial of five day chronomodulated infusion of 5-fluorouracil and I-folinic acid in patients with metastatic colorectal cancer. *Eur J Cancer* 1997;33(10):1566–1571.
81. Curé H, Chevalier V, Adenis A, et al. Phase II trial of chronomodulated infusion of high-dose 5-fluorouracil and *l*-folinic acid in previously untreated patients with metastatic colorectal cancer. *J Clin Oncol* 2002;20(5):1175–1181.
82. Jolivet J, Létourneau Y. Colorectal cancer chronotherapy: implementation in general hospitals and clinical results. In: *Biological Clocks Mechanisms and Applications.* Proc. Intl. Cong. Chronobiol, Paris, 7–11 Sept. 1997, Y. Touitou Ed, Elsevier Science BV, Amsterdam, 1998, pp. 483–490.
83. Caussanel JP, Lévi F, Brienza S, et al. Phase I trial of 5-day continuous venous infusion of oxaliplatin at circadian rhythm-modulated rate compared with constant rate. *J Natl Cancer Inst* 1990;82:1046–1050.
84. Lévi F, Misset JL, Brienza S, et al. A chronopharmacologic phase II clinical trial with 5-fluorouracil, folinic acid and oxaliplatinum using an ambulatory multichannel programmable pump: high antitumor effectiveness against metastatic colorectal cancer. *Cancer* 1992;69(4):893–900.
85. Giacchetti S, Perpoint B, Zidani R, et al. for the International Organization of Cancer: Phase III multicenter randomized trial of oxaliplatin added to chronomodulated fluorouracil – leucovorin as first line treatment of metastatic colorectal cancer. *J Clin Oncol* 2000;18(1):136–147.
86. Focan C, Kreutz F, Focan-Henrard D, Moeneclaey N. Chronotherapy with 5-fluorouracil, folinic acid and carboplatin for metastatic colorectal cancer; an interesting therapeutic index in a phase II trial. *Eur J Cancer* 2000;36(3):341–347.
87. Garufi C, Dogliotti L, D'Attino RM, et al. Irinotecan and chronomodulated infusion of 5-fluorouracil and folinic acid in the treatment of patients with advanced colorectal carcinoma. A Phase I study. *Cancer* 2001;91:712–720.
88. Curé H, Forestier D, Chevalier V, et al. Phase II trial of chronomodulated (CM) quadritherapy combining 5-fluorouracil (5-FU), L-folinic acid (L-FA), oxaliplatin (L-OHP) and irinotecan (CPT11) in previously untreated patients with metastatic colorectal cancer (MCC). *Proc Am Ass Cancer Res* 92nd Ann. Meeting, March 24–28 2001, New-Orleans USA, 2001, 42: abstr # 3334.
89. Lévi F, Zidani R, Coudert B, et al. Chronomodulated irinotecan (I) – fluorouracil (F) – leucovorin (L) – oxaliplatin (O) (chrono IFLO) as salvage therapy in patients with heavily pretreated metastatic colorectal cancer (MCC). *Proc Am Soc Clin Oncol* 2001;abstr. 552.
90. Marsh RD, Chu NM, Vauthey JN, et al. Preoperative treatment of patients with locally advanced unresectable rectal adenocarcinoma utilizing continuous chronobiologically shaped 5-fluorouracil infusion and radiation therapy. *Cancer* 1996;78(2):217–225.
91. Penberthy D, Rich T, Shelton III C, Adams R, Minasi J, Jones RS. A pilot study of chronomodulated infusional 5-FU chemoradiation for pancreatic cancer. *Ann Oncol* 2001;12(5):681–684.
92. Lévi F, Zidani R, Vannetzel JM, et al. Chronomodulated versus fixed infusion rate delivery of ambulatory chemotherapy with oxaliplatin, 5-fluorouracil and folinic acid in patients with colorectal cancer metastases. A randomized multiinstitutional trial. *J Natl Cancer Inst* 1994;86:1608–1617.
93. Lévi F, Zidani R, Misset JL. for the International Organization for Cancer Chronotherapy: Randomized multicentre trial of chronotherapy with oxaliplation, fluorouracil, and folinic acid in metastatic colorectal cancer. *Lancet* 1997;350:681–686.
94. Bertheault-Cvitkovic F, Jami A, Ithzaki M, et al. Biweekly intensified ambulatory chronomodulated chemotherapy with oxaliplatin, 5-fluorouracil and folinic acid in patients with metastatic colorectal cancer. *J Clin Oncol* 1996;14(11):2950–2958.
95. Lévi F, Zidani R, Brienza S, et al. International Organization for Cancer Chronotherapy: A multicenter evaluation of intensified ambulatory chronomodulated chemotherapy with oxaliplatin, fluorouracil and leucovorin as initial treatment of patients with metastatic colorectal cancer. *Cancer* 1999;85(12):2532–2540.

96. Bismuth H, Adam R, Lévi F, et al. Resection of nonresectable liver metastases from colorectal cancer after neoadjuvant chemotherapy. *Ann Surg* 1996;224(4):509–522.
97. Giacchetti S, Itzhaki M, Gruia G, et al. Long term survival of patients with unresectable colorectal liver metastases following infusional chemotherapy with 5-fluorouracil, folinic acid, oxaliplatin and surgery. *Ann Oncol* 1999;10:1–7.
98. Buyse M, Thirion P, Carlson RW, Burzykowski T, Molenberghs G, Piedbois P: Relation between tumour response to first-line chemotherapy and survival in advanced colorectal cancer: a meta-analysis. Meta-Analysis Group in Cancer. *Lancet* 2000;356:373–378.
99. Rivard G, Infante-Rivard C, Hoyeux C, Champagne J. Maintenance chemotherapy for childhood acute lymphoblastic leukemia: better in the evening. *Lancet* 1985;i.i.:1264–1266.
100. Schmiegelow K, Glomstein A, Kristinsson J, Salmi T, Schroder H, Bjork O. Impact of morning versus evening schedule for oral methotrexate and 6-mercaptopurine on relapse risk for children with acute lymphoblastic leukemia. Nordic Society for Pediatric Hematology and Oncology (NOPHO). *J Pediatr Hematol Oncol* 1997;19:102–109.
101. Serin D, Curé H, Laplaige P, et al. Is there any advantage in chronomodulating 5–FU combined with taxol in second or third-line treatment of metastatic breast cancer (MBC)? Results of two french multicenter studies. *Proc Am Soc Clin Oncol* 36th Ann. Meeting, May 20–23 2000, New-Orleans, LA, 2000;19:431.
102. Bruguerolle B. Chronopharmacokinetics. Current status. *Clin Pharmacokinet* 1998;35:83–94.

8 Relevance of Scheduling to the Efficacy of 5-Fluorouracil Alone and in Combination with Other Agents

Alberto F. Sobrero, MD, *and Ornella Belvedere,* MD

CONTENTS

1. INTRODUCTION

Until 4–5 years ago the hot topics in clinical colorectal cancer research were scheduling of 5-fluorouracil (5-FU) and its biochemical modulation. The long series of clinical failures on one side and the lack of strong evidence for something new coming up soon, generated the feeling that several years should pass before seeing appreciable progress in the clinical management of this disease. The situation has changed dramatically. Recently, in the last few years, a series of well-designed, well-conducted, randomized studies have demonstrated the value of CPT-11 as second line treatment of patients with advanced colorectal cancer *(1,2)* and subsequently the value of CPT-11 + 5-FU in the front line treatment of this disease *(3–5)*. Oxaliplatin is somewhat behind CPT-11, but it elicits similar optimism among oncologists, particularly in Europe *(6,7)*. although from a research perspective the small improvements afforded by the two new agents, particularly CPT-11, must be greeted as major breakthroughs, caution must be exercised from a broader perspective. The very small (< 3 mo) advantage in survival for CPT-11 + 5-FU combination vs 5-FU alone must be weighed against the increased toxicity and cost of the combinations. It is thus a pity that most of the research aimed at defining the best 5-FU schedule and modulation has been dropped: first,

From: *Fluoropyrimidines in Cancer Therapy*
Edited by: Y. M. Rustum © Humana Press Inc., Totowa, NJ

because the issue whether the new agents are most effective when given in combination or sequentially after 5-FU failure is still not solved; second, because it is likely that each of the new agents produces different effects depending on the schedule of 5-FU used when given in combination.

For these reasons, despite the declining popularity of the topic, these authors believe that attention should still be paid to appropriate scheduling of the fluoropyrimidine and its modulation. This is true not only for the relevance of scheduling to combination studies with CPT-11 and oxaliplatin, but also for combinations with the new target based therapies *(8–10)*. The basic reasoning behind this consideration is that there is ample evidence that 5-FU behaves differently when given as a bolus or as continuous infusion (CI) and that it may indeed be considered two different drugs depending on the schedule of administration *(11)*.

2. PRECLINICAL EVIDENCE FOR A SCHEDULE-DEPENDENT MECHANISM OF ACTION OF 5-FU

Several lines of evidence support the notion that infusional 5-FU kills cells predominantly by a DNA-related mechanism, whereas bolus 5-FU works primarily by incorporation of fraudulent nucleotides into nucleic acids *(11)*.

1. Pharmacokinetics. Conventional iv bolus doses (400–600 mg/m^2) result in peak plasma concentrations in the Millimolor range (0.1–1 m*M*) followed by a rapid decline *(12)*. Plasma levels above the threshold for cytotoxic effects (1 μ*M*) *(13)* are thus maintained for only a few hours. Given the tight S-phase dependence of thymidylate synthetase (TS) inhibition, it is unlikely that this enzyme represents a major site of action under conditions of short-term, high-dose exposure. Conversely, the relative independence of 5-FU incorporation into RNA from a specific cell cycle phase is compatible with significant cytotoxicity even in conditions of short-term administration *(14)*.
2. Thymidine protection experiments. Long-term, low-dose fluoropyrimidine exposure produces cytotoxicity that is prevented by thymidine, whereas, in general, short-term, high-dose fluoropyrimidine administration results in growth inhibition refractory to thymidine protection *(15–20)*.
3. Apoptosis. p53-dependent cell death of intestinal epithelial crypt cells induced by the administration of bolus 5-FU was inhibited only by administration of uridine:thymidine abrogated apoptosis induced by the pure TS inhibitor Tomudex, but it had no effect on bolus 5-FU-induced apoptosis *(21)*.
4. Deoxyuridine accumulation following 5-FU treatment. Deoxyuridylate increases as a consequence of TS inhibition. In vivo murine studies showed that short-term exposure to 5-FU produced no elevation of deoxyuridine with substantial antiproliferative toxicity, while prolonged infusion of the fluoropyrimidine did elevate the level of the indicator nucleoside without major toxicity *(22)*.
5. Slopes of the dose-response curves. Long-term exposure to 5-FU (but not pulse) produces a lack of a shoulder and tail in dose-response curves in colorectal carcinoma cell lines *(23,24)*. In addition, while sensitivity to pulse 5-FU shows a significant variability even within the same tumor type (adenocarcinoma of the colon), longer exposure times result in more uniform levels of sensitivity to this agent *(20)*.
6. Mechanisms of resistance. Long-term, repeated exposures to 5-FU resulted in resistance due to decreased TS inhibition, while short-term, high-dose exposures were associated with selection of resistant cells showing a decreased uptake of the fluoropyrimidine into RNA in HCT-8 cells *(25)*. In addition, Pizzorno et al. *(26)*, suggested that the schedule of 5-FU administration determines the mode of metabolic activation and resistance to this agent.

7. Lack of cross resistance between pulse and prolonged exposure 5-FU. Cells resistant to pulse 5-FU still retain sensitivity to a prolonged exposure to the fluoropyrimidine *(27)*. Cells resistant to CI 5-FU were only partially sensitive to pulse 5-FU.
8. Synergism between bolus and CI 5-FU. The finding that sequential pulse and prolonged exposures to 5-FU produce more than additive cytotoxicity on HCT-8 cells in vitro *(27)* further supports the contention that 5-FU may be considered to have two different mechanisms of action depending on the dose and schedule of administration.

3. CLINICAL EVIDENCE FOR A SCHEDULE-DEPENDENT MECHANISM OF ACTION OF 5-FU

1. Different dose-response curves. Unmodulated bolus 5-FU appears to have a threshold dose intensity, 500–600 mg/m^2/wk, which produces marginal activity against colorectal cancer, but little or no advantage is gained by increasing its dose intensity. The same is true for modulated bolus 5-FU at a dose reduced by 20%. The threshold dose for clinical activity of CI 5-FU is likely in the range of 1500 mg/m^2/wk, whereas there is probably no therapeutic gain in giving more than 2600 mg/m^2/wk. The concept of different threshold doses for activity is quite evident *(11)*.
2. Different achievable dose intensities. As noted very early in the clinical development of this fluoropyrimidine, the dose intensity achieved for CI 5-FU is 3–4 times higher than that of bolus 5-FU. Achievable dose intensities range between 500 *(27)* and 750 *(28)* mg/m^2/wk for the bolus schedules and 1625 *(29)* and 2875 *(30)* mg/m^2/wk for the CI schedules. It is remarkable that within each type of administration modality the differences in dose intensities achievable are minimal.
3. Different toxicities. Bolus schedules mainly produce leukopenia, mucositis, and diarrhea, while CI schedules are complicated primarily by stomatitis and dermatitis *(11)*.
4. Different activities. Unmodulated bolus 5-FU is less active than CI 5-FU and the survival of infusional regimen is slightly, but significantly, longer than bolus regimens as evidenced by a meta-analysis on six studies *(31)*.

4. CLINICAL CONSEQUENCES OF THE DUAL NATURE OF 5-FU

There are four clinically relevant consequences of the hypothesis that 5-FU is indeed two different drugs: first, CI 5-FU should still work in patients failing bolus 5-FU; Second, the two administration modalities could be combined; third, biochemical modulation of 5-FU should be schedule specific; fourth, combinations of 5-FU plus CPT-11 or oxaliplatin should take into consideration the schedule of 5-FU administration.

4.1. Partial Lack of Cross Resistance

A few reports clearly indicate that 10–15% of patients achieve a partial response to infusional regimens after failing treatment with bolus 5-FU and another 20% obtain disease stabilization that often lasts as long as a partial response *(32–34)*. Data on the opposite sequence, that is, activity of 5-FU bolus on CI 5-FU-resistant patients, are not available to our knowledge.

Finally, MTX → 5-FU still retains marginal activity in patients failing front line treatment with bolus 5-FU plus LV *(35)*.

4.2. Combined Bolus + Infusional 5-FU

The De Gramont regimen *(36)* is a good example of hybrid regimen with modulated 5-FU because it combines bolus 5-FU 400 mg/m^2 with CI 5-FU, 600 mg/m^2 Biochemical modulation of this regimen is not "schedule specific" in that high-dose LV is intended to modulate bolus and CI 5-FU. Unfortunately, the initial high response rates, around 40%, and long progression-free survivals, around seven mo, of this regimen *(37)* have not been confirmed by other authors *(38–40)* or by the same author when this regimen was used as comparator arm in randomized studies testing the addition of oxaliplatin *(41)*. This decline in activity, coupled with the very low toxicity of this regimen, allows speculation that while the bolus 5-FU dose intensity is more than adequate, i.e., 400 mg/m^2/wk, that of CI 5-FU, i.e., 600 mg/m^2/wk is well below the threshold for activity (optimal dose intensity for LV modulated CI 5-FU is 1400 mg/m^2/wk) *(42)*.

4.3. Schedule-Specific Biochemical Modulation of 5-FU

4.3.1. Preclinical Data

If it is true that CI 5-FU works primarily via a TS-related mechanism and that bolus 5-FU works primarily by incorporation into nucleic acids, biochemical modulators should be used in a schedule-specific manner to achieve maximal potentiation. Maximal enhancement of bolus 5-FU is more likely obtained with drugs that enhance the RNA effect of this fluoropyrimidine such as methotrexate (MTX), trimetrexate, phosphon-acetyl-L-aspartate, 6-methylmercaptopurine ribosyde, and so on, than with LV. On the other hand, enhancement of 5-FU cytotoxicity with LV might be greater when the fluoropyrimidine is administered as a CI. This concept has not been tested directly in preclinical studies, but indirect evidence is there to support it.

In vitro, the importance of prolonged 5-FU exposures to obtain optimal potentiation with LV is underscored by studies on human colorectal (WiDr), bladder (T24), breast MCF-7, and erythroleukemia cancer cells showing that major potentiation was only achieved when prolonged exposures to FU were used *(43–46)*.

Fewer data are available for the combination MTX→FU. Synergistic cytotoxic interactions were demonstrated with the sequence MTX→FU in a series of studies using short-term exposures to the fluoropyrimidine while in general, longer exposures to 5-FU, with the same sequence of administration, only resulted in additive interactions, lending some support to the concept of schedule-specific biochemical modulation *(47–49)*.

Murine in vivo studies in this area are complicated by the high plasma folate and thymidine levels in mice, with consequent tumor salvage. The combination 5-FU + LV given by repeated bolus injections produced only modest delays in tumor growth *(50–52)* while, enhancement of 5-FU antitumor activity by LV was obtained with CI 5-FU *(53)* but not with repeated daily bolus injections *(54)*.

4.3.2. Clinical Data

The regimen consisting of a single high-dose bolus of 5-FU (1000 mg/m^2 given every 3 wk) modulated by LV was dropped for inactivity by the GITSG from their four-arm randomized study in 1989 *(55)*.

CI 5-FU plus MTX was ineffective as first line chemotherapy in a small phase II study *(56)*. In addition, a number of small studies done just prior the to advent of CPT-11 and oxaliplatin indicated high activity of CI 5-FU plus LV when protracted 5-FU infusion times (longer than

5 d) are used *(57–59)*. In addition, a recently reported EORTC showed superiority of infusional 5-FU + LV over infusional 5-FU alone in terms of response rate and progression free survival *(60)*. In the mid 1990s, when biochemical modulation of 5-FU was still dominating the scene of colorectal (CRC) treatment, we tested the activity of a hybrid regimen based on the hypothesis that biochemical modulation is schedule specific. The regimen alternates two biweekly cycles of 5-FU bolus (600 mg/m^2), preceded by (24-h interval) MTX (200 mg/m^2) with a 3-wk continuous infusion of 5-FU (200 mg/m^2/d) modulated by low-dose 6-S-leucovorin (20 mg/m^2 bolus, weekly) *(61)*. This sequence and not the reverse was chosen because in vitro cells resistant to bolus FU were still sensitive to CI 5-FU but not the reverse. Three complete and 13 partial responses were obtained among 33 consecutive patients (RR = 48%, 95% confidence limits, 31–66%) at the cost of very low toxicity. The addition of natural beta interferon to the above regimen, based upon in vitro studies *(62)*, did not improve the therapeutic outcome in a second phase II study in 57 patients *(63)*. Accordingly, we randomized 216 advanced colorectal cancer patients to receive our new schedule-specific regimen or modulated bolus FU as first line treatment *(64)*. Almost three times higher response rate was obtained in the experimental arm with a significantly longer PFS (6 vs 4 mo), and a very good MST (15 mo). It was also reassuring that the high response rates and long PFS that our group obtained in the previous phase II studies *(61,63)* were confirmed in this phase III trial.

As we will see in the next session, the recent studies using chronomodulated 5-FU *(65,66)* or combinations of 5-FU plus oxaliplatin *(41,67)* or irinotecan *(3,4)* have shown response rates in the 30–50% range and PFS values in the 6–9 mo range in randomized settings. The results of our experimental arm fall into these ranges at the cost of very low toxicity and expenses. Furthermore, the survival data in our study are similar to those obtained with the latest regimens mentioned above (range 14–17 mo).

A word of caution and criticism is needed. Our data may in fact also be interpreted under a different perspective. Considering that the survival was similar in the two arms and that quality of life during these first line regimens was also similar, one wonders if it is better to use the two methods of 5-FU administration upfront as in our schedule-specific modulation regimen, or to use them sequentially, i.e., starting with modulated bolus 5-FU and upon progression using CI 5-FU. Our study suggests that the two approaches are ultimately equivalent in terms of overall survival. Nevertheless, this also strengthens our hypothesis that 5-FU is indeed two different drugs and that both should be used either in an alternating or in a sequential fashion or even back to back, if one tries to get the most out of this agent.

We are still pursuing the first of these potentially valuable approahes, i.e., alternating bolus–infusional 5-FU. Our plans of development are to conduct a series of phase II studies that incorporate the other active new agents in our alternating regimen in an effort to further potentiate the activity of the bolus or the infusional part, since toxicity appears to allow so. Based on a British report *(68)*, mitomycin C has been added to the infusional part of our regimen in a large phase II study that showed a moderate response rate (37%) but very long PFS and OS *(69)*. Since the bolus part needs more "work" of refinement, oxaliplatin is added to MTX→5-FU in the ongoing phase II study and we plan to substitute MTX with trimetrexate in the bolus part and will consider adding irinotecan as well.

We think that our regimen of schedule-specific biochemical modulation represents one of the most active ways of giving 5-FU presently available, and it should serve as the basis for the development of combination regimens with the new active compounds that are now so promising in this disease.

Table 1

	5-FU regimen	FU CI duration hr	I-OHP or CPT-11 dose (mg/m^2)	LV	Phase	Pts n	RR (%)	PFS (mo)	OS (mo)	TOX(gr 3/4) Neutro (%)	Diarrhea (%)	Mucositis (%)	Vomiting (%)	Neuro (%)	First author
Infusional 5-FU + I-HOP	I-OHP (50 mg/m^2) → LV 500 mg/m^2) → 24h 5-FU (2500 mg/m^2)day 1, 8, 15, 22, 29, 36 q50	24	50	Y	II	32	13	3	9	10	54	3	28	0	Janinis *(70)*
	I-OHP (85 mg/m^2) + LV (200mg/m^2) → 5-FU bolus (400 mg/m^2) → 22h 5-FU (600 mg/m^2) day 1,2 q14	44	85	Y	III	210	50.7	9	16.2	41.7	11.9	5.8		18.2	de Gramont *(41)*
	I-OHP (100 mg/m^2) day 1 + LV (200 mg/m^2) → 5-FU bolus (400 mg/m^2) → 22h 5-FU (600 mg/m^2) day 1,2 q14	44	100	Y	II	33	30.5	N/A	N/A	48	3	3	N/A	6	Souglakos *(71)*
	I-OHP (100 mg/m^2) d 1 + LV (500 mg/m^2) → 22h 5-FU (1750 mg/m^2) day 1, 2 q14	44	100	Y	II	41	17	11	12	41	N/A	N/A	N/A	N/A	Kouroussis *(73)*
	I-OHP (85 mg/m^2) + LV (350 mg/m^2) → 5-FU bolus (400 mg/m^2) → 46hr 5-FU (2400 mg/m^2) day 1 q14	46	85	Y	II	36	23	4.5	10	19	5	N/A	3	N/A	Cheeseman *(72)*
	I-OHP (85 mg/m^2) day 1 and 48hr 5-FU (2500 mg/m^2) day 1, 8 q14	48	85	N	II	31	46	N/A	N/A	0	20	3	N/A	N/A	Abad *(74)*
Bolus 5-FU + I-OHP	I-OHP (85 mg/m^2) day 1, 15 and LV (20 mg/m^2) + 5-FU (500 mg/m^2) bolus day 1, 8, 15 q28	bolus	85	Y	II	31	14	N/A	N/A	N/A	6	N/A	N/A	9.6	Giornelli *(75)*
	I-OHP (85 mg/m^2) day 1, 15 and LV (20 mg/m^2) → 5-FU bolus (500 mg/m^2) day 1, 8, 15 q28	bolus	85	Y	II	II	100	N/A	N/A	9	9	N/A	N/A	9	Hochster *(76)*
Infusional 5-FU + CPT-11	CPT-11 (125 mg/m^2) → LV (500 mg/m^2) + 5-FU 24hr i.c. (1800 mg/m^2) day 1, 8, 15 q42	24	125	Y	II	18	57	N/A	N/A	22	44	5	22	0	Vazquez *(77)*
	CPT-11 (80 mg/m^2) → LV (500 mg/v) + 24hr 5-FU (2300 mg/m^2) day 1 q7	24	80	Y	III	54	39.6	7.2	N/A	28.8	44.4	0	11.1	0	Douillard *(3)*
	CPT-11 (180 mg/m^2) day 1 and 5-FU bolus (400 mg/m^2) → LV (200 mg/m^2) and 22hr 5-FU (600 mg/m^2) day 1, 2 q14	44	180	Y	III	145	33.1	6.5	17.4	46.2	46.2	4.1	2.8	0	Douillard *(3)*
Bolus 5-FU + CPT-11	CPT-11 (125 mg/m^2) → LV (20 mg/m^2) → 5-FU (500 mg/m^2) bolus day 1, 8, 15, 22 q42	bolus	125	Y	III	231	50	7	14.8	53.8	22.7	22.2	9.7	0	Saltz *(4)*
	CPT-11 (125 mg/m^2) → LV (20 mg/m^2) → 5-FU (500 mg/m^2) bolus day 1, 8, 15 22 q42	bolus	125	Y	II	24	43	4.2	8.7	33.3	9.5	0	19	N/A	Salgado *(78)*

5. CLINICAL RELEVANCE OF 5-FU SCHEDULING IN COMBINATION WITH IRINOTECAN AND OXALIPLATIN

Table 1 represents a comparison of the different doublets (5-FU + CPT-11 and 5-FU + oxaliplatin) analyzed as a function of 5-FU scheduling.

Too few patients have been treated with bolus 5-FU + oxaliplatin to draw even preliminary conclusions. Conversely, some speculations are possible on infusional 5-FU + oxaliplatin. The most widely tested regimen is De Gramont's and several variations have been investigated. It appears that even small changes to the original regiment (such as omitting the second 5-FU bolus) result in dicreased activity. With the 48-infusional regimen (Spanish regimen), the dose of 5-FU is crucial as it must be maintained above 2500 mg/m^2 every week for good activity.

No reliable data are available for the protracted infusion of 5-FU (Lokich regimen). The general conclusion is that the best 5-FU regimen to be combined with oxaliplatin is probably infusional 5-FU, but which type of infusional 5-FU is still to be determined.

The same general concept seems to hold true for combinations of 5-FU with CPT-11 where the weekly infusional schedule seems to be a bit inferior to the bi-monthly de Gramont regimen.

ACKNOWLEDGMENTS

Supported by grants AIRC, CNR Bridge 2000, and CNR Biotechnology 2000.

REFERENCES

1. Cunningham D, Pyrrhonen S, James RD, et al. Randomised trial of irinotecan plus supportive care versus supportive care alone after fluorouracil failure for patients with metastatic colorectal cancer. *Lancet* 1998; 352:1413–1418.
2. Rougier P, Van Custem E, Bajetta E, et al. Randomised trial of irinotecan versus fluorouracil by continuous infusion after fluorouracil failure in patients with metastatic colorectal cancer. *Lancet* 1998; 352:1407–1412.
3. Douillard JY, Cunningham D, Roth AD, et al. Irinotecan combined with fluorouracil alone as first-line treatment for metastatic colorectal caner: a multicentre randomised trial. *Lancet* 2000; 355:1041–1047.
4. Saltz LB, Cox JV, Blanke C, et al. Irinotecan plus fluorouracil and leucovorin for metastatic colorectal cancer. *New Engl J Med* 2000; 343:905–914.
5. Saltz JB, Douillard J, Pirotta N, et al. Combined analysis of two phase III randomized trials comparing irinotecan, fluorouracil, leucovorin vs fluororuacil alone as first-line therapy of previously untreated metastatic colorectal cancer. *Proc Am Soc Clin Oncol* 2000; 19:938.
6. Maindrault-Goebel F, Louvet C, Andre T, et al. Oxaliplatin added to the simplified bimonthly leucovorin and 5-fluorouracil regimen as second-line therapy for metastatic colorectal cancer (FOLFOX6). GERCOR *Eur J Cancer* 1999; 35:1338–1342.
7. Giachetti S, Perpoint B, Zidani R, et al. Phase III multicenter randomized trial of oxaliplatin added to chronomodulated fluorouracil-leucovorin as first line treatment of mletastatic colorectal cancer. *J Clin Oncol* 2000; 18:136–147.
8. Rosen PJ, Amado R, Hecht JR, et al. A phase I/II study of SU5416 in combination with 5-FU/leucovorin in patients with metastatic colorectal cancer. *Proc Am Soc Clin Oncol* 2000; 19:5D.
9. Bergsland E, Hurwitz H, Fehrenbacher L. A randomized phase II trial comparing rhuMAb VEGF (recombinant humanized monoclonal antibody to vascular endothelial cell growth factor) plus 5-fluorouracil/leucovorin (FU/LV) to FU/LV alone in patients with metastatic colorectal cancer. *Proc Am Soc Clin Oncol* 2000; 19:936.
10. Reid T, Galanis E, Abbruzzese J, et al. Hepatic artery infusion of onyx-015, a selectively-replicanting adenovirus in combination with 5-FU/leucovorin for gastrointestinal carcinoma metastatic to the liver *Proc Am Soc Clin Oncol* 2000; 19:953.
11. Sobrero AF, Aschele C, Bertino JR. Fluorouracil in colorectal cancer: a tale of two drugs. Implications for biochemical modulation. *J Clin Oncol* 1997; 15:368–381.

12. Fraile RJ, Baker LH, Buroker TR, et al. Pharmacokinetics of 5-fluorouracil administered orally, by rapid intravenous and by slow infusion. *Cancer Res* 1980; 40:2223–2228.
13. Grem JL. Fluorinated pyrimidines, in Chabner BA, Collins JM (eds): Cancer Chemotherapy. Principles and practice. Philadelphia, PA, Lippincott, 1990,pp.180–224.
14. Nord LD, Stolfi RL, Martin DS. Biochemical modulation of 5-fluorouracil with leucovorin or delayed uridine rescue: correlation of antitumor activity with dosage and FUra incorporation into RNA. *Biochem Pharmacol* 1992; 43:2543–2549.
15. Evans RM, Laskin JD, Hakala MT. Assessment of growth-limiting events caused by 5-fluorouracil in mouse cells and in human cells. *Cancer Res* 1980; 40:4113–4122.
16. Wilkinson D, Crumly J. The mechanism of 5-fluorouridine toxicity in Novikoff hepatoma cells. *Cancer Res* 1976; 36:4032–4038.
17. Maybaum J, Ullman B, Mandel HG, et al. Regulation of RNA- and DNA-directed actions of 5-fluoropyrimidines in mouse T-lymphoma (S-49) cells. *Cancer Res* 1980; 40:4209–4215.
18. Radparvar S, Houghton PJ, Germain G, Pennington J, Rahman A, Houghton JA. Cellular pharmacology of 5-fluorouracil in a human colon adenocarcinoma cell line selected for thymidine kinase deficiency. *Biochem Pharmacol* 1990; 39:1759–1765.
19. Piper AA, Fox RM Biochemical basis for the differential sensitivity of human T- and B-lymphocyte lines to 5-fluorouracil. *Cancer Res* 1982; 42:3753–3760.
20. Washtien WL. Comparison of 5-fluorouracil metabolism in two human gastrointestinal tumor cell lines. *Cancer Res* 1984; 44:909–914.
21. Pritchard DM, Watson AJM, Potten CS, Jackman AL, Hickman JA. Inhibition by uridine but not thymidine of p53-dependent intestinal apoptosis initiated by 5-fluorouracil: evidence for the involvment of RNA perturbation. *Proc Natl Acad Sci USA* 1997; 94:1795–1799.
22. Jackman AL, Ford HE, Farrugia DC, et al. The effects of Raltitrexed ('Tomudex'), ZD9331 ('Vamidex') and 5-FU on plasma dUrd, a surrogate marker of thymidylate synthase inhibition. *Proc Am Soc Clin Oncol* 2000; 19:183a.
23. Santelli G, Valeriote F. Schedule-dependent cytotoxicity of 5-fluorouracil in mice. *J Natl Cancer Inst* 1986; 76:159–164.
24. Calabro-Jones PM, Byfield JE, Ward JF, et al. Time-dose relationships for 5-fluorouracil cytotoxicity against human epithelial cancer cells in vitro. *Cancer Res* 1982; 42:4413–4420.
25. Aschele C, Sobrero A, Faderan MA, et al. Novel mechanism(s) of resistance to 5-fluorouracil in human colon cancer (HCT-8) sublines following exposure to two different clinically relevant dose schedules. *Cancer Res* 1992; 52:1855–1864.
26. Pizzorno G, Handschumacher RE. Effect of clinically modeled regimens on the growth response and development of resistance in human colon carcinoma cell lines. *Biochem Pharmacol* 1995; 49:559–565.
27. Wooley P, Ayoob M, Smith FP. A controlled trial of the effect of 4-hydroxypyrazolopyrimidine (Allopurinol) on the toxicity of a single bolus dose of 5-fluorouracil. *J Clin Oncol* 1985; 3:103–109.
28. Herrmann R, Knuth A, Kleeberg U, et al. Sequential methotrexate and 5-fluorouracil vs 5-fluorouracil alone in metastatic colorectal cancer. *Ann Oncol* 1992; 3:539–543.
29. Seifert P, Baker LH, Reed ML, et al. Comparison of continuously infused 5-fluorouracil with bolus injection in treatment of patients with colorectal adenocarcinoma. *Cancer* 1975; 36:123–128.
30. Trump DL, Egorin MJ, Forrest A. Pharmacokinetic and pharmacodynamic analysis of fluorouracil during 72-hour continuous infusion with and without dipyridamole. *J Clin Oncol* 1991; 11:2027–2035.
31. Efficacy of intravenous continuous infusion of fluorouracil compared with bolus administration in advanced colorectal cancer. Meta-analysis Group In Cancer. *J Clin Oncol* 1998; 16:301–308.
32. Mori A, Bertoglio S, Guglielmi A, et al. Activity of continuous infusion 5-fluorouracil in patients with advanced colorectal cancer clinically resistant to bolus 5-fluorouracil. *Cancer Chemother Pharmacol* 1993; 33:179–180.
33. Izzo J, Zarba JJ, Rougier P, et al. Low dose 5-FU continuous infusion in advanced colorectal cancer: clinical evidence for reversal of acquired/intrinsic resistance to 5-FU or 5-FU folinic acid. *Proc Am Ass Cancer Res* 1992; 33:217.
34. Hartmann H, Kennsinger A, Lemon H. Five days continuous infusion 5-fluorouracil for advanced colorectal gastric and pancreatic adenocarcinomas. *J Surg Oncol* 1979; 11:227–238.
35. Zaniboni A, Labianca R, Martignoni G, et al. Sequential methotrexate and 5-fluorouracil as second line chemotherapy for advanced colorectal cancer pretreated with 5-fluorouracil and leucovorin: a GISCAD study. *J Chemother* 1996; 8:82–84.
36. De Gramont A, Krulik M, Cady J, et al. High-dose folinic acid and 5-fluorouracil bolus and continuous infusion in advanced colorectal cancer. *Eur J Cancer Clin Oncol* 1998; 24:1499–1503.

37. De Gramont A, Bosset JF, Milan C et al. Randomized trial comparing monthly low-dose leucovorin and fluorouracil bolus with bimonthly high-dose leucovorin and fluorouracil bolus plus continuous infusion for advanced colorectal cancer: A French intergroup study. *J Clin Oncol* 1997; 15:808–815.
38. Jodrell DI, Murray LS, Reed NS, et al. Bolus/infusional 5-fluorouracil and folinic acid for metastatic colorectal carcinoma: are suboptimal dosages being used in the UK? *Br J Cancer* 1994; 70:749–752.
39. Seymour MT, Slevin M, Cunningham D, et al. A randomized trial to assess the addition of interferon alpha 2a to 5-fluorouracil and leucovorin in advanced colorectal cancer. *Br J Cancer* 1994; 69:24.
40. Hanna CL, Mc Kinna FE, Williams LB, et al. High dose folinic acid and 5-fluorouracil bolus and continuous infusion in advanced colorectal cancer. *Br J Cancer* 1995; 72:774–776.
41. De Gramont A, Figer A, Seymour M, et al. Leucovorin and fluorouracil with or without oxaliplatin as first-line treatment in advanced colorectal cancer. *J Clin Oncol* 2000; 18:2938–2947.
42. Leichman CG, Leichman L, Spears CP, et al. Prolonged infusion of fluorouracil with weekly bolus leucovorin: a phase II study in patients with disseminated colorectal cancer. *J Natl Cancer Inst* 1993; 85:41–44.
43. Beck A, Etienne MC, Chéradame S, et al. Wide range for optimal concentration of folinic acid in fluorouracil modulation-Experimental data on human tumour cell lines. *Eur J Cancer* 1994; 30A:1522–1526.
44. Jolivet J. Role of leucovorin dosing and administration schedule. *Eur J Cancer* 1995; 31A:1311–1315.
45. Moran RG, Scanlon KL. Schedule-dependent enhancement of the cytotoxicity of fluoropyrimidines to human carcinoma cells in the presence of folinic acid. *Cancer Res* 1991; 51:4618–4623.
46. Waxman S, Bruckner H. The enhancement of 5-fluorouracil antimetabolic activity by leucovorin, menadione and a-tocopherol. *Eur J Cancer Clin Oncol* 1982; 18:685–692.
47. Sobrero AF, Bertino JR. Sequence-dependent synergism between dichloromethotrexate and 5-fluorouracil in a human colon carcinoma cell line. *Cancer Res* 1983; 43:4011–4013.
48. van der Wilt CL, Braakhuis BJM, Pinedo HM, et al. Addition of leucovorin in modulation of 5-fluorouracil with methotrexate: potentiating or reversing effect? *Int J Cancer* 1995; 61:672–678.
49. Sobrero AF, Romanini A, Russello et al. Sequence-dependent enhancement of HCT-8 cell kill by trimetrexate and fluoropyrimidines: implications for the mechanism of this interaction. *Eur J Cancer Clin Oncol* 1989; 25:977–982.
50. van der Wilt CL, Peters GJ. New targets for pyrimidine antimetabolites in the treatment of solid tumours. *Pharm World Sci* 1994; 16:84–103.
51. Nadal JC, Van Groeningen CJ, Pinedo HM, et al. In vivo potentiation of 5-fluorouracil by leucovorin in murine colon carcinoma. *Biomed Pharmacother* 1988; 42:387–393.
52. Houghton JA, Williams LG, Loftin SK, et al. Factors that influence the therapeutic activity of 5-fluorouracil [6RS]leucovorin combinations in colon adenocarcinoma xenografts. *Cancer Chemother Pharmacol* 1992; 30:423–432.
53. Rustum YM. Selective modulation of 5-fluorouracil action in patients with colorectal carcinoma. *Chemioterapia* 1985; 4:377–382.
54. Cao S, Duranni F, Rustum YM: Antitumor activity of fluorouracil/6-(RS)-leucovorin (FUra/LV) in rats bearing colon carcinoma: role of dose and schedule. *Proc Am Assoc Cancer Res* 1992; 33:422.
55. Petrelli N, Douglass OH Jr, Herrera L, et al. The modulation of fluorouracil with leucovorin in metastatic colorectal carcinoma: a prospective randomized phase III trial. *J Clin Oncol* 1989; 7:1419–1426.
56. Lokich JJ, Phillips D, Green R, et al. 5-fluorouracil and methotrexate administered simultaneously as a continuous infusion, a phase I study. *Cancer* 1985; 56:2395–2398.
57. Loeffler TM, Weber FW, Hausamen TU. Protracted continuous infusion 5-fluorouracil with intermittent high dose leucovorin in advanced and metastatic colorectal cancer: a pilot study. in Pinedo HM, Rustum YM (eds): Leucovorin modulation of fluoropyrimidines: a new frontier in cancer chemotherapy. London, Royal Society of Medicine Services Limited, 1989, pp 65–69.
58. Ardalan B, Chua L, Tian E, et al. A phase II study of weekly 24 hour infusion with high dose 5-fluorouracil with leucovorin in colorectal carcinoma. *J Clin Oncol* 1991; 9:625–630.
59. Tempero M, Berg A, Block M, et al. A phase II trial of protracted therapy with 5-fluorouracil and leucovorin in metastatic colorectal cancer. *Proc Am Soc Clin Oncol* 1992; 11:189.
60. Schmoll HJ, Kohne CH, Lorenz M, et al. Weekly 24 hour infusion of high dose fluorouracil with or without folinic acid vs. bolus Fu/FA (NCCTG/Mayo) in advanced colorectal cancer (CRC): a randomized phase III study of the EORTC GITCCG and the AIO. *Proc Am Soc Clin Oncol* 2000; 19:241a.
61. Sobrero AF, Aschele C, Guglielmi A, et al. Schedule-selective biochemical modulation of 5-fluorouracil: a phase II study in advanced colorectal cancer. *Clin Cancer Res* 1995; 1:955–960.
62. Guglielmi A, Aschele C, Mori A, et al. In vitro synergism between 5-fluorouracil and natural beta interferon in human colon carcinoma cells. *Clin Cancer Res* 1995; 1:334–341.

63. Aschele C, Guglielmi A, Frassineti GL, et al. Schedule selective biochemical modulation of 5-fluorouracil in advanced colorectal cancer: a multicentric phase II study. *British J Cancer* 1998; 77:341–346.
64. Sobrero A, Zaniboni A, Frassineti GL, et al. Schedule specific biochemical modulation of 5-fluorouracil in advanced colorectal cancer: a randomized study *Ann Oncol* 2000; 11:1413–1428.
65. Lévi F, Zidani R, Misset JL, et al. Randomized multicentre trial of chronotherapy with oxaliplatin, fluorouracil, and folinic acid in metastatic colorectal cancer. *Lancet* 1997; 350:681–686.
66. Lévi FA, Zidani R, Vannetzel J-M, et al. Chronomodulated versus fixed-infusion-rate delivery of ambulatory chemotherapy with oxaliplatin, fluorouracil, and folinic acid (leucovorin) in patients with colorectal cancer metastases: a randomized multi-institutional trial. *J Natl Cancer Inst* 1994; 86:1608–1617.
67. Bertheault-Cvitkovic F, Jami A, Ithzaki M, et al. Biweekly intensified ambulatory chronomodulated chemotherapy with oxaliplatin, fluorouracil, and leucovorin in patients with metastatic colorectal cancer. *J Clin Oncol* 1996; 14:2950–2958.
68. Ross P, Norman A, Cunningham D, et al. A prospective randomized trial of protracted venous infusion fluorouracil with or without mitomycin C in advanced colorectal cancer. *Ann Oncol* 1997; 8:995–1001.
69. Sobrero A, Guglielmi A, Cirillo M, et al. Highly effective, low cost chemotherapy for advanced colorectal cancer: a multicentric phase II study. *Brit J Cancer* 2001; in press.
70. Janinis J, Papakostas P, Samelis G, Skarlos D, Papagianopoulos P, Fountzilas G. Second-line chemotherapy with weekly oxaliplatin and high-dose 5-fluorouracil with folinic acid in metastatic colorectal carcinoma: a Hellenic Cooperative Oncology Group (HeCOG) phase II feasibility study. *Ann Oncol* 2000; 11:163–167.
71. Souglakos J, Kouroussis C, Ziras N, et al. First line treatment with 5-fluorouracil (5-FU), leucovorin (LV), and oxaloplatin (1-OHP) in advanced colorectal cancer (ACC): a multicenter phase II study. *Proc Am Soc Clin Oncol* 2000, 302a.
72. Cheeseman SL, Crosse B, Chester JD, Richards FJ, Seymour MT. Second-line combination Oxaliplatin, Leucovorin, and 5FU ("OxMdG) in patients with 5FU-resistant colorectal cancer (CRC). *Proc Am Soc Clin Oncol* 2000; 19:282.
73. Kouroussis C, Souglakos J, Giannakanis T, et al. Biweekly oxaliplatin (1-OHP) with high-dose leucovorin (LV) and 5-fluorouracil (5-FU) in irinotecan pretreated patients with advanced colorectal cancer (ACC). *Proc Am Soc Clin Oncol* 2000; 19:282.
74. Abad A, Navarro M, Sastre J, et al. Biweekly oxaliplatin (OXA) plus weekly 48hr continuous infusion (ci)5FU (TTD regimen) in first line treatment of advanced colorectal cancer (ACC). *Proc Am Soc Clin Oncol* 2000; 19:300a.
75. Giornelli G, Roca E, Chacon M, Martin C, Wasserman E. Bimonthly oxaliplatin (1-OHP) and weekly bolus 5-fluorouracil (5-FU) and folinic acid (FA) in patients (Pts) with metastatic colorectal cancer (CRC): a feasible and active regimen. *Proc Am Soc Clin Oncol* 2000; 19:295a.
76. Hochster HS, Chachoua A, Wernz J, Escalon J, Martinez S, Muggia F. Oxaliplatin with weekly bolus 5FU and low-dose leucovorin (LV): early report of high activity in first line therapy of advanced colorectal cancer (ACRC). *Proc Am Soc Clin Oncol* 2000; 19:289a. 2000.
77. Vazquez S, Mel J, Sabin P, Alvarez E, Quintero G. Irinotecan (CPT-11) in combination with 5-fluorouracil/folinic acid (5-FU/FA) as a weekly schedale in previously untreated patients with metastatic colorectal cancer (MCRC). *Proc Am Soc Clin Oncol* 2000; 19:316a.
78. Salgado M, Firida J, Mata J, et al. A phase II study of weekly irinotecan (CPT-11) combinated with folinic acid and 5-FU in pretreated advanced colorectal cancer (CRC) patients. *Proc Am Soc Clin Oncol* 2000; 19:296a.

9 Noninvasive Studies of Fluoropyrimidines

Walter Wolf, PhD, *Cary A. Presant,* MD, FACP,
and Victor Waluch, PhD, MD

Contents

1. INTRODUCTION

Fluoropyrimidines occupy a unique niche in the noninvasive studies of drugs. For one, 5-fluorouracil (5-FU), which was introduced by Heidelberger in the late 1950s as an anticancer agent, continues to be used widely for chemotherapy of colorectal and other cancers. And the physical properties of the fluorine atom make fluorinated drugs highly suitable for studies by two of the key imaging technologies. The 2-h ^{18}F isotope allows fluorinated drugs to be studied using positron emission tomography (PET) methods, whereas the natural, 100% abundant ^{19}F nuclide allows the use of nuclear magnetic resonance methods, including NMR spectroscopy (MRS) and imaging (MRI). Such noninvasive studies have been providing a unique insight into the fate of fluoropyrimidines at their target sites and are allowing us to gain a much better understanding of their mechanism of action. These noninvasive methods will allow, when properly used in clinical settings, objective assessments of whether the fluoropyrimidine chosen is likely to be effective in a given patient, as well as the development of a proper strategy for *individualizing* the dose and the dose regimen that is required to *optimize* chemotherapy for a given patient. Furthermore, these same methods can also provide an evidence-based evaluation of fluorinated pyrimidines in development, as well as assess the potential effect of any modulators. And finally, the noninvasive methods and techniques developed for the study of fluoropyrimidines are likely to document the potential of these methodologies for other noninvasive studies that can monitor and assist in the development of other drugs in oncology as well as in other areas of medicine.

From: *Fluoropyrimidines in Cancer Therapy*
Edited by: Y. M. Rustum © Humana Press Inc., Totowa, NJ

Table 1
Comparative Characteristics of Noninvasive ^{18}F and ^{19}F Studies

	^{18}F	^{19}F
Characteristics	Radioactive $t_{1/2}$: 108 min β^+	Natural (stable) 100% abundance Spin 1/2 84% of the NMR sensitivity of ^{1}H at constant field
Method of measurement	PET	MRS
Biological considerations	Best spatial resolution of the commonly used PET radionuclides	Absence of naturally occurring fluorinated compounds
Chemical considerations	No chemical information	Wide chemical shift range (>200 ppm)
Key advantages	Very high sensitivity Ability to quantitate concentrations of products	Exquisite chemical resolution
Main limitations	Products must be radiolabeled In vivo studies are limited to an upper limit of ~12 h Radioactive exposure to patient	Like all NMR methods, poor sensitivity. Compounds must be present in concentrations above 0.1 m*M* to be detectable Macromolecules are "NMR invisible" Very difficult to measure concentrations of products

The readers are also referred to a recent theme issue on Noninvasive Drug Monitoring published in the March 15, 2000 issue of *Advanced Drug Delivery Reviews* 41(1), where many of these issues have been discussed.

The need for measurements using noninvasive imaging methods is based on both theoretical and practical considerations. The rates of change of processes can vary significantly from individual to individual, and even within the same individual, be measurably affected by changes in their physiopathological functions. Thus, measuring such rates of change (kinetics) should be done under conditions that do not *perturb* the process being measured. The second theoretical consideration is that tissues are not necessarily homogeneous, and hence, a small biopsy may, or may not, be properly representative of the tissue being analyzed. And on a practical basis, obtaining serial tissue samples (e.g., biopsies) from patients can be both logistically difficult and traumatic.

Without entering into all the technical details of PET and MRS/MRI studies (the reader will be referred to the relevant publications where pertinent), Table 1 summarizes the relevant characteristics of the two nuclides of fluorine discussed in this chapter. Although both MRS and PET have unique advantages (and limitations), they are two highly complementary techniques, both allowing for the noninvasive studies of the fluorinated drugs in a unique manner.

It is expected that the principles and the methods being developed with the study of fluorinated drugs will be extended, in the not too distant future, to the study of many other drugs.

2. NONINVASIVE STUDIES WITH ^{18}F-5-FU

The idea of studying radiolabeled drugs using the newly developing imaging methods of nuclear medicine evolved when, after the start of the USC Radiopharmacy program in 1968, one of us (W.W.) started considering what noninvasive imaging studies, other than for diagnostic imaging, could or should be done with radioactive nuclides. Labeling biochemicals and drugs with radioactive isotopes of the elements they contain was at the very origin of the biomedical use of radionuclides.

In studies that helped to usher in modern concepts of biochemistry, Calvin et al. (in ref. *1*) used ^{11}C (the isotope of carbon with a half-life of 20 min) to study the process of photosynthesis. Because of the very short half-life of ^{11}C, Kamen et al. *(1)* searched for a longer-lived isotope of carbon and discovered ^{14}C, whose half-life is 5618 yr. Since then, the two most common radioisotopes used in biochemical and pharmacological studies have been ^{14}C and ^{3}H (the radioactive isotope of hydrogen with a half-life of 12.5 yr). However, both these radionuclides are pure β-emitters, a fact that does not allow direct in vivo measurements (using noninvasive imaging) of compounds (drugs, biochemicals) radiolabeled with these β-emitters.

Noninvasive nuclear imaging studies require the use of gamma or positron (β^+) emitters. One choice for the study of drugs was to return to using the short-lived ^{11}C. There are two limitations in the use of this short-lived radionuclide: Its $t_{1/2}$ of 20 min limits the observations to those processes that can be measured during the first approx 2 h ($6 \times t_{1/2}$), and it also requires an in-house cyclotron, in order for the synthesis of the radiolabeled drug to be performed at the same site as where the drug will be studied. In the case of fluorinated drugs, there was the option of using ^{18}F, the 108-min radioisotope of fluorine, also a positron emitter. Discussions with oncologists suggested that studies with a brand new drug then (in the late 1960s) being introduced into cancer treatment and which is, 30 yr later, still widely in use as an antimetabolite, 5-fluorouracil (5-FU) *(2)*, could be of interest. The questions that our oncology colleague Joseph Bateman asked in 1969 were:

1. Why is 5-FU active in some of my patients and not in others?
2. How can I know whether a given patient will respond to treatment with 5-FU?
3. How much 5-FU do I need to give to achieve maximal effect?

It is of some interest that 30 yr later the questions have not changed dramatically. As will be seen in this chapter, noninvasive imaging methods are contributing to generate some of the answers, but have not yet answered all the fundamental questions that need to be understood in order to use this drug (and most others) most effectively.

Having decided to radiolabel 5-FU with ^{18}F, it was obvious that the original synthesis of 5-FU, by Dushinksy and Heidelberger *(3)*, which started with a fluorinated substrate and took over 2 d from start of synthesis to the isolation of the final, pure product, was clearly unsuitable for preparing a compound to be radiolabeled with a nuclide whose $t_{1/2}$ is 108 min. After various attempts in our laboratory and others to introduce ^{18}F into uracil had failed, the Brookhaven group achieved a suitable synthesis of ^{18}F-5-FU *(4)*, which was improved further to allow a 45% yield in 45 min of a sterile, pyrogen-free product of > 99% purity, ready for human use *(5)*. Using this material, Shani and Wolf *(6)* observed that there was a significant difference in the targeting of ^{18}F to the responsive variant of an experimental tumor model, the L-1210 lymphocytic leukemia, over that of the refractory variant of the same tumor model. This observation was the first documented evidence of a direct association, in an animal tumor model, between the degree of targeting of an antitumor drug to a tumor mass and the ability of such tumors to respond to treatment with that drug. The logical conclusion one could draw was that this finding might allow a prediction of whether a given patient would—or would not—be responsive to such chemotherapy.

This initial observation was then followed by extensive animal biodistribution studies *(7,8)* and human imaging studies by our laboratory and in others *(9–16)*. An excellent summary of the current status of human studies using ^{18}F-5-FU has recently been presented by Saleem, Aboagye, and Price *(17)*. As these authors state, following administration of the radiotracer, the serial PET images acquired represent quantitative maps of the concentration of radioactivity (kBq/mL or C) in the tissue, and allow calculation of pharmacokinetic parameters such as peak concentrations (C_{max}), time to reach peak concentrations (T_{max}), area under the concentration–time curve (AUC), and uptake (standardized uptake value; SUV). One study showed that colorectal liver metastases with a higher uptake of 5-FU at 2 h (SUV > 3) had a negative growth rate, whereas those with SUV < 2 showed disease progression. The importance of drug delivery in the initial drug uptake and its retention up to 1 h was underlined by a significant correlation between tumor blood flow and its exposure to ^{18}F radioactivity at 8 and 60 min. Blood flow to the tumor and hence its exposure to ^{18}F activity decreased significantly ($p < 0.05$) after modulation with PALA and a nonsignificant increase was seen with interferon-α. On the other hand, no changes in tumor pharmacokinetics were seen with folinic acid biomodulation.

Although these ^{18}F-studies have (and are) providing a unique insight into the fate of the fluorine-containing compounds in living systems under different conditions, they fail to allow a direct differentiation of which chemical specie(s) is present at any given target site. This is because PET studies measure the total fluorine rather than distinguish between fluorinated compounds. And inasmuch as the metabolism of 5-FU leads to both catabolites and anabolites in varying amounts, a knowledge of which of these chemical compounds is present and of its kinetics is desirable. Because of some of these inherent limitations in the use of ^{18}F for the study of 5-FU, it was desirable to consider alternate methods that would allow noninvasive studies of this drug in living systems. The development of methods, in the late 1970s and early 1980s that allowed the use of the NMR techniques in human studies spurred us to consider the possible use of ^{19}F as a tool to study 5-FU.

3. THE DEVELOPMENT OF THE ^{19}F-MRS METHODS

The natural nuclide of fluorine, ^{19}F, has uniquely suitable NMR properties, as shown in Table 1. The first demonstration that ^{19}F could be used in the study of living animal systems was presented by Stevens et al. *(18)* in 1984, and the first human studies were reported by Wolf et al. shortly thereafter *(19–21)*, as well as by others *(22,23)*. A recent review article summarizes many of technical aspects of the ^{19}F-MRS method *(24)*.

A brief summary of the clinical protocol used in our human ^{19}F-MRS studies of human tumors is as follows:

1. Patient eligibility: Patients with imageable breast, colorectal or other tumors scheduled to receive a fluorinated drug (5-FU, FUR, UFT, capecitabine, gemcitabine, and so on.)
2. Patient exclusions: Patients with pacemakers or ferromagnetic clips, or patients who are claustrophobic.

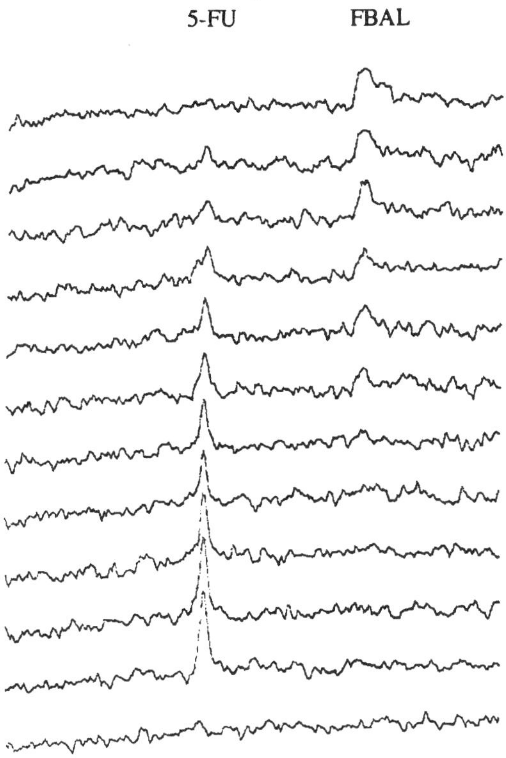

Fig. 1. [9]F-NMR serial spectra of the tumor of a 48-y-old male patient with colorectal cancer metastasized to the liver, following IV administration of a bolus of 5-FU, 600 mg/m^2. A 7-cm diameter surface coil was used to localize the tumor and avoid ^{19}F signals from most of the surrounding nontumoral tissue. The peak at 5.6 ppm is 5-FU and the at –13.5 ppm is that of FBAL (2-fluoro-β-alanine). The external reference peak (not shown), 1,2-difluorobenzene, is at 36.0 ppm.

3. Procedure: Following placement of an IV line to allow for drug administration while in the magnet, patients are positioned in the magnet (e.g., Siemens Magnetom 2T) and imaged to locate their tumor in the isocenter of the magnet.
4. The surface coil, tuned to ^{19}F, whose size is most suitable for the desired tumor to be studied, is selected and placed on the patient as close to the tumor as possible.
5. The frequency is switched to ^{1}H and shimming is performed at 50 Hz or better.
6. The frequency is switched to ^{19}F and background spectra are acquired to determine the presence of any fluorinated products present before drug administration.
7. A bolus of 5-FU (600 mg/m^2) is administered and sequential spectra (256 FIDs, TR = 1000 ms) are acquired for at least 30–60 min. This allows the determination of the tumoral $t_{1/2}$ of 5-FU in that tumor.
8. The peak heights and the peak areas are measured, and suitable curve-fitting programs analyze their kinetics.

For studies at other organ or tissue sites, such as the liver, the surface coil is placed over that organ. Figure 1 illustrates the time course of the ^{19}F-NMR signals obtained from a patient with colorectal cancer metastasized to the liver.

4. NONINVASIVE STUDIES OF 5-FU IN THE LIVER

The initial human studies using the ^{19}F-MRS method had shown that fluorinated drugs could be readily measured in the liver of patients treated with 5-FU. Subsequent studies revealed that the metabolism of 5-FU in human livers differed significantly from that of 5-FU in rodents *(25)*. Figure 2 illustrates the metabolism of 5-FU using a compartmental model approach. Kinetically, most of the administered drug is cleared rapidly from the blood *(26)* and taken up by the liver. A study by Li et al. *(27)* demonstrated the ability to quantitate the kinetics of 5-FU and of its metabolites in the livers of patients, allowing for better correlation of 5-FU catabolism with drug toxicity. A recent study *(28)* has documented the importance of the functional status of the gallbladder in understanding the catabolism of 5-FU in patients. It is of interest that we had previously suggested, in our first human noninvasive studies of 5-FU using ^{18}F *(8,10)*, that an enterohepatic recirculation of 5-FU could be observed in some patients.

The growing interest in modulation of 5-FU using metabolic blockers, such as ethynyluracil *(29)*, strengthens the desirability of using either or both ^{18}F-PET and ^{19}F-MRS to measure noninvasively in patients the role of liver metabolism of 5-FU in that specific patient and thereby to achieve a better control of the potential toxicity of this drug.

5. PHARMACOKINETIC IMAGING OF 5-FU: BASIC CONSIDERATIONS

The most relevant information obtained in the initial ^{18}F-animal studies was that there was, potentially, a direct correlation between the level of 5-FU and its metabolites that had targeted to the tumor mass with the antitumor effectiveness of the administered drug. However, because such noninvasive PET methods measure the sum of all the fluorinated compounds present in a given region-of-interest (ROI), further analysis of PET data required the estimations using various types of models. Figure 2 is a representation, using a compartmental model approach, of the key aspects of the metabolism and the biodistribution of 5-FU. It must be stressed that although the model illustrated in Fig. 2 is a simplification, it also is much too complex for its use in compartmental analysis. Further simplifications are required to allow for models where meaningful parameters can be estimated.

When 5-FU is administred by the iv route, whether as a bolus or as an infusion, it enters into the systemic blood pool, represented as compartment **[1]**. The free drug will then be transported, as the free drug, to the tumor **[2–4]**, to the liver **[7]**, to the kidneys **[11]**, and to a number of other organs and tissues **[8]**. Although these transport processes appear to be reversible, the exact mechanisms regulating 5-FU transport are not yet fully understood. In a simplified manner, one can state that the fate of 5-FU in the liver is primarily catabolic, whereas in the tumor 5-FU may be converted to its active, cytotoxic anabolites. And the tumor is itself a complex environment with at least three distinct environments: the tumoral blood pool, the interstitial fluid space, and the intracellular space. Again, using a simplified approach, free 5-FU in the systemic blood pool moves into the tumoral blood pool **[2]** and from there into the tumoral interstitial fluid space **[3]**. The flux of 5-FU is illustrated more specifically in Fig. 3. Jain et al. *(30–33)* have highlighted the importance and the uniqueness of the interstitial fluid space in the tumor. The absence of lymphatic drainage results in significant variability of osmotic pressure in the tumor that affects the movement of drugs, such as 5-FU, and the active anaerobic glycolysis of tumors results in a significant degree of lactic acidosis in the interestitial fluid space *(34)*, the known "acidification" of tumors *(35)*. Work by Stubbs et al. *(36)*, using in vivo ^{31}P-NMR, has documented this by showing that the intracellular space is at physiological or even slightly basic pH.

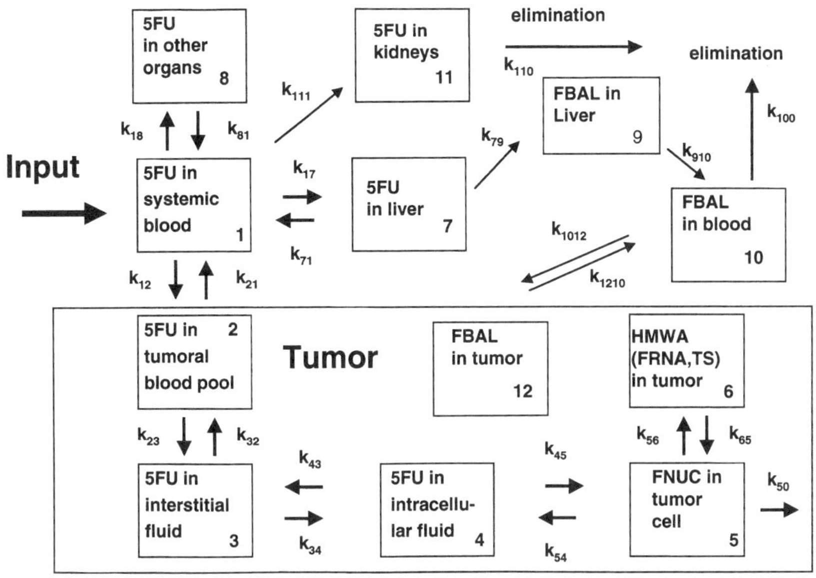

Fig. 2. 12-compartment Flow Chart for 5FU; systemic input, 22 rates. This conceptual, simplified diagram highlights the fate of free 5-FU in tumor patients.

The transport of free 5-FU from the interstitial fluid space into the cellular space appears to be an active process *(37–40)*, apparently by using the EI nucleoside transporter *(41)*. A better knowledge of the transport mechanism may be very useful in enhancing the activity of 5-FU in selected tumors by the use of suitable modulators of drug transport.

The two noninvasive methods of measurement, using ^{18}F-PET and ^{19}F-MRS, provide different data. ^{18}F-PET measures the sum of all the fluorinated compounds present in the tumor, and because of the relatively high sensitivity of nuclear measurements, allows quantitation of the sum of products down to the submicromolar level, provided proper care is taken in such measurements *(42)*. ^{19}F-MRS measurements are both much more selective but much less sensitive. The concentrations of fluorinated compounds need to be near the millimolar level to be detected in a given ROI.

6. TUMORAL PHARAMACOKINETICS OF 5-FU USING ^{18}F MEASUREMENTS

A different conceptual 12-compartment model of describing the transport and the metabolism of 5-FU was proposed by Kissel et al. *(43)*. Their model assumes that the concentration of 5-FU in systemic plasma and in the microvascular space of the tumor is equivalent, an assumption that may not be entirely correct depending on the degree of interstitial pressure in a particular tumor mass. Using the data obtained from a noninvasive PET study following administration of 8–23 mCi of ^{18}F-5FU, Kissel et al. *(43)* estimated various pharmacokinetic parameters by using a simplified six-compartment model with 10 parameters. They estimated the hepatic and extrahepatic clearance of 5-FU, the rate of conversion of 5-FU into FBAL, as well as the rates of transport of the fluorinated materials into and out of the metastatic sites measured. They concluded that the latter two parameters (k_{in} and k_{out}) were the most sensitive to predict response to chemotheraphy, and that trapping occurs when k_{in} is high and k_{out} is low.

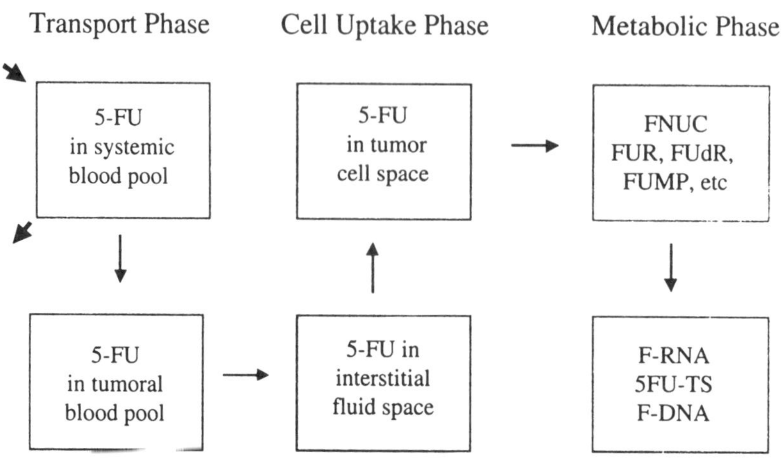

Fig. 3. Schematic representation of the flux of free 5-FU to and inside a solid tumor and of its biotransformation products in the tumor mass.

Other studies using ^{18}F-5-FU have been discussed by Saleem et al. *(17),* and their work on the effect of modulators on the pharmacokinetics of 5-FU will be discussed below.

The main limitation in the use of ^{18}F-5-FU for pharmacokinetic studies is that all the in vivo measurements provide a sum of various products (5-FU and all its metabolites), with no distinction whether the product(s) detected are active or inactive materials. Nevertheless, the sensitivity of the use of ^{18}F-labeled products suggests that their combined use with the chemical information provided by the much less sensitive ^{19}F-MRS method may, at some time, allow for the direct estimate of the tumoral pharmacokinetics of the active anabolites of 5-FU.

7. TUMORAL PHARMACOKINETICS OF 5-FU USING ^{19}F MEASUREMENTS

While very suitable for measuring, current NMR spectroscopic methods make it very difficult to measure accurately absolute drug concentrations because of the shape of the field-of- view seen by the surface coils, that of an inverted cone *(44).* This precluded the ability to estimate drug concentrations directly and suggested that measuring the *rates of change* of the ^{19}F-signals would yield more robust data. The work from our group focused on determining those kinetic parameters that could be estimated when the exact values of concentrations were not measurable.

There are two main features that require kinetic measurements to be performed noninvasively, rather than making them only desirable and convenient:

1. Kinetic measurements will only be reliable when the system is not perturbed during the process of measurement.
2. When measuring the effect of modulators (activators or inhibitors), interpatient variability is such that kinetic measurements will only be reliable when each patient serves as his/her own control.

The initial studies measuring the kinetics of ^{19}F-5-FU in tumors suggested that there was a bimodal distribution in the kinetics of 5-FU. Some patients exhibited a long tumoral $t_{1/2}$ of 5-FU—e.g., appeared to retain or trap 5-FU—whereas in others the tumoral $t_{1/2}$ was much shorter. The current data on the association between clinical response to 5-FU bolus treat-

Table 2
Association Between the Tumoral $t_{1/2}$ of 5-FU and Clinical Response to 5-FU Bolus Treatment

Tumoral $t_{1/2}$ of 5-FU	*Responders*	*Nonresponders*
$t_{1/2} < 20$ min (Nontrappers)	0	31
$t_{1/2} \geq 20$ min (Trappers)	17	12

ment and response are shown in Table 2, where response is measured using the criterion of a 50% reduction in bidimensionally measured tumor area *(45)*. The association between trapping and response $p < 0.000001$, using Fisher's exact tables *(46)*. And in a related study where, following the long-term infusion of 5-FU, Findlay et al. *(22)* measured the long-term retention of free 5-FU in tumors, a similar association was observed between the retention parameter and response, albeit with a lower probability value ($p = 0.017$).

What are the potential consequences that can be drawn from such an association between trapping and response? For one, that patients who do not trap 5-FU following administration of 5-FU as a bolus of 600 mg/m^2 do not appear to respond to chemotherapy using 5-FU or 5-FU plus leucovorin. Thus, this appears to be a necessary, but apparently not a sufficient condition. As can be seen from the data of Table 2, some of the patients who trapped 5-FU did not respond. What could be the reasons? We have proposed *(24)* that for 5-FU to be effective in a given tumor mass three conditions need to be met concurrently:

1. The molecular nature of the tumor cell needs to be suitable for response to 5-FU.
2. The perfusion of the tumor mass needs to be sufficient so as to allow an adequate amount of 5-FU to reach the tumor cells.
3. The pharmacokinetics of free 5-FU in the tumor need to be sufficiently long (e.g., with a $t_{1/2}$ of 20 min or longer) for 5-FU to have a sufficient presence to allow its conversion to its active anabolites (FdUMP, F-RNA, and so on).

Although the ^{19}F-MRS method is currently the only technique that allows for a direct measure of the tumoral pharmacokinetics of free 5-FU, we have proposed the use of MRI contrast agents as a means of measuring the initial blood flow/perfusion of tumors, and thereby, whether a sufficient and necessary amount of drugs such as 5-FU will be deliverable to the tumor mass. These dynamic MRI studies using the DEMRI (Dynamic Enhanced MRI) method *(47,48)* have documented the significant functional heterogeneity of human tumors and allow a simple measurement of whether a given tumor mass in a given patient is perfused—whether well or poorly.

The third condition that needs to be met, that the molecular nature of the tumor is suitable for response to 5-FU, has not been measured noninvasively at this time owing to the low concentrations of the target molecules. Methods need to be developed to make this possible inasmuch as reliance on biopsy specimens has severe limitations. Biopsy specimens are not always readily available, they do not generally provide data on the spatial heterogeneity inside a tumor mass, and they do not allow measures of how a given treatment has affected the expression of various enzymes inside a rapidly changing tumor mass.

Notwithstanding these limitations, pharmacokinetic imaging studies using ^{19}F-MRS do provide useful information on the pathophysiology of a given tumor mass, and should be used much more widely to identify those patients likely to respond and those highly unlikely to do so, as well as those patients whose tumors may be modified by suitable modulations.

8. STUDIES ON THE MODULATION OF 5-FU

Experimental studies had shown that certain agents would enhance the action of 5-FU, and a number of such drug combinations are used clinically. Methotrexate (MTX) is a drug that has been used widely as a modulator of the action of 5-FU *(49)*. Its putative mode of action as a modulator was to inhibit the formation of purines, thereby making more phospho-ribosyl-pyrophosphate available for the conversion of 5-FU into of 5-FUR and 5-FdUR and their nucleotides *(50)*. We had shown in animal studies that while the rate of conversion of 5-FU into its nucleotides increased 2.5 times in tumors of rats having been administered MTX 5 h before, the rate of transfer of 5-FU changed by more than three orders of magnitude *(51)*. Others *(52,53)* obtained similar results. These results suggest that the modulatory action of MTX on 5-FU occurred both at the transport and at the metabolic phases, rather than solely at the metabolic phase. The modulatory effect of MTX to enhance the transport process has now also been documented in human studies *(52)*.

Table 3 summarizes our studies measuring the modulatory effect of MTX, interferon, and trimetrexate (TMTX) in a limited number of patients (pilot studies). These results indicate a prolongation of the $t_{1/2}$ of 5-FU in the human tumors studied induced by interferon, MTX, and in two of the five patients treated with TMTX. In order to understand the possible role of modulators of 5-FU, it is important to consider the flux of 5-FU into and inside the tumor, as illustrated in Fig. 3. Free 5-FU, whether administered systemically or absorbed orally, will enter the tumoral space throught the vascular space of the tumor, diffuse into the interstitial fluid space, and then be transported into the tumor cell. Agents that alter blood flow and perfusion can affect (modulate) the delivery of 5-FU to the tumoral space, agents that affect membrane transport can modulate the entry of 5-FU into the tumoral space, and agents that affect the metabolism of 5-FU will modulate its conversion and the stability of its active anabolites. We have recently shown that leucovorin has no apparent effect on the tumoral pharmacokinetics of 5-FU *(53)*, presumably because its effect on the stabilization of the 5-FU-TS ternary complex does not affect the kinetics of free 5-FU in the tumor.

The mechanism by which the interferons modulate the action of 5-FU is not yet clear. Although it has been postulated that the mechanism of the modulatory action of IFN-α is on 5-FU-mediated DNA damage, no mechanism of action of IFN-gamma could be determined in colon cancer cell studies *(54)*. Inasmuch as studies by ourselves and by the Royal Marsden group have shown significant variations in the tumoral pharmacokinetics of 5-FU following interferon treatment, it would appear that interferon may affect, by processes still not identified, the transport into and/or the retention of 5-FU in the tumor cell. Further noninvasive studies should therefore help in understanding the mechanism of modulation and whether such an effect, and the extent thereof, occurs in a specific patient.

The importance of the effect of how 5-FU is delivered to tumors is illustrated further by studies performed measuring the effect of a loco-regional administration of 5-FU *(55)*. The intralesional injection of 30 mg of 5-FU into basal cell tumors resulted in a very significant local concentration of the tumor, whose retention in the tumor mass could be enhanced further by the coadministration of a vasoconstrictor (epinephrine), thereby retaining 5-FU in the tumor mass for a considerably long time. The report by Menei et al. *(56)* that 5-FU could be delivered to the cerebrospinal space and retained there for a long time is another observation that highlights the importance of drug delivery processes in ensuring proper availability of 5-FU at its target site(s).

Table 3
Comparative Tumoral Pharmacokinetic Parameters of Cancer Patients Treated Either with 5-FU+interferon-α2a, with 5-FU and MTX (High Dose) and with tr TMTX

Patient Number	*Sex and age*	*Primary metastases*	*Site of tumor metastases*	*Modulator used*	*$T_{1/2}$ of 5-FU control (min)*	*$T_{1/2}$ of 5-FU after modulator (min)*	*Change in $T_{1/2}$*	*Clinical response*	*Time to progression (mo)*	*Survival (mo)*
57	F 49	Colon	Liver	IFα2a	18.8	26.5	41.0%	Partial	5	11
68	M 80	Colon	Liver	IFα2a	42.0	54.7	30.2%	Partial	4	6
73	F 68	Colon	Liver	IFα2a	36.0	38.0	5.6%	Progression	1	4
42	M 59	Gastric	Liver	MTX	29.2*	28.6*	13.5%	Progression	1	3
60	F 64	Gastric	Liver	MTX	42.3	60.0	41.8%	Progression	1	2
129	M76	Colon	Liver	TMTX	15.6	30.1	93%	Partial	7	12
132	M48	Colon	Liver	TMTX	14.8	26.2	77%	Progression	2.5	9
133	M74	Colon	Liver	TMTX	28.3	27.7	NSD	Progression	4	14
135	M48	Tailgut	Liver	TMTX	13.9	14.4	NSD	Stable	4	5.5
138	M71	Gastric	Liver	TMTX	19.3	20.2	NSD	Stable	4	19

* The α-half lives for patient #42 were 2.9 and 7.3 min, with a change of 150% in the $t_{1/2}$.

9. OVERALL CONCLUSIONS AND FUTURE DIRECTIONS

The results summarized in this chapter illustrate some of the achievements to date using noninvasive methods. Both noninvasive methods (^{19}F-MRS and ^{18}F-PET) have advantages and limitations. Both methods should be used more actively in clinical research and in clinical practice. The strength of the ^{18}F-PET studies lies in its very high sensitivity and ability to quantitate, whereas that of ^{19}F-MRS in its ability to identify the specific chemical species present at any time in the study.

The noninvasive methods provide objective (evidence-based) measurements on the fate of 5-FU in a given subject. They can therefore help in understanding the mechanisms of action of this drug, thereby guiding its proper use. They can assess whether a combination of 5-FU and other drugs act synergistically or additively, and the degree to which the targeting of 5-FU to tumors occurs in a given individual. And, perhaps most importantly, they can be used to predict whether a given patient is likely to respond to chemotherapy and to monitor whether the effect of treatment is changing the tumoral characteristics and how long a given tumor remains responsive to treatment with 5-FU.

Noninvasive methods may thereby both help to individualize chemotherapy and to enhance the effectiveness of this drug by allowing administration of the correct dose and dose rate needed by a given patient.

REFERENCES

1. Kamen MD, *Isotopic Tracers in Biology*, Academic Press, New York, 1957.
2. Ansfield FJ, Ramirez G, Mackman S, Bryan GT, Curreri AR. *Cancer Res* 1969;29:1062–1066.
3. Duschinsky R, Pleven E, Heidelberger C. The synthesis of 5- Fluoropyrimidines. *J Am Chem Soc* 1959;79:4559–4560.
4. Fowler JS, Finn RD, Lambrecht RM, Wolf AP. The synthesis of ^{18}F-5-Fluorouracil *J Nucl Med* 1973;14:63–64.
5. Vine EN, Young D, Vine WH, Wolf W. An Improved Synthesis of ^{18}F-5-Fluorouracil. *Int J Appl Radn Isotop* 1979;30:401–405.
6. Shani J, Wolf W. A Model of Prediction of Chemotherapy Response to 5-FU in Sensitive versus Resistant Lymphocytic Leukemia in Mice. *Cancer Res* 1977;37:2306–2308.
7. Shani J, Wolf W, Schlesinger T, et al. Distribution of ^{18}F-5-Fluorouracil in Tumor Bearing Mice and Rats. Int. *J Nucl Med Biol* 1978;5:19–28.
8. Young D, Vine E, Ghanbarpour A, Shanti J, Siemsen JK, Wolf W, et al. Metabolic and Distribution Studies with Radiolabeled 5-Fluorouracil. *Nucl Med* 1982;21:1–7.
9. Lieberman LM, Wessels BW, Wiley AL, Jr et al. ^{18}F-5-fluorouracil studies in human's and animals. *International Journal of Radiation Oncology, Biology, Physics* 1980;6:505–509.
10. Young D. Radiopharmacokinetic Model Development and Structural Identification Ph.D. Dissertation, University of Southern California, Los Angeles, CA. 1983.
11. Shani J, Young D, Siemsen JK, et al. (1982) Dosimetry and Preliminary Human Studies of ^{18}F-5FU. *Int J Nucl Med Biol* 1982;9:25–35.
12. Port RE, Strauss LG, Clorius JH. Positron emission tomography following brief infusion of 5-[18F]uracil: linear model for the kinetics of ^{18}F radioactivity in tumors. *Onkologie* 1989;12 Suppl 1:51–52.
13. Dimitrakopoulou A, Strauss LG, Clorius JH, et al. Studies with positron emission tomography after systemic administration of fluorine-18-uracil in patients with liver metastases from colorectal carcinoma. *J Nucl Med* 1993;34:1075–1081.
14. Kissel J, Brix G, Bellemann ME, et al. Pharmacokinetic analysis of 5-[^{18}F]fluorouracil tissue concentrations measured with positron emission tomography in patients with liver metastases from colorectal adenocarcinoma. *Cancer Res* 1997; 57:3415–3423.
15. Harte RJ, Matthews JC, O'Reilly, SM, et al. Tumor, normal tissue, and plasma pharmacokinetic studies of fluorouracil biomodulation with N-phosphonacetyl-L-aspartate, folinic acid, and interferon alfa. *J Clin Oncol* 1999; 17:1580–1588.
16. Saleem A, Yap J, Osman S, et al. Modulation of fluorouracil tissue pharmacokinetics by eniluracil: in-vivo imaging of drug action. *Lancet* 2000; 355:2125–2131.

17. Saleem A, Aboagye EO, Price PM. In Vivo Monitoring of Drugs Using Radiotracer Techniques. *Adv Drug Deliv Revs* 2000; 41:21–39.
18. Stevens, AN, Morris, PG, Iles, RA, Sheldon, PW, Griffiths, JR 5-Fluorouracil metabolism monitored *in vivo* by ^{19}F NMR *Br J Cancer* 1984; 50:113–117.
19. Wolf W, Griffiths JR, Silver MS Bruckner H Can NMR Contribute to the Radiopharmacokinetics of 5-Fluorouracil (5-FU) in Man?. *J Nucl Med* 1986; 27:737.
20. Wolf W, Albright MJ, Silver MS, et al. Fluorine-19 NMR Spectroscopic Studies of the Metabolism of 5-Fluorouracil in the Liver of Patients Undergoing Chemotherapy Mag *Reson Imaging,* 1987; 5:165–169.
21. Wolf W, Presant CA, Servis KL, et al. Tumor Trapping of 5-Fluorouracil: in vivo ^{19}F-NMR Spectroscopic Pharmacokinetics in Tumor-bearing Humans and rabbits.. *Proc Natl Acad Sci* 1990; 87:492–496.
22. Findlay MPN, Leach MO, Cunningham D, et al. The noninvasive monitoring of low-dose, infusional 5-Fluorouracil and its modulation by interferon-alpha using in vivo F-19 Magnetic Resonance Spectroscopy in Patients with Colorectal Cancer. A Pilot study. *Ann Oncol,* 1993; 4:597–602.
23. Schlemmer HP, Bachert P, Semmler W, et al. Drug monitoring of 5-fluorouracil: in vivo ^{19}F NMR study during 5-FU chemotherapy in patients with metastases of colorectal adenocarcinoma. *Magn Reson Imaging* 1994; 12:497–511.
24. Wolf W, Presant CA, Waluch V. ^{19}F-MRS Studies of Fluorinated Drugs in Humans. *Adv Drug Deliv Revs* 2000; 41:55–74.
25. El-Tahtawy A, Wolf W. Tumor Pharmacokinetics of 5-Fluorouracil (5FU) in rats using noninvasive ^{19}F NMR spectroscopy (NMRS). *Proc AACR* 1990; 31:383 (#2273).
26. Cohen J, Irwin LE, Marshall JG. et al. Clinical Pharmacology of Oral and Intravenous 5-Fluorouracil (NSC 19893). *Cancer Chemo Repts* 1974; 58:723–731.
27. Li CW, Negendank WG, Padavic-Shaller KA, et al. Quantitation of 5-fluorouracil catabolism in human liver in vivo by three-dimensional localized ^{19}F magnetic resonance spectroscopy. *Clin Cancer Res* 1996; 2:339–345.
28. Dzik-Jurasz ASK, Collins DJ, Leach MO, et al. Gallbladder localization of ^{19}F MRS Catabolite Signals in Patients Receiving Bolus and Protracted Venous Infusional 5-Fluorouracil. *Mag Reson Med* 2000; 44:516–520.
29. Adams ER, Leffert JJ, Craig DJ, Spector T, Pizzorno G. *In vivo* effect of 5-ethynyluracil on 5-fluorouracil metabolism determined by ^{19}F nuclear magnetic resonance spectroscopy. *Cancer Res* 1999; 59:122–127.
30. Leu AJ, Berk DA, Lymboussaki A, et al. Absence of functional lymphatics within a murine sarcoma: a molecular and functional evaluation. *Cancer Research* 2000; 60:4324–4327.
31. Stohrer M, Boucher Y, Stangassinger M, et al. Oncotic pressure in solid tumors is elevated. *Cancer Research* 2000; 60:4251–4255.
32. Swartz MA, Kaipainen A, Netti PA, et al. Mechanics of interstitial-lymphatic fluid transport: theoretical foundation and experimental validation. *J Biomech* 1999; 32:1297–1307.
33. Hobbs SK, Monsky WL, Yuan F, et al. Regulation of transport pathways in tumor vessels: role of tumor type and microenvironment. *Proc Nat Acad Sci* 1998; 95:4607–4612.
34. Vallabhajosula S, Harwig JF, Wolf W. Effect of pH on Tumor Uptake of Gallium *in vitro* and *in vivo.* European *J Nucl Med* 1982; 7:462–468.
35. Gerweck LE. Tumor pH: implications for treatment and novel drug design. *Seminars Radiat Oncol* 1998; 8:176–182.
36. McCoy CL, Parkins CS, Chaplin DJ, Griffiths JR, Rodrigues LM, Stubbs M. The effect of blood flow modification on intra- and extracellular pH measured by ^{31}P magnetic resonance spectroscopy in murine tumours. *Brit J Cancer* 1995; 72:905–911.
37. Wohlhuetter RM, McIvor RS, Plagemann PGW. Facilitated transport of uracil and 5-fluorouracil, and permeation of orotic acid into cultured mammalian cells. *J. Cell. Phys.* 1980; 104:309–319.
38. Yamamoto S, Kawasaki T. Active Transport of 5-Fluorouracil and Its Energy Coupling in Ehrlich Ascites Tumor Cells. *J Biochem* 1981; 90:635–642.
39. AS, McSheehy PM, Stubbs M, Alder G, et al. Influence of pH on the uptake of 5-fluorouracil into isolated tumour cells. *Brit J Cancer* 1998; 77:873–879.
40. Ikonte C, Wolf W. The transport of 5-Fluorouracil (5-FU) into tumor cells as an active process: studies with Walker 256 tumor cells. *Proc Am Assoc Cancer Res* 2000; 41:492.
41. Ikonte C, Wolf W. Mechanism of the active transport of 5-Fluorouracil (5-FU) into Walker 256 tumor cells. *Proceeding AACR:*294 (#1585), 2001.
42. Harte RJ, Matthews JC, O'Reilly SM Price PM. Sources of error in tissue and tumor measurements of 5-[^{18}F]fluorouracil. *J Nucl Med* 1998; 39:1370–1376.

43. Kissel J, Brix G, Bellemann ME, et al. Pharmacokinetic analysis of 5-[^{18}F]fluorouracil tissue concentrations measured with positron emission tomography in patients with liver metastases from colorectal adenocarcinoma. *Cancer Res* 1997; 57:3415–3423.
44. Schnall M. Probes tuned to multiple frequencies for *in-vivo* NMR. In *In-Vivo Magnetic Resonance Spectroscopy I. Probeheads and Radiofrequency Spectrum Analysis.* Springer Verlag, Berlin, Heidelberg, New York.
45. Green SJ, Weiss GR. Southwest Oncology Group standard response criteria, endpoint definitions and toxicity criteria. *Investigational New Drugs* 1992; 10:239–253.
46. AE Maxwell, "Analysing Quantitative Data", Methuen & Co., London, 1971.
47. Taylor JS, Reddick WE. Evolution from Empirical Dyamic Contrast-Enhanced Magnetic Resonance Imaging to Pharmacokinetic MRI. *Adv Drug Deliv Revs* 2000; 41:91–110.
48. Wolf W, Waluch V, Kim HK, Presant CA, Dowell JA, Sancho AR. DEMRI and Pharmacokinetic Analysis in the Study of Blood Flow/ Perfusion: its Potential for Measuring Drug Targeting and Angiogenesis/Antiangiogenesis. *Proc Am Assoc Cancer Res* 1999; 40:419 (#2769).
49. Machov D. The pharmacological modulation of 5-FU with folinic acid methotrexate trimetrexate and m-phosphonacetyl-1-aspartic acid (PALA) mechanisms of the interactions and clinical data. *Bull Cancer 9 Supp* 1994; 2:74s–78s.
50. Cadman E, Heimer R, Davis L. Enhanced 5-FU nucleotide formation after MTX administration: explanation for drug synergism. *Science* 1979; 205:1135–1137.
51. El-Tahtawy A, Wolf W. *In Vivo* Measurements of the Intratumoral Metabolism, Modulation and Pharmacokinetics of 5-Fluorouracil, using ^{19}F-Nuclear Magnetic Resonance Spectroscopy. *Cancer Research* 1991; 51:5806–5812.
52. Presant CA, Wolf W, Waluch V, Wiseman CL, Weitz I, Shani J. Enhancement of 5-Fluorouracil Uptake in Human Colorectal and Gastric Cancers, by Interferon or by High-Dose Methotrexate – An *In Vivo* Human Study Using Noninvasive ^{19}F-Magnetic Resonance Spectroscopy. *J Clin Oncol* 2000; 18:255–261.
53. Presant CA, Jacobson J, Wolf W, Waluch V, Weitz I, Macdonald J. Does leucovorin alter the intratumoral pharmacokinetics of 5-Fluorouracil (5-FU)? A Southwest Oncology Group Study. Submitted for publication.
54. van der Wilt CL, Smid K, Aherne GW, Noordhuis P, Peters GJ. Biochemical mechanisms of interferon modulation of 5-fluorouracil activity in colon cancer cells. *Europ J Cancer* 1997; 33:471–478.
55. Wolf W, Waluch V, Kim HK, et al. Noninvasive ^{19}F Magnetic Resonance Spectroscopy to Evaluate Tumoral Pharmacokinetics of AccuSite™ (Fluorouracil/ Epinephrine) Injectable Gel for Treatment of Human Basal Cell Carcinoma. *AACR Proceedings* 1995; 36:365 (#2174).
56. Menei P, Venier M-C, Gamelin E, et al. Local and Sustained Delivery of 5-Fluorouracil from Biodegradable Microspheres for the Radiosensitization of Glioblastoma A Pilot Study *Cancer* 1999; 86:325–330.

10 Comparative Antitumor Activity of 5-Fluorouracil (5-FU) Prodrugs in Preclinical Model Systems

Role of Leucovorin and Dihydropyrimidine Dehydrogenase Inhibitors

Shousong Cao, MD, *Gunnar Hapke,* PhD, MD, *and Youcef M. Rustum,* PhD

Contents

1. INTRODUCTION

Over the last two decades, attempts have been made to improve the efficacy of 5-fluorouracil (5-FU) by either schedule or biochemical modulation. Among the changes of particular importance in schedule of administration has been the use of prolonged infusion *(1)*. Several studies have investigated different schedules for 5-FU administration including bolus administration up to 5 d, protracted infusion over weeks, continuous infusion over a period of 24 h, or a combination of both continuous and bolus administration *(2)*. A meta-analysis was carried out on all randomized trials and have shown that if 5-FU is used alone, continuous infusion induces more tumor regression than bolus regimens, prolongs the time to disease progression, but the difference on the impact on survival is not significant *(3)*. Clinical data, however, demonstrated similar results when protracted infusion of 5-FU was compared (historically) with 5-FU modulated by leucovorin (LV).

Several drugs have been used as biochemical modulators in order to increase the therapeutic index of 5-FU. This includes LV, methotrexate, 5-enyluracil, and 5-chlorodihydropyrimidine. Overall the results indicated greater tumor regression compared to 5-FU alone. However, this has not been translated clinically into significant survival benefit *(4)*.

The survival benefit achieved with the current 5-FU-based regimens is modest and thus investigations are ongoing to identify more effective agents with novel mechanisms of action. Recently, new cytotoxic drugs are emerging with antitumor activity similar or superior to 5-FU-based chemotherapy. Two agents, namely oxaliplatin and CPT-11 (irinotecan),

From: *Fluoropyrimidines in Cancer Therapy*
Edited by: Y. M. Rustum © Humana Press Inc., Totowa, NJ

are used together with 5-FU and LV and improved treatment results in patients with advanced colorectal cancer were reported. In addition, a rationally designed 5-FU prodrug, Xeloda (capecitabine) was recently developed and evaluated in several preclinical model systems. Also, it was FDA approved in patients with either breast or colorectal cancer. 5-FU prodrugs were designed based on differential expression of metabolic enzymes associated with activation of prodrugs, namely, thymidine/uridine phosphorylase and catabolic enzyme, dihydropyrimidine dehydrogenase (DPD). The levels of the enzymes as well as the target enzyme, thymidylate synthase have been associated with response to 5-FU based therapy *(5,6)*. Oral 5-FU prodrugs appear to have the same activity as 5-FU and LV and may replace the intravenous administration in certain patients *(7)*.

1.2. Thymidylate Synthase (TS)

TS catalyzes intracellular the *de novo* formation of thymidine-5′-monophosphate from dioxyuridine monophosphate (dUMP). During this process a methyl group is transferred from the reduced folate cofactor 5, 10-methylene tetrahydrofolate to the carbon 5 position of uracil moiety. Inhibition of TS leads to depletion of deoxythymidine triphosphate (dTTP) thus interfering with DNA synthesis and repair *(8)*. In contrast to the interaction between TS and its physiological substrate, the TS–FdUMP–folate complex is only slowly reversible *(9)*. The stability of the ternary complex is influenced by the intracellular levels of folate.

1.3. Dihydropyrimidine Dehydrogenase (DPD)

Dihydropyrimidine dehydrogenase (also known as dihydrouracil dehydrogenase, dihydrothymidine dehydrogenase, uracil reductase) is the initial rate-limiting enzymatic step in the catabolism of not only the naturally occurring pyrimidines but also the widely used antimetabolite, 5-FU. It converts over 85% of the administrated 5-FU to dihydrofluorouracil, which is an inactive metabolite *(10)*. It has recently been shown to play a critical role in determining the clinical pharmacology of 5-FU. It also accounts for the variability that has been noted in clinical studies with 5-FU whether intrapatient or inpatient. DPD activity was found to follow a circadian rhythm in both animals and humans.

Although most patients tolerate 5-FU reasonably well, a number of patients have developed severe, life-threatening toxicities after standard doses of 5-FU. Subsequent studies showed that many of these patients might have an enzyme deficiency *(11)*. The variability in DPD levels may provide a basis to consider either altering the dose of fluoropyrimidines or inhibiting DPD. So, the presence of increased tumor DPD levels might lead to increasing the level of 5-FU to overcome the increased catabolism within the tumor. Another approach is to use a DPD inhibitor in combination with fluoropyrimidines *(12)*.

1.4. Thymidine Phosphorylase (TP)

TP is a key enzyme for the phosphorylation of pyrimidine in DNA synthesis. TP catalyzes the reversible phosphorylation of thymidine and subsequent production of thymidine and 2′-deoxy-D-ribose in the salvage pathway of pyrimidine synthesis *(13)*. Higher activity of the enzyme has been found in malignant cells compared with normal tissue cells *(14)*. Furthermore, it exerts a significant influence on the effects of 5-FU. In vitro data suggest that high level of TP correlate with the enhanced response to fluoropyrimidines *(15)*. TP is identical to platelet-derived endothelial cell growth factor, the enzymatic function of which promotes both angiogenic and cell motility function necessary for growth and progression of malignancy *(16)*. The association of TP expression with increased intratumoral angiogenesis; microvessel density and vascular endothelial growth factor (VEGF) has been verified in studies in breast,

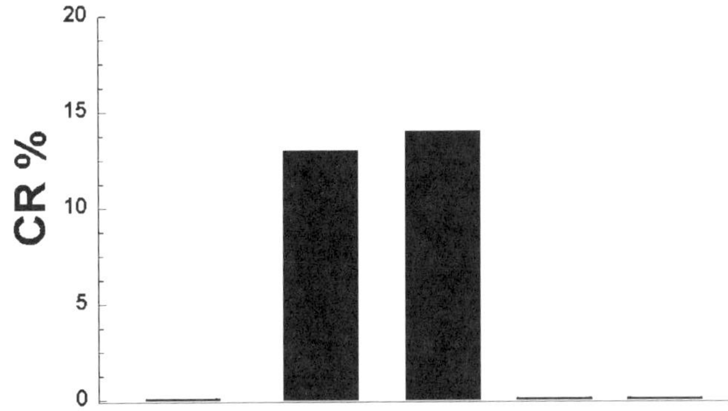

Fig. 1. Antitumor activity of different 5-FU schedules in rats bearing Ward colon tumor. Shown is the induction of complete remission (CR) using five different schedules at their maximal tolerated dosages (MTD): **(A)** 35 mg/kg/day, d 1–5 iv push (d × 5); **(B)** 100 mg/kg/week, once weekly iv push for 3 consecutive weeks (wk × 3); **(C)** 35 mg/kg/day, continuous infusion day 1–4 (c.i. × 4 d); **(D)** 15 mg/kg/d, continuous infusion day 1–14 (c.i. × 14 d); **(E)** 12.5 mg/kg/d, continuous infusion day 1–28 (c.i. × 28d). The animals were observed for at least 2 more months after induction of CR. The data are combined from three to five independent experiments, 12–20 rats in total for each experimental group.

lung, and colorectal cancer. Also, it has been suggested that TP may confer aggressive tumor behavior through pathways not necessarily linked to the intratumoral vascularization, so the role of this enzyme in defining prognosis and response is multifactorial *(17)*.

1.5. Role of 5-FU Treatment Schedule

For nearly three decades 5-FU-based chemotherapy has been the mainstay of choice for the systemic and/or regional treatment of patients with advanced colorectal and gastrointestinal cancers *(18–20)*. Three schedules of 5-FU administration have been utilized clinically: daily, weekly and 4d continuous iv infusion schedules *(1,21–25)*. These schedules were evaluated at their respective maximum tolerated doses (MTD) against rats bearing advanced colorectal cancer (3 gm). The data in Fig. 1 indicate that complete tumor remission (CR) was only achieved with the weekly and 5 d continuous iv infusion. With all other schedules, partial responses (>50%, reduction in the original tumor weight) were achieved (data not shown).

1.6. Role of Leucovorin in Modulation of the Antitumor Activity of 5-FU and FU Prodrugs

A number of phase II clinical trials using 5-FU plus leucovorin (LV) vs 5-FU alone have demonstrated the superiority of the 5-FU combination *(26–30)*. The important therapeutic role of LV in modulation of the therapeutic selectivity of 5-FU was confirmed in rats bearing advanced colorectal cancer *(28)*. The data in Fig. 2 are an outline of the effects of LV on the therapeutic efficacy of the 5-FU prodrugs: UFT, S-1, and Xeloda. Although LV potentiated the tumor growth inhibition of Xeloda and 5-FU (data not shown), increased CR was achieved with UFT. The antitumor activity was compared using similar schedules, 28 d of treatment and route of administration (po except for iv infusion of 5-FU) using MTDs of each treatment. Since S-1 can produce 100% CR in this model system, the effect of LV on this drug could not be accurately assessed under these conditions.

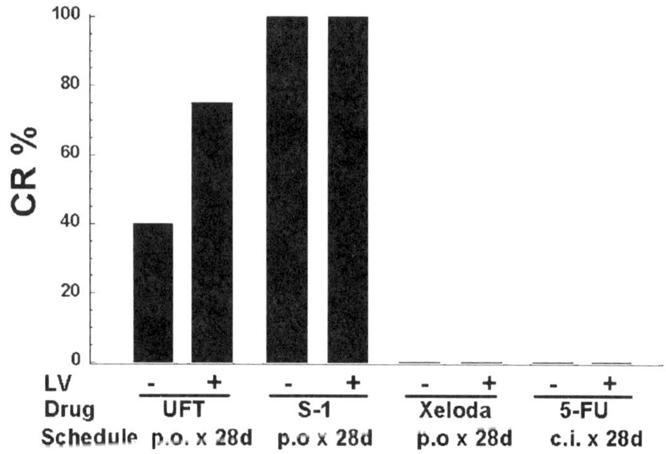

Fig. 2. Antitumor activity of 5-FU and 5-FU prodrugs in rats bearing Ward colon tumor: Role of Leukovorin (LV). Shown is the induction of complete remission (CR) using 5-Fu (12.5 mg/kg/d) and three different 5-FU prodrugs (UFT: 60 mg/kg/d; S-1: 22.5 mg/kg/d, and Xeloda: 200 mg/kg/d) with and without LV. The prodrugs were given orally for 28 consecutive days (p.o. × 28d) and 5-FU as a continuous iv infusion for 28 d (c.i. × 28d) at their MTDs. The data are combined from three to five independnet experiments, 12–20 rats in total for each experimental group.

1.7. Role of Dihydropyrimidine Inhibitors

The role of DPD in response to fluoropyrimidines based therapy in colorectal cancer has been implicated *(31–35),* confirming studies were carried out with capecitabine (Xeloda) using the ward rat tumor model system (Fig. 3). The ward colon tumor contains high levels of DPD. In this tumor, although FT and Xeloda are inactive (no CR), in combination with noncytotoxic concentration of uracil or Eniluracil, 100% CR similar results were obtained with S-1 and UFT, drugs with DPD inhibitors. Collectively, these data clearly demonstrate the important role of DPD inhibitors in combination of fluoropyrimidine prodrugs.

1.8. Combination of CPT-11/5-FU

CPT-11 as a single agent is clinically active in the treatment of colorectal cancer with no crossresistance to prior therapy of 5-FU with or without LV modulation, with reported response rates of 15–32% in chemonaive and 18–27% in 5-FU-pretreated patients *(36–40).* The combination of CPT-11 with 5-FU is highly active with manageable toxicities in clinical trials *(36–41).* However, the optimal dose sequence relationship between CPT-11 and 5-FU has not been fully defined. The data in Table 1 are a summary of results of CPT-11/5-FU alone at 50% of MTD (50 mg/kg) using a weekly schedule and in combination, simultaneously, and with 5-FU or CPT-11 separated by 24-h intervals. The MTDs of the drug alone did not result in increased CR rates. The results in Table 1 demonstrated the superiority of CPT-11 administered 24 h prior to 5-FU in both rats bearing ward colon tumors and in nude mice bearing human colon carcinoma (HCT-8) xenograft. More extensive studies have been published *(42).*

To determine the relationship between drug dose ratios and antitumor efficacy with CPT-11/5-FU combinations, a wide range of doses of CPT-11 followed 24 h later by 5-FU were used (Table 2). Similar CR rates were observed when the dose of CPT-11 was escalated from

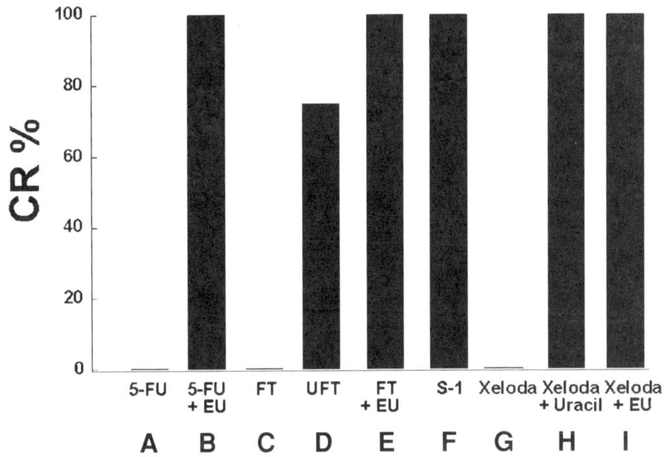

Fig. 3. Antitumor activity of 5-FU and 5-FU prodrugs in rats bearing Ward colon tumor: Role of DPD inhibitors. Shown is the induction of complete remission (CR). 5-FU and different 5-FU prodrugs were administered with and without different DPD inhibitors at their MTD's using the following comparable schedules: **(A)** 5-FU (35 mg/kg/d, iv push d 1–5); **(B)** 5-FU (10 mg/kg/d, iv push d 1–5) + Eniluracil (EU 1 mg/kg/day, ip dl, d6, d7); **(C)** Ftorafur (FT 200 mg/kg/d, po d1–7); **(D)** UFT (80 mg/kg/d, po. d 1–7); **(E)** FT (5 mg/kg/day, po d 1–7) + EU (1 mg/kg/d, ip d1–7); **(F)** S-1 (31.5 mg/kg/d, po d 1–7); **(G)** Xeloda (600 mg/kg/d, po d 1–7); **(H)** Xeloda (300 mg/kg/d, po d 1–7) + Uracil (800 mg/kg/d, po d 1–7); **(I)** Xeloda (100 mg/kg/d, po d 1–7) + Eniluracil (1 mg/kg/day, ip d 1–7). The data are combined from three to five independent experiments, 12–20 rats in total for each experimental group.

Table 1
Comparative Antitumor Activity of CPT-11 and 5-FU Alone and in Combination Against Rodents Bearing Tumors

	CR Rate (% Total)	
Treatment (mg/kg/wk × 4)	*Ward Tumor (in rat)*	*HCT-8 (in nude mice)*
CPT-11 (50)	0	20
CPT-11 (100[a])	0	20
5-FU (50)	25	0
5-FU (100[a])	31	0
CPT-11 (50) × 5-FU (50)	62	20
5-FU (50) 24 h →CPT-11 (50)	38	10
CPT-11 (50) 24 h →5-FU (50)	95[b]	80[b]

[a] MTD; [b]There are significant differences from other groups in CR rate ($p < 0.01$). The data are combined from two to five independent experiments, 12–20 rats and 10–20 nude mice in total for each experimental group.

12.5 to 100 mg/kg (i.e., in combination with a fixed dose of 50 mg/kg of 5-FU $^1/_2$ MTD). While CPT-11 at 6.25 mg/kg (< 10% MTD) still potentiated the antitumor activity of 5-FU, CPT-11 doses above 50% of the MTD did not further increase the antitumor activity but resulted in severe toxicity. When 5-FU was administered at its MTD (100 mg/kg), the doses of CPT-11 as low as 6.25% MTD was highly toxic while the antitumor activity was completely lost when 5-FU doses were decreased to 25% or below (Table 2). The results indicate that the 5-FU dose is more important and should be kept at 50–75% of the MTD.

Table 2
Antitumor Activity and Toxicity of Sequential Combination of CPT-11 24 h Later Followed by 5-FU in Rats Bearing Advanced Colorectal Carcinoma: Role of Drug Dose[a]

Drug (mg/kg/wk × 4)		*Antitumor Activity (%)*		*Toxicity (%)*	
CPT-11	*5-FU*	*PR*	*CR*	*MWL[a]*	*Death*
100[b]	0	69	31	12.8 ± 2.4[c]	0
0	100[b]	0	0	11.8 ± 2.4	0
6.25	50	62	38	7.5 ± 1.6	0
12.5	50	25	75	8.6 ± 2.4	0
25	50	25	75	11.4 ± 2.2	0
50	**50**	**5**	**95**	**9.0 ± 1.8**	**0**
75	50	31	69	14.2 ± 2.5	0
100	50	25	75	15.2 ± 2.2	0
6.25	75	58	42	8.8 ± 1.8	0
12.5	75	25	75	11.2 ± 2.6	0
25	75	25	75	11.6 ± 2.2	0
50	75	40	60	21.5 ± 3.8	38
100	12.5	0	0	11.8 ± 2.0	0
100	25	50	0	13.6 ± 3.0	0

[a] Maximum weight loss (MWL) of percentage of pretreatment body weight; [b]MTD; [c]Mean ± SD. The data are combined from three to five independent experiments, 12–20 rats in total for each experimental group. 100% of treated animals died when 5-FU was given at a dose of 100 mg/kg in the combination.

2. DISCUSSION

Although 5-FU has been widely employed as a single agent in varying doses and schedules for the treatment of advanced colorectal carcinoma and other malignancies, response rates have been limited; objective tumor responses in patients with advanced colorectal cancer generally range from 10% to 20% *(18,24)*. The search for improved response rates and survival has fueled research on drug administration schedule and/or biochemical modulation as a means of enhancing the efficacy of 5-FU. We evaluated three clinically relevant treatment schedules, namely, daily intravenous push, weekly intravenous push, and continuous infusion with 5-FU. Although the total doses of 5-FU per course were similar in the daily and continuous infusion treatment schedules, it was possible to deliver up to three times more drug with the weekly schedule. The dose-limiting toxicities were stomatitis (mucositis) and diarrhea with the daily and continuous infusion schedules and diarrhea with the weekly schedule (data not shown). For antitumor activity, CR was only achieved with weekly and 4 d infusion (Fig. 1). The daily ×5 iv push schedule induced only partial tumor response. Interestingly, prolonged infusion (14–28 d) with 5-FU produced only temporarily tumor growth inhibition, neither PR nor CR. The reason may be due to low 5-FU plasma concentrations that were not sufficient to produce significant antitumor activity. For 5-FU therapy, the balance between peak concentrations of 5-FU and drug duration is important. We also observed that 5-FU had no significant antitumor activity with single iv push at doses as high as 300 mg/kg (MTD) in the same model system (data not shown).

Improving therapeutic efficacy and selectivity are the major goals of anticancer drug development and biochemical modulation. Attempts to enhance the effectiveness of 5-FU have been based on consideration of both the biochemical pathway of 5-FU activation and the site of 5-FU action. One direction is to develop oral fluoropyrimidine prodrugs with greater threapeutic efficacy and selectivity than 5-FU. UFT is a combination of ftorafur (FT) and uracil in a molar ratio of 1:4, which is the optimal therapeutic ratio determined in in vitro and in vivo studies *(43)*. The antitumor activity of UFT has been demonstrated in patients with colorectal and gastric cancers *(44)*. S-1 is a combination of FT, 5-chloro-2,4-dihydropyridine (CDHP), and potassium oxonate (Oxo) in a fixed molar ratio of 1:0.4:1, predetermined for optimal selective tissue distribution *(45)*. CDHP is a potent inhibitor of DPD and Oxo is an inhibitor of phosphoribosylpyrophosphate transferase, an enzyme that metabolizes 5-FU to 5-FUMP. Results from our laboratory indicate that high antitumor efficacy achieved with S-1 is directly associated with high and sustained levels of treatment-induced apoptosis, which could not be produced with 5-FU *(46)*. Xeloda (capecitabine) is a new oral fluoropyrimidine carbamate, converted to 5-FU by three enzymatic steps. Xeloda is absorbed intact in the gastrointestinal tract and metabolized in the liver by carboxylesterase to 5′-deoxy-5-fluorocytidine, then metabolized to 5′-deoxy-5-fluorouridine by cytidine deaminase, and is finally converted to 5-FU by TP, which is present at higher levels in the tumor than in normal tissue *(47)*. Xeloda is not active against Ward tumor because of the low level of carboxylesterase in rat. However, it is much more active than 5-FU against several human colon cancer xenografts *(46,48)*.

LV is a source of intracellular reduced folates that increase the inhibition of TS by FdUMP through the stabilization of a ternary complex of the enzyme, reduced folate, and FdUMP. Phase III clinical trials demonstrated that the antitumor activity of the 5-FU/LV combination against colorectal carcinoma is significantly greater than the response rate obtained with 5-FU administered as a single agent at the maximum tolerated dose *(1,18–26,28,29,49)*. The data in Fig. 2 indicate that LV potentiated only the antitumor activity if the drug itself was active (such as UFT and S-1). LV could not enhance the antitumor efficacy of nonactive drugs or schedules (Xeloda and 5-FU) at the MTD in this model system (Fig. 2). However, LV did increase the antitumor activity (CR rates) of 5-FU given as a 4-d infusion or as a weekly schedule which are more active schedules in the same tumor model system *(42)*.

In clinical and preclinical model systems, 5-FU is eliminated rapidly from the plasma with a $t_{1/2}$ α of less than 10 min *(50,51)*. Furthermore, more than 85% of the injected dose of 5-FU is inactivated by DPD in normal and tumor tissues *(52)* and of the remaining 15% of 5-FU, activated via the anabolic pathway, a major fraction is incorporated into cellular RNA *(53)*.

In our study, several DPD inhibitors, such as uracil, CDHP, and Eniluracil (5-ethynyluracil), were used. All of the DPD inhibitors increased significantly the antitumor activity of 5-FU and 5-FU prodrugs without enhancing the host toxicity (Fig. 3). Uracil increased the CR rates from 0% to 75% with FT and from 0% to 100% with Xeloda, while CDHP (S-1) and Eniluracil achieved 100% cure rate with either 5-FU, FT, or Xeloda (Fig. 3).

Although the combination of CPT-11 with 5-FU/LV under clinical evaluation are showing significant antitumor activity and toxicity *(41,54,55)*, the optimal dose-sequence relationship has not been fully defined. In several tested tumor models, we found that a 24-h interval between CPT-11 and 5-FU was the most active treatment when compared to CPT-11 at different times (0, 6, 24, 48, and 72 h) before 5-FU (unpublished data). Both antitumor activity and toxicity were significantly higher with this sequence compared to the others. However, when the drug doses were reduced, the toxicity was decreased while maintaining high antitumor efficacy (cure). In other words, reduction of the CPT-11 dose resulted in an increased selectivity of the drug combination with improved therapeutic index. Cell cycle kinetic studies demonstrated that 24 h following CPT-11 administration, the conditions are optimal for sensitizing the tumor to S-phase-specific drugs such as 5-FU (unpublished data). The role of the individual drug dose used appears also to be an important factor for the CPT-11/5-FU combination. CPT-11 and 5-FU appear to play different roles for the antitumor efficacy of the combination. CPT-11 could be used as low as 12.5% of the MTD and still be equally highly curative in the combination as compared to the MTD, whereas 5-FU had to be used at least at 50% of the MTD to maintain the antitumor activity of the combination, increasing the dose of 5-FU to the level of MTD did not translate into additional therapeutic benefit but was associated with increased toxicities (Table 2). The antitumor activity was completely lost when 5-FU was used at 25 mg/kg (25% MTD) or below. In the combination, 5-FU doses appear to be critical for the antitumor activity while CPT-11 doses appear to play a modulatory role in sensitizing the tumor cells for the subsequent (24 h) 5-FU treatment.

In summary, in order to enhance the maximum antitumor efficacy without increasing the toxicities of 5-FU and 5-FU prodrugs, studies should assess the optimal administration schedules of 5-FU and its modulators (LV, uracil, CDHP, EU) which interfere with the anabolic and catabolic pathways of 5-FU. 5-FU and 5-FU prodrugs should be combined with other drugs with different mechanisms of action (i.e., topoisomerase I inhibitors, platinum compounds, EGF and VEGF inhibitors) and their interactions should be studied further. Finally, biochemical and molecular markers that are associated with antitumor response to 5-FU and 5-FU prodrugs need to be identified.

REFERENCES

1. de Gramont A, Bosset JF, Milan C, et al. Randomized trial comparing monthly low dose leucovorin and 5-FU bolus with biomonthly high dose leucovorin and 5-FU bolus plus continuous infusion for advanced colorectal cancer. *J Clin Oncol* 1997;15:808–815.
2. Meta-analysis Group in Cancer. Efficacy of intravenous continuous infusion of fluorouracil compared with bolus administration in advanced colorectal cancer. Meta-analysis Group in Cancer. *J Clin Oncol* 1998;16:301–308.
3. Borner MM, Castiglione M, Bacchi M. The impact of adding low dose leucovorin to monthly 5-FU in advanced colorectal cancer: results of phase III randomized trial. *Ann Oncol* 1998;9:535–541.
4. Advanced Colorectal Cancer: meta-analysis project. Meta-analysis of randomized trials testing the biochemical modulation of 5-FU by methotrexate in metastatic colorectal cancer. *J Clin Oncol* 1994;12:960–969.
5. Leichman CG, Lenz HJ, Leichman L, et al. Quantitation of intratumoral thymidylate synthase expression predicts for disseminated colorectal cancer response and resistance to protracted-infusion fluorouracil and weekly leucovorin. *J Clin Oncol* 1997;15:3223–3229.
6. Johnston PG, Fisher ER, Rockette HE, et al. The role of thymidylate synthase expression in prognosis and outcome of adjuvant chemotherapy in patients with rectal cancer. *J Clin Oncol* 1994;12:2640–2647.
7. Twelves C, Harper P, Custem EV. A phase III trial of xeloda (capecitabine) in previously untreated advanced metastatic colorectal cancer. *Proc Am Soc Clin Oncol* 1999;18:1010.
8. Daher GC, Harris BE, Diasio RB. Metabolism of pyrimidine anologues and their nucleotides in metabolism and reaction of anticancer drugs, volume 1: the international encyclopedia of pharmacology and therapeutics, chapter 2. 1994.
9. Grem JL. Biochemical modulation of 5-FU in systematic treatment of advanced colorectal cancer. *Oncology* 2001;15:13–19.
10. Takimoto CH, Lu Z-H, Zhang R. Severe neurotoxicity following 5-Fu based chemotherapy in a patient with dihydropyrimidine dehydrogenase deficiency. *Clin Cancer Res* 1996;2:477–481.
11. Harris BE, Carpenter JT, Diasio RB. Severe 5-FU toxicity secondary to dihydropyrimidine dehydrogenase deficiency: a potentially more common pharmacogenetic syndrome. *Cancer* 1991;68:499–501.
12. Diasio RB. Oral administration of 5-FU: a new approach utilizing modulators of dihydropyrimidine dehydrogenase. *Cancer Therapeutics* 1999;2:97–106.
13. Friedkin M, Roberts D. The enzymatic synthesis of nucleosides. Thymidine and related pyrimidines neucleosides. *J Biol Chem* 1954;207:257–266.
14. Luccioni C, Beaumatin J, Bardot V. Pyrimidine nucleotide metabolism in human colon carcinomas. Comparison of normal tissue, primary tumors and xenografts. *Int J Cancer* 1994;58:517.
15. Schwartz EL, Baptiste N, Wadler S, Makower D. Thymidine phosphorylase mediates the sensitivity of human colon carcinoma cells to 5-fluorouracil. *J Biol Chem* 1995;270:19073–19077.

16. Moghaddam A, Zhang HT, Fan T, et al. Thymidine phosphorylase is angiogenic and promotes tumor growth. *Proc Nat Acad Sci* 1995;92:998–1002.
17. Toi M, Hoshina S, Taniguchi T. Vascular endothelial growth factor and platelet derived endothelial cell growth factor are frequently co-expressed in highly vascularized human breast cancer. *Clin Cancer Res* 1995;1:961–964.
18. Moertel CG. Chemotherapy of gastrointestinal cancer. *N Engl J Med* 1978;229:1049–1052.
19. Davis HL. Chemotherapy of large bowel cancer. *Cancer* 1982;50:2638–2646.
20. Kemeny N, Daly J, Reichman B, et al. Intrahepatic or systemic infusion of fluorodeoxyuridine in patients with liver metastases from colorectal carcinoma. *Ann Intern Med* 1987;107:459–465.
21. Lokich JJ, Ahlgren JD, Gullo JJ, et al. A prospective randomized comparison of continuous infusion fluorouracil with a conventional bolus schedule in metastatic colorectal carcinoma: a Mid-Atlantic Oncolology Program Study. *J Clin Oncol* 1989;7:425–432.
22. Buroker TR, O'Connell MJ, Wieand HS, et al. Randomized comparison of two schedules of fluorouracil and leucovorin in the treatment of advanced colorectal cancer. *J Clin Oncol* 1994;12:14–20.
23. Nobile MT, Rosso R, Sertoli MR, et al. Randomized comparison of weekly bolus 5-fluorouracil with or without and leucovorin in metastatic colorectal carcinoma. *Eur J Cancer* 1992;28A:1823–1827.
24. Creaven PJ, Rustum YM, Petrelli NJ, et al. Phase I and pharmacokinetic evaluation of floxuridine/leucovorin given on the Roswell Park weekly regimen. *Cancer Chemo & Pharm.* 1994;34:261–265.
25. Loffler TM, Weber FW, Hausamen TU. Protracted continuous infusion 5-fluorouracil with intermittent high-dose leucovorin in advanced and metastatic colorectal cancer: a pilot study. *London Royal Society of Medicine Services Ltd* 1989; 65–77.
26. Di Costanzo F, Bartolucci R, Calabresi F, et al. Fluorouracil-alone versus high-dose folinic acid and fluorouracil in advanced colorectal cancer: a randomized trial of the Italian Oncology Group for Clinical Research (GOIRC). *Ann Oncol* 1992;3:371–376.
27. Petrelli N, et al. The modulation of fluorouracil with leucovorin in metastatic colorectal carcinoma: a prospective randomized Phase III trial. *J Clin Oncol* 1989;7:1419–1426.
28. Piedbois P, Buyse M, Rustum Y, et al. Modulation of fluorouracil by leucovorin in patients with advanced colorectal cancer:evidence in terms of response rate. *J Clin Oncol* 1992;10:896–903.
29. Poon MA, O'Connell MJ, Wieand HS, et al. Biochemical modulation of fluorouracil with leucovorin: confirmatory evidence of improved therapeutic efficacy in advanced colorectal cancer. *J Clin Oncol* 1991;9:1967–1972.
30. Mansoni S. Efficacy of adjuvant fluorouracil and folinic acid in colon cancer. *Lancet* 1995;345:939–949.
31. Cao S, Frank C, Rustum YM. Role of fluoropyrimidine Schedule and (6R,S)leucovorin dose in a preclinical animal model of colorectal carcinoma *J Natl Cancer Inst* 1996;88(7):430–436.
32. Porter DJT, Chestnut WG, Merrill BM, Spector T. Mechanism-based inactivation of dihydropyrimidine dehydrogenase by 5-ethynyluracil. *J Biol Chem* 1992;267:5236–5242.
33. Beck A, Etienne MC, Cheradame JL, et al. A role for dihydropyrimidine dehydrogenase and thymidylate synthase in tumor sensitivity to fluorouracil. *Europ J Cancer* 1994;10:1517–1522.
34. Cao S, Rustum YM Spector T. 5-Ethynyluracil (776C85): modulation of 5-fluorouracil efficacy and therapeutic index in rats bearing advanced colorectal carcinoma. *Cancer Res* 1994;54(6):1507–1510.
35. Fischel JL, Formento P, Etienne MC, et al. Dual modulation of 5-fluorouracil cytotoxicity using folic acid with a dihydropyrimidine dehydrogenase inhibitor. *Biochem Pharm* 1997;53:1703–1709.
36. Conti JA, Kemeny NE, Saltz LB, et al. Irinotecan is an active agent in untreated patients with metastatic colorectal cancer. *J Clin Oncol* 1996;14:709–715.
37. Rougier P, Bugat R, Douillard JY, et al. Phase II study of irinotecan in the treatment of advanced colorectal cancer in chemotherapy-naive patients and patients pretreated with fluorouracil-based chemotherapy. *J Clin Oncol* 1997;15:251–260.
38. Pitot HC, Wender DB, O'Connell MJ, et al. Phase II trial of irinotecan in patients with metastatic colorectal carcinoma. *J Clin Oncol* 1997;15:2910–2919.
39. Rothenberg ML, Eckardt JR, Kuhn JG, et al. Phase II trial of irinotecan (CPT-11) in patients with progressive or rapidly recurrent colorectal cancer. *J Clin Oncol* 1996;14:1128–1135.
40. Saltz LB, Kanowitz J, Kemeny NE, et al. Phase I clinical and pharmacokinetic study of irinotecan, fluorouracil, and leucovorin in patients with advanced solid tumors. *J Clin Oncol* 1996;14(11):2959–2967.
41. Vanhoefer U, Harstrick A, Kohne CH, et al. Phase I study of a weekly schedule of irinotecan, high-dose leucovorin, and infusional fluorouracil as first-line chemotherapy in patients with advanced colorectal cancer. *J Clin Oncol* 1999;17(3):907–913.
42. Cao S Rustum YM. Synergistic antitumor activity of irinotecan in combination with 5-fluorouracil in rats bearing advanced colorectal cancer: role of drug sequence and dose. *Cancer Res* 2000;60(14):3717–3721.

43. Fujii S, Kitano S, Ikenaka K, Shirasaka T. Effect of coadministration of uracil or cytosine on the antitumor activity of clinical dose of 1-(2-tetrahydrofuryl)-5-fluorouracil and levelof 5-fluorouracil in rodents. *Gann* 1979;70:209–214.
44. Malik STA, Talbot D, Clarke PI, et al. Phase II trial of UFT in advanced colorectal and gastric cancer. *Br J Cancer* 1990;62:1023–1025.
45. Shirasaka T, Nakano K, Takechi T, et al. Antitumor activity of 1M tegafur-0.4 M 5-chloro 2-4-dihydroxypyrimidine-1M potassium oxonate (S-1) against human colon carcinoma orthotopically implanted into nude rats. *Cancer Res* 1996;56:2602–2606.
46. Cao S, Lu K, Ishitsuka H, Rustum YM. Antitumor efficacy of capecitabine against fluorouracil-sensitive and-resistant tumors. *Proc Am Soc Clin Oncol* 1997;16:226.
47. Ishikawa T, Utoh M, Sawada N, et al. Tumor selective delivery of 5-fluorouracil by capecitabine, a new oral fluoropyrimidine carbamate, in human cancer xenografts. *Biochem Pharmacol* 1998;55:1091–1093.
48. Ishikawa T, Utoh M, Sawada N, Sekiguchi F, Ishitsuka H. Zeloda (capecitabine): an orally available tumor-sensitive fluoropyrimidine carbamate. *Proc Am Soc Clin Oncol* 1997;16:208.
49. Petrellli N. The modulation of fluorouracil with leucovorin in metastatic colorectal carcinoma: a prospective randomized Phase III trial. *J Clin Oncol* 1989;7:1419–1426.
50. Fraile RJ, Baker LH, Buroker TR, et al. Pharmacokinetics of 5-fluorouracil administered orally, by rapid intravenous and by slow infusion. *Cancer Res* 1980;40:2223–2228.
51. Hegie GD, Sommadoss JP, Gross DS, et al. Clinical pharmacokinetics of 5-fluorouracil and its metabolites in plasma, urine, and bile. *Cancer Res* 1987;47:2203–2206.
52. Diasio RB, Harris BE. Clinical pharmacology of 5-fluorouracil. *Clin Pharmacokinet* 1989;16:215–237.
53. Nord LD, Stolfi RL Martin DS. Biochemical modulation of 5-fluorouracil with leucovorin or delayed uridine rescure: correlation of antitumor activity with dosage and FUra incorporation into RNA. *Biochem Pharmacol* 1992;43:2543–2549.
54. Saltz LB, Locker PK, Pirotta N, et al. Weekly irinotecan (CPT-11), leucovorin (LV), and fluorouracil (FU) is superior to daily × 5 LV/FU in patients with previously untreated metastatic colorectal cancer. *Proc Am Soc Clin Oncol Abstr* 1999;18:1999.
55. Ducreux M, Ychou M, Seitz JF, et al. Irinotecan combined with bolus fluorouracil, continuous infusion fluorouracil, and high-dose leucovorin every two weeks (LV5FU regimen): a clinical dose-finding and pharmacokinetic study in patients with pretreated metastatic colorectal cancer. *J Clin Oncol* 1999;17:2901–2901.

11 Bimonthly 48-h Leucovorin and 5-Fluorouracil-Based Regimens in Advanced Colorectal Cancer

Aimery de Gramont, MD,
and Christophe Louvet, MD

CONTENTS

1. INTRODUCTION

5-Fluorouracil (5-FU) has been the mainstay of systemic therapy for metastatic colorectal cancer since its introduction into clinical practice more than four decades ago and remains the agent of choice in the treatment of this malignancy. However, objective responses are observed in less than 20% of patients treated with single-agent 5-FU administered as a bolus, with a median survival of less than 9 mo.

During the last two decades, several 5-FU dosing schedules have been evaluated in an attempt to improve the outcome of treatment with this agent. Clinical trials have demonstrated that both tumor response rates and patient survival are increased following continuous infusion of 5-FU compared with bolus administration *(1,2)*. Because 5-FU is an antimetabolite and therefore only active in dividing cells, a longer exposure time results in enhanced uptake of 5-FU by tumors with a relatively slow doubling time, such as colorectal cancers. The administration of 5-FU by continuous infusion has been shown to produce an altered toxicity profile compared with bolus administration, changing the dose-limiting toxicities from myelosuppression or stomatitis to skin toxicities, in particular the hand-foot syndrome *(1,3)*. In most published reports, the toxicity of 5-FU administered by continuous infusion is less than with bolus administration *(1,4–6)*. As a result, the use of continuous infusion permits an increase in the total tolerated dose of 5-FU compared with other methods of administration. These data may explain the superior clinical results that are observed with this approach compared with bolus administration *(1,4–6)*.

From: *Fluoropyrimidines in Cancer Therapy*
Edited by: Y. M. Rustum © Humana Press Inc., Totowa, NJ

A meta-analysis of six randomized trials of continuous infusion vs bolus administration of 5-FU showed that while significantly higher response rates were achieved with continuous infusion compared with bolus administration (22% vs 14%, respectively), median survival was only marginally improved (12.1 mo vs 11.3 mo, respectively) *(2)*.

Furthermore, clinical research has demonstrated that patients with progressive disease following bolus treatment can achieve partial responses and disease stabilization in response to the administration of 5-FU by continuous infusion *(7)*.

The limited impact of single-agent 5-FU on the overall survival of patients with advanced colorectal cancer has prompted the investigation of biochemical modulation of 5-FU as a means of improving the outcome of treatment.

2. BIOMODULATION OF 5-FU

Biomodulation is a strategy that involves the alteration of tumor cell susceptibility to anticancer drugs through the modification of biochemical pathways to produce an accentuated or selective action on the cancer cells. This approach differs from that of combination chemotherapy because the biomodulator is not a cytotoxic agent. The most widespread use of biomodulation involves the use of leucovorin (LV) to increase intracellular folate cofactors and, thus, enhance the binding of fluorodeoxyuridylate to thymidylate synthase (TS), the enzyme involved in the biosynthesis of nucleic acids *(8–10)*. This enhanced binding leads to increased cytotoxicity of 5-FU, and clinical trials have demonstrated that the response to 5-FU in colorectal cancer can be increased by concomitant administration of LV.

The first LV/5-FU protocol to be clinically evaluated involved the administration of high-dose LV (500 mg/m^2) plus weekly 5-FU (600 mg/m^2), administered for 6 wk with a 2-wk rest, to 343 patients with previously untreated metastatic colorectal cancer *(11)*. The combination was associated with significantly improved tumor response rates compared with 5-FU alone (30.3% vs 12.1%), although there was no significant difference in overall survival. A second LV/5-FU regimen has been developed by researchers at the Mayo Clinic in conjunction with the North Central Cancer Treatment Group (NCCTG) *(12)*. This is a monthly regimen involving 5-d courses of 5-FU bolus therapy (425 mg/m^2) plus low-dose LV (20 mg/m^2). In a large study of 429 patients, the clinical efficacy of several 5-FU-based regimens were compared with that of 5-FU alone. The NCCTG–Mayo Clinic regimen was associated with significantly higher tumor response rates compared with 5-FU alone (43% vs 10%, respectively) and this was reflected in a significant increase in median survival among patients treated with LV/5-FU (12.0 mo vs 7.7 mo, respectively, $p = 0.05$).

A meta-analysis of nine randomized clinical trials, involving 1381 patients, also demonstrated significantly improved response rates following combination therapy with LV/5-FU, compared with 5-FU alone (23% vs 11%, respectively), although there was no significant impact on survival (11.5 mo vs 11.0 mo, respectively) *(13)*.

3. THE BIMONTHLY LV/5FU REGIMENS

The bimonthly LV/5-FU regimens combine 5-FU continuous infusion and biomodulation by LV. In addition, based on the different mechanisms of action of 5-FU depending on the dose and schedule of administration, the bimonthly regimens also combine 5-FU bolus and continuous infusion. This combination is supported by the in vitro demonstration of a synergism between 5-FU administered by bolus and continuous infusion *(14)*. Lastly, the

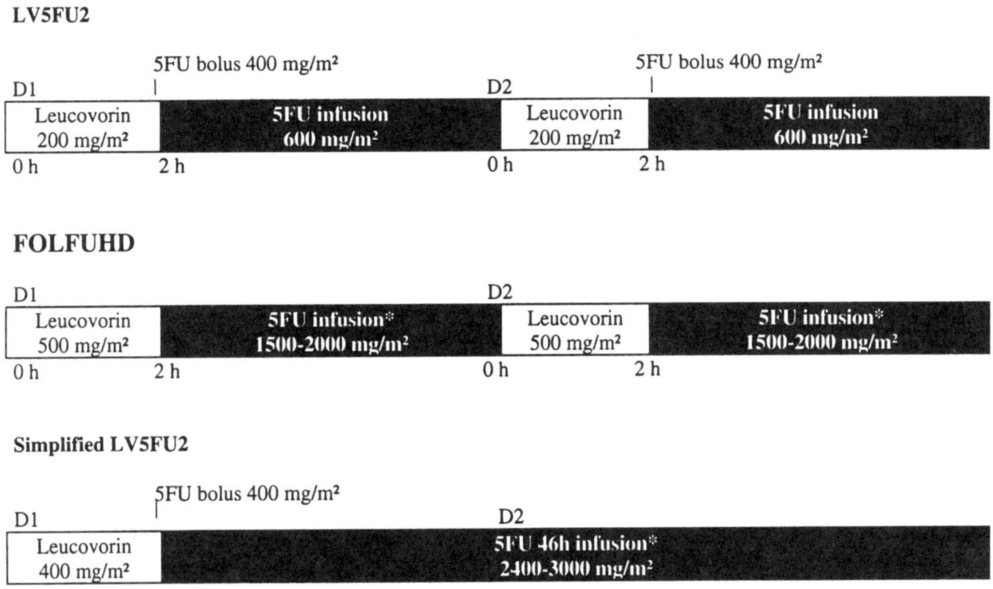

Fig. 1. Outline of the three main LV/5-FU bimonthly regimens that have been investigated in patients with advanced colorectal cancer. Treatment cycles were repeated every 2 wk.
*The dose was administered at the lower level for two cycles, then at the higher level for subsequent cycles, if toxicity < WHO grade 2.

bimonthly schedule, which is also in accordance with the in vitro optimal TS inhibition duration, was selected as the optimal method to keep the toxicity at a low level.

After a preliminary study which showed that a bimonthly 48-h schedule was well tolerated, the first bimonthly regimen to be investigated was administered to 37 chemotherapy-naive patients with advanced colorectal cancer *(15)*. This approach permitted a doubling of the total administered dose of 5-FU compared with the monthly NCCTG–Mayo Clinic regimen (4.0 g/m^2 vs 2.1 g/m^2 per month, respectively). Furthermore, the bimonthly regimen produced encouraging clinical results, with tumor responses occurring in 54% of patients, and a median survival of 18 mo.

Further evaluation of the bimonthly schedule, performed by the French Intergroup, has confirmed the favorable toxicity profile of this treatment regimen compared with monthly 5-FU/LV. In a randomized trial of 433 previously untreated patients, a bimonthly regimen of high-dose LV plus 5-FU bolus and infusion of low-dose 5-FU (2-h infusion of LV, 200 mg/m^2, followed by iv bolus of 5-FU, 400 mg/m^2/d, then 22-h infusion of 5-FU, 600 mg/m^2/d, the LV/5-FU2 regimen, Fig. 1) was compared with the monthly NCCTG–Mayo Clinic regimen *(16)*. Tumor response rates were significantly higher among patients who received LV/5-FU2 compared with the NCCTG–Mayo Clinic regimen (32.6% vs 14.4%, respectively, $p = 0.0004$). In addition, the median progression-free survival was significantly improved by the bimonthly regimen (27.6 wk vs 22 wk, p=0.001). Median survival was not significantly increased compared with the monthly regimen (62.0 wk vs 56.8 wk respectively, p=0.067). However, crossovers between treatment groups and the use of second line therapies were permitted during the study, and this may have reduced any differences that could be detected between the original treatment groups. Importantly, the bimonthly regimen was associated with lower toxicity than the monthly regimen, with World Health Organization (WHO) grade 3–4 toxicities occurring in 11.1% of patients who received LV/5-FU2, compared with 23.9% for the NCCTG–Mayo Clinic regimen (*p*=0.0004).

In view of these promising findings, a modified bimonthly regimen was subsequently investigated in 101 patients with advanced colorectal cancer (The FOLFUHD study; *FOL*inic acid, 5-*FU H*igh *D*ose) *(17)*. The regimen consisted of high-dose LV (500 mg/m^2) plus a 2-h infusion of high-dose 5 FU (1500–2000 mg/m^2/d for 2 d), repeated every 2 wk until there was evidence of disease progression (Fig. 1). An overall response rate of 33.7% was reported, with five complete responses (5%) and 29 partial responses (28.7%). Survival rates were also encouraging, with median progression-free and overall survival rates of 8 and 18 mo, respectively. The efficacy of this bimonthly regimen was not affected by treatment status and was equivalent among previously treated and chemotherapy-naive patients. In addition, the low toxicity of bimonthly LV/5-FU2 was confirmed; 15.2% of patients experienced no toxic effects with the bimonthly regimen, and a further 28.3% had only grade 1 toxicity.

On the basis of the assumption that high-dose 5-FU infusion has equivalent activity to 5FU bolus plus low-dose 5-FU infusion, the LV/5-FU2 regimen has recently been simplified so that, instead of requiring patients to be admitted to the hospital for two consecutive days every 2 wk, the procedure requires only 2 h at the hospital. A single, 2-h LV infusion (400 mg/m^2) is given immediately before the bolus of 5-FU (400 mg/m^2), followed by a 46-h infusion of 5-FU (2400–3000 mg/m^2), administered via a disposable pump, which is fitted before the patient is discharged (Fig. 1) *(18)*. In a study involving 93 patients, the new simplified regimen demonstrated antitumor efficacy combined with low toxicity and, interestingly, this regimen appears to be even more active than the first two bi-monthly regimens to be investigated, with an overall response rate of 41%, a median progression-free survival of 9.4 mo (personal communication).

4. BIMONTHLY LV/5-FU IN COMBINATION WITH NOVEL CYTOTOXIC AGENTS

The efficacy and low toxicity of the LV/5-FU2 regimen provides the opportunity to add other antitumor agents to the regimen with the aim of improving patient survival, and combination regimens with LV/5-FU2 have been extensively investigated.

4.1. Oxaliplatin

Oxaliplatin is the first platinum compound to demonstrate significant activity in colorectal cancer *(19)*. In clinical studies, single-agent oxaliplatin produces objective responses in 20–24% of patients with previously untreated advanced colorectal cancer *(20,21)* and 10% of those with tumors that are resistant to 5-FU, *(21,22)*. Strong synergistic cytotoxic activity has been demonstrated with oxaliplatin and 5-FU, both in vitro and in vivo, and this synergism is maintained even in 5-FU-resistant cell lines *(23)*.

The value of adding oxaliplatin to LV/5-FU2 (Fig. 1) has been evaluated recently in a large study of the first-line treatment of colorectal cancer. The full-dose regimen was administered when toxicity remained at a tolerable level, and treatment was continued until the development of unacceptable toxicity or in the event of disease progression. In 420 patients with previously untreated advanced colorectal cancer, the addition of oxaliplatin, 85 mg/m^2, to LV/5-FU2 was associated with substantially enhanced activity compared with the bimonthly regimen alone *(24)*. Patients allocated to oxaliplatin plus LV/5-FU2 showed significantly longer progression-free survival (median, 9.0 mo vs 6.2 mo, *p*=0.0003) and improved response rates (50.7% vs 22.3%, $p = 0.001$) compared with those who received LV/5-FU2 alone. In this study, where crossovers between treatment groups were permitted, there was also a trend toward increased overall survival in the oxaliplatin group, although this did not reach statistical significance (median 16.2 mo vs 14.7 mo, $p = 0.12$). The incidence of toxicities was higher with the combination regimen than LV/5-FU2 alone; grade 3–4 neutropenia, diarrhea, and grade 3 neurosensory toxicity were all observed more frequently among patients treated with oxaliplatin than those who were not ($p < 0.05$). However, as this did not result in impairment of quality of life, the small survival benefit observed with the combination regimen may be considered to be of value. Importantly, multivariate analysis revealed that oxaliplatin was a strong independent predictor of overall survival. Furthermore, metastectomy was possible in twice as many patients who received oxaliplatin than among those who received LV/5-FU2 alone (6.7% vs 3.3%), raising the possibility of potentially curative surgery for metastatic disease.

The efficacy of various doses of oxaliplatin in combination with 48-h bimonthly regimens of LV/5-FU has also been evaluated in the second-line setting, among patients with tumors that had demonstrated resistance to treatment with LV/5-FU alone (the FOLFOX studies; *FOL*inic acid,5-*FU*,*OX*aliplatin). The doses and schedules of administration were modified with the aim of minimizing the incidence of toxicity while enhancing the efficacy of oxaliplatin. With the exception of FOLFOX 7, all of the regimens were administered until disease progression or the development of unacceptable toxicity.

A feasibility study (FOLFOX 1) evaluated the bimonthly FOLFUHD regimen with oxaliplatin (130 mg/m^2) added at every other treatment cycle (Fig. 2) *(25)*. An encouraging response rate of 31% was observed in 13 patients who received the FOLFOX 1 regimen, with median and progression-free survival times of 6 and 11 mo, respectively (Table 1). The low level of toxicity associated with the FOLFOX 1 regimen led to the design of FOLFOX 2, in which the total dose of oxaliplatin was increased to 100 mg/m^2, administered at every treatment cycle to 46 patients (Fig. 2) *(26)*. The dose of 5-FU was 1500 mg/m^2/d for the first two treatment cycles and this was increased to 2000 mg/m^2/d in subsequent cycles if maximal toxicity remained below WHO grade 2. The major dose-limiting toxicities were neutropenia and peripheral neuropathy. The FOLFOX 2 regimen produced a high response rate of 46%, with median and progression-free survival times of 7 and 17 mo, respectively. The high response rate was attributed to an effective synergy between the FOLFUHD regimen and oxaliplatin, given that patients had tumors that were already refractory to LV/5-FU regimens.

These findings prompted further trials in which the dose of the 5-FU infusion was reduced to 1500 mg/m^2/d, and that of oxaliplatin to 85 mg/m^2 (FOLFOX 3) *(27,28)*. The FOLFOX 4 regimen used the LV/5-FU2 regimen in combination with oxaliplatin (85 mg/m^2). Both regimens were administered to patients whose disease had progressed while receiving the LV/5-FU regimen alone and the studies provided further clinical confirmation of the synergistic effects of oxaliplatin and LV/5-FU. However, the response rates and survival times were lower than those observed with the FOLFOX 2 regimen (Table 1). Subsequent trials have used the new simplified LV/5-FU2 regimen, which retains the low toxicity of the standard LV/5-FU2 regimen and demonstrates at least equivalent efficacy *(18)*. In FOLFOX 6, oxaliplatin 100 mg/m^2 was added to the simplified regimen *(29)*. A higher dose intensity of oxaliplatin (130 mg/m^2) was added in FOLFOX 7 and treatment was suspended after eight cycles, in an attempt to limit toxicity *(30)*. Patients were then evaluated every 2 mo and the FOLFOX 7 regimen as resumed in the event of disease progression. Among the 34 patients treated, a high response rate of 44% was observed and the regimen was well tolerated.

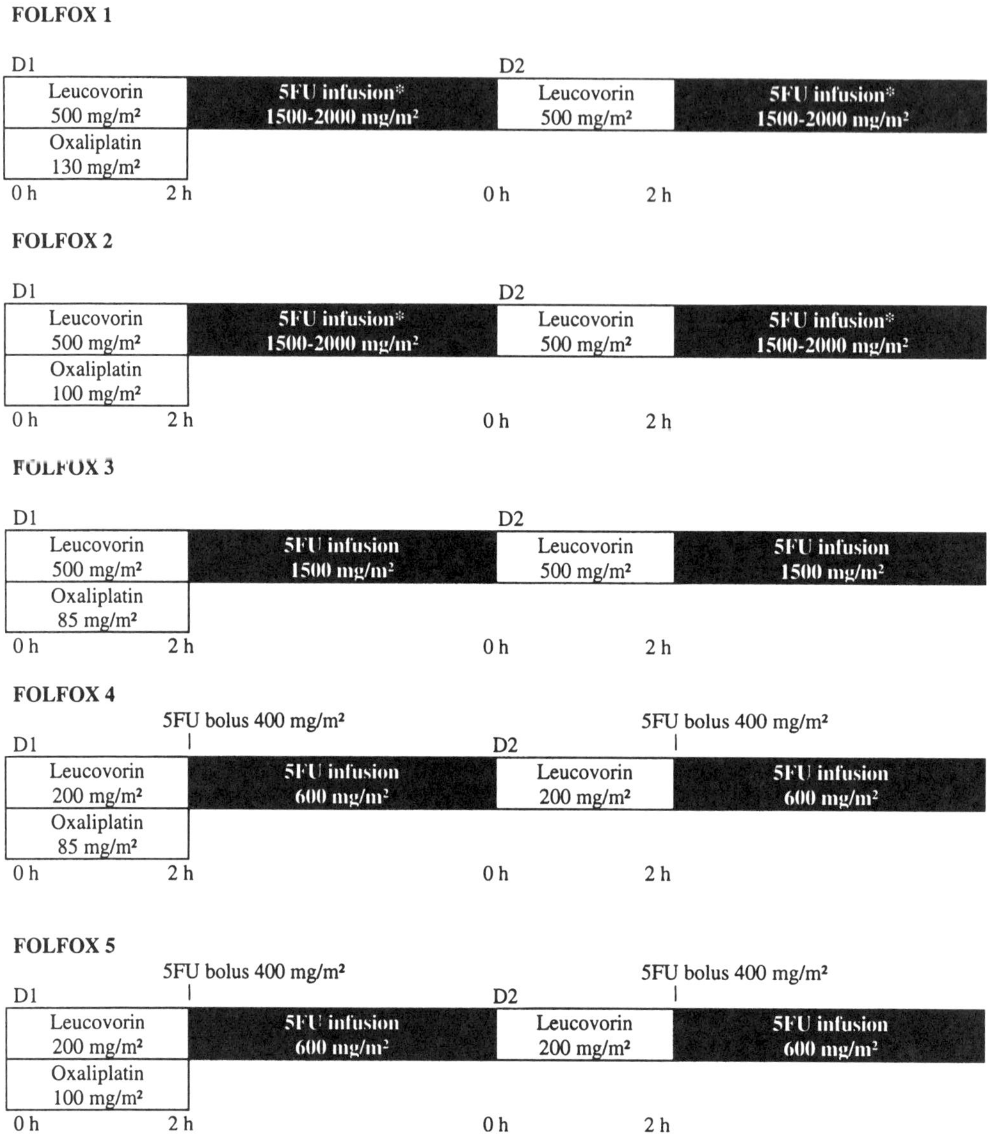

Fig. 2. Regimens used in FOLFIRI and the FOLFOX 1–7 studies. Treatment cycles were repeated every two weeks. Oxaliplatin was administered at every other cycle in FOLFOX 1, and at every cycle in FOLFOX 2–6.
*The dose was administered at the lower level for two cycles, then at the higher level for subsequent cycles, if toxicity < WHO grade 2.
Hy: hydroxyurea

Furthermore, median and progression-free survival (12.6 mo and 6.2 mo, respectively) were not adversely affected by the break in therapy.

Taken together, the FOLFOX trials indicate that the dose intensity of oxaliplatin may be important in determining the efficacy of the triple agent regimen *(31)*. No other factors, such as age, number of metastatic sites, carcinoembryonic antigen level, or response to first-line therapy, have been shown to influence the response to second-line therapy. The FOLFOX 7

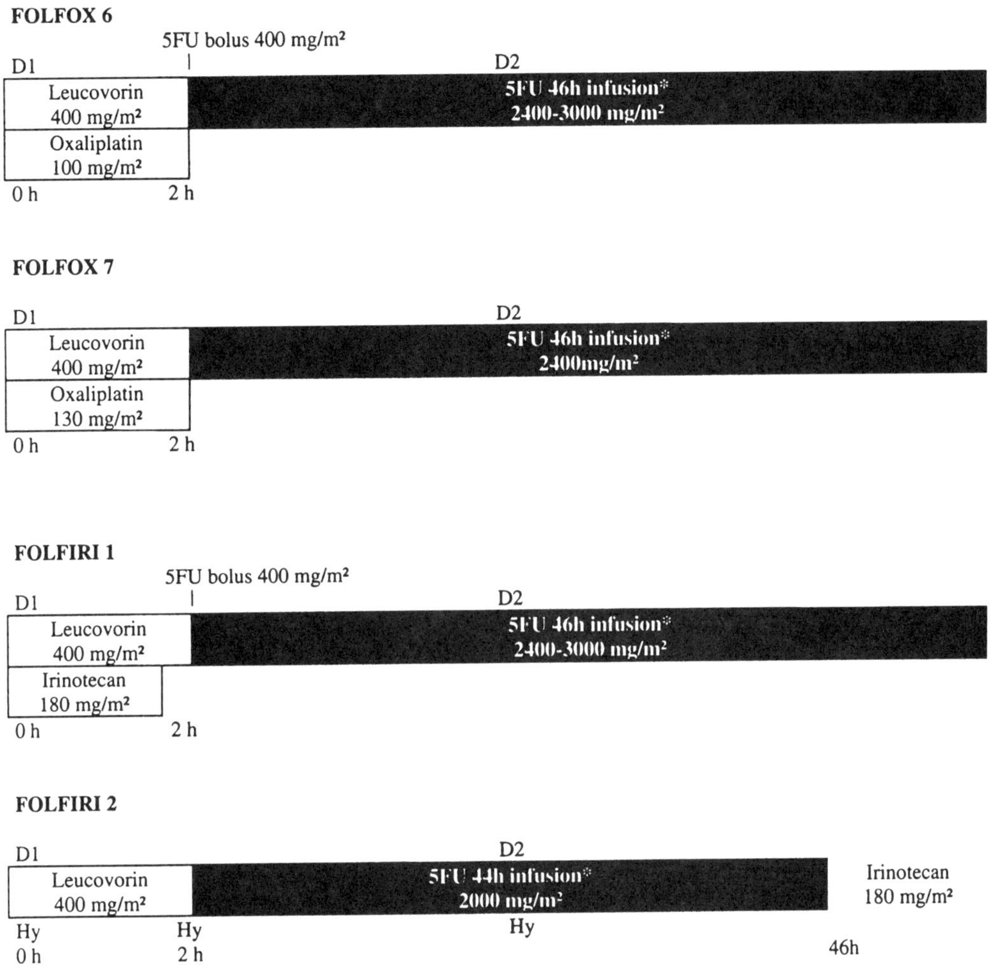

Fig. 2. *Continued.*

Table 1
Summary of the Findings of the FOLFOX Studies, in which LV/5-FU Are Administered with Oxaliplatin in the Second-Line Therapy of Advanced Colorectal Cancer[a]

Regimen	*n*	*Response rate (%)*	*Median PFS[b] (mo)*	*Median survival (mo)*
FOLFOX 1	13	31	6	11
FOLFOX 2	46	46	7	17
FOLFOX 3	30	20	6	10
FOLFOX 3	40	18	4.6	10.6
FOLFOX 4	57	23	5.1	11.1
FOLFOX 6	60	27	5.3	10.8
FOLFOX 7	34	44	6.2	12.6

[a] There were two FOLFOX 3 studies and FOLFOX 5 was not conducted.

[b] PFS = progression-free survival.

regimen is currently being evaluated in the first-line setting; the OPTIMOX study (aimed at identifying the *optim*al FOLF*OX* regimen) is comparing the efficacy of FOLFOX 7 with FOLFOX 4 in previously untreated patients with advanced colorectal cancer. In addition, the combination of oxaliplatin with LV/5-FU2 is to be evaluated in the adjuvant treatment of patients with this disease (the Multicenter International Study of Oxaliplatin in the Adjuvant treatment of Colon Cancer study).

4.2. Irinotecan

Irinotecan (or CPT-11) is a topoisomerase inhibitor that is active against colorectal cancer cells *(32)*. The drug does not demonstrate crossresistance with 5-FU and is active via a novel molecular mechanism *(33)*. In phase II clinical trials, irinotecan has shown antitumor activity in patients with colorectal cancer, including those whose disease had progressed on 5-FU-based therapy *(34–36)*. The first large phase III trial of irinotecan demonstrated a significant survival advantage among patients who received the drug in addition to supportive care, compared with those who received supportive care alone (overall 1-yr survival 36.2% vs 13.5%, respectively, $p = 0.001$) *(37)*. In another phase III trial, irinotecan was associated with significantly improved survival, compared with continuous infusion of 5-FU (overall 1-yr survival 45% vs 32%, respectively, $p = 0.035$), among patients with metastatic colorectal cancer who had failed to respond to first-line 5-FU-based regimens *(38)*. Importantly, the irinotecan regimens were well tolerated and the survival advantages reported in these two trials were not gained at the expense of quality of life.

Preclinical data have indicated a potential synergy between irinotecan and LV/5-FU *(39)*. This synergy appears to be sequence-dependent. In view of the potential clinical benefit of this combination, the addition of irinotecan to the simplified bimonthly LV/5-FU2 regimen has been investigated. A recent phase II study has demonstrated that this combination is active even in heavily pretreated patients *(28)*. The FOLFIRI-1 trial (*FOL*inic acid, 5*FU*, *IRI*notecan) evaluated LV/5-FU in combination with irinotecan as third-line therapy in 33 patients with advanced colorectal cancer. Patients received a twice weekly schedule of irinotecan, 180 mg/m^2, as a 90-min infusion on day 1, at the same time as a 2-h infusion of LV, 400 mg/m^2. This was immediately followed by a bolus of 5-FU, 400 mg/m^2, and a 46-h continuous infusion of 5-FU, 2400–3000 mg/m^2. Treatment was continued until disease progression, unless significant toxicity occurred. Diarrhea and neutropenia were the main limiting toxicities. Overall, 30% of patients experienced grade 3–4 toxicities which resolved with treatment or dose reduction, and the tolerability of the regimen was regarded as acceptable. Although the overall response rate was low (6%), with median and progression-free survival times of only 9.9 mo and 4.1 mo respectively, the FOLFIRI-1 trial nonetheless indicates that third-line therapy can be of benefit for some patients with metastatic colorectal cancer.

Following this study, a further attempt was made to improve the regimen in the FOLFIRI-2 study *(40)*. Hydroxyurea was added to enhance the 5-FU RNA pathway, based on the assumption that the inhibition of TS is not of primary importance in patients with tumors that are refractory to 5-FU, and that 5-FU-RNA and hydroxyurea can impair cellular repair mechanisms after irinotecan exposure. The FOLFIRI-2 regimen consisted of hydroxyurea, 1500 mg, administered on d 1–3, plus LV, 400 mg/m^2, as a 2-h infusion on day 1, immediately followed by a 46-h continuous infusion of 5-FU, 2000 mg/m^2, and irinotecan, 180 mg/m^2 as a 90-min infusion on d 3. The regimen was repeated every 2 wk. Twenty-nine patients with metastatic colorectal cancer, who had received at least two previous chemotherapy regimens including LV/5-FU and oxaliplatin, received the FOLFIRI-2 regimen. Partial responses were obtained in five patients (17%), while 15 patients (51%)

achieved disease stabilization, three patients (10%) showed disease progression, and six (21%) were withdrawn from the study due to toxicity or absence of clinical benefit. Median progression-free survival was 4.1 mo and median survival was 9.7 mo. Grade 3–4 neutropenia was observed in 52% of patients (febrile neutropenia in 7%), while other grade 3–4 toxicities were diarrhea (21%), nausea and mucositis (10%). In spite of the dose-limiting hematological toxicity, the FOLFIRI-2 regimen produced higher rates of response and disease stabilziation than the FOLFIRI-1 regimen.

A phase III trial has recently shown promising results in 387 patients with advanced disease *(41)*. In this multicenter study of the first-line treatment of metastatic colorectal cancer, patients received LV/5-FU, either with or without irinotecan, in a once or twice weekly regimen (according to local clinical practice or preference). The once weekly regimen involved 5-FU, 2300–2600 mg/m^2 by 24-h infusion and LV, 500 mg/m^2, with or without irinotecan, 80 mg/m^2. In the bimonthly regimen 5-FU, 400 mg/m^2, was administered on d 1 as an iv bolus followed by a 22-h infusion of 5-FU, 600 mg/m^2, and LV, 200 mg/m^2, on d 1 and 2, with or without irinotecan. Treatment was continued until disease progression or the occurrence of unacceptable toxicity. The addition of irinotecan to LV/5-FU was associated with improved tumor response rates (35% vs 22%, $p < 0.005$, in the intention-to-treat population), progression-free survival (6.7 mo vs 4.4 mo, $p < 0.001$) and overall survival (17.4 mo vs 14.1 mo, $p = 0.031$), compared with LV/5-FU alone. Furthermore, the combination had acceptable tolerability and although the incidence of grade 3–4 neutropenia, leukopenia, diarrhea, and asthenia was higher in the irinotecan group ($p < 0.05$), these effects were reported to be predictable, reversible, manageable, and noncumulative.

The combination FOLFOX-6 and FOLFIRI-1 regimens are currently being evaluated in another randomized study which aims to determine whether FOLFIRI followed by FOLFOX (arm A), or vice versa (arm B), is the most desirable sequence in the treatment of advanced colorectal cancer. Preliminary results are promising, with response rates of 55% observed for both arms *(42)*.

5. CONCLUSIONS

Since its introduction into clinical practice more than four decades ago, 5-FU has been used in the treatment of a range of cancers. For much of this time, this agent has formed the cornerstone of therapy for colorectal cancer, although tumor response rates and overall survival remain disappointing with 5-FU monotherapy. Extensive experimental and clinical evaluation of 5-FU have indicated that this drug has two mechanisms of action depending on the schedule of administration. This observation has led to the novel concept of schedule-specific modulation of 5-FU, and modulated hybrid regimens incorporating bolus and infusional 5-FU appear to produce the most promising results in advanced colorectal cancer.

The addition of LV to 5-FU schedules results in potentiation of the antitumor activity of 5-FU, and this combination is generally regarded as standard therapy for advanced colorectal cancer. The use of continuous infusions permits the administration of high doses of LV and 5-FU, leading to enhanced antitumor efficacy of the combination, with acceptable toxicity. The relatively low toxicity of bimonthly LV/5-FU regimens has allowed the addition of other agents, such as oxaliplatin and irinotecan, which further improves the response rates. Several studies of LV/5-FU regimens are currently in progress with the aim of identifying chemotherapeutic regimens that can improve both tumor response rates and overall survival. The addition of novel chemotherapeutic agents to LV/5-FU regimens is being evaluated in the first- and second-line treatment of advanced colorectal cancer, and also in the adjuvant setting.

ACKNOWLEDGMENT

The authors wish to thank all the GERCOR investigators who participated in the different studies reported in this chapter.

REFERENCES

1. Lokich JJ, Ahlgren JD, Gullo JJ, Philips JA, Fryer JG. A prospective randomized comparison of continuous infusion fluorouracil with a conventional bolus schedule in metastatic colorectal carcinoma: a Mid-Atlantic Oncology Program study. *J Clin Oncol* 1989; 7:425–32.
2. Meta-analysis Group in Cancer. Efficacy of intravenous continuous infusion of fluorouracil compared with bolus administration in advanced colorectal cancer. *J Clin Oncol* 1998; 16:301–8.
3. hansen RM, Quebbeman E, Anderson T. 5-Fluorouracil by protracted venous infusion. A review of current progress. *Oncology* 1989; 46:245–50.
4. Hansen RM, Ryan L, Anderson T, et al. Phase III study of bolus versus infusion fluorouracil with or without cisplatin in advanced colorectal cancer. *J Natl Cancer Inst* 1996; 88:668–74.
5. Leichman CG, Fleming TR, Muggia FM, et al. Phase II study of fluorouracil and its modulation in advanced colorectal cancer: a Southwest Oncology Group study. *J Clin Oncol* 1995; 13:1303–11.
6. Rougier PH, Paillot B, Laplanche A, et al. End results of a multicenter randomized trial comparing 5-FU in continuous systemic infusion (CI) to bolus administration (B) in measurable metastatic colorectal cancer. *Proc Am Soc Clin Oncol* 1992; 11:163.
7. Mori A, Bertoglio S, Guglielmi A, et al. Activity of continuous-infusion 5-fluorouracil in patients with advanced colorectal cancer clinically resistant to bolus 5-fluorouracil. *Cancer Chemother Pharmacol* 1993; 33:179–80.
8. Evans RM, Laskin JD, Hakala MT. Effects of excess folates and deoxyinosine on activity and site of action of 5-fluorouracil. *Cancer Res* 1981; 41:3288–95.
9. Houghton JA, Maroda SJ, Philips JO, Houghton PJ. Biochemical determinants of responsiveness to 5-fluorouracil and its derivatives in xenografts fo human colorectal adenocarcinoma in mice. *Cancer Res* 1981; 41:144–9.
10. Rustum YM, Trave F, Zakrzewski SF, et al. Biochemical and pharmacologic basis for potentiation of 5-fluorouracil action by leucovorin. *NCI Monogr* 1987; 5:165–70.
11. Petrelli N, Douglass HO Jr, Herrera L, et al. for the Gastrointestinal Tumor Study Group. The modulation of fluorouracil with leucovorin in metastatic colorectal carcinoma: a prospective randomized phase III trial. *J Clin Oncol* 1989; 7:1419–26.
12. Poon MA, O'Connell MJ, Moertel CG, et al. Biochemical modulation of fluorouracil: evidence of significant improvement of survival and quality of life in patients with advanced colorectal carcinoma. *J Clin Oncol* 1989; 7:1407–18.
13. Advanced Colorectal Cancer Meta-analysis Project. Modulation of fluorouracil by leucovorin in patients with advanced colorectal cancer: evidence in terms of response rate. *J Clin Oncol* 1992; 10:896–903.
14. Sobrero AF, Aschele C, Guglielmi AP, et al. Synergism and lack of cross-resistance between short-term and continuous exposure to fluorouracil in human colon adenocarcinoma cells. *J Natl Cancer Inst* 1993; 85:1937–44.
15. de Gramont A, Krulik M, Cady J, et al. High dose-folinic acid and 5-fluorouracil bolus and continuous infusion in advanced colorectal cancer. *Eur J Cancer Clin Oncol* 1988; 24:1499–1503.
16. de Gramont A, Bosset JF, Milan C, et al. Randomized trial comparing monthly low-dose leucovorin and fluorouracil bolus with bimonthly high-dose leucovorin and fluorouracil bolus plus continuous infusion for advanced colorectal cancer: a French intergroup study. *J Clin Oncol* 1997a; 15:808–15.
17. Beerblock K, Rinaldi Y, André T, et al. Bimonthly high dose leucovorin and 5-fluorouracil 48-hour continuous infusion in patients with advanced colorectal carcinoma. Groupe d'Etude et de Recherche sur les Cancers de l'Ovaire et Digestifs (GERCOD). *Cancer* 1997; 79:1100–15.
18. Tournigand C, de Gramont A, Louvet C, et al. for the GERCOR. A simplified bimonthly regimen with leucovorin and 5FU for metastatic colorectal cancer. *Proc Am Soc Clin Oncol* 1998; 17:274.
19. Raymond E, Faivre S, Woynarowski JM, Chaney SG. Oxaliplatin: mechanism of action and antineoplastic activity. *Semin Oncol* 1998a; 25(suppl 5)4–12.
20. Becouarn Y, Ychou M, Ducreux M, et al. A phase II trial of oxaliplatin as first-line chemotherapy in metastatic colorectal cancer patients. *J Clin Oncol* 1998; 8:2739–44.
21. Diaz-Rubio E, Sastre J, Zaniboni A, et al. Oxaliplatin as single agent in previously untreated colorectal carcinoma patients: a phase II multicentric study. *Ann Oncol* 1998;9:105–8.

22. Lévi F, Perpoint B, Garufi C, et al. Oxaliplatin activity against metastatic colorectal cancer. A phase II study of five-day continuous venous infusion at circadian rhythm modulated rate. *Eur J Cancer* 1993; 9(29A):1280–4.
23. Raymond E, Chaney SG, Taamma A, Cvitkovic E. Oxaliplatin: a review of preclinical and clinical studies. *Ann Oncol* 1998b; 9:1053–71.
24. de Gramont A, Figer A, Seymour M, et al. Leucovorin and fluorouracil with or without oxaliplatin as first-line treatment in advanced colorectal cancer. *J Clin Oncol* 2000; 18:2938–47.
25. de Gramont A, Gastiaburu J, Tournigand C, et al. Oxaliplatin with high-dose folinic acid and 5-fluorouracil 48 hour infusion in pretreated metastatic colorectal cancer. *Proc Am Soc Clin Oncol* 1994; 13:220.
26. de Gramont A, Vignoud J, Tournigand C, et al. Oxaliplatin with high-dose leucovorin and 5 fluorouracil 48 hour continuous infusion in pretreated metastatic colorectal cancer. *Eur J Cancer* 1997b; 33:214–19.
27. André T, Louvet C, Raymond E, Tournigand C, de Gramont A. Bimonthly high-dose leucovorin, 5-fluorouracil infusion and oxaliplatin (FOLFOX3) for metastatic colorectal cancer resistant to the same leucovorin and 5-fluorouracil regimen. *Ann Oncol* 1998; 9:1–3.
28. André T, Louvet C, Maindrault-Goebel F, et al. on behalf of GERCOR. CPT-11 (Irinotecan) addition to bimonthly, high-dose leucovorin and bolus and continuous-infusion 5-fluorouracil (FOLFIRI) for pretreated metastatic colorectal cancer. *Eur J Cancer* 1999; 35:1343–7.
29. Maindrault-Goebel F, Louvet C, André T, et al. for the GERCOR. Oxaliplatin added to the simplified bimonthly leucovorin and 5 fluorouracil regimen as second-line therapy for metastatic colorectal cancer (FOLFOX6). *Eur J Cancer* 1999a; 35:1338–42.
30. Maindrault-Goebel F, de Gramont A, Louvet C, Andre T, for the GERCOR. High-dose intensity oxaliplatin added to the simplified bimonthly leucovorin and 5-fluorouracil regimen as second-line therapy for metastatic colorectal cancer (FOLFOX7). *Proc Am Soc Clin Oncol* 1999b; 18:265.
31. de Gramont A, Maindrault-Goebel F, Louvet C, et al. for the GERCOR. Evaluation of oxaliplatin dose-intensity with the bimonthly 48h leucovorin and 5 fluorouracil regimens (FOLFOX) in pretreated metastatic colorectal cancer. *Proc Am Soc Clin Oncol* 1999; 18:265a.
33. Creemers GJ, Lund B, Verweij J. Topoisomerase I inhibitor: topotecan and irinotecan. *Cancer Treat Res* 1994; 20:73–96.
34. Ducreux M, Ychou M, Seitz JF, et al. Irinotecan combined with bolus fluorouracil, continuous infusion fluorouracil, and high-dose leucovorin every two weeks (LV5FU2 regimen): a clinical dose-finding and pharmacokinetic study in patients with colorectal cancer. *J Clin Oncol* 1999; 17:2901–8.
35. Pitot HC, Wender DB, O'Connell MJ, et al. Phase II trial of irinotecan in patients with metastatic colorectal carcinoma. *J Clin Oncol* 1997; 5:2910–19.
32. Shimada Y, Rothenberg M, Hilsenbeck SG, Burris HA 3rd, Degen D, Von Hoff DD. Activity of CPT-11 (irinotecan hydrochloride), a topoisomerase inhibitor, against human tumour colony-forming units. *Anticancer Drugs* 1994; 5:20–6.
36. Rougier P, Bugat R, Douillard Y, et al. Phase II study of irinotecan in the treatment of advanced colorectal cancer in chemotherapy-naïve patients and patients pretreated with fluorouracil-based chemotherapy. *J Clin Oncol* 1997; 15:251–60.
37. Cunningham D, Pyrhonen S, James RD, et al. Randomized trial of irinotecan plus supportive care versus supportive care alone after fluorouracil failure for patients with metastatic colorectal cancer. *Lancet* 1998; 352:1413–8.
38. Rougier P, Van Cutsem E, Bajetta E, et al. Randomised trial of irinotecan versus fluorouracil by continuous infusion after fluorouracil failure for patients with metastatic colorectal cancer. *Lancet* 1998; 352:1407–12.
39. Mullany S, Svingen PA, Kaufmano SH, Erlichman C. Effect of adding the topoisomerase 1 poison 7-ethyl 10-hydroxycamptothecin (SN 38) to 5-fluorouracil and folinic acid in HCT8 cells: elevated dTTP pools and enhanced cytotoxicity. *Cancer Chemother Pharm* 1998; 42:391–99.
40. Mabro M, André T, Louvet Carola E, Beerblock K, Krulik M, de Gramont A. Bimonthly leucovorin, 5-fluorouracil infusion and hydroxyurea followed by CPT-11 (FOLFIRI-2) in pretreated patients with metastatic colorectal cancer. *Proc Am Soc Clin Oncol* 2000; 19:294a.
41. Douillard JY, Cunningham D, Roth AD, et al. Irinotecan combined with fluorouracil compared with fluorouracil alone as first-line treatment for metastatic colorectal cancer: a multicentre randomised trial. *Lancet* 2000; 355:1041–7.
42. Tournigand C, Achille E, Lledo G, et al. FOLFIRI followed by FOLFOX or FOLFOX followed by FOLFIRI in metastatic colorectal cancer (MCRC). Preliminary results of a randomized phase III study of the GERCOR. ESMO meeting, Hamburg, October 2000.

12 Review on the Combination of Systemic and Locoregional Treatment for Colorectal Liver Metastases

Roberto Labianca, MD*, Gianfranco Pancera,* MD*,*
Marinella Mastore, MD*, Marina Garassino,* MD*,*
Giordano D. Beretta, MD*, Paola Poletti,* MD*,*
and M. Adelaide Pessi, MD

CONTENTS

1. INTRODUCTION

Colorectal cancer is one of the most frequent malignancies of both men and women in Western countries. In the United States about one person out of 20 is affected by adenocarcinoma of the large bowel, which represents 15% of all cancers and therefore constitutes a major public health problem.

In the early stages this neoplasm is highly curable by surgical treatment with minimal morbidity and mortality, but in advanced (unresectable or recurrent) disease an additional therapy is required *(1)*.

The occurrence of hepatic metastates implies a poor prognosis, regardless of whether or not the tumor has spread at the time of primary diagnosis. In autopsy series patient survival was inversely correlated with the degree of liver involvement: widespread metastases involving both lobes of the liver determine a 1-yr survival rate of 5.6% only. If, on the contrary, metastatic disease involves a segment or a lobe only, 1-yr survival rate increases to 27% and rises to 60% in case of single localizations *(2,3)*. It is well known that about 20% of patients with primary colon cancer present synchronous liver metastases and that the overall probability to develop them during the disease natural history is nearly 50%, with metastatic disease con-

From: *Fluoropyrimidines in Cancer Therapy*
Edited by: Y. M. Rustum © Humana Press Inc., Totowa, NJ

fined to the liver in half of cases. Surgical resection represents the best choice to cure patients with metastatic disease confined to the liver, but a radical resection is possible in less than 25% of cases. A number of studies reported a 2-yr overall survival of 55–65% and a 5-yr percentage of 25–30%: after this period, patients can reasonably be considered as cured.

2. NATURAL HISTORY OF COLORECTAL LIVER METASTASES

The venous system of colon and upper rectum drains into the portal circulation: since 1938, the importance of tumor vascular invasion has been recognized and this is differentiated in "intramural" (when blood vessels within the bowel wall are involved) and "extramural" (if pericolonic fat or adventitia are involved) *(4)*. As expected, the incidence of blood vessel invasion varies widely in relation to several prognostic factors, such as pathological stage of disease and histologic grading. A very important issue is that normal hepatocytes and also micrometastases derive their blood supply from both the portal vein and hepatic artery, whereas liver metastases larger than 0.5 cm in their main diameter receive most of their supply from hepatic artery *(5)*. This evidence led to the development of cytotoxic therapy with hepatic arterial infusion (HAI) of antiproliferative agents: this approach was first experimented on in 1959 by Sullivan et al. *(6)*, who evaluated the intrahepatic administration of the 5-fluorouracil (5-FU) analog fluorodeoxyuridine (FUDR) because of its favorable pharmacodynamics (with a nearly complete intrahepatic extraction and therefore a minimal systemic exposure). As a matter of fact, at the first passage the liver clearance of the drug varies from 94 to 99%, as compared with 19–55% of 5-FU or even lower percentage of other agents, such as mitomicyn C, cisplatin, and doxorubicin. The rationale for hepatic arterial chemotherapy includes also the concept of a stepwise pattern of metastatic progression: according to this theory hematogenous spread occurs first through the portal vein to the liver, then to the lungs, and finally to other organs. Therefore, an aggressive treatment of metastases confined to the liver (resection, whenever possible, or HAI or both) could increase the survival of a number of patients and possibly be curative in selected cases *(7–9)*.

3. HEPATIC ARTERY INFUSION: FEASIBILITY AND RESULTS

At present HAI is usually delivered by means of implantable devices (catheters, port-a-caths, or totally implantable pumps, which are much more expensive). In the last 15–20 yr these devices were usually placed through a surgical approach (laparotomy), but now the angiographic technique is frequently used (see below).

The major side-effects of HAI are represented by gastroduodenal ulceration and by hepatic toxicity. Ulceration is usually caused by drug perfusion of stomach and duodenum through small collateral branches from hepatic artery, whereas hepatic injury [clinically evidenced by increase of alanine aminotransferase (ALT), alkaline phosphatase, and bilirubin] is probably the result of a combination of ischemic and inflammatory effect on the bile ducts. Alteration of ALT is an early indication of toxicity, whereas a rise of alkaline phosphatase or bilirubin usually indicates more severe and advanced damage. Sometimes, in the early stages of toxicity, drug discontinuation or the adoption of a more prolonged interval period may be enough to reduce liver enzymes to normal values. If, on the contrary, toxicity is in a more advanced stage, endoscopic retrograde cholanges pancreatography (ERCP) can demonstrate lesions resembling those of the idiopathic sclerosing cholangitis. The sensitivity of bile ducts to intraarterial chemotherapy is explained by their physiologic perfusion by hepatic artery *(10)*.

Myelosuppression is not frequent using HAI, with the exception of thrombocytopenia in case of mitomicyn C or carmustine administration. Nausea and emesis usually do not occur with HAI of FUDR. If diarrhea does occur, shunting to the bowel should be suspected, investigated by abdomen radiography, and eventually corrected.

The addition of heparin to FUDR solution prevents the risk of arterial thromboembolism and the administration of dexamethasone in the pump together with FUDR is able to decrease the risk of liver toxicity *(11,12)*. Also the use of a circadian rhythm of FUDR administration could decrease the risk of hepatic damage.

The activity of HAI is clearly documented in many trials and confirmed by systematic revisions. Two meta-analyses published in 1996 and including 7–8 phase III trials with several hundred patients demonstrated that tumor response rate in patients with unresectable liver metastases from colorectal cancer was 41% for hepatic infusion therapy with FUDR as compared with 14% for systemic chemotherapy. Analysis of impact on survival is less clear and an objective and quantitative appraisal of the benefits of HAI in terms of overall patient survival is still required. Because of development of extrahepatic sites of metastatic disease left untreated by regional chemotherapy, controlled trials have generally failed to achieve a significant survival benefit compared with the use of systemic therapy. In spite of a trend toward a better survival in the HAI group of patients and the observation that the number of patients surviving more than 2 yr was higher in the HAI group, the comparison with the intravenous chemotherapy group showed that the benefit appeared to be small and not statistically significant *(13,14)*.

4. COMBINED LOCOREGIONAL AND SYSTEMIC CHEMOTHERAPY

The rationale for combining locoregional and systemic chemotherapy in advanced colorectal cancer with metastases to the liver only is based on the following issues:

1. Locoregional chemotherapy has a well-defined activity in these patients and is possibly superior, as reported above, to systemic treatment (at least when traditional agents are administered intravenously).
2. The two therapeutic modalities have nonoverlapping side-effects (liver toxicity for intraarterial therapy, chiefly when FUDR is employed; mucositis, diarrhea, and myelotoxicity with the most frequently used intravenous agents such as biomodulated 5-FU, irinotecan and oxaliplatin).
3. From a theoretical point of view, the addition of a systemic treatment should be able to reduce the occurrence of extra-hepatic relapse or progression.
4. Recently, significant progress have been registered in the availability of innovative compounds able to obtain (when given through the intravenous route) a higher objective response rate and an increased survival in comparison with the conventional agents: this should permit a more active combination with the standard locoregional treatments (FUDR or modulated 5-FU) or a promising evaluation of these new agents in the intraarterial route.

A number of phase II trials have been conducted recently with the aim of evaluating the activity of a combined locoregional × systemic treatment for patients with metastatic disease limited to the liver. However, owing to the small number of included patients and the lack of homogeneity of the therapeutic regimens, only general indications can be drawn from these experiences. A brief outline of these trials follows:

1. In Germany, Lorenz et al. *(15)* treated 20 patients with intraarterial FUDR (at a reduced dose of 0.2 mg/kg/d × 14 d every 4 wk) and intravenous 5-FU (700 mg/sqm/d × 3 d every 4 wk) and reported a satisfactory objective response rate, but a high percentage of extrahepatic relapse (62%), very close to the figure of 56% observed by Kemeny with locoregional treatment only

(FUDR: 0.3 mg/kg/d × 14 d every 4 wk) *(16)* and to the 73% reported by Niederhuber *(17)* with a similar regimen.

2. Again in Germany, Safi et al. *(18)* included 45 cases in a small controlled clinical trial in which a combination of intraarterial FUDR (0.2 mg/kg/d × 14 d every 4 wk) and the same drug given intravenously (0.09 mg/kg/d in the same period) was evaluated in comparison with FUDR administered only intraarterially at the same dose as above. In this study a response rate of 48% was obtained with the combined strategy and the percentage of extrahepatic spread of cancer during therapy seemed of interest in comparison to that observed with locoregional treatment only (33% vs 61%, even though without statistical significance due to the low power of the study). Of course, the limited number of patients and the questionable statistical design prevented any definitive conclusion about the possible superiority of the intraarterial/intravenous chemotherapy vs the locoregional approach.
3. The Mayo Clinic group performed a trial presented by O'Connell *(19)* in which the reduced dose of intraarterial FUDR (0.2 mg/kg/d × 14 d) was associated, after a 1-wk rest period, with the low-dose daily-times five regimen of 5-FU (425 mg/m^2/d) and LV (20 mg/m^2/d) every 4 wk; the combined treatment was administered until maximal regression of hepatic metastases, whereas a maintenance therapy with intravenous 5-FU and LV was continued until disease progression. In a group of 40 evaluable patients (out of 57 enrolled in the trial) the extrahepatic relapse, once again, was quite high (45%) even though the global response rate was 62% and the overall median survival was 18 mo, with a tolerable toxicity and no cases of biliary sclerosis.
4. At the Memorial Sloan-Kettering Cancer Center (MSKCC), Kemeny *(20)* conducted a pilot study of hepatic arterial infusion and systemic chemotherapy in order to establish the correct doses for concurrent treatment in patients with resected disease. 5-FU was administered for 5 d as an intravenous bolus of 325 mg/m^2, preceded each day by a 30-min infusion of LV at the dose of 200 mg/m^2; two weeks later the first dose of FUDR (0.25 mg/kg/d) was instilled into the pump for 14 d in combination with 20 mg of dexamethasone and 50,000 IU of heparin. The treatment was recycled after a 1 wk rest for six courses. This regimen was thereafter employed in the following phase III trial (see below).
5. At the S.Carlo Borromeo Hospital (Milano, Italy) Pancera et al. *(21)* pioneered a monoinstitutional trial with intraarterial FUDR at intermediate dosage (0.25 mg/kg/d × 14 d on third and fourth week) combined with 5FU (370 mg/m^2 d 1 to 4) and levo-LV (100 mg/m^2 d 1 to 4) on first week; the treatment was recycled every five weeks. In a group of 27 patients, a response rate of 69.2% was obtained with a median TTP of 17 mo, a median survival of 20 mo and 35% patients alive at 2 yr; even more interestingly, a low percentage of extrahepatic relapse (23% only) was observed and toxicity was acceptable, without toxic deaths, allowing the administration of the whole treatment program on an outpatient basis. These promising data generated the successor phase III trial performed in the nineties by GISCAD (Gruppo Italiano per lo Studio dei Carcinomi dell'Apparato Digerente = Italian Group for the Study of Digestive Tract Cancer), reported below.

The phase III trials in this field are very rare and this is due to several reasons: difficult collaboration among medical oncologists, surgeons, and interventional radiologists; legal and commerical obstacles to drug supply, chiefly for FUDR; an increased role for systemic chemotherapy in this disease and a reduction of interest for locoregional treatment by the vast majority of medical oncologists. On the other hand, the availability of new implant techniques should allow an easier inclusion of patients in trials evaluating the role of intraarterial chemotherapy in combination or in comparison with an optimal systemic treatment. As a matter of fact, whereas the surgical method has some potential advantages (it is well established, permits a complete intraoperative staging, and is particularly suitable for synchronous metastases) there are also important drawbacks for this approach (it appears too aggressive for metachronous metastases and the economic costs can be too high). On the contrary, the radiological percutaneous techniques *(22,23)*, even though more recent, are minimally invasive, require much lower costs, and allow an easier catheter substitution when necessary: The main disadvantage is the possibility of only performing an instrumental staging. On the basis of these technological improvements, the conduction of large-scale cooperative trials on this topic should be more feasible than in the last years.

The most important phase III trial evaluating the role of combined locoregional and systemic chemotherapy was published by Kemeny et al. in 1999 *(24)*. The MSKCC team randomly assigned 156 patients resected for liver metastases from colorectal cancer to receive six courses of hepatic arterial infusion with FUDR and dexamethasone plus systemic 5-FU (usually biomodulated by LV) or six cycles of intravenous therapy alone. A stratification was performed on the basis of a previous treatment and on the number of liver metastases detected at the moment of operation. The results of this unique trial showed a significant advantage in overall survival at 2 yr for patients receiving combined chemotherapy in comparison to those treated with systemic drugs alone (86% vs 72%, $p = 0.03$). Also the rate of survival free from hepatic relapse was in favor of the group assigned to the associated treatment (90% vs 60%, $p<0.001$) and the tolerability of the two regimens was similar, except for a higher frequency of diarrhea and liver toxicity in the combined treatment arm. Therefore, the outcome at 2 yr for this selected population (patients amenable to liver resection for limited hepatic involvement) appears to be increased through the addition of a combined (locoregional + systemic) chemotherapy to the standard surgical resection. Of course, a longer observation is needed to confirm this advantage at 5 yr, when no more than 25–30% of resected only patients are expected to be alive.

Another important trial concerning the possible usefulness of a combined therapy in this setting was conducted by ECOG (Eastern Cooperative Oncology Group) and SWOG (Southwest Oncology Group) *(25)*. Also in this experience (comparing patients treated after liver resection with intraarterial + intravenous chemotherapy vs resected only patients) an advantage for chemotherapy was detected, but it is noteworthy that a 9-yr period was needed to enroll 109 cases only.

What is the future for trials in this field? In our opinion they are still needed and we want to remind that in his editorial in the *Journal of Clinical Oncology (26)*, commenting on a three-arm trial by Lorenz (in which a comparison among systemic therapy and two different regimens of intra-arterial treatment was performed) *(27)*, Daniel Haller said that we are still waiting for the definitive trial on this matter: This can be true not only for the comparison between locoregional chemotherapy and "the" (or, at least, "an") optimal systemic treatment but also for the combination of the two modalities vs one or each of them.

5. THE "GISCAD" PHASE III TRIAL

In May 1993, GISCAD began a randomized trial (no. C-04) with the aim of evaluating the role of combined locoregional + systemic chemotherapy vs locoregional chemotherapy only in the treatment of advanced colorectal cancer with unresectable liver metastases and without concomitant involvement of extrahepatic organs. The purpose of this study was to confirm the interesting observation coming from the previous single-center trial and concerning the possible decrease in extrahepatic disease relapse; another issue was to evaluate whether the combined treatment was more active (in terms of response rate) and/or more effective (in terms of TTP and overall survival) in comparison with locoregional chemotherapy alone without an unacceptable increase in toxicity. Of course, a third arm with systemic therapy alone could have been warranted in such a trial (and this was the original GISCAD project) but after a long discussion inside the group we decided to delete this arm for the following reasons:

1. Most centers with expertise in intraarterial delivery of chemotherapy and with a primary involvement of surgeons did not trust in systemic treatment.
2. In the early 1990s intravenous therapy of advanced colorectal cancer was mainly based on regimens including biomodulated bolus 5-FU (such as the "Mayo Clinic" or the "Machover" combination), as 5-FU continuous infusion was used only in a very limited number of institutions and the new drugs (such as irinotecan, oxaliplatin, raltitrexed, and the oral compounds) were not available at that time: with those "standard" treatments the median overall survival did not exceed 1 yr.
3. In the selected population of patients with unresectable but "limited" (< 50% organ involvement) liver metastases, locoregional chemotherapy had been demonstrated very active (response rate about 50–70% and median survival approaching 2 yr) in several phase II trials.
4. The first results of at least 7–8 phase III studies favored the use of intraarterial administration of drugs, even though with the methodological concerns discussed before and therefore this route of delivery was considered by many of us the best therapy for this particular subset of patients.

The inclusion criteria for the trial were: unresectable liver metastases with hepatic involvement less than 50%; no evidence of disease outside the liver (a complete staging, including an accurate intraoperative assessment, was mandatory, with biopsy of every suspected lesion); no concomitant serious disease (at the hepatic, renal, cardiac, or metabolic level); a good performance status (PS), 0–2 according to ECOG score; a satisfactory bone marrow function; no major contraindication to laparotomy, when required (during a long period of this trial the percutaneous catheter insertion was not yet available); no previous chemotherapy for advanced disease (adjuvant treatment was allowed if terminated at least 1 yr before the occurrence of metastases); no previous tumour (with the exception of basocellular skin cancer and early cervical carcinoma); oral informed consent, and, lastly, geographic accessibility (of particular importance for this complex treatment).

A complete staging (pre- and intraoperative) was required and an accurate clinical and hematological evaluation was programmed before each drug administration. The objective response evaluation was planned after three courses of treatment and therapy was continued until disease progression or heavy toxicity or patient decision. The protocol included detailed recommendations to prevent and/or to treat the most important side-effects (with particular emphasis on hepatoxicity from FUDR) and to optimize the patient management.

The treatment regimens were:

**Arm A* (experimental):

levo-LV: 100 mg/m^2/iv d 1 to 4 on first week
5-FU: 400 mg/m^2 iv 15 min d 1 to 4 on first week
FUDR: 0.25 mg/kg/ia × 14 d on third and fourth wk
Dexamethasone: 20 mg in the pump together with FUDR
Heparin (sodic): 20,000 IU in the pump together with FUDR
Recycle every 5 wk

* *Arm B* (standard):

FUDR: 0.25 mg/kg/ia × 14 d every 4 wk
Dexamethasone: 20 mg in the pump together with FUDR
Heparin (sodic): 20,000 IU in the pump together with FUDR

A sample of at least 120 patients was calculated assuming a 2-yr survival of 20% in the standard arm and of 38% in the experimental one (with a relative reduction of 40%), with an alpha error of 0.05 and a beta error of 0.20 (two-tailed test).

From May 1993 to November 1999 127 patients were included in the trial: this prolonged period indicates, once again, the difficulty on both sides of the Atlantic in performing these trials. However, this case list was the one planned by our group and permitted us to observe that the tolerability of both regimens was acceptable, with an increased incidence of gastroenteric side-effects (nausea and vomiting, diarrhea, and mucositis) for arm A, in which patients received also systemic chemotherapy. The data on activity and efficacy of this trial are reported in an original paper submitted for publication to a major oncology journal and, for this reason, they cannot be quoted in this book, even though a report was made at ASCO Meeting in 2000 *(28)*.

In 2001, GISCAD is involved in further research on the topic of locoregional (+/– systemic) treatment of colorectal liver metastases. The ongoing trial is evaluating, on a phase II basis, a combination of intravenous FOLFOX-4 regimen (I-LV: 100 $mg/m^2/2$ h infusion. + 5-FU: 400 mg/sqm/iv bolus + 5-FU: 600 $mg/m^2/22$ h infusion, all the drugs given on d 1 and 2, with oxaliplatin: 85 $mg/m^2/2$ h infusion on d 1 only) with intraarterial FUDR (0.25 mg/kg/d from d 15 to 28), recycling every 5 wk. Out of six patients treated by November 30, 2000, an objective response was observed in three.

REFERENCES

1. Adson MA. Diagnosis and surgical treatment of primary and secondary solid tumors in the adult. *Surg Clin North Am* 1981; 61:1181–1192.
2. Lokich JJ. Primary and metastatic liver cancer. *Semin Oncol* 1983; 10:227–233.
3. Welch JP, Donaldson GA. Clinical correlation of an autopsy study of recurrent colorectal cancer. *Ann Surg* 1979; 189:496–506.
4. Brown CE, Warren S. Visceral metastases from rectal carcinoma. *Surg Gynecol Obst* 1938; 66:611–619.
5. Breedis C, Young C. The blood supply of neoplasm in the liver. *Am J Pathol* 1954; 30:969–978.
6. Sullivan RD, Miller E, Skyes MP. A clinical-pharmacological evaluation of hepatic arterial infusion of 5-fluoro-2-deoxyuridine and 5-fluorouracil. *Cancer Res* 1959; 38:3784–3792.
7. Ackermann NB, Lien WM, Kondi ES, et al. The blood supply of experimental liver metastases. The distribution of hepatic artery and portal vein blood to "small" and "large" tumors. *Surgery* 1969; 66:1067–1074.
8. Weiss L, Grundmann E, Torhorst J, et al. Hematogenous metastatic patterns in colonic carcinoma: an analysis of 1541 necropsies. *J Pathol* 1986; 150:195–203.
9. Weiss L. Metastatic inefficiency and regional therapy for liver metastases from colorectal carcinoma. *Reg Cancer Treat* 1989; 2:77–85.
10. Northover JM, Terblanche J. A new look at the arterial supply of the bile duct in man and its surgical implications. *Br J Surg* 1979; 66:379–386.
11. Kemeny N, Sigurdson E. Intra-arterial chemotherapy for liver tumours. In: Blumgart LH, ed. Surgery of liver and biliary tract. Edinburgh; Churchill and Livingstone, 1994.
12. Kemeny N, Conti JA, Cohen A, et al. Phase II study of hepatic arterial floxuridine, leucovorin and dexamethasone for unresectable liver metastases from colorectal carcinoma. *J Clin Oncol* 1994; 12:2288–2295.
13. Meta-Analysis Group In Cancer. Reappraisal of hepatic arterial infusion in the treatment of nonresectable liver metastases from colorectal cancer. *J Natl Cancer Inst* 1996; 88:252–259.
14. Harmantas A, Rotstein LE, Langer B. Regional versus systemic chemotherapy in the treatment of colorectal carcinoma metastatic to the liver. Is there a survival difference? Meta-analysis of the published literature. *Cancer* 1996; 78:1639–1645.
15. Lorenz M, Hottenrott C, Maier P, et al. Continuous regional treatment with fluoropyrimidines for metastases from colorectal carcinomas. Influence of modulation with leucovorin. *Semin Oncol* 1992 (Suppl 3); 19:163–170.
16. Kemeny N, Daly J, Reichmann B, et al. Intrahepatic or systemic infusion of fluorodeoxuridine in patients with liver metastases from colorectal carcinoma. *Ann Intern Med* 1987; 107:459–465.

17. Niederhuber JE, Ensminger W, Gyvers J, et al. Regional chemotherapy of colorectal cancer metastatic to the liver. *Cancer* 1984; 53:1336–1343.
18. Safi F, Bittner R, Roscher R, et al. Regional chemotherapy for hepatic metastases of colorectal carcinoma (continuous intraarterial versus continuous intraarterial/intravenous therapy). *Cancer* 1989; 64:379–387.
19. O'Connell MJ, Nagorney DM, Bernath AM, et al. Sequential intrahepatic fluorodeoxyuridine and systemic fluorouracil plus leucovorin for the treatment of metastatic colorectal cancer confined to the liver. *J Clin Oncol* 1998; 16:2528–2533.
20. Kemeny N, Conti JA, Sigurdson E, et al. A pilot study of hepatic artery floxuridine combined with systemic 5-fluorouracil and leucovorin: a potential adjuvant program after resection of colorectal hepatic metastases. *Cancer* 1993; 71:1964–1971.
21. Pancera (fase II)
22. Grosso M, Zanon C, Zanon E, et al. The percutaneous placement of intra-arterial catheters with "reservoirs" for subcutaneous infusion. The technique and preliminary results. *Radiol Med* 1997; 94:226–232.
23. Herrmann KA, Waggershauser T, Sittek H, et al. Liver intra-arterial chemotherapy: use of the femoral artery for percutaneous implantation of catheter-port systems. *Radiology* 2000; 215:294–299.
24. Kemeny N, Huang Y, Cohen AM, et al. Hepatic arterial infusion of chemotherapy after resection of hepatic metastases from colorectal cancer. *N Engl J Med* 1999; 341:2039–2048.
25. Kemeny MM, Adak S, Lipsitz S, et al. Results of the intergroup ECOG and SWOG prospective randomized study of surgery alone versus continuous hepatic artery infusion FUDR and continuous systemic infusion of 5FU after hepatic resection of colorectal liver metastases. *Proc Am Soc Clin Oncol* 1999; 18:1012 (abstract).
26. Haller DG. Waiting for the definitive trial of hepatic arterial chemotherapy for colorectal cancer (editorial). *J Clin Oncol* 2000; 18:239–242.
27. Lorenz M, Muller HH for the German Cooperative Group on Liver Metastases. Randomized, multicenter trial of fluorouracil plus leucovorin administered either via hepatic arterial or intravenous infusion versus fluorodeoxyuridine administered via hepatic arterial infusion in patients with nonresectable liver metastases from colorectal carcinoma. *J Clin Oncol* 2000; 18:243–254.
28. Pancera G. Randomized trial of intraarterial vs combination CT in unresectable liver metastases from colorectal cancer: a multicentric GISCAD-SITILO study. *Proc Am Soc Clin Oncol* 2000; 19:986 (abstract).

13 Fluoropyrimidines in Advanced Colorectal Cancer

A Review of Six Consecutive Meta-Analyses

Pascal Piedbois, MD, and Marc E. Buyse, ScD

CONTENTS

1. INTRODUCTION

Management of patients with advanced colorectal cancer (ACC) has been based for 40 yr on fluoropyrimidines, and despite the recent introduction of new and active drugs, such as CPT-11 (irinotecan) and oxaliplatin, most effective chemotherapy regimens still include fluoropyrimidines. In the last decade, the *Meta-Analysis Group In Cancer* (formerly *Advanced Colorectal Cancer Meta-Analysis Project*) has systematically addressed through a meta-analytic approach the efficacy of various fluoropyrimidine regimens in ACC. This chapter reviews the evidence accumulated in this work.

2. METHODS

Meta-analysis aims to combine all trials addressing a similar question into a single analysis. Such combination permits the ascertainment of treatment benefits too small or too erratic to be demonstrated in individual trials *(1)*. Meta-analysis of randomized clinical trials is widely considered a major tool in "evidence-based medicine," especially meta-analyses based on individual patient data, which are more powerful and more reliable than overviews based on published or summary data *(2–4)*. Moreover, meta-analysis can generate hypotheses to be addressed in future trials.

The *Meta-Analysis Group In Cancer* has conducted six meta-analyses in ACC, exploring the modulation of 5-fluorouracil (5-FU) by leucovorin *(5)*, by methotrexate *(6)*, or by inter-

From: *Fluoropyrimidines in Cancer Therapy*
Edited by: Y. M. Rustum © Humana Press Inc., Totowa, NJ

feron *(7)*, and the administration of fluoropyrimidines by continuous infusion *(8)* or by hepatic arterial infusion *(9)*. All meta-analyses used individual patient data, and were performed by intention to treat, without any patient exclusion. Each meta-analysis was conducted in close collaboration with principal investigators of individual trials. End-points evaluated in these meta-analyses are necessarily limited to those addressed by individual trials, often performed in the 1980s. Consequently tumor response evaluation is based on WHO criteria *(10,11)* rather than the recently proposed RECIST criteria *(12)*. Time to progression and quality of life data were seldom available. Tumor response, overall survival, and simple prognostic factors such as the patient's age and performance status, the primary tumor location, the number and sites of metastases, were available in over 7000 patients. In some cases toxicity data were also available *(13)*. The benefits of experimental treatments were expressed in terms of response odd ratios (OR) and survival hazard ratios (HR), with the convention that ORs and HRs smaller than one indicate treatment benefit, while ORs and HRs larger than one indicate treatment harm *(5)*.

3. MODULATION OF 5-FU

5-Fluorouracil (5-FU) alone, given as a bolus intravenous injection, has a modest activity in ACC. Attempts of combining 5-FU with cytotoxic agents, such as cisplatin or nitrosoureas, have either failed to improve these results significantly or have been associated with an unacceptable increase in morbidity.

Several compounds have been shown to modulate the cytoxicity of 5-FU in vitro, and three of them have been extensively explored in randomized clinical trials: Leucovorin, methotrexate, and interferon.

3.1. 5-FU Plus Folinic Acid

Fluorodeoxyuridylate (FdUMP), one of the metabolites of 5-FU, binds to thymidylate synthase in the presence of 5–10-methylene tetrahydrofolate (CH_2FH_4). This interaction leads to the formation of a covalent ternary complex, and to the inhibition of thymidylate synthase. In some human tumors, the amount of folate may be insufficient to permit optimal cytotoxicity of 5-FU *(14)*. Folinic acid (leucovorin), a mixture of stereoisomers [(6R,S)-5-formyltetrahydrofolate], can increase the intracellular concentration of CH_2FH_4 and thereby stabilize the ternary complex *(15)*. Finally, in vitro studies confirmed that the cytotoxic activity of 5-FU can be potentiated by folinic acid *(15–17)*.

The meta-analysis of randomized trials comparing 5-FU alone to intravenous leucovorin and 5-FU (5-FU/LV) was published in 1992 *(5)*. The analysis included 1381 patients randomized in nine trials. Objective tumor response rates were 11% in patients allocated to 5-FU, and 23% in patients allocated to 5-FU/LV (Table 1). The overall response odds ratio was 0.45 (95% CI: 0.34–0.60; $p < 10^{-7}$). Interestingly enough, the tests for treatment effect were highly significant in favor of 5-FU/LV both in the trials adding weekly leucovorin ($p<10^{-5}$) and in those adding monthly leucovorin ($p<10^{-5}$), but far from significant in the trials using a higher 5-FU dose as control (p=0.71). These results suggest a dose effect of 5-FU in ACC, and were subsequently observed in the other meta-analyses performed by our group.

The important advantage in tumor response of 5-FU/LV over 5-FU alone did not translate into a significant survival difference between the two treatment arms, even when trials with a crossover were excluded from the analysis. Median survival was 11.0 mo for 5-FU, and 11.5 mo for 5-FU/LV (Table 2). The overall survival hazard ratio was 0.97 (95% CI: 0.86–1.09; p=0.57).

Table 1
Tumor Response Rates Reported in the Meta-Analyses of Fluoropyrimidines in Advanced Colorectal Cancer

Meta-analysis	*Tumor response rates*		*Treatment comparison*
5FU vs 5FU/LV *(5)*	5FU bolus	5FU/LV	OR=0.45 (95% CI=
1381 patients	11%	23%	0.34–0.60; $p < 10^{-7}$)
5FU vs 5FU/MTX *(6)*	5FU bolus	5FU/MTX	OR=0.51 (95% CI=
1178 patients	10%	19%	0.37–0.70; $p < 10^{-4}$)
5FU ± LV vs 5FU ± LV + α-IFN *(7)*	5FU ± LV	5FU ± LV + α-IFN	RR=1.02(95%C.I=
1766 patients	25%	24%	0.87–1.2; p=0.8)
5FU + LV vs 5FU + α-IFN *(7)*	5FU + LV	5FU + α-IFN	RR=1.26 95%C.I=
1488 patients	23%	18%	(1.00–1.58; p=0.042)
5FU bolus vs 5FU continuous	5FU bolus	5FU C.I.	OR=0.55 (95% CI,
infusion *(8)*			0.41–0.75; p=0.0002)
1219 patients	22%	14%	
IV FP vs HAI FUDR *(9)*	IV FP	HAI FUDR	OR=0.25 (95% CI,
654 patients	14%	41%	0.16–0.40; $p < 10^{-10}$)

OR = Odds Ratio; RR = relative risk; CI = confidence interval; IV = intravenous; FP = fluoropyrimidines; HAI = hepatic artery infusion; FUDR = 5-fluoro-2′deoxyuridine

Table 2
Overall Survival Reported in the Meta-Analyses of Fluoropyrimidines in Advanced Colorectal Cancer

Meta-analysis	*Median survivals*		*Treatment comparison*
5FU vs 5FU/LV *(5)*	5FU bolus	5FU/LV	HR=0.97 (95% CI:
1381	11mo	11.5 mo	0.86–1.09; p=0.57)
5FU vs 5FU/MTX *(6)*	5FU bolus	5FU/MTX	HR=0.76 (95% CI,
1178 patients	9.1 mo	10.7 mo	0.59–0.98; p=0.024)
5FU ± LV vs 5FU ± LV + α-IFN *(7)*	5FU ± LV 1	5FU ± LV + α-IFN	HR = 0.95 (95% C.I=
1766 patients	1.4 mo	11.5 mo	0.86–1.05; p=0.33)
5FU + LV vs 5FU + α-IFN *(7)*	5FU + LV	5FU + α-IFN	HR=1.11 (95%C.I=
1488 patients	11.7 mo	11.3 mo	0.99–1.24; p=0.066)
5FU bolus vs 5FU continuous	5FU bolus	5FU C.I.	HR=0.88 (95% CI,
infusion *(8)*			0.78–0.99; p=0.04)
1219 patients	11.3 mo	12.1 mo	
IV FP vs HAI FUDR *(9)*	IV FP	HAI FUDR	HR=0.73 (95% CI,
654 patients	10.1 mo	14.5 mo	0.61–0.88; p=0.0009)

HR = Hazard Ratio; CI = confidence interval; IV = intravenous; FP = fluoropyrimidines; HAI = hepatic artery infusion; FUDR = 5-fluoro-2′deoxyuridine

Randomized treatment was the only prognostic factor for tumor response, whereas performance status was the only prognostic factor for overall survival (Table 3).

The *Meta-Analysis Group In Cancer* is now conducting an update of this work, which will include all trials performed after the publication of this meta-analysis.

3.2. 5-FU Plus Methotrexate

Synergistic antitumor activity after sequential administration of methotrexate (MTX) and 5FU has been observed in vitro *(18,19)*.

Table 3
Prognostic Factors for Tumor Response and Overall Survival (Multifactorial Analysis)

Meta-analysis	*Prognostic factors for tumor response*	*Prognostic factors for overall survival*
5FU vs 5FU/LV *(5)* 1381 patients	Randomized treatment	Performance status
5FU vs 5FU/MTX *(6)* 1178 patients	Performance status Randomized treatment	Performance status Randomized treatment
5FU ± LV vs 5FU ± LV + α-IFN *(7)*		Performance status
5FU + LV vs 5FU + α-IFN *(7)* 3254 patients	Primary rectal tumor Metastases confined to the liver	Primary rectal tumor Metastases confined to the liver or to the lung
5FU bolus vs 5FU continuous infusion *(8)* 1219 patients	Performance status Randomized treatment	Performance status Randomized treatment Primary rectal tumor
IV FP vs HAI FUDR *(9)* 654 patients	Randomized treatment	Performance status Randomized treatment Percentage of liver involvement

IV = intravenous; FP = fluoropyrimidines; HAI = hepatic artery infusion; FUDR = 5-fluoro-2′-deoxyuridine

In addition to the inhibition of DNA synthesis, 5-FU can also inhibit RNA synthesis. 5-FU is anabolized to 5FUMP after direct conversion by orotic acid phosphoribosyl transferase in the presence of a cosubstrate, 5-phosphoribosyl-1-pyrophosphate (PRPP), or after intermediate conversion to a ribonucleoside, 5FUR, followed by formation of 5FUMP by uridine kinase. 5FUMP is subsequently phosphorylated to 5FUTP, and incorporated into RNA to alter its maturation and induce cytotoxicity *(20)*. MTX inhibits purine synthesis, leading to intracellular accumulation of PRPP, which leads to an increased formation of FUTP. This increases incorporation of FUTP into RNA.

The meta-analysis of randomized trials comparing 5-FU alone to MTX and 5-FU (5-FU/MTX) was published in 1994 *(6)*. All trials having started patient recruitment before January 1990 were considered.

The analysis included 1128 patients randomized in eight trials. The objective tumor response rate was 10% for patients allocated to 5-FU alone and 19% for patients allocated to 5-FU/MTX. The overall response OR was 0.51 (95% CI, 0.37–0.70; $p < 10^{-4}$). The median overall survival time was 9.1 mo in the 5-FU alone group and 10.7 mo in the 5-FU/MTX group (Table 2). The overall survival advantage of 5-FU/MTX cover 5-FU alone was small but statistically significant (HR = 0.76, 95% CI, 0.59–0.98; $p = 0.024$).

As in the 5-FU/LV meta-analysis, the 5-FU/MTX meta-analysis suggested that the dose of 5-FU played an important role. In trials using a higher dose of 5-FU in the 5-FU alone arm, neither tumor response nor overall survival appeared to be better for patients allocated to 5-FU/MTX compared to patients allocated to 5-FU alone.

Performance status and randomized treatment were the only two significant predictors of tumor response and survival (Table 3).

3.3. 5-FU Plus Interferon

Alpha interferon (α-IFN) increases in vitro the cytotoxicity of 5-FU in a variety of tumor cell lines *(21,22)*. The enzyme thymidylate synthase might be a target for the interaction between 5-FU and α-IFN *(21)*, and the presence of thymidine in the culture medium tends to block the synergic effect *(23)*. Interferon may also modify the plasma pharmacokinetics of 5-FU *(24,25)*, and 5-FU may influence the immunomodulatory actions of interferon *(23)*.

The *Meta-Analysis Group In Cancer* has recently conducted two meta-analyses addressing the place of α-IFN in ACC *(7)*. The first one considered all properly randomized trials comparing 5-FU with or without folinic acid (5-FU ± LV) to the same 5-FU ± LV regimen plus α-IFN (5FU ± LV + α-IFN). The second one considered all properly randomized trials comparing 5-FU + LV to 5-FU + α-IFN. In both meta-analyses, α-IFN must have consisted of α-2a-interferon or α-2b-interferon, and patients must have been included in the trial before July 1996.

One thousnad seven hundred and sixty-six patients were included in the 5-FU ± LV vs 5-FU ± LV + α-IFN meta-analysis. After exclusion of patients with nonmeasurable disease, 1683 patients were eligible for tumor response comparisons. Response rates were 25% for patients allocated to 5-FU ± LV, and 24% for 5-FU ± LV + α-IFN (RR = 1.02; 95%CI=0.87–1.2; p = 0.8), showing no advantage for α-IFN administration. Median survivals were 11.4 mo for patients treated without α-IFN, and 11.5 mo for patients treated with α-IFN, and overall survival hazard ratio was 0.95 (95%CI=0.86–1.05; p=0.33), showing no advantage for α-IFN administration.

One thousand four hundred and eighty-eight patients were included in the 5-FU + LV vs 5-FU + α-IFN meta-analysis. After exclusion of patients with nonmeasurable disease, 1305 patients were eligible for tumor response assessment. Tumor response rate was significantly higher in patients allocated to 5-FU + LV than in patients allocated to 5-FU + α-IFN (23% vs 18%; RR=1.26;95%CI=1.01–1.59; p=0.042). However, the heterogeneity between trials in this meta-analysis was rather important (p-value for heterogeneity, p=0.001), and analyses stratified by type of 5-FU administration showed that the advantage of 5-FU + LV over 5-FU + α-IFN was limited to the group of trials using the same 5-FU schedules in both treatment arms (RR=1.80; 95%C.I.=1.29–2.51; p=0.0005). Median survivals were 11.7 mo for patients allocated to 5-FU + LV and 11.3 mo for patients allocated to 5-FU + α-IFN (HR=1.11; 95%CI=0.99–1.24; p=0.066). The survival difference between treatment groups reached statistical significance in the group of trials using the same 5-FU schedules in both treatment arms (HR=1.29; 95%CI 1.07–1.57; p=0.008).

Individual patient data used for these two meta-analyses were combined to identify prognostic factors for response and survival (3254 patients). Metastases confined to the liver ($p<10^{-4}$), and primary rectal tumors were the independent favorable prognostic factors for tumor response, whereas good performance status ($p < 10^{-4}$), metastases confined to the liver or confined to the lung (p=0.0002 and p =0.004, respectively), and primary tumor in the rectum (p=0.003) were the favorable prognostic factors for survival.

4. 5-FU CONTINUOUS INTRAVENOUS INFUSION

There are several theoretical reasons for giving 5-FU by continuous intravenous infusion rather than by rapid bolus injection. 5-FU is relatively S-phase dependent, and its half-life in the serum is short. Prolonged infusion may therefore expose a larger proportion of tumor cells to 5-FU *(26,27)*. It has also been suggested that bolus administration of 5-FU inhibits RNA synthesis, whereas continuous infusion may be more cytotoxic via inhibition of thymidilate synthase *(28)*. Finally, delivering 5-FU by continuous infusion allows more drug to be given, and changes the limiting toxicity from myelosuppression to stomatitis, and hand-foot syndrome *(27,29)*.

The meta-analysis of randomized trials comparing 5-FU bolus to 5-FU continuous infusion was published in 1998 *(8)*. All trials having accrued patients between 1984 and 1989 were considered in the meta-analysis.

The analysis included 1219 patients randomized in six trials. One hundred and sixteen patients with nonmeasurable disease were excluded from the tumor response analysis.

Tumor response rate were 22% for patients assigned to 5-FU continuous infusion and 14% for patients assigned to 5-FU bolus (OR=0.55; 95% CI, 0.41–0.75; p=0.0002). This is equivalent to a risk reduction of 45% with a standard error of 12%.

Median survivals were 11.3 mo in the 5-FU bolus group vs 12.1 mo in the 5-FU CI group (HR=0.88; 95% CI, 0.78–0.99; p=0.04).

In this meta-analysis, data were also collected on acute treatment toxicities *(13)*. Hand-foot syndrome, and grade 3 or 4 hematological or nonhematological toxicities were analyzed; 31% of patients allocated to 5-FU bolus experienced an hematological toxicity (mainly neutropenia) vs 4% of those allocated to 5-FU continuous infusion (p<0.0001). Hand-foot syndrome was less frequent with 5-FU bolus than with 5-FU CI (respectively 13% and 34%; p<0.0001), and there was no difference between the two treatment groups in terms of other nonhematological toxicities.

5. HEPATIC ARTERY INFUSION

Liver is the most frequent site of metastasis of patients with colorectal cancer. In patients with disease confined to the liver, surgery must be performed whenever possible, but most of the patients have nonresectable lesions. Hepatic artery infusion (HAI) chemotherapy is an attempt to deliver high dose chemotherapy directly to the liver without toxicity due to systemic effects of the drug that is eliminated by the liver. HAI of fluoropyrimidines leads to a high concentration of fluorouracil in the tumor bed *(30)*, and the concentration of fluoropyrimidines in the liver is even higher with 5-fluoro-2′-deoxyuridine (FUDR) than with 5-FU *(31)*.

The meta-analysis of randomized trials comparing HAI to intravenous 5-FU was published in 1996 *(9)*, and included all trials having started accruing patients before January 1989. Five trials (391 patients) compared HAI and IVC. FUDR was used in both the HAI and IV arms in three trials. The other two trials compared HAI FUDR to intravenous 5-FU. Two trials (263 patients) did not compare HAI to intravenous chemotherapy, but HAI FUDR to *no* HAI. The *no* HAI group, depending on the physician and patient choice, was either observation only or systemic 5-FU.

Among trials comparing HAI to IVC, the objective tumor response rates were 41% for patients allocated to HAI and 14% for patients allocated to intravenous chemotherapy (HR=0.25; 95% CI, 0.16–0.40; $p < 10^{-10}$).

When all trials were taken into consideration, median survival times were 10.1 mo in the control group vs 14.5 mo in the HAI group (HR=0.73; 95% CI, 0.61–0.88; p=0.0009). However, the difference between treatment groups was not statistically significant when the analysis was restricted to trials comparing strictly HAI to intravenous chemotherapy (median survivals 12.2 mo vs 16 mo, HR=0.81; 95% CI, 0.62–1.05, p=0.14).

6. CONCLUSION

Our meta-analyses confirmed that the antitumoral effect of fluoropyrimidines can be enhanced either through modulation by leucovorin or methotrexate, but not by interferon, or by continuous infusion of 5-FU or by hepatic artery infusion. The benefits of experimental fluoropyrimidines regimens were much more impressive in terms of response rates than in terms of overall survival. Survival benefits were in most cases too small to be of clinical relevance, even when response rates were doubled by experimental regimens. One reason for the small impact of tumor response improvements of overall survival is that many patients receive second line therapies that may have diluted any benefits of first line therapy. Another reason is that response rates remain modest (under 30%), and short lived even in the most successful randomized trials with few complete responses (under 5%). These results suggest, however, that it may be important to give optimal first line therapy to patients with advanced colorectal cancer, since treatment that induce higher response rate may ultimately be expected to prolong survival *(32)*. They also provide some indirect justification to the policy of bringing to the adjuvant setting treatments that demonstrate superior response rates, even if these treatments fail to improve survival in advanced disease. A case in point is leucovorin modulated 5FU which has been shown to double the response rate to 5-FU alone, with survival benefit too small to reach statistical significance in advanced disease *(5)*. As an adjuvant for resected colon cancer, this treatment has been shown to improve survival as compared with an untreated control group, whereas in this situation the benefit of 5-FU alone remained uncertain *(33)*.

ACKNOWLEDGMENTS

This study was supported in part by the European Association for Research in Oncology (AERO) (Paris, France)

REFERENCES

1. Buyse M, Piedbois P, Piedbois Y, Carlson R. Meta-analysis: methods, strengths and weaknesses. *Oncology* 2000; 14:437–443.
2. Piedbois P, Buyse M. Meta-analyses need time, collaboration, and funding. *J Clin Oncol* 1994; 12:878–879.
3. Buyse M, Carlson R, Piedbois P. Meta-analyses of published results are unreliable. *J Clin Oncol* 1999; 17:1646–1647.
4. Piedbois P, Buyse M, Pignon JP. Critical issues in colorectal cancer randomized trials and meta-analyses. Management of Colorectal Cancer, (Harry Bleiberg, Philippe Rougier, Hans-Joachim Wilke, Publisher Martin Dunitz, eds.) ISBN 1-85317-377-0, 1998, pp. 375–386.
5. Advanced Colorectal Cancer Meta-analysis Project. Modulation of fluorouracil by leucovorin in patients with advanced colorectal cancer: evidence in terms of response rate. *J Clin Oncol* 1992; 10:896–903.
6. Advanced Colorectal Cancer Meta-analysis Project. Meta-analysis of randomized trials testing the biochemical modulation of 5-fluorouracil by methotrexate in metastatic colorectal cancer. *J Clin Oncol* 1994; 12:960–969.
7. Meta-Analysis Group In Cancer. Alpha-interferon does not increase the efficacy of 5-fluorouracil in advanced colorectal cancer. *Br J Cancer* 2001; 84:611–620.
8. Meta-Analysis Group In Cancer. Efficacy of intravenous continuous infusion of 5-Fluorouracil compared with bolus administration in advanced colorectal cancer. *J Clin Oncol* 1998; 16:301–308.
9. Meta-Analysis Group In Cancer. Reappraisal of hepatic arterial infusion in the treatment of non resectable liver metastases from colorectal cancer. *J Natl Cancer Inst* 1996; 88:252–258.
10. WHO Handbook for reporting results of cancer treatment. WHO offsets publication No 48, World Health Organization, Geneva, 1979.
11. Miller AB, Hoogstraten B, Staquet M, Winkler A: Reporting results of cancer treatment. *Cancer* 1981; 47:207–214.
12. Therasse P, Arbuck SG, Eisenhauer EA, et al. New guidelines to evaluate the response to treatment in solid tumors. *J Natl Cancer Inst* 2000; 92:205–216.
13. Meta-Analysis Group In Cancer. Toxicity of 5-fluorouracil in patients with advanced colorectal cancer: effect of administration schedule and prognostic factors. *J Clin Oncol* 1998; 16:3537–3541.
14. Machover D, Goldschmidt E, Chollet P, et al. Treatment of advanced colorectal and gastric adenocarcinomas with 5-fluorouracil and high-dose folinic acid. *J Clin Oncol* 1986; 4:685–696.

15. Evans RM, Laskin JD, Hakala MT: Effect of excess folates and deoxyinosine on the activity and site of action of 5-fluorouracil. *Cancer Res* 1981; 41:3288–3295.
16. Berger SH, Hakala MT: Relationship of dUMP and free FdUMP pools to inhibition of thymidilate synthetase by 5-fluorouracil. *Mol Pharmacol* 1984; 25:303–309.
17. Waxman S, Bruckner H: The enhancement of 5-fluorouracil antimetabolic activity by leucovorin, menadione and alpha-tocopherol. *Eur J Cancer Clin Oncol* 1982; 18:685–692.
18. Bertino JR, Sawicki WL, Linquist CA, et al: Schedule-dependent antitumor effects of methotrexate and 5-fluorouracil. *Cancer Res* 1977; 37:327–328.
19. Allegra CJ. Methotrexate and fluorouracil following tamoxifen and premarin in advanced breast cancer. *Semin Oncol* 1983; 10 (suppl 2):23–28.
20. Curt GA, Allegra CJ, Fine RL, et al: Antimetabolites. In Cancer Chemotherapy Ann. 6, chapter 1, Elsevier Publ., 1984.
21. Elias L, Crissman HA. Interferon effects upon the adenocarcinoma 38 and HL-60 cell lines: antiproliferative responses and synergistic interactions with halogenated pyrimidine antimetabolites *Cancer Res* 1988; 48:4868–4873.
22. Wadler S, Wersto R, Weinberg V, et al. Interaction of fluorouracil and interferon in human colon cancer cell lines: cytotoxic and cytokinetic effects. *Cancer Res* 1990; 50:2653–2665.
23. Neefe JR, John W. Mechanisms of interaction of interferon and 5-fluorouracil in solid tumors. *Semin Oncol* 1991; 18 (suppl 7):77–82.
24. Lindley C, Bernard B, Gavlan M, et al. Interferon-alpha increases 5-luorouracil levels 16-fold within 1 hour: results of a phase I study. *J Interferon Res* 1990; 10:9–5.
25. Danhauser L, Gilchrist T, Friemann J et al. Effect of recombinant interferon-alpha-2b on the plasma pharmacokinetics of fluorouracil in patients with advanced cancer. *Proc Am Assoc Cancer Res* 1991; 32:1052 (abstr).
26. Myers CE, Diasio R, Eliot HM, et al. Pharmacokinetics of the fluoropyrimides: implications for their clinical use. *Cancer Treat Rev* 1975; 3:175–183.
27. Fraile RJ, Baker LH, Buroker TR, et al. Pharmacokinetics of 5-fluorouracil administered orally, by rapid intravenous and by slow infusion. *Cancer Res* 1980; 40:2223–2228.
28. Aschele C, Sobrero A, Faderan MA, Bertino JR. Novel mecanism(s) of resistance to 5-fluorouracil in human colon cancer (HCT-8) sublines following exposure to two different clinically relevant dose schedules. *Cancer Res* 1992; 52:1855–1864.
29. Carlson R. Continuous intravenous infusion chemotherapy. In: The Chemotherapy Source Book. Ed. Michael C. Perry, Williams and Wilkin, Baltimore, 1996.
30. Chen GHG, Gross JF. Intra-arterial infusion of anticancer drugs: theoretic aspects of drug delivery and review of responses. *Cancer Treat Rep* 1980; 64:31–40.
31. Ensminger WD, Gyves JW. Regional chemotherapy of neoplastic diseases. *Pharmacol Ther* 1983;21:277–293.
32. Buyse M, Thirion P, Carlson RW, Burzykowski T, Molenberghs G, Piedbois P. for the *Meta-Analysis Group In Cancer.* Relation between tumor response to first-line chemotherapy and survival in advanced colorectal cancer: a meta-analysis. *Lancet* 2000;356:373–378.
33. Buyse M, Zeleniuch-Jacquotte A, Chalmers TC. Adjuvant therapy of colorectal cancer: Why we still don't know. *JAMA* 1988;259:3571–3578.

14 The Mayo/NCCTG Experience with 5-Fluorouracil and Leucovorin in Adjuvant Advanced Colorectal Cancer

Charles Erlichman, MD *Richard M. Goldberg,* MD, *and Daniel J. Sargent,* PhD

CONTENTS

1. INTRODUCTION

Hundreds of studies have evaluated the activity of fluorinated pyrimidines in the treatment of colorectal and other cancers. The background data regarding the mechanisms of action of these agents is discussed elsewhere and will be mentioned here only briefly to provide historical context. Fluorinated pyrimidines, of which 5-fluorouracil (5-FU) is the most commonly used, exert their antineoplastic effect in part by inhibiting the activity of the enzyme thymidylate synthase (TS) critical in the *de novo* synthesis of DNA. They also are incorporated into RNA and DNA, which may contribute to their cytotoxic effects. A number of different fluorinated pyrimidines have been administered as single agents and as a part of combinations with other cytotoxic drugs. Biochemical modulation of fluorinated pyrimidines designed to improve their therapeutic index has been evaluated extensively. Leucovorin is the most common biochemical modulator used with fluorinated pyrimidines.

From 1956 to the early 1980s 5-FU was administered as a single agent with predictable but limited activity and moderate toxicity in patients with metastatic colorectal cancer. Tumor shrinkage was observed in a very small proportion of patients treated with bolus or infusion schedules of single agent 5-FU. Approximately 11% of patients with metastatic colorectal cancer had measurable tumor shrinkage and responses were short lived, lasting a few months *(1)*. 5-FU is metabolized to 5-flourodeoxyuridylate (FdUMP) which binds TS and inhibits DNA synthesis. This inhibition of TS is increased 10^6-fold in the presence of excess reduced folate cofactor—5, 10-methylene tetrahydrofolate. The understanding of this bio-

From: *Fluoropyrimidines in Cancer Therapy*
Edited by: Y. M. Rustum © Humana Press Inc., Totowa, NJ

chemical interaction led to the hypothesis that 5-FU activity could be enhanced if tumor cell reduced folates could be increased.

In the 1970s laboratory investigators reported that leucovorin (5-formyltetrahydrofolate) potentiated the cytotoxicity of 5-FU in vitro and in human tumor xenografts *(2–4)*. The addition of leucovorin led to the formation of stable, covalently bound, ternary complexes of TS–FdUMP–5,10-methylene tetrahydrofolate. In the absence of sufficient folate the ternary complexes were weak resulting in only transient TS inhibition. In tumor model systems, the optimal concentrations of leucovorin ranged from 1 to 20 mmol/L *(6–9)*. These studies supported the clinical leucovorin doses ranging from 10 to 600 mg/m^2 to achieve tissue concentrations ranging from 1 to 20 mmol/L in patients. Further experiments were designed to determine the optimum dose, schedule of administration, and intracellular concentration of leucovorin when administered with 5-FU. These studies indicated that the interplay between 5-FU, leucovorin, and cellular replicative machinery depended, at least in part, on the cell lines employed in the experiments. For example, in H630 colon carcinoma cells, the highest concentrations of the ternary complex were noted when leucovorin preceded administration of 5-FU by 18 h *(10)*. In contrast, the optimal conditions for ternary complex formation occurred when 5-FU was administered 4 h after leucovorin exposure in MCF-7 breast cancer cells. In a study done in Ward colorectal carcinomas, 5-FU was administered with or without leucovorin in three different schedules at different leucovorin doses in a factorial design *(9)*. The three leucovorin doses were high (200 mg/m^2), low (20 mg/m^2), and none. The administration schedules were:

1. A 96-h infusion of 5-FU with leucovorin given daily over 2 h.
2. A daily 5-FU bolus for four consecutive days given midway through a 2-h leucovorin infusion.
3. Three consecutive weekly bolus injections of 5-FU given midway through a 2-h infusion of leucovorin.

The administration of high-dose leucovorin resulted in more complete tumor responses in these studies than did low-dose or no leucovorin regardless of schedule. Studies such as these indicated that different schedules of drug administration and different doses of the combination may achieve the same effect depending on the tumor model. Considering the heterogeneity of tumors in patients and variable drug pharmacokinetics, in hindsight perhaps these laboratory investigations were predicting that no single fixed-dose schedule of 5-FU and leucovorin would be optional for all tumors *(11)*.

2. THE MAYO/NCCTG REGIMEN IN ADVANCED COLORECTAL CANCER

Machover and colleagues were among the first investigators to evaluate the biochemical modulation of 5-FU with leucovorin in the treatment of colorectal and gastric cancers *(12,13)*. The Machover regimen consisted of high-dose leucovorin at a dose of 200 mg/m^2/d administered prior to 5-FU at a dose of 370 mg/m^2/d. Both drugs were given for five consecutive days repeated every 28 d. This dose of leucovorin is associated with blood levels of 10–20 μmol/L *(14)*. A randomized trial of this regimen compared to 5-FU alone demonstrated a significant improvement in response for the combination *(15)*. The Mayo/NCCTG regimen was originally devised to replace the high-dose leucovorin with a lower dose of 20 mg/m^2/d as the biochemical modulator of 5-FU. The 5-FU dose and schedule were identical to that used in the Machover regimen, i.e., 370 mg/m^2/d for five consecutive days. The scientific rationale for this treatment program was to test whether a low-dose leucovorin regimen projected to achieve systemic leucovorin concentrations of 1–2 μmol/L would provide sufficient biochemical modulation of 5-FU to augment the response rate and survival of patients with metastatic colorectal cancer compared to 5-FU alone. This was stimulated in part by the lower cost of the low-dose leucovorin regimen.

In the initial study of this regimen, patients with advanced unresectable colorectal cancer were randomized to one of six chemotherapy regimens *(16)*. Only three of the treatment arms will be considered further in this discussion:

1. 5-FU alone administered at a dose of 500 mg/m^2/d by IV bolus for five consecutive days every five wk.
2. 5-FU 370 mg/m^2/d with 200 mg/m^2/d of leucovorin administered for five consecutive days repeated 4 wk, 8 wk, and every 5 wk thereafter.
3. 5-FU 370 mg/m^2/d combined with 20 mg/m^2/d of leucovorin given for five consecutive days, repeated at 4 wk, 8 wk, and every 5 wk thereafter.

A 5-wk interval between courses after the third set of treatments was chosen because of concern about the cumulative nature of the toxicity. The initial 4-wk interval allowed initial dose intensive treatment, with the dose intensity then reduced for patients with stable or responsive disease over time. Upon analysis of the toxicity patterns of the first 100 patients, the starting dose of 5-FU for the low-dose leucovorin (Mayo) regimen was increased to 425 mg/m^2/d *(17)*. Dose escalation of 5-FU on all treatment arms occurred in this study if no significant myelosuppression or nonhematologic toxicity were observed during the previous treatment course. The protocol change was made upon observation that in this trial the majority of patients treated with the Mayo/NCCTG regimen were dose escalating per protocol. The dosage adjustment to 425 mg/m^2/d was made to produce definite but tolerable toxicity that was of similar magnitude between the six treatment programs.

At the conclusion of the study, 208 eligible patients had been entered on the three study arms of interest. The overall response rates were 10% for 5-FU alone, 26% for 5 FU 370 mg/m^2/d + leucovorin 200 mg/m^2/d, and 43% for the 5-FU 425 mg/m^2/d combined with 20 mg/m^2/d—the Mayo regimen. The response rates for the two leucovorin-modulated regimens were significantly better than 5-FU alone ($p = 0.04$ and 0.001, respectively). Survival was also significantly longer for the two leucovorin modulated regimens at 12.2 mo (high-dose leucovorin) and 12.0 mo (low-dose leucovorin) as compared to 7.7 mo for single agent 5-FU (p=0.037 and 0.05, respectively).

Petrelli et al. at Roswell Park Memorial Cancer Institute (RPMI) devised a weekly high-dose regimen of leucovorin 500 mg/m^2/d with 5-FU 600 mg/m^2/d given for six consecutive weeks followed by a 2 wk rest period *(18)*. This RPMI regimen has also been shown to significantly improve the response rate when compared to single agent 5-FU with a response rate of 30% for the RPMI regimen vs 12% for 5-FU alone (p<0.01). Based on these results, the RPMI and Mayo/NCCTG regimens were compared in a randomized trial of 366 patients performed by the NCCTG *(19)*. The observed objective tumor response rates were similar (35% for the Mayo/NCCTG regimen, 31% for the RPMI regimen) and no survival difference between regimens was observed.

Goldberg et al. *(20)* undertook a randomized trial in which 5-FU was combined with L-leucovorin or oral leucovorin or standard racemic leucovorin in patients with metastatic colorectal cancer. Nine hundred twenty-six patients were randomized to 5-FU 370 mg/m^2 combined with either 500 mg/m^2 of oral (D, L) leucovorin in four divided doses, (D, L) leucovorin 200 mg/m^2 intravenously, or L-leucovorin 100 mg/m^2. Each was given on a daily × 5 schedule every 4 wk for three cycles then every 5 wk. The overall response was 32%, and there was no difference in response between arms (28% vs 34% vs 34%) in time to tumor progression, or in overall survival. This data indicated that leucovorin could be given orally but in divided doses and that L-leucovorin did not add any further benefit.

The Mayo/NCCTG Regimen in the Adjuvant setting: The activity of leucovorin modulated 5-FU in the metastatic setting naturally led to the evaluation of the various regimens in the treatment of patients with stage II and III colon cancer *(21)*. Patients with resected stage II or III colon cancer were randomized to the Mayo/NCCTG 5-FU leucovorin regimen for 6 mo or to a no treatment control arm. The study was suspended after accrual of 317 patients when the results of the GI intergroup trial of 5-FU plus levamisole were released, establishing that effective treatment was available in this setting *(22)*. In the 317 patients enrolled before suspension, the 5-yr survival for treated patients was 74% compared to 63% in the control group (p=0.02). This trial clearly supported the efficacy of the Mayo/NCCTG 5-FU plus leucovorin regimen in the adjuvant setting.

Subsequently, a large trial sponsored by the GI intergroup (INT-0089) randomized 3759 stage II and III colon cancer patients to one of four 5-FU and leucovorin and/or levamisole programs. The regimens included the Mayo/NCCTG 5-FU plus leucovorin regimen for 6 mo, 5-FU plus levamisole for 12 mo, 5-FU with high-dose leucovorin (the RPMI regimen) for 8 mo, or 5-FU plus leucovorin plus levamisole for 12 mo *(23)*. The outcomes were similar for the Mayo/NCCTG, the RPMI 5-FU plus leucovorin, and the 5-FU plus both leucovorin and levamisole regimens. These three regimens resulted in a 65–67% 5-yr overall survival. With essentially identical activity profiles at this present time, the choice of 5-FU leucovorin regimens relates to patient preference, cost, toxicity profile, and the clinician's preference.

3. MAYO/NCCTG REGIMEN: TOXICITY

Substantial data exist regarding the adverse events rate associated with the Mayo/NCCTG regimen. Toxicity data from several of the initial trials of Mayo/NCCTG regimen *(16,19,24)* are summarized in Table 1. The rates of severe (grade ≥3) toxicity were consistent in the early studies, with diarrhea rates from 10 to 18%, nausea/vomiting observed in 5–10% of patients, leukopenia in 17–29%, and thrombocytopenia rarely observed. In all of these trials stomatitis was common, with rates ranging from 12 to 26% grade ≥3. However, Mahood et al. *(25)* reported that holding ice chips in the mouth during 5-FU treatment significantly reduced the incidence of stomatitis with the Mayo/NCCTG regimen. The prophylactic use of ice chips has since been standard practice for patients enrolled on Mayo/NCCTG clinical trials and also those treated off study at the Mayo Clinic with the Mayo/NCCTG regimen. In many comparative trials done by other investigators this supportive care measure is not standard practice.

Several recent reports have indicated high levels of neutropenia with the Mayo/NCCTG regimen *(26–29)*. The studies included in Table 1 were conducted before routine collection of neutropenia data. To estimate the rate of febrile neutropenia from these early studies, using data from the studies of Poon et al. *(16)* and Buroker et al. *(19)*, and a conservative assumption that every patient with fever or infection was also neutropenic, we may calculate an upper boundary on the rate of febrile neutropenia in these trials. Of 343 patients with advanced disease treated with the Mayo/NCCTG regimen on these trials, 13 patients had grade ≥3 fever or infection, resulting in a worse case rate of febrile neutropenia of 3.8%.

The Buroker study *(19)* randomized patients between the Mayo/NCCTG and Roswell Park regimens, allowing a direct toxicity comparison in advanced disease. In that study stomatitis was significantly worse on the Mayo regimen (24% vs 2% grade ≥3), whereas diarrhea was significantly worse on the Roswell Park regimen (32% vs 18% grade ≥3). Leukopenia was more common on the Mayo Regimen, but was rarely accompanied by fever

Table 1
Toxicity of Mayo/NCCTG Regimen: Initial Reports

Toxicity	*Poon* (16) (n=*68)*	*Buroker* (19) (n=*183)*	*Leichman* (24) (n=*85)*
Diarrhea			
Any	64	64	48
Severe	14	18	10
Stomatitis			
Any	80	71	49
Severe	26	24	12
Vomiting			
Any	46	43	31
Severe	9	8	5
Nausea			
Any	76	60	
Severe	10	9	
Leukopenia (/µL)			
<4,000	83	78	51
<2,000	21	29	17
Granulocytopenia (/µL)			
<2,000			54
<1,000			40
Thrombocytopenia (/µL)			
<LLN		21	12
<50,000		3	2

(Number shown is the percentage with each toxicity)

or infection. Other toxicities were similar between the two arms. In this study, significantly more patients on the RPMI regimen required hospitalization than on the Mayo/NCCTG regimen (31% vs 21% respectively, $p=0.02$) and the proportion of toxic deaths did not differ between the two arms (5 deaths on the Mayo/NCCTG regimen, 2 on the RPMI regimen, $p=0.26$).

The toxicity profile of the Mayo/NCCTG regimen in the advanced disease setting was also documented in the abstracts from five large randomized trials reported at meetings. Four of these trials *(26–29)* compared the Mayo/NCCTG regimen to an oral 5-FU-based regimen using an equivalence trial design. Comparative toxicity was thus a primary focus of the trials. The remaining trial *(30)* compared the Mayo/NCCTG regimen to a three-drug regimen containing 5-FU, LV, and CPT-11 and was designed with response rate and overall survival as the primary endpoints. Toxicity data from three of the abstracts is sufficient to summarize in tabular form in Table 2. These data are similar to the data shown in Table 1. The high frequency of neutropenia cannot be compared in the two tables as it was not collected in studies of Poon and Buroker.

In comparing results between the initial trials and the recent reports *(23,27,29,30)* it should be noted that in the most recent studies, the 5-FU leucovorin regimen was given every 4 wk rather than increasing the treatment interval to 5 wk after two cycles. In addition, the use of ice chips, which have been demonstrated to significantly reduce stomatitis *(25)* was not clearly stated.

Representative toxicity data from the Mayo/NCCTG regimen in the adjuvant setting for the two studies mentioned above (*21,23* [toxicity data kindly provided by Dr. Dan Haller, PI]) is

Table 2
Toxicity of Mayo/NCCTG Regimen: Recent Reports

Toxicity	*Carmichael* (28) (n=*190*)	*Pazdur* (26) (n=*408*)	*Saltz* (30) (n=*221*)
Diarrhea			
Any	60	76	
Severe	11	16	13
Stomatitis/Mucositis			
Any	55	75	
Severe	16	20	10
Nausea/Vomiting			
Any	58	75	
Severe	9	10	4
Neutropenia			
Any	67	77	
Severe	31	56	37
Neutropenic Fever			
Any			
Severe			13
Thrombocytopenia (/μL)			
Any	28	31	
Severe	2	2	
Anemia			
Any	89	87	
Severe	4	7	

(Number shown is the percentage with each toxicity)

Table 3
Toxicity of Mayo/NCCTG Regimen: Adjuvant Setting

Toxicity	*O'Connell* (21) (n=*158*)	*Haller* (23) (n=*984*)
Diarrhea		
Any	73	–
Severe	21	21
Stomatitis/Mucositis		
Any	75	–
Severe	34	18
Vomiting		
Any	31	–
Severe	6	3
Nausea		
Any	56	–
Severe	8	4
Leukopenia		
Any	69	–
Severe	14	12
Thrombocytopenia		
Any	13	–
Severe	0	1
Granulocytopenia		
Any		–
Severe		25

(Number shown is the percentage with each toxicity)

summarized in Table 3. No toxic deaths were observed in the O'Connell study *(21)*, while 5 of 984 patients (0.5%) expired due to treatment related causes on the Mayo/NCCTG regimen in INT-0089 *(23)*. These rates are consistent with the rates shown in Table 1 in the advanced disease setting. In addition, while explicit data on febrile neutropenia is not available in INT-0089, the rate of grade ≥3 infection was 2%, and of grade ≥3 fever without infection ≤1%. Taken together, it is predicted that the rate of febrile neutropenia is therefore ≤3%.

SUMMARY

The Mayo/NCCTG regimen of 5-FU and leucovorin has demonstrated clinical activity in both the treatment of metastatic colorectal cancer and in the adjuvant setting. If used with ice chips its toxicity pattern is tolerable with a lower incidence of diarrhea than that seen with the RPMI schedule. Although severe leukopenia and neutropenia are common, the risk of febrile neutropenia is ≤3% and treatment related deaths are rare (≤1%). This profile has made the Mayo/NCCTG regimen the "standard" by which new therapies are compared *(28,31)*. Although irinotecan combined with 5-FU and leucovorin has been reported to be more effective in treatment of metastatic colorectal cancer *(30)*, the Mayo/NCCTG regimen of 5-FU and leucovorin remains a reasonable option in older patients with metastatic colorectal cancer and other comorbidities. Pending the results of ongoing clinical trials (CALGB 89803), the Mayo/NCCTG regimen remains a standard of care in the adjuvant setting.

REFERENCES

1. Advanced Cancer Meta-Analysis Project. Modulation of fluorouracil by leucovorin in patients with advanced colorectal cancer: Evidence in terms of response rate. *J Clin Oncol* 1992; 10:896–903.
2. Ullman B, Lee M, Martin DW Jr. Santi DV. Cytotoxicity of 5-fluoro-2-deoxyuridine: equirement for reduced folate co-factors and antagonism by methotrexate. *Proc Natl Acad Sci USA* 1978; 75:980–983.
3. Evans RM, Laskin JD, Hakala MT. Effect of excess folates and deoxyinosine on the activity and site of action of 5-fluorouracil. *Cancer Res* 1981; 41:3288–3295.
4. Waxman S, Bruckner H. The enhancement of 5-fluorouracil antimetabolic activity by leucovorin, menadione, and alpha-tocopherol. *Eur J Cancer Clin Oncol* 1982; 18:685–692.
5. Keyomarsi K, Moran RG, Folinic augmentation of the effects of fluoropyrimidines on murine and human leukemic cells. *Cancer Res* 1986; 46:5229–5235.
6. Houghton JA, Williams LG, Loftin SK, et al. Relationship between the dose rate of [6RS] leucovorin administration, plasma concentrations of reduced folates, and pools of 5,10 methylenetetrahydrafolates and tetrahydrafolates in human colon adenocarcinoma xenografts. *Cancer Res* 1990; 50:3493–3502.
7. Houghton JA, Williams LG, Loftin SK, et al. Factors that influence the therapeutic activity of 5-fluorouracil[6RS] leucovorin combinations in colon adenocarcinoma xenografts. *Cancer Chemother Pharmacol* 1992; 30:423–432.
8. Houghton JA, Williams LG, Cheshire PJ, et al. Influence of the dose of [6RS] leucovorin on reduced folate pools and 5-fluorouracil-mediated thymidylate synthase inhibition in human colon adenocarcinoma xenografts. *Cancer Res* 1990; 50:3940–3946.
9. Cao S, Frank C, Rustum YM. Role of fluoropyrimidine scheduling and (6R,S) leucovorin dose in a preclinical animal model of colorectal carcinoma. *J Natl Cancer Inst* 1996; 88:430–436.
10. Drake JC, Voeller DM, Allegra CJ, et al. The effect of dose and interval between 5-fluorouracil and leucovorin on the formation of thymidylate synthase ternary complex in human cancer cells. *Br J Cancer* 1990; 71:1145–1150.
11. Machover D. A comprehensive review of 5-fluorouracil and leucovorin in patients with metastatic colorectal carcinoma. *Cancer* 1997; 80:1179–1187.
12. MachoverD, Goldschmidt E, Chollet P, et al. Treatment of advanced colorectal and gastric adenocarcinomas with 5-fluorouracil and high-dose folinic acid. *J Clin Oncol* 1986; 4:685–696.
13. Machover D, Schwartenberg L, Goldschmidt E, et al. Treatment of advanced colorectal and gastric adenocarcinomas with 5-FU combined with high-dose folinic acid: A pilot study *Canc Treat Rep* 1982; 66:1803–1807.

14. Rustum YM, Trave F, Zakrzewski SF, et al. Biochemical and pharmacologic basis for potentiation of 5-Fluoruracil action by leucovorin. *NCI Monogr* 1987; 5:165–170.
15. Erlichman C, Fine S, Wong A, Elhakin R. a randomized Treal of Flourornacil and Folinic Acid in Patients with Metastatic Colorectal Carcinoma. *J Clin Oncol* 1988; 6:469–475.
16. Poon MA, O'Connell MJ, Moertel CG, et al. Biochemical modulation of fluorouracil: Evidence of significant improvement in survival and quality of life in patients with advanced colorectal carcinoma. *J Clin Oncol* 1989; 7:1407–1418.
17. O'Connell MJ. A phase III trial of 5-fluoruracil and leucovorin in the treatment of advanced colorectal cancer: A Mayo Clinic/North Central Cancer Treatment Group study. *Cancer* 1989; 63:1026–1030.
18. Petrelli N, Herrara L, Rustum Y, et al. A prospective randomized trial of 5-fluorouracil vs. 5-fluoruracil and high dose leucovorin + 5-fluorouracil and methotrexate in previously untreated patients with advanced colorectal carcinoma. *J Clin Oncol* 1987; 5:1559–1565.
19. Buroker TR, O'Connell MJ, Wieand HS, et al. Randomized comparison of two schedules of fluorouracil and leucovorin in the treatment of advanced colorectal cancer. *J Clin Oncol* 1994; 12:14–20.
20. Goldberg RM, Hatfield AR, Kahn M. et al. Prospectively indomized North Central Cancer Treatment Group trial of intensive – course combined with the L-isomer of intravenous leucovorin, oral leucovorin, or intravenous leucovorin for the treatment of advanced colorectal cancer. *J Clin Oncol* 1997; 15:3320–3329.
21. O'Connell MJ, Mailliard JA, Kahn MJ, et al. Controlled clinical trial of fluorouracil and low-dose leucoovrin given for 6 months as postoperative adjuvant therapy for colon cancer. *J Clin Oncol* 1997; 15:246–250.
22. Moertel CG, Fleming TR, Macdonald JS, et al. Levamisole and fluorouracil for adjuvant therapy of resected colon carcinoma. *N Engl J Med* 1990; 322:352–358.
23. Haller DG, Catalano PJ, Macdonald JS, et al. Flourouracil (FU), leucovorin (LV), and levamisole (LEV) adjuvant therapy for colon cancer: Five-year final report of INT-0089. *Proc Am Soc Clin Oncol* 1998; 17:256a.
24. Leichman CG, Fleming TR, Muggia FM, et al. Phase II study of fluorouracil and its modulation in advanced colorectal cancer: A Southwest Oncology Group Study. *J Clin Oncol* 1995; 13:1303–1311.
25. Mahood DJ, Dose AM, Loprinzi CL, et al. Inhibition of fluorouracil-induced stomatitis by oral cryotherapy. *J Clin Oncol* 1991; 9:449–452.
26. Pazdur R, Douillard J-Y, Skillings JR, et al. Multicenter phase III study of 5-flourouracil (5-FU) or UFT® in combination with leucovorin (LV) in patients with metastatic colorectal cancer. *Proc Am Soc Clin Oncol* 1999; 18:263a.
27. Twelves C, Haper P, Van Cutsem E, et al. A phase III trial (S014796) of Xeloda® (Capecitabine) in previously untreated advanced/metastatic colorectal cancer. *Proc Am Soc Clin Oncol* 1999; 18:263a.
28. Carmichael J, Popiela T, Radstone D, et al. Randomized comparative study of ORZEL® (Oral Uracil/Tegafur (UFT®) plus Leucovorin (LV) versus parenteral 5-fluorouracil (5-FU) plus LV in patients with metastatic colorectal cancer. *Proc Am Soc Clin Oncol* 1999; 18:264a.
29. Cox JV, Pazdur R, Thibault A, et al. A phase III trial of XELODA™ (Capecitabine) in previously untreated advanced/malignant colorectal cancer. *Proc Am Soc Clin Oncol* 1999; 18:265a.
30. Saltz LB, Locker PK, Pirotta N, et al. Weekly irinotecan (CPT-11), leucovorin (LV), and fluorouracil (FU) is superior to daily × 5 LV/FU in patients with previously untreated metastatic colorectal cancer (CRC). *Proc Am Soc Clin Oncol* 1998; 19:233a.
31. Douillard JY, Cunningham D, Roth AD, et al. A randomized phase III trial comparing irinotecan (IRI) + 5FU/folinic acid (FA) to the same schedule of 5FU/FA in patients (pts) with metastatic colorectal cancer (MCRC) as front line chemotherapy (CT). *Proc Am Soc Clin Oncol* 1998; 18:233a.
32. De Gramont A, Figer A, Seymour M, et al. A randomized trial of leucovorin (LV) and 5-flourouracil (5FU) with or without oxaliplatin in advanced colorectal cancer (CRC). *Proc Am Soc Clin Oncol* 1998; 17:257a.

15 Fluoropyrimidines for the Adjuvant Treatment of Colorectal Cancer

The NSABP Experience

Roy E. Smith, MD, *Eleftherios P. Mamounas*, MD, *and Norman Wolmark*, MD

CONTENTS

1. INTRODUCTION

Early hypotheses for the use of adjuvant chemotherapy in colorectal cancer focused on the consequences of local tumor perturbation, and efforts were directed toward the elimination of circulating tumors cells dislodged during surgery *(1,2)*. Early trials eventually led to the postoperative administration of fluoropyrimidines, in the hope of eradicating micrometastatic foci *(3,4)*. At the time of the initiation of the National Surgical Adjuvant Breast and Bowel Project's (NSABP) first adjuvant colon cancer and rectal cancer trials (1977), despite evidence that the postoperative administration of these agents caused a modest prolongation in survival, there was no consensus that they were appropriate for the treatment of patients with resected early-stage carcinoma of the colon and rectum.

By the mid-1970s, some studies had indicated that a combination of nitrosoureas + fluoropyrimidines might offer benefit to patients with early stage colorectal cancer. Murine colon cancer models suggested that this combination had synergistic activity against colon tumors *(5,6)*. The agent fluorouracil, a fluoropyrimidine, had been used to treat patients with early or advanced stage colorectal cancer since 1957. Three randomized clinical trials in the 1970s indicated that in combination with MeCCNU it produced response rates superior to those obtained with when it was used alone *(7–9)*.

From: *Fluoropyrimidines in Cancer Therapy*
Edited by: Y. M. Rustum © Humana Press Inc., Totowa, NJ

Coincident with the evolution of a rationale for the use of nitrosourea + fluoropyrimidine combinations in the adjuvant setting was the development of nonspecific immunostimulatory agents such as bacille Calmette Guérin (BCG). The results of nonrandomized trials investigating BCG alone and with chemotherapy in patients with advanced colon and rectal cancer had a profound influence on the development of randomized adjuvant trials and led to the development of the first NSABP adjuvant trials for patients with cancer of the colon and rectum *(10,11)*.

2. NSABP COLON CANCER ADJUVANT TRIALS

The NSABP historically has included Stage II and Stage III colon cancer patients in all its adjuvant chemotherapy trials. Four such trials (C-01, C-02, C-03, and C-04) are described below.

2.1. NSABP Protocol C-01

From November 1977 through February 1983, 1166 patients were entered into the NSABP's first randomized adjuvant clinical trial for patients with resected Stage II and Stage III colon cancer *(12)*. Patients were stratified by stage, gender, and age to receive either MOF (MeCCNU, vincristine, and fluorouracil), BCG, or no further treatment. At 5 yr, disease-free survival (DFS) and survival for patients who received MOF were better than for patients treated by surgery alone (58% vs 51%, p=0.02; and 67% vs 59%, p=0.05, respectively). When patients who received BCG alone were compared to those who were treated with surgery alone, there was no significant difference in 5-yr DFS (56% vs 51%, p=0.09), but there was a 5-yr survival advantage in the BCG-treated group (67% vs 59%, p=0.03). Subsequent analysis revealed that this difference in survival was likely due to an imbalance in the number of cardiovascular-related events, and when this imbalance was taken into account, there was no statistically significant difference between the two groups (p=0.40). NSABP C-01 was the first adjuvant colon cancer trial to demonstrate that a significant DFS and survival benefit could be achieved with postoperative adjuvant chemotherapy in patients with Stage II and Stage III carcinoma of the colon.

2.2. NSABP Protocol C-02

Protocol C-02 was designed to evaluate the immediate postoperative infusion of fluorouracil into the portal vein of patients with Stages I, II, or III carcinoma of the colon *(13)*. Between March 1984 and July 1988, a total 1158 patients with such cancers were entered into the study. Since ascertainment of the correct stage of disease could not be confirmed until surgery, all patients entered were randomized, but the subsequent analysis was based on findings in the 901 eligible patients who were found to have Stages I, II, or III tumors. Patients were stratified by age and gender and were assigned to either surgery alone or surgery plus portal vein infusion. Those assigned to portal vein infusion received fluorouracil and sodium heparin over 24 h beginning no later than 6 h after the completion of surgery and continuing for a total of 7 d. At 4 yr, a comparison between the two groups indicated both improved DFS (74% vs 73%, p=0.02) and a survival advantage (81% vs 73%, p=0.07) in the chemotherapy-treated group. Those who had undergone surgery alone were 1.26 times more likely to die after 4 yr; in 32.9% (27) of the 82 patients in the control group who had documented recurrence, the liver was the first site of treatment failure, compared to 46.3% (31/67) of patients with documented recurrences in the portal-vein infusion group. Reanalysis after a mean time on study of 65 mo demonstrated a benefit in both DFS (p=0.03) and overall survival (*p*=0.01) in the patients treated with chemotherapy. Tests for the interaction of outcome with age, gender, and stage were carried out for DFS and overall survival; results were not statistically significant. Specific interaction between treatment and age, treatment and gender, or treatment and stage were also not significant for either DFS or overall survival. Although this study failed to demonstrate a benefit for intraportal infusion of fluorouracil and heparin for the prevention of recurrences involving the liver, it did demonstrate an unexpected advantage in both DFS and overall survival, leading to the speculation that benefit derived from the intraportal infusion of fluorouracil and heparin was the result of a systemic effect.

2.3. NSABP Protocol C-03

At the time of this protocol's initiation in August 1987, there was considerable interest in the efficacy of leucovorin-modulated fluorouracil in the adjuvant setting. Phase I and II trials conducted on patients with advanced colon cancer provided information to suggest benefit from a leucovorin + fluorouracil regimen. A meta-analysis of nine studies indicated an objective response rate of 23% in patients who had received this combination, compared to 11% in those who had received fluorouracil alone *(14)*. Although this benefit did not translate into a survival advantage, its finding supported the contention that there was a useful pharmacologic modulation of fluorouracil by leucovorin. Such modulation is thought to occur as the result of an increase in the formation and stability of the fluorodeoxyuridylate-thymidylate synthase complex. This is turn results in a covalent ternary complex, with the consequent inhibition of thymidylate synthase, which affects the cytotoxic activity of the fluorouracil. NSABP protocol C-03 was a two-arm study comparing MOF (identical to the treatment arm of C-01) with fluorouracil + leucovorin for the first 6 wk of each 8-wk cycle, for a total of six cycles *(15)*. Between August 1987 and April 1989, 1081 patients similar to those studied in protocol C-01 were stratified by age, stage, tumor location, and number of involved lymph nodes and were randomized between the two arms. At 3 yr of follow-up, DFS (73% vs 64%, *p*=0.0004) and overall survival (84% vs 77%, *p*=0.007) were better for the patients assigned to weekly fluorouracil + leucovorin. Based on a cumulative odds ratio of 1.48, this represents a 32% reduction in mortality risk in favor of the fluorouracil + leucovorin-treated group. In addition, none of the tests for interaction for individual stratification variables were significant. Since the results of the C-01 trial demonstrated that the MOF regimen showed activity in the adjuvant setting, it is likely that the results of trial C-03 underestimate the efficacy of weekly fluorouracil + leucovorin. If one reviews the 3-yr DFS and overall survival data from the untreated control arm of protocol C-01, the control arm of C-03 (MOF), and the treatment arm of C-03 (weekly fluorouracil + leucovorin), the value of fluorouracil + leucovorin can be placed into perspective more easily. While the 3-yr DFS of untreated controls in protocol C-01 was 60%, in C-03 it was 73% for the fluorouracil + leucovorin regimen. Likewise, 3-yr overall survival was increased from 72% to 84%. These results established six cycles of weekly fluorouracil + leucovorin as an acceptable choice for the adjuvant treatment of patients with Stage II or III colon cancer.

2.4. NSABP Protocol C-04

This protocol evolved from the results of protocols C-01 and C-03. Its purpose was to compare the weekly fluorouracil + leucovorin regimen used in protocol C-03 with fluorouracil + levamisole and to ascertain whether the addition of levamisole to the C-03 fluorouracil + leucovorin combination added benefit *(16)*. This study accrued 2151 patients between July 1989 and December 1990 who were assigned to receive either

1. Weekly fluorouracil + leucovorin (as in C-03);
2. The same chemotherapy + levamisole; or
3. Fluorouracil (daily for 5 d and then weekly starting on d 29) + levamisole (for three consecutive days every 2 wk) for 1 yr.

A pairwise comparison between patients treated with fluorouracil + leucovorin and those treated with fluorouracil + levamisole disclosed a prolongation in 5-yr DFS in the fluorouracil + leucovorin group (60% vs 65%, p=0.04). There was also a small prolongation in overall survival in the latter group that was of borderline significance (70% vs 74%, p=0.07). There were no differences when a pairwise comparison was done of patients who received weekly fluorouracil + leucovorin and those who received fluorouracil + leucovorin + levamisole, for either 5-yr DFS (65% vs 64%, p=0.67) or 5-yr overall survival (74% vs 73%, p=0.99). There was no significant interaction between the effect of treatment and stage of disease with either regimen. In summary, this study showed that treatment with weekly fluorouracil + leucovorin conferred a small DFS advantage and a borderline prolongation in overall survival when compared to treatment with fluorouracil + levamisole. The addition of levamisole to weekly fluorouracil + leucovorin did not provide benefit beyond that achieved with fluorouracil + leucovorin alone. The results from this study established weekly fluorouracil + leucovorin as an acceptable therapeutic standard for the treatment of patients with Stage II or III carcinoma of the colon.

2.5. NSABP Protocol C-05

Based on the results of protocol C-03 and preclinical data that suggested that interferon alpha-2a enhanced the activity of fluorouracil, the NSABP initiated protocol C-05 to test the proposition that the addition of interferon alpha-2a would increase the efficacy of adjuvant fluorouracil + leucovorin *(17)*. The fluorouracil + leucovorin regimen used in this study was a departure from that used in protocols C-03 and C-04 and reflects the results of early pharmacokinetic studies performed in patients with colon cancer which showed that coadministration of fluorouracil and interferon alpha-2a decreased fluorouracil clearance, prolonged fluorouracil half-life, and resulted in a 1.5-fold increase in fluorouracil exposure *(18, 19)*. Between October 1991 and February 1994, 1176 patients were entered into this trial and randomly assigned to the control group (fluorouracil + leucovorin daily for the first 5 d of each of six 28-d cycles) or to the treatment group fluorouracil + leucovorin daily + subcutaneous interferon alpha-2a. At 4 yr follow-up there was no statistically significant difference between the groups, either in DFS (control, 69%; treatment, 70%) or overall survival (control, 80%; treatment 81%). Patients who received interferon alpha-2a experienced more grade 3+ adverse events (72% vs 62%), and fewer of these patients completed protocol-mandated treatment (77% vs 89%). Protocol C-05 established that the addition of interferon alpha-2a to fluorouracil + leucovorin resulted in an increase in the frequency of adverse events and did not confer a benefit in either DFS or overall survival.

2.6. NSABP Protocol C-06

In protocol C-06, the NSABP compared three cycles of weekly fluorouracil + leucovorin (as in protocol C-03) to five cycles of an oral regimen of UFT (tegafur and uracil) (300 mg/m^2 daily) + leucovorin (90 mg/m^2) daily for 28 d of a 35-d cycle. UFT is a 5-fluorouracil (5-FU) prodrug. Preclinical studies have shown that uracil + UFT enhanced the concentration of 5-FU in tumors and increased antineoplastic activity (A–E). In patients with advanced cancer and metastatic colon cancer in Phase I and II trials, UFT + calcium folinate (a biochemical modulator) for more than 28 d resulted in response rates of 25–43% and an acceptable toxicity profile for the adjuvant setting (F–H). Between February 1997 and March 1999, 1608 patients were stratified (by age and stage) and randomly assigned to one of the two treatments. The mean time of follow-up is currently too short to yield analyzable results. This study, however, should definitively ascertain the role of UFT + leucovorin in the adjuvant treatment of patients with carcinoma of the colon.

2.7. NSABP Protocol C-07

Protocol C-07 was initiated February 1, 2000, and is still accruing. The aim of this study is to ascertain whether the addition of three once-per-week administrations of oxaliplatin, given in weeks 1, 3, and 5, of a 6-wk regimen confers a benefit in DFS and overall survival for patients with Stage II or III disease beyond that which is seen with weekly fluorouracil + leucovorin alone. Oxaliplatin, a platinum compound, is a relatively recent agent in the treatment of colorectal cancer. It has been shown to have synergistic effect with 5-FU, even in 5-FU-resistant tumors. Oxaliplatin has an outstanding safety profile, a unique mechanism of action, and a lack of crossresistance with other agents used in the treatment of colorectal cancer. The target accrual for this study is 2472 patients. It is projected that the final analysis for the DFS endpoint will occur in August 2005.

3. NSABP RECTAL CANCER ADJUVANT TRIALS

3.1. NSABP Protocol R-01

This protocol was designed to explain the role of postoperative chemotherapy and radiotherapy in the treatment of patients with resected Stage II or III rectal cancer *(20)*. Between November 1977 and October 1986, 555 eligible patients with follow-up entered. They were stratified by age, gender, and stage and randomized to receive entirely no further treatment, MOF (as in the treatment arm of C-01 and control arm of C-03), or radiation therapy. At 5 yr of follow-up, patients who received MOF demonstrated an overall improvement in DFS (p=0.006) and in survival (p=0.05) compared to the group treated by surgery alone. Gender was the primary stratification variable contributing to the DFS and survival benefit from chemotherapy; however, to a lesser extent, age and stage also interacted. The benefit for chemotherapy, both in DFS (29% vs 47%, p<0.001) and survival (37% vs 60%, p=0.001) was restricted to males, with the greatest benefit occurring in the younger age groups. This age benefit was not evident among women. When the outcome of the group treated with radiation therapy was compared to that of the group that underwent surgery alone, there was an overall reduction in local-regional recurrence (16% vs 25%, p=0.06) in the group that received radiation but no significant benefit in overall DFS (p=0.4) or survival (p=0.7). The global test for interaction to identify heterogeneity of response to radiation within subsets of patients was not significant. This study demonstrated that patients with selected Stage II or III rectal cancer derived a DFS and survival benefit from fluoropyrimidine-containing chemotherapy (MOF) and that postoperative radiation therapy reduced local-regional recurrence but failed to affect overall disease-free survival or survival.

3.2. NSABP Protocol R-02

The aim of this study was to evaluate the role of postoperative radiation therapy and to determine whether adjuvant treatment with fluorouracil + leucovorin is superior to adjuvant MOF in patients with Stage II or III carcinoma of the rectum *(21)*. From September 1987 through December 1992, 694 eligible patients were stratified according to age, gender, stage, and number of involved lymph nodes. Male patients received either MOF with or without radiation therapy or weekly fluorouracil + leucovorin (as in protocol C-03) with or without radiation therapy. Because NSABP protocol C-01 demonstrated that MOF did not benefit women, all female patients received either fluorouracil + leucovorin alone or the same chemotherapy with radiation therapy. At an average 93 mo on study, there was no benefit from postoperative radiation therapy either in DFS (p=0.90) or survival (p=0.89), regardless of the type of chemotherapy delivered. However, radiation therapy reduced the cumulative incidence of locoregional relapse (from 13% to 8% at 5 yr of follow-up, p=.02). The benefit of radiation therapy appeared to be limited to patients younger than 60 yr or those who had undergone an abdominoperineal resection. Males who received fluorouracil + leucovorin demonstrated a benefit in DFS at 5 yr compared to those treated with MOF (55% vs 47%, p=0.009), but not in 5-yr survival (65% vs 62%, p=0.17). The results of this study indicate that

1. Radiation therapy was effective in reducing locoregional recurrence regardless of the type of chemotherapy used.
2. Chemotherapy reduced both locoregional and distant recurrence.
3. Neither radiation therapy nor chemotherapy had an impact on survival.

4. COMPARATIVE EFFICACY OF CHEMOTHERAPY IN STAGE II VS STAGE III COLON CANCER: THE NSABP EXPERIENCE

Although several large prospective randomized trials *(12–16,22)*, have demonstrated benefit from the administration of adjuvant chemotherapy for Stage III colon cancer patients, the value of such therapy is still debated for patients with Stage II disease. The US National Institutes of Health (NIH) Consensus Development Conference on colorectal adjuvant therapy in 1990 recommended that patients with Stage III colon cancer receive adjuvant chemotherapy with 5-fluorouracil and levamisole (5-FU + LEV) *(23)* but did not recommend any specific adjuvant therapy for those with Stage II colon cancer outside of clinical trials. The recommendation was based mainly on results from Intergroup Study 0035, which demonstrated a significant survival improvement with adjuvant 5-FU + LEV in patients with Stage III colon cancer but no such improvement in patients with Stage II disease *(22)*. The lack of survival benefit in Stage II patients was confirmed in a subsequent update of this trial *(24,25)*, although a reduction in recurrence similar to that documented for Stage III patients was seen.

Since the time of the last NIH Consensus Development Conference, results from NSABP studies (see above) suggest that leucovorin-modulated 5-fluorouracil (5-FU + LV) is also effective in improving DFS and overall survival both in patients with Stage III and patients with Stage II colon cancer *(15,16)*. The NSABP trials showed no evidence of a differential treatment effect between Stage II and Stage III patients, indicating that adjuvant chemotherapy was effective in both groups. A likely explanation for the discrepancy between the NSABP C-03 and C-04 results and those from the Intergroup trial is that the Intergroup trial was by design underpowered to demonstrate significant survival differences in the subset of Stage II patients who had a lower event rate.

When one reviews the results from the NSABP C-01, C-02, C-03, and C-04 trials, either by themselves or in combined analysis, there is significant evidence that the relative efficacy of adjuvant chemotherapy in Stage II patients is comparable to that seen in Stage III patients.

The relatively large proportion of patients with Stage II tumors in NSABP studies provides the opportunity to address whether Stage II patients benefit from adjuvant chemotherapy and, if so, to what extent, compared to Stage III patients. Results from the comparison in

Table 1
Five-Year Overall Survival (S) Results in NSABP C-01, C-02, C-03, and C-04, According to Stage of Disease

	All			*Stage II*			*Stage III*		
Study	*N*	*% 5-year survival*	p-*value*	*N*	*% 5-year survival*	p- *value*	*N*	*% 5-year survival*	p-*value*
C-01									
Operation	375	60	0.07	166	72	0.73	209	50	0.05
MOF	351	67		150	75		201	59	
C-02									
Operation	343	67	0.08	201	76	0.005	142	56	0.81
PVI	340	74		188	88		152	58	
C-03									
MOF	516	66	0.0008	141	84	0.03	375	59	0.003
5-FU + LV	513	76		149	92		364	70	
C-04									
5-FU + LEV	690	70	0.06	285	81	0.25	405	63	0.21
5-FU + LV	692	75		285	85		407	67	

benefit have been reported in both an abstract *(26)* and a manuscript *(27)* and will be summarized here.

In all four of the NSABP trials described above, patients were classified as having Stage II tumors if on pathologic examination the tumor demonstrated full thickness penetration of the bowel wall (through the serosa or into the pericolic fat) with no regional lymph node involvement *(28)*. Patients were classified as having Stage III tumors if on pathologic examination there was evidence of regional lymph node involvement. In all four trials, patients who had obstruction or contained perforation were eligible, but patients with free perforation were not. The four studies included 3820 patients available for analysis; 1565 (41%) presented with Stage II and 2255 (59%) with Stage III tumors. Five-year follow up results in the four trials demonstrated a difference in overall survival for all patients for at least two of the arms, as described above (Table 1).

Five-year survival results according to stage of disease showed in all four studies that the observed difference in overall survival was in the same direction for Stage II and Stage III patients (Table 1). In *C-01,* the administration of MOF compared to surgery alone resulted in a 3% absolute improvement in survival for Stage II patients (p=0.73) and a 9% absolute improvement in survival in Stage III patients (p=0.05). In *C-02,* perioperative portal venous infusion of 5-FU compared to surgery alone resulted in a 12% improvement in survival for Stage II patients (p=0.005) and a 2% improvement for Stage III patients (p=0.81). In *C-03,* 5-FU + LV compared to MOF resulted in an 8% improvement in survival in Stage II patients (p=0.03) and an 11% improvement in Stage III patients (p=0.003). In *C-04,* when 5-FU + LV was compared to 5-FU + LEV, there was a 4% improvement in survival in Stage II patients (p=0.25) and a 4% improvement in Stage III patients in those who received the former regimen (p=0.21).

Regardless of stage of disease, these studies always showed a reduction in mortality, recurrence, or DFS event rate with chemotherapy, and in most cases, the reduction was as great as or greater in Stage II patients than in Stage III patients (Fig. 1). However, because of the limited number of Stage II and Stage III patients in each of these trials, one cannot rule out with

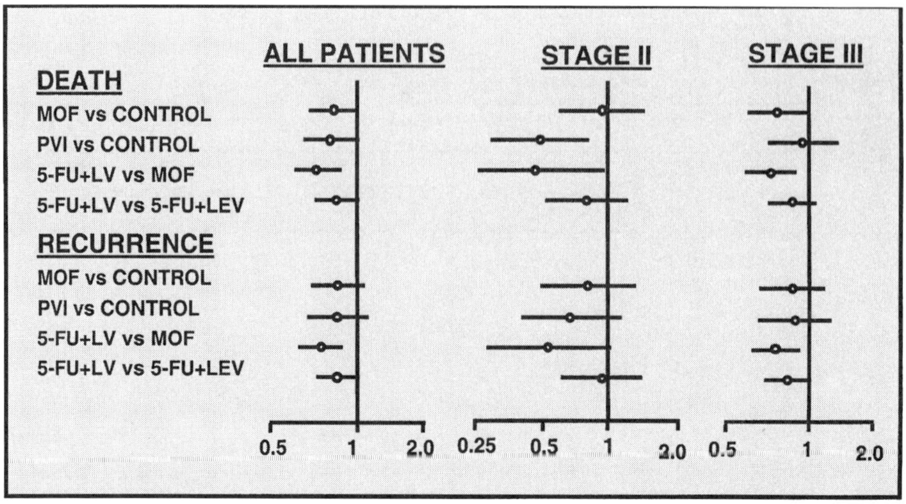

Fig. 1. Reduction in cumulative odds of death and recurrence according to stage for four NSABP adjuvant colon trials (with 95% confidence intervals).

confidence a substantial difference in treatment effect according to stage for any one trial. To address this question, data from all four of these trials were combined into two treatment groups. *Combined Group 1* included the patient groups from each trial that received treatment that resulted in the inferior outcome (surgery alone groups in C-01 and C-02, MOF group in C-03, and 5-FU + LEV group in C-04). *Combined Group 2* included the patient groups from each trial that received treatment that resulted in the superior outcome for all patients (MOF group in C-01, perioperative PVI of 5-FU in C-02, and 5-FU + LV in C-03 and C-04).

To estimate the differential effect of treatment according to stage, the cumulative odds of death were calculated in the "better outcome" group *(Combined Group 2)* relative to the "worse outcome" group *(Combined Group 1)* both for Stage II and Stage III patients. The cumulative odds of death in Stage II patients were 0.70 (indicating a 30% reduction in death rate for Stage II patients in *Combined Group 2* compared to Stage II patients in *Combined Group 1*). In comparison, at 5 yr, the cumulative odds of death in Stage III patients were 0.82 (indicating an 18% reduction in death rate for Stage III patients in *Combined Group 2* compared to Stage III patients in *Combined Group 1*). When the mortality reduction in Stage II patients was examined according to the presence or absence of clinical adverse prognostic factors such as obstruction, contained perforation, or direct extension to adjacent organs, the efficacy of adjuvant chemotherapy was evident whether patients presented with or without any of the adverse prognostic factors. Patients with none of the high-risk characteristics had a 32% reduction in mortality rate (cumulative odds: 0.68); those with one or more high-risk characteristics had a 20% reduction in mortality rate (cumulative odds: 0.80). This reduction in mortality rate was translated into an absolute improvement in survival of 5% in each risk category (*Combined Group 2:* 87% vs *Combined Group 1:* 82% in the low-risk category, and *Combined Group 2:* 75% vs *Combined Group 1:* 70% in the high-risk category).

These NSABP findings demonstrate that the 5-yr survival of patients with Stage II colon cancer treated with surgery alone is such that effective adjuvant chemotherapy is desirable in such cases. Even those who oppose the routine administration of adjuvant chemotherapy in all Stage II patients agree that such therapy may be indicated in a subset of patients, viz., those with adverse clinical prognostic factors such as obstruction, contained perforation, or extension into adjacent organs. However, our results indicate that the benefit from adjuvant chemotherapy in Stage II patients is independent of the presence or absence of such adverse prognostic factors. Furthermore, the 5-yr survival for patients in *Combined Group 1* who received less effective therapy and who did not have any of the adverse prognostic factors was only 82%, emphasizing the point that even in this group of patients withholding adjuvant chemotherapy is unwarranted. With the emergence of new molecular and genetic prognostic markers such as 18q chromosomal deletion *(29),* DNA mismatch repair gene mutations *(30,31),* thymidylate synthase levels *(32),* and p53 mutations *(33,34),* in the future it may be possible to identify subgroups of Stage II patients who have such a good prognosis that adjuvant chemotherapy can be avoided. However, until such biomarkers become validated in prospective studies, Stage II patients should be considered for adjuvant chemotherapy after discussion of the risks and benefits from such treatment.

5. CONCLUSION

Over the last three decades, considerable progress has been made in the treatment of carcinoma of the colon and rectum with adjuvant chemotherapy. NSABP Protocols C-01 and R-01 established the importance of fluoropyrimidine-containing adjuvant treatments for patients with either rectal or colon cancer. Protocols C-03 and R-02 established fluorouracil + leucovorin as a logical choice for the adjuvant treatment of these two diseases. Protocol C-04 demonstrated fluorouracil + leucovorin to be a rational alternative to fluorouracil + levamisole, and protocol C-05 put to rest the speculation that interferon alpha-2a might improve the efficacy of leucovorin-modulated fluorouracil. Protocol R-02 demonstrated that fluoropyrimidine-containing chemotherapy reduced locoregional and distant recurrence, and that neither chemotherapy (fluorouracil + levamisole or MOF) nor regional radiation therapy has a beneficial impact on survival. Recent analysis of the NSABP experience has confirmed that fluoropyrimidine-based chemotherapy is effective for patients with either Stage II or III carcinoma of the colon. Future directions in the treatment of colorectal cancer include the introduction of novel agents such as irinotecan, oxaliplatin, and oral fluoropyrimidines or prodrugs of fluoropyrimidines.

REFERENCES

1. Mrazek R, Economou S, McDonald G, et al. Prophylactic and adjuvant use of nitrogen mustard in the surgical treatment of cancer. *Ann Surg* 1959; 150:745.
2. Holden WD, Dixon WJ, Kuzma JW. The use of triethylenethiophosphamide as an adjuvant to the surgical treatment of colorectal carcinoma. *Ann Surg* 1967; 165:481.
3. Higgins GA, Dwight RW, Smith JV, Keehn RJ. Fluorouracil as an adjuvant to surgery in carcinoma of the colon. *Arch Surg* 1971; 102:339–343.
4. Higgins GA, Humphrey E, Juler G, LeVeen HH, McCaughan J, Keehn RJ. Adjuvant chemotherapy in the surgical treatment of large bowel cancer. *Cancer* 1976; 38:1461–1467.
5. Corbett TH, Griswold DP Jr, Roberts BJ, et al. A mouse colon-tumor model for experimental therapy. *Cancer Chemother Rep (Part 2)* 1975; 5:169–186.
6. Corbett TH, Griswold DP Jr, Roberts BJ, Peckham JC, Schabel FM Jr. Evaluation of single agents and combinations of chemotherapeutic agents in mouse colon carcinomas. *Cancer* 1977; 40:2660–2680.
7. Moertel CG, Schutt AJ, Hahn RG, Reitemeier RJ. Therapy of advanced colorectal cancer with a combination of 5-fluorouracil, methyl-1, 3-cis(2-chloroethyl)-1-nitrosourea and vincristine. *J Natl Cancer Inst* 1975; 54:69–71.
8. Baker LH, Talley RW, Matter R, et al. Phase III comparison of the treatment of advanced gastrointestinal cancer with bolus weekly 5-FU vs. methyl-CCNU plus bolus weekly 5-FU. *Cancer* 1976; 38:1–7.
9. Falkson G, Falkson HC. Fluorouracil, methyl CCNU, and vincristine in cancer of the colon. *Cancer* 1976; 38:1468–1470.

10. Mavligit GM, et al. Clinical immunotherapy as adjuvant therapy for colon and rectal cancer. In: Enker WE, ed. Carcinoma of the colon and rectum. *Chicago: Year Book Medical Publishers Inc.* 1978; 133–171.
11. Mavligit GM, Gutterman JU, Malahy MA, Burgess MA, McBride CM, Jubert A, Hersh EM. Adjuvant immunotherapy and chemoimmunotherapy in colorectal cancer. (Dukes' Class C): Prolongation of disease-free interval and survival. *Cancer* 1977; 40:2726–2730.
12. Wolmark N, Fisher B, Rockette H, et al. Postoperative adjuvant chemotherapy or BCG for colon cancer: Results from NSABP Protocol C-01. *J Natl Cancer Inst* 1988; 80:30–36.
13. Wolmark N, Rockette H, Wickerham DL, et al. Adjuvant therapy of Dukes' A, B, and C adenocarcinoma of the colon with portal-vein fluorouracil hepatic infusion: Preliminary results of National Surgical Adjuvant Breast and Bowel Project Protocol C-02. *J Clin Oncol* 1990; 8:1466–1475.
14. Piedbois P, Buyse M, Rustum Y, et al. Modulation of fluorouracil by leucovorin in patients with advanced colorectal cancer: Evidence in terms of response rate. *J Clin Oncol* 1992; 10:896–903.
15. Wolmark N, Rockette H, Fisher B, et al. The benefit of leucovorin-modulated fluorouracil as postoperative adjuvant therapy for primary colon cancer: Results from National Surgical Adjuvant Breast and Bowel Project Protocol C-03. *J Clin Oncol* 1993; 11:1879–1887.
16. Wolmark N, Rockette H, Mamounas EP, et al. Clinical trial to assess the relative efficacy of fluorouracil and leucovorin, fluorouracil and levamisole, and fluorouracil, leucovorin, and levamisole in patients with Dukes B and C carcinoma of the colon: Results from National Surgical Adjuvant Breast and Bowel Project C-04. *J Clin Oncol* 1999; 17:3553–3559.
17. Wolmark N, Bryant J, Smith R, et al. Adjuvant 5-fluorouracil and leucovorin with or without interferon alfa-2a in colon carcinoma: National Surgical Adjuvant Breast and Bowel Project Protocol C-05. *J Natl Cancer Inst* 1998; 90:1810–1816.
18. Grem JL, Jordan E, Robson ME, et al. Phase II study of fluorouracil, leucovorin, and interferon alfa-2a in metastatic colorectal carcinoma. *J Clin Oncol* 1993; 9:1737–1745.
19. Schuller J, Czejka MJ, Schernthaner G, Fogl U, Jager W, Micksche M. Influence of interferon alfa-2b with or without folinic acid on pharmacokinetics of fluorouracil. *Semin Oncol* 1992; 19 (2 Suppl 3):93–97.
20. Fisher B, Wolmark N, Rockette H, et al. Postoperative adjuvant chemotherapy or radiation therapy for rectal cancer: Results from NSABP Protocol R-01. *J Natl Cancer Inst* 1988; 80:21–29.
21. Wolmark N, Wieand HS, Hyams DM, et al. Randomized trial of postoperative adjuvant chemotherapy with or without radiotherapy for carcinoma of the rectum: National Surgical Adjuvant Breast and Bowel Project Protocol R-02. *J Natl Cancer Inst* 2000; 92:388–396.
22. Moertel CG, Fleming TR, MacDonald JS, et al. Levamisole and fluorouracil for adjuvant therapy of resected colon carcinoma. *N Engl J Med* 1990; 322:352–358.
23. NIH Consensus Conference: Adjuvant therapy for patients with colon and rectal cancer. *J Am Med Assoc* 1990; 246:1444–1450.
24. Moertel CG, Fleming TR, MacDonald JS, et al. Fluorouracil plus levamisole as effective adjuvant therapy after resection of stage III colon carcinoma: A final report. *Ann Intern Med* 1995; 122:321–326.
25. Moertel CG, Fleming TR, MacDonald JS, et al. Intergroup study of fluorouracil plus levamisole as adjuvant therapy for stage II/Stage III colon cancer. *J Clin Oncol* 1995; 13:2936–2943.
26. Mamounas EP, Rockette H, Jones J, et al. Comparative efficacy of adjuvant chemotherapy in patients with Dukes' B vs. Dukes' C colon cancer: Results from four NSABP adjuvant studies (C-01, C-02, C-03, and C-04). *Proc Am Soc Clin Oncol* 1996; 15:205 (#461).
27. Mamounas E, Wieand S, Wolmark N, et al. Comparative efficacy of adjuvant chemotherapy in patients with Dukes' B vs. Dukes' C colon cancer: Results from four NSABP adjuvant studies (C-01, C-02, C-03, and C-04). *J Clin Oncol* 1999; 17:1349–1355.
28. Dukes CE. The classification of cancer of the rectum. *J Pathol* 1932; 35:323–332.
29. Jen J, Kim H, Piantatosi S, et al. Allelic loss of chromosome 18q and prognosis in colorectal cancer. *N Engl J Med* 1994; 331:213–221.
30. Bronner CE, Baker SM, Morrison PT, et al. Mutation in the DNA mismatch repair gene homologue hMLH1 is associated with hereditary non-polyposis colon cancer. *Nature* 1994; 368:258–261.
31. Nicolaides NC, Papadopoulos N, Liu B, et al. Mutations in two PMS homologues in hereditary nonpolyposis colon cancer. *Nature* 1994; 371:75–80.
32. Johnston PG, Fisher ER, Rockette HE, et al. The role of thymidylate synthase expression in prognosis and outcome of adjuvant chemotherapy in patients with rectal cancer. *J Clin Oncol* 1994; 12:2640–2647.
33. Bosari S, Viale G, Possi P, et al. Cytoplasmic accumulation of p53 protein: An independent prognostic indicator in colorectal adenocarcimomas. *J Natl Cancer Inst* 1994; 86:681–687.
34. Zeng ZS, Sarkis AS, Zhang ZF, et al. P53 nuclear overexpression: An independent predictor of survival in lymph node positive colorectal cancer patients. *J Clin Oncol* 1994; 12:2043–2050.

16 Clinical Trials of UFT Leucovorin in Gastrointestinal Malignancies

Paulo M. Hoff, MD, *and Everardo D. Saad,* MD

CONTENTS

1. INTRODUCTION AND PHASE I STUDIES OF UFT/LEUCOVORIN

The combination of tegafur and uracil (UFT) plus leucovorin has been used extensively in Japan and Europe for the treatment of a variety of malignancies. Extensive clinical trials of UFT/leucovorin have also been conducted in the United States and Europe. This chapter reviews the studies of UFT/leucovorin in the treatment of patients with gastrointestinal malignancies. Studies of UFT/leucovorin in combination with other agents are also briefly discussed. Clinical studies of UFT/leucovorin in other malignancies are reviewed by Dr. Lembersky in Chapter X. In Chapter 17, Dr. Blijham addresses the basic pharmacology and preclinical development of UFT.

After the demonstration of the unacceptably high toxicity of intravenous tegafur in the early U.S. studies *(1),* further clinical development of orally administered tegafur and later UFT took place mainly in Japan (reviewed in ref. *2*). The addition of leucovorin enhanced the antitumor activity of UFT in animal models *(3)* and augmented the inhibition of thymidylate synthase in gastric tumors in humans *(4).* Following these studies, clinical development of the UFT/leucovorin combination was pursued in the West. Six phase I studies of the combination were reported from Spain and the United States (Table 1). Daily doses of UFT ranging from 200 to 600 mg/m^2, administered once, twice, or three times daily, were given either continuously *(5)* for 14 d every 4 wk *(7,9)* or for 28 d every 5 *(8,10)* or 6 wk *(6).* Leucovorin doses used in the studies ranged from 30 to 150 mg/d. Dose-limiting toxic effects were diarrhea, mucositis, vomiting, fatigue, leukopenia, abdominal pain, and abnormal liver function tests. The recommended UFT dose for phase II studies in the United States was 300 mg/m^2 per day, administered in three divided doses for 28 d every 5 wk *(10).*

From: *Fluoropyrimidines in Cancer Therapy*
Edited by: Y. M. Rustum © Humana Press Inc., Totowa, NJ

Table 1
Phase I Studies of UFT/Leucovorin Conducted in Europe and the United States

Study	*No. of patients*	*UFT dose (per day) and schedule*	*Leucovorin dose (per day) and schedule*	*UFT maximum tolerated dose (per day)*
Spicer *(6)*	14	300–400 mg/m² × 28 d every 6 wk	20 mg/m² IV on days 1, 8, 15, 22	300 mg/m²
Nogué *(5)*	9	200–600 mg/m²	30–60 mg	10 mg/kg
González-Báron *(7)*	26	200–440 mg/m² in 2 doses × 14 d every 4 wk	500 mg/m² IV on day 1, then 30 mg orally × 13	390 mg/m²
Meropol *(8)*	26	200–350 mg/m² in 3 doses × 28 d every 5 wk	150 mg × 28 days every 5 wk	350 mg/m²
Pazdur *(9)*	14	350–400 mg/m² × 14 d every 4 wk	150 mg × 14 days every 4 wk	350 mg/m²
Pazdur *(10)*	18	220–350 mg/m² × 28 d every 5 wk	150 mg × 28 days every 5 wk	350 mg/m²

Abbreviation: IV = Intravenously

Because of the saturable oral absorption of leucovorin *(11),* the recommended dose for further clinical trials was 90 mg/d, delivered in three divided doses. At doses near the maximum tolerated doses determined in the phase I studies (i.e., UFT 350 mg/m^2 per day and leucovorin 150 mg/d), UFT/leucovorin had a favorable toxicity profile. Furthermore, the ability to deliver an oral regimen of the leucovorin-modulated 5-fluorourocil (5-FU) prodrug UFT offered logistical and patient convenience, leading investigators in Europe and the United States to pursue additional clinical development of the combination.

2. CLINICAL TRIALS OF UFT/LEUCOVORIN IN COLON CANCER

Many patients treated in the phase I studies of UFT/leucovorin had colorectal cancer. However, the vast majority of these patients had failed previous 5-FU therapy, and very few patients showed objective responses to UFT/leucovorin. The poor activity of UFT/leucovorin in 5-FU-refractory disease has been confirmed in recent phase II trials of the drug combination in patients with advanced disease previously treated with 5-FU *(12,13).* The next logical step in the development of the combination was to test the regimen in the setting of advanced, previously untreated colorectal cancer.

Phase II studies of UFT/leucovorin as front-line chemotherapy in patients with advanced colorectal cancer are summarized in Table 2. Except for one study that enrolled only patients with rectal cancer *(14),* the studies were designed for patients with either colon or rectal tumors *(15–20).* Two of the seven studies specifically assessed the efficacy and safety of UFT/leucovorin in elderly patients *(18,19),* a subject reviewed by Dr. Abad in Chapter 18. In all but one of these studies *(19),* UFT was administered intermittently, either for 14 d every 4 wk *(14,17)* or for 28 d every 5 wk *(15,16,18,20).* Leucovorin doses used in the studies ranged from 15 to 150 mg/d and were administered orally, except in two studies from Spain in which leucovorin was initially given as a 500 mg/m^2 intravenous injection on d 1 *(17,18).*

Front-line chemotherapy with UFT/leucovorin produced objective responses in 16% to 42% of patients with advanced colorectal cancer (Table 2). Pooling the results from all phase II trials

Table 2
Phase II Studies of UFT/Leucovorin as Front-Line Therapy for Advanced Colorectal Cancer

Study	*No. of evaluable patients*	*UFT dose (per day) and schedule*	*Leucovorin dose (per day) and schedule*	*Response rate (%)*	*95% CI*	*Median Overall Survival (months)*
Pazdur *(15)*	45	300–350 mg/m^2 × 28 d every 5 wk	150 mg × 28 d every 5 wk	42	28–58	NR[a]
Sanchiz *(14)*	52	600 mg/m^2 × 14 d every 4 wk	90 mg/m^2 × 14 d every 4 wk	40	27–55	NR
Saltz *(16)*	20	350 mg/m^2 × 28 d every 5 wk	15 mg × 28 d every 5 wk	25	6–44	12+
González-Báron *(17)*	75	390 mg/m^2 × 14 d every 4 wk	500 mg/m^2 IV on day 1 and 30 orally days 2–14	38.7	27.8–50	13.5
Feliu *(18)*	38	390 mg/m^2 × 14 d every 4 wk	500 mg/m^2 IV on day 1 and 30 orally d 2–14	29	15–46	12.5
Abad *(19)*	77	400 mg/m^2 continuously	45 mg continuously	16.8	9–27	14.4[b]
Aranda *(20)*	111	300 mg/m^2 × 28 d every 5 wk	150 mg × 28 d every 5 wk	20.7	13.7–29.7	13[b]

[a] An updated analysis showed a median overall survival of 15.8 mo; [b]Actuarial survival; Abbreviations: IV = Intravenously; NR = Not reported.

shows that major responses were documented in 121 (28.9%) of 418 patients. Although most of the responses (100 of 121) were partial, 21 complete responses were reported. Among the studies reporting time-dependent variables, the median duration of response ranged from 4.4 to 10 mo *(14,17,18,20)*, and the median overall survival ranged from 12.5 to 14.4 mo *(16–20)*.

The phase I and phase II toxicity profiles of UFT/leucovorin were similar. The most common toxic effects were diarrhea, nausea/vomiting, abdominal pain, and fatigue. World Health Organization (WHO) grade 3 or 4 toxicity was infrequent and included diarrhea (approx 15% of patients), nausea/vomiting (approx 6% of patients), mucositis (approx 4% of patients), and fatigue (approx 3% of patients). Hematologic toxicity was minimal, and hand-foot syndrome and neurotoxicity were not observed.

The results obtained with UFT/leucovorin in phase II trials were comparable to historical data for 5-FU. The 23% response rate determined in a meta-analysis of randomized trials of bolus 5-FU/leucovorin regimens *(21)* falls within the range of response rates to UFT/leucovorin in phase II trials (16% to 42%). Furthermore, the range of overall median survival times for the UFT/leucovorin studies (12.5 to 14.4 mo) was comparable to the median survival time seen in a recent trial assessing a variety of 5-FU-containing regimens (14 mo), *(22)* as well as to the median survival times seen in a large randomized trial of commonly used bolus 5-FU/leucovorin regimens *(23)*. The toxicity profile of UFT/leucovorin compared favorably with historical data for continuous infusion 5-FU, except that hand-foot syndrome was seen in approx 34% of patients treated with the latter regimen *(24)* and virtually absent in those treated with UFT/leucovorin. On the basis of these results, UFT/leucovorin was evaluated in phase III trials, both in the setting of advanced disease and as adjuvant treatment after surgery.

Two large, randomized phase III trials published in abstract form compared the effects of UFT/leucovorin with those of bolus 5-FU/leucovorin in the treatment of patients with advanced colorectal cancer *(25,26)*. In both trials, patients in the experimental arm received UFT 300 mg/m^2 per day given orally for 28 d every 5 wk in combination with oral leucovorin 75 mg/d or 90 mg/d, both given in three divided doses, and patients in the control arm received 5-FU 425 mg/m^2 per day and leucovorin 20 mg/m^2 per day, both given intravenously for five consecutive days, every 4 *(25)* or 5 *(26)* wk.

The main findings of these two large trials are summarized in Table 3. In advanced colorectal cancer, the response rates and survival duration obtained with UFT/leucovorin were comparable to those obtained with bolus 5-FU/leucovorin. However, the UFT/leucovorin combination exhibited a more favorable toxicity profile, with significantly less frequent WHO grade 3 or 4 hematologic toxicity, mucositis, and infectious complications. The incidences of grade 3 or 4 diarrhea in the separate analyses were not significantly different, but a combined analysis demonstrated a slightly higher incidence of diarrhea after UFT/leucovorin treatment that was statistically significant. Hyperbilirubinemia was also more common with UFT/leucovorin, but no other liver function abnormalities were observed in either group.

Many workers regarded the combined results of these two large trials as evidence that UFT/leucovorin is a suitable alternative to 5-FU/leucovorin as first-line therapy for advanced colorectal cancer. However, as of this writing, UFT/leucovorin has not been approved by the FDA for use in patients with colorectal cancer.

The UFT/leucovorin combination is also being investigated in the adjuvant setting. The ONCOPAZ Cooperative Group in Spain evaluated 269 patients with Dukes' stage B2 and C colon cancer who received UFT 390 mg/m^2 per day for 14 d every 4 wk plus leucovorin 500 mg/m^2 intravenously on d 1 followed by 15 mg/d orally on d 2–14. *(27)* With a median follow-up of 36 mo, the relapse rates for patients with Dukes' stages B2 and C colon cancer were 11% and 30%, respectively. Disease-free survival rates were 83% for patients with

Table 3
Summary Results of Phase III Trials of UFT/Leucovorin in Advanced Colorectal Cancer

	Pazdur (25) n=*802*		*Carmichael* (26) n=*373*		*Combined Total* n=*1175*	
	UFT/LV	*5-FU/LV*	*UFT/LV*	*5-FU/LV*	*UFT/LV*	*5-FU/LV*
Toxicity[a]						
Diarrhea (%)	21	16	18	11	20[b]	14
Nausea/vomiting (%)	13	10	9	9	12	10
Anemia (%)	3[b]	7	5	4	4	6
Neutropenia (%)	1[b]	56	3[b]	31	1[b]	48
Febrile neutropenia (%)	0[b]	13	1[b]	8	<1[b]	11
Mucositis (%)	1[b]	19	2[b]	16	2[b]	18
Efficacy parameters						
Response rate (%)	12	15	11	9	—	—
Median overall survival (months)	12.4	13.2	12.2	11.9	—	—

[a] Toxicity refers to World Health Organization grade 3 or 4 toxic effects; [b]Statistically significant differences ($p<0.05$, Fisher's exact test for individual studies and Cochran-Mantel-Haenszel test for combined total).

Abbreviations: 5-FU = 5-fluorouracil; LV = Leucovorin; UFT = Uracil plus tegafur.

stage B2 and 62% for patients with stage C disease, and overall survival rates for these patients were 94% and 87%, respectively. These results compare favorably with those of large randomized trials of adjuvant 5-FU-based therapies *(28–30)*. Diarrhea was the primary toxic effect in the ONCOPAZ study, and 42% of patients required dose reductions owing to toxicity. The National Surgical Adjuvant Breast and Bowel Project (NSABP) is conducting a large phase III trial comparing UFT/leucovorin with 5-FU/leucovorin as adjuvant therapy for resected colon cancer (NSABP C-06). Patients are randomly assigned to receive five courses of UFT 300 mg/m^2 per day and leucovorin 90 mg/d, both given for 28 d every 5 wk, or three courses of leucovorin 500 mg/m^2 followed by 5-FU 500 mg/m^2, both given intravenously once a week for 6 wk. Accrual to this study closed in March 1999, and preliminary results demonstrate that both regimens show similar toxicity and are well tolerated *(31)*.

3. CLINICAL TRIALS OF UFT/LEUCOVORIN IN RECTAL CANCER

Most of the studies described in the preceding section included patients with colon tumors and patients with rectal tumors, but the results were not reported according to the site of the primary tumor. A phase II study from Spain evaluated UFT/leucovorin exclusively for the treatment of patients with advanced rectal cancer *(14)*. Fifty-two patients received UFT 600 mg/m^2 and leucovorin 90 mg/m^2 daily for 14 d every 4 wk, and 21 partial responses were seen (40%). Lack of response to treatment correlated with previous chemotherapy; 7 (22%) of 32 patients who had previously received chemotherapy had an objective response to UFT/leucovorin, whereas 14 (70%) of 20 patients with no previous chemotherapy achieved a partial response.

Used as adjuvant treatment, protracted infusion of 5-FU plus external beam radiation therapy has yielded promising results in Tumor Node Metastasis (TNM) stages II and III rectal cancer *(32)*. Thus, the use of oral UFT/leucovorin in combination with radiation therapy warrants testing. An oral regimen could represent a convenient means of delivering effective adjuvant treatment without central venous catheters or portable infusion pumps. Furthermore, radiosensitization through orally administered drugs would have many potential applications in oncology.

Two phase I studies of UFT/leucovorin as radiation sensitizers for patients with operable rectal cancer have been conceived. In the study by Minsky and colleagues from Memorial Sloan-Kettering Cancer Center and the University of Pennsylvania, Patients who have undergone surgical resection of TNM stage II and III rectal tumors receive adjuvant chemoradiation with UFT/leucovorin beginning 4–6 wk after surgery *(33)*. This study is open to accrual as of this writing. We have conducted a phase I study in which oral UFT/leucovorin was administered concurrently with radiation therapy in a preoperative setting in patients with TNM stages II and III rectal cancer as confirmed by endoscopic ultrasound *(34)*. Fifteen patients were treated Mondays through Fridays with escalating doses of UFT/leucovorin given concurrently with a 5-wk course of preoperative radiation totaling 4500 cGy. Surgery was performed 4–6 wk after radiation and was followed by four 35-d courses of fixed doses of UFT/leucovorin. The maximum tolerated dose of UFT with this radiation schedule was 350 mg/m^2 per day with 90 mg/d of leucovorin. Diarrhea was the dose-limiting toxic effect. This schedule allowed for delivery of higher daily doses of UFT (350 mg/m^2) than those usually recommended (300 mg/m^2), possibly because of the 2-d rest each weekend. In our study sphincter-sparing surgery was performed in 12 of the 14 patients who had surgery. Pathologic evaluation of the 14 resected specimens showed a complete response in three cases. We concluded that preoperative chemoradiation with oral UFT plus leucovorin is feasible and well tolerated and should be further investigated.

Given the feasibility and good results of preoperative 5-FU-based chemoradiation *(35)* and the lack of randomized trials comparing preoperative and postoperative chemoradiation for the treatment of operable rectal cancer, most investigators currently believe that the two approaches are equally effective. Protocol NSABP R-03, *(36)* designed to answer the question of which strategy might be superior, was recently closed owing to slow accrual. Most physicians treating these patients developed personal preferences regarding the timing of adjuvant chemoradiation and were unwilling to randomize the patients. The NASBP is considering a randomized phase III trial of oral UFT/leucovorin vs intravenous 5-FU/leucovorin, both combined with radiation therapy, for patients with operable rectal cancer.

UFT/leucovorin has also been investigated in the setting of locally advanced rectal cancer. Spanish investigators reported the preliminary results of a phase II study in which patients with locally advanced disease were given either UFT/leucovorin concurrently with radiation therapy before surgery or UFT/leucovorin alone for six courses after surgery *(37)*. The regimen consisted of UFT 300 or 350 mg/m^2 per day for 14 d every 4 wk and leucovorin 500 mg intravenously on day 1 and 30 mg/d orally on d 2–14. In 53% of cases, treatment resulted in tumor downstaging, allowing for more conservative surgical procedures. In another study from Spain, patients with unresectable or recurrent rectal cancer received UFT/leucovorin concomitantly with pelvic irradiation. Among 32 patients evaluable for clinical response, 4 (13%) had a complete response and 22 (69%) had a partial response. Pathologic analysis showed a complete response in three cases *(38)*.

4. CLINICAL TRIALS OF UFT/LEUCOVORIN IN OTHER GASTROINTESTINAL MALIGNANCIES

Given the role of 5-FU in the treatment of several noncolorectal gastrointestinal malignancies, UFT/leucovorin was a logical choice for clinical trials among patients with cancers of the stomach, esophagus, pancreas, and hepatobiliary system.

4.1. Stomach

In a phase II study from France, UFT 300 mg/m^2 per day and leucovorin 90 mg/d, both given for 28 d every 5 wk, produced 4 (15.3%) major responses among 26 evaluable patients with previously untreated metastatic gastric cancer *(39)*. The toxicity profile was similar to that seen in other clinical trials of UFT/leucovorin. In a smaller phase II trial from Korea *(40)*, UFT starting at 480 mg/m^2 per day and escalated according to tolerance and leucovorin at the fixed dose of 25 mg/m^2 per day, both given for 21 d every 4 wk, produced 4 (28.6%) major responses among 14 evaluable patients with advanced gastric cancer. Toxicity was acceptable, with the most serious toxic effects being grade 3 nausea/vomiting and diarrhea in 12.5% and 43.8% of patients, respectively, and grade 3 or 4 stomatitis/mucositis in 12% of patients. The median survival in this small cohort of patients was 25 wk, leading the authors to conclude that UFT/leucovorin is a reasonable alternative for advanced gastric cancer. The same investigators reported preliminary results of a phase II study of UFT/leucovorin combined with cisplatin and epirubicin: 20 (54%) of 37 patients with locally advanced or metastatic gastric cancer achieved a major response *(41)*. In this trial, grade 3 or 4 toxic events also included leukopenia in 37.8% of patients, an expected finding given that the drug combination is known to be myelotoxic.

Japanese investigators have also conducted studies of UFT in combination with other agents. In a series of studies among patients with advanced gastric cancer utilizing UFT in combination with cisplatin, etoposide, mitomycin C, and doxorubicin, response rates ranged from 38% to 55% *(42–45)*. The Spanish ONCOPAZ group has conducted a phase II study of UFT/leucovorin combined with etoposide *(46)*. Forty-six patients with advanced gastric cancer not previously treated with chemotherapy received a regimen that included oral UFT and oral and intravenous etoposide and leucovorin. Among the 46 patients, 4 achieved a complete response and 12 achieved a partial response, for an overall response rate of 35%. The toxicity of this regimen was relatively mild, with infrequent grade 3 or 4 toxic effects. The median overall survival was 9 mo for all patients and 13 mo for patients who responded to chemotherapy.

4.2. Esophagus

The combination of chemoradiation with cisplatin and 5-FU yields survival rates superior to those achieved with radiation therapy alone in the nonsurgical treatment of esophageal cancer *(47)*; a combined modality approach that includes surgery is being evaluated *(48)*. In addition, investigators at the Oregon Health Sciences University and the Vanderbilt Cancer Center have designed a phase I trial to evaluate UFT/leucovorin in combination with cisplatin and radiation therapy among patients with potentially resectable esophageal cancer *(49)*. Patients receive preoperative and postoperative chemotherapy with cisplatin 80 mg/m^2 for two cycles and leucovorin 90 mg/d from d 1 through 35 preoperatively and d 1 through 21 and d 29 through 50 postoperatively. UFT is given, along with leucovorin, in escalating doses starting at 200 mg/m^2 per day before and 300 mg/m^2 per day after surgery.

4.3. Pancreas and Liver

At the University of Alabama at Birmingham, the same concept of oral radiosensitization was explored in a phase I study *(50)* in which 12 patients with resected (*n*=5) or unresectable (*n*=7) locally advanced pancreatic cancer were treated with escalating doses of UFT and fixed doses of leucovorin (90 mg/d) with concomitant radiation therapy (4500 cGy at 180 cGy/d). The treatment regimen was extremely well tolerated, and the maximum tolerated dose of UFT was not reached in this trial. Two of the three episodes of grade 3 or 4 toxic events were not thought to be secondary to the experimental regimen. Of the seven patients with unresectable disease, radiography documented a complete response in one case, and four patients had stable disease following treatment. The authors will conduct a similar, larger phase I/II study starting with UFT doses of 300 mg/m^2 per day, thus refining the evaluation of the toxicity, efficacy, and pharmacokinetic parameters of this drug combination.

Despite the encouraging results of UFT/leucovorin-based chemoradiation for locally advanced disease *(50)*, the use of UFT/leucovorin chemotherapy without radiation therapy produced no objective responses among 14 patients with advanced pancreatic cancer in a phase II trial from the University of Chicago *(51)*. The same group of investigators reported similarly discouraging results among patients with advanced hepatocellular *(52)* or biliary carcinoma *(53)*, none of whom responded to UFT/leucovorin given according to the schedule typically used in the United States studies *(10)*.

5. CONCLUSIONS

Clinical trials of UFT/leucovorin have demonstrated its favorable toxicity profile and its activity in colorectal cancer, suggesting that this oral regimen represents an alternative to intravenous bolus 5-FU/leucovorin regimens. However, as of this writing, UFT/leucovorin has not been approved by the FDA for use in patients with colorectal cancer.

In addition to the potential role in the treatment of metastatic disease, UFT/leucovorin may prove to be a suitable alternative to intravenous 5-FU/leucovorin for the adjuvant treatment of colorectal cancer. Recent work also suggests that administration of UFT/leucovorin concurrently with radiation therapy yields encouraging results in a variety of gastrointestinal malignancies.

REFERENCES

1. Valdivieso T, Bodey GP, Gottlieb JA, Freireich EJ. Clinical evaluation of ftorafur (pyrimidine-deoxyribose N1-2′-furanidyl-5-fluorouracil). *Cancer Res* 1976; 36:1821–1824.
2. Sulkes A, Benner SE, Canetta RM. Uracil-ftorafur: an oral fluoropyrimidine active in colorectal cancer. *J Clin Oncol* 1998; 16:3461–3475.
3. Okabe H, Toko T, Saito H, et al. Augmentation of the chemotherapeutic effectiveness of UFT, a combination of tegafur (1-(2-tetrahydrofuryl)-5-fluorouracil) with uracil, by oral l-leucovorin. *Anticancer Res* 1997; 17:157–164.
4. Ichikura T, Tomimatsu S, Okusa Y, et al. Thymidylate synthase inhibition by an oral regimen consisting of tegafur-uracil (UFT) and low-dose leucovorin for patients with gastric cancer. *Cancer Chemother Pharmacol* 1996; 38:401–405.
5. Nogué AM, Saigui GE. Protracted treatment with UFT and leucovorin by oral way. *Oncologia (Spain)* 1992; 15:114–116.
6. Spicer D, Muggia F, Tulpule A, et al. Phase I circadian dosing of daily oral uracil (U) plus 1-(tetrahydro-2-furanyl)-5-fluorouracil (FT) with leucovorin (LV) (abstract). *Proc Am Assoc Cancer Res* 1991; 10:342.
7. González-Báron M, Feliu J, Ordonez A, et al. Phase I study of UFT plus leucovorin in advanced colorectal cancer: a double modulation proposal. *Anticancer Res* 1993; 13:759–762.
8. Meropol NJ, Rustum YM, Petrelli NJ, et al. A phase I and pharmacokinetic study of oral uracil, ftorafur, and leucovorin in patients with advanced cancer. *Cancer Chemother Pharmacol* 1996; 37:581–586.
9. Pazdur R, Lassere Y, Diaz-Canton E, et al. Phase I trial of uracil-tegafur (UFT) plus oral leucovorin: 14-day schedule. *Invest New Drugs* 1997; 15:123–128.
10. Pazdur R, Lassere Y, Diaz-Canton E, Ho DH. Phase I trial of uracil-tegafur (UFT) plus oral leucovorin: 28-day schedule. *Cancer Invest* 1998; 16:145–151.
11. Priest D, Schmitz J, Bunni M, Stuart R. Pharmacokinetics of leucovorin metabolites in human plasma as a function of dose administered orally and intravenously. *J Natl Cancer Inst* 1991; 83:1806–1812.
12. Pazdur R, Patt Y, Ajani J, et al. Phase II/pharmacology study of UFT (BMS-200604) and leucovorin in refractory colorectal cancer patients (abstract). *Proc Am Soc Clin Oncol* 1997; 16:270a.
13. Meropol NJ, Sonnichsen DS, Birkhofer MJ, et al. Bioavailability and phase II study of oral UFT plus leucovorin in patients with relapsed or refractory colorectal cancer. *Cancer Chemother Pharmacol* 1999; 43:221–226.

14. Sanchiz F, Milla A. Tegafur-uracil (UFT) plus folinic acid in advanced rectal cancer. *Jpn J Clin Oncol* 1994; 24:322–326.
15. Pazdur R, Lassere Y, Rhodes V, et al. Phase II trial of uracil and tegafur plus oral leucovorin: an effective oral regimen in the treatment of metastatic colorectal carcinoma. *J Clin Oncol* 1994; 12:2296–2300.
16. Saltz LB, Leichman CG, Young CW, et al. A fixed-ratio combination of uracil and ftorafur (UFT) with low dose leucovorin. An active oral regimen for advanced colorectal cancer. *Cancer* 1995; 75:782–785.
17. Gonzalez-Baron M, Feliu J, de la Gandara I, et al. Efficacy of oral tegafur modulation by uracil and leucovorin in advanced colorectal cancer. A phase II study. *Eur J Cancer* 1995; 31A:2215–2219.
18. Feliu J, González-Báron M, Espinosa E, et al. Uracil and tegafur modulated with leucovorin: an effective regimen with low toxicity for the treatment of colorectal carcinoma in the elderly. *Cancer* 1997; 79:1884–1889.
19. Abad A, Navarro M, Sastre J, et al. Phase II continuous UFT plus folinic acid in elderly patients with colorectal cancer (CRC) (abstract). *Proc Am Soc Clin Oncol* 1997; 16:280a.
20. Aranda E, Antón-Torres A, Sastre J, et al. UFT plus leucovorin (LV) in advanced colorectal cancer (CRC). A phase II trial (abstract). *Proc Am Soc Clin Oncol* 1999; 18:245a.
21. Advanced Colorectal Cancer Meta-Analysis Project. Modulation of fluorouracil by leucovorin in patients with advanced colorectal cancer: evidence in terms of response rate. *J Clin Oncol* 1992; 10:896–903.
22. Leichman CG, Fleming TR, Muggia FM, et al. Phase II study of fluorouracil and its modulation in advanced colorectal cancer: a Southwest Oncology Group study. *J Clin Oncol* 1995; 13:1303–1311.
23. Buroker TR, O'Connell MJ, Wieand HS, et al. Randomized comparison of two schedules of fluorouracil and leucovorin in the treatment of advanced colorectal cancer. *J Clin Oncol* 1994; 12:14–20.
24. Meta-Analysis Group In Cancer. Toxicity of fluorouracil in patients with advanced colorectal cancer: effect of administration schedule and prognostic factors. *J Clin Oncol* 1998; 16:3537–3541.
25. Pazdur R, Douillard J-Y, Skillings JR, et al. Multicenter phase III study of 5-fluorouracil (5-FU) or UFT in combination with leucovorin (LV) in patients with metastatic colorectal cancer (abstract). *Proc Am Soc Clin Oncol* 1999; 18:263a.
26. Carmichael J, Popiela T, Radstone D, et al. Randomized comparative study of ORZEL (oral uracil/tegafur (UFT) plus leucovorin (LV) versus parenteral 5-fluorouracil (5-FU) plus LV in patients with metastatic colorectal cancer (abstract). *Proc Am Soc Clin Oncol* 1999; 18:264a.
27. Espinosa E, González-Báron M, Feliu J, et al. UFT-leucovorin as adjuvant treatment for Dukes' B2-C colon cancer (abstract). *Proc Am Soc Clin Oncol* 1998; 17:275a.
28. Laurie JA, Moertel CG, Fleming TR, et al. Surgical adjuvant therapy of large bowel carcinoma: an evaluation of levamisole and the combination of levamisole and fluorouracil. *J Clin Oncol* 1989; 7:1447–1456.
29. International Multicentre Pooled Analysis of Colon Cancer Trials (IMPACT) investigators. Efficacy of adjuvant fluorouracil and folinic acid in colon cancer. *Lancet* 1995; 345:939–944.
30. O'Connell MJ, Maillard JA, Kahn MJ, et al. Controlled trial of fluorouracil and low-dose leucovorin given for 6 months as postoperative adjuvant therapy for colon cancer. *J Clin Oncol* 1997; 15:246–250.
31. Smith R, Wieand H, Mamounas E. UFT plus calcium folinate vs 5-FU plus calcium folinate in colon cancer. *Oncology (Huntingt)* 1999; 13(Suppl 3):44–47.
32. O'Connell M, James M, Martenson JA, et al. Improving adjuvant therapy for rectal cancer by combining protracted infusion fluorouracil with radiation therapy after curative surgery. *N Engl J Med* 1994; 331:502–507.
33. Minsky B. Adjuvant postoperative combined-modality therapy for rectal cancer. *Oncology (Huntingt)* 1999; 13(7 Suppl 3):132–135.
34. Hoff PM, Janjan NA, Saad ED, et al. Phase I study of preoperative oral uracil and tegafur plus leucovorin and radiation therapy in rectal cancer. *J Clin Oncol* 2000; 18:3529–3534.
35. Janjan NA, Khoo VS, Abbruzzese J, et al. Tumor downstaging and sphincter preservation with preoperative chemoradiation in locally advanced rectal cancer: the M. D. Anderson Cancer Center experience. *Int J Radiat Oncol Biol Phys* 1999; 44:1027–1038.
36. Hyams DM, Mamounas EP, Petrelli N, et al. A clinical trial to evaluate the worth of preoperative multimodality therapy in patients with operable carcinoma of the rectum: a progress report of National Surgical Breast and Bowel Project Protocol R-03. *Dis Colon Rectum* 1997; 40:131–139.
37. Feliu J, Calvillo J, Escribano A, et al. Neoadjuvant therapy of rectal carcinoma with UFT-folinic acid (LV) plus radiotherapy (RT) (abstract). *Proc Am Soc Clin Oncol* 1999; 18:239a.
38. de la Torre A, Ramos S, Valcarcel F, et al. Phase II study of radiochemotherapy with UFT and low-dose oral leucovorin in patients with unresectable rectal cancer. *Int J Radiat Oncol Biol Phys* 1999; 45:629–634.
39. Ravaud A, Borner M, Schellens JH, et al. UFT and oral calcium folinate as first-line chemotherapy for metastatic gastric cancer. *Oncology (Huntingt)* 1999; 13(7 Suppl 3):61–63.
40. Kim YH, Cheong SK, Lee JD, et al. Phase II trial of oral UFT and leucovorin in advanced gastric carcinoma. *Am J Clin Oncol* 1996; 19:212–216.

41. Kim YH, Kim BS, Seo JH, et al. Epirubicin, cisplatin, oral UFT, and calcium folinate in advanced gastric carcinoma. *Oncology (Huntingt)* 1999; 13(7 Suppl 3):64–68.
42. Tadaoka N, Yoshinaga K, Nakamura Y, et al. Phase II trial of UFT and cisplatinum (CDDP) in advanced gastric cancer (GC) with primary foci (abstract). *Proc Am Soc Clin Oncol* 1998; 17:303a.
43. Sato A, Hasegawa K, Kurihara M, et al. Combination chemotherapy with tegafururacil (UFT) and cisplatin (CDDP) for advanced gastric cancer. *Gan To Kagaku Ryoho* 1995; 22:1355–1362.
44. Hayakawa M, Morise K, Chin K, et al. Combination chemotherapy with Tegafur Uracil (UFT), etoposide, adriamycin and cisplatinum (UFT-EAP) for advanced gastric cancer. *Jpn J Clin Oncol* 1994; 24:282–288.
45. Sawa T, Kinoshita K, Takekawa S, et al. Effect of PMUE therapy (CDDP, MMC, UFT, etoposide) for terminal gastric cancer. *Gan To Kagaku Ryoho* 1990; 17:2381–2386.
46. Feliu J, González-Báron M, García-Gíron C, et al. Treatment of patients with advanced gastric carcinoma with the combination of etoposide plus oral tegafur modulated by uracil and leucovorin: a phase II study of the ONCOPAZ Cooperative Group. *Cancer* 1996; 78:211–216.
47. Herskovic A, Martz K, al-Sarraf M, et al. Combined chemotherapy and radiotherapy compared with radiotherapy alone in patients with cancer of the esophagus. *N Engl J Med* 1992; 326:1593–1598.
48. Minsky BD. Carcinoma of the esophagus. Part 1: primary therapy. *Oncology (Huntingt)* 1999; 13:1225–1232.
49. Blanke CD, Teng M, Choy H. The role of UFT in combined-modality therapy *Oncology (Huntingt)* 1999; 13(10 Suppl 5):47–54.
50. Childs HA, III, Spencer SA, Raben DR, et al. A phase I study of combined UFT plus leucovorin and radiotherapy for pancreatic cancer. *Int J Radiat Oncol Biol Phys* 2000; 47:939–944.
51. Mani S, Kugler JW, Sciortino DF, et al. Phase II trial of uracil/tegafur (UFT) plus leucovorin in patients with advanced pancreatic carcinoma: a University of Chicago phase II consortium study. *Ann Oncol* 1998; 9:1035–1037.
52. Mani S, Schiano T, Garcia JC, et al. Phase II trial of uracil/tegafur (UFT) plus leucovorin in patients with advanced hepatocellular carcinoma. *Invest New Drugs* 1999; 16:279–283.
53. Mani S, Sciortino D, Samuels B, et al. Phase II trial of uracil/tegafur (UFT) plus leucovorin in patients with advanced biliary carcinoma. *Invest New Drugs* 1999; 17:97–101.

17 The Development of Oral UFT with and without Leucovorin

Geert H. Blijham, MD, PhD

Contents

1. INTRODUCTION

The fluoropyrimidines are among the most active classes of anticancer agents used in the chemotherapy of colorectal cancer. More than 40 yr after its introduction, intravenous 5- fluorouracil (IV 5-FU) therapy remains a fundamental treatment for this disease. Results, however, are moderate at best and IV 5-FU is typically associated with significant toxicity.

The efficacy of 5-FU can be improved through biomodulation. Biomodulation of 5-FU by non cytotoxic agents increases the antitumor effect while reducing the toxicity. The most intensively studied biomodulator of 5-FU is leucovorin (LV). In patients with metastatic colorectal cancer, 5-FU/LV combination therapy has resulted in significantly improved response rates and prolonged survival compared to 5-FU monotherapy. Thus, for many years iv 5-FU/LV has been considered the most established treatment regimen for patients with metastatic colorectal cancer.

5-FU has a short half-life of approx 10–20 min. However the length of exposure of tumor cells to 5-FU can be improved with prolonged infusion, and evidence suggests that prolonged infusion of 5-FU appears to be more effective in inhibiting DNA synthesis in tumor cells. Prolonged exposure is particularly relevant in colorectal cancer cells, which typically have a slow doubling time.

From: *Fluoropyrimidines in Cancer Therapy*
Edited by: Y. M. Rustum © Humana Press Inc., Totowa, NJ

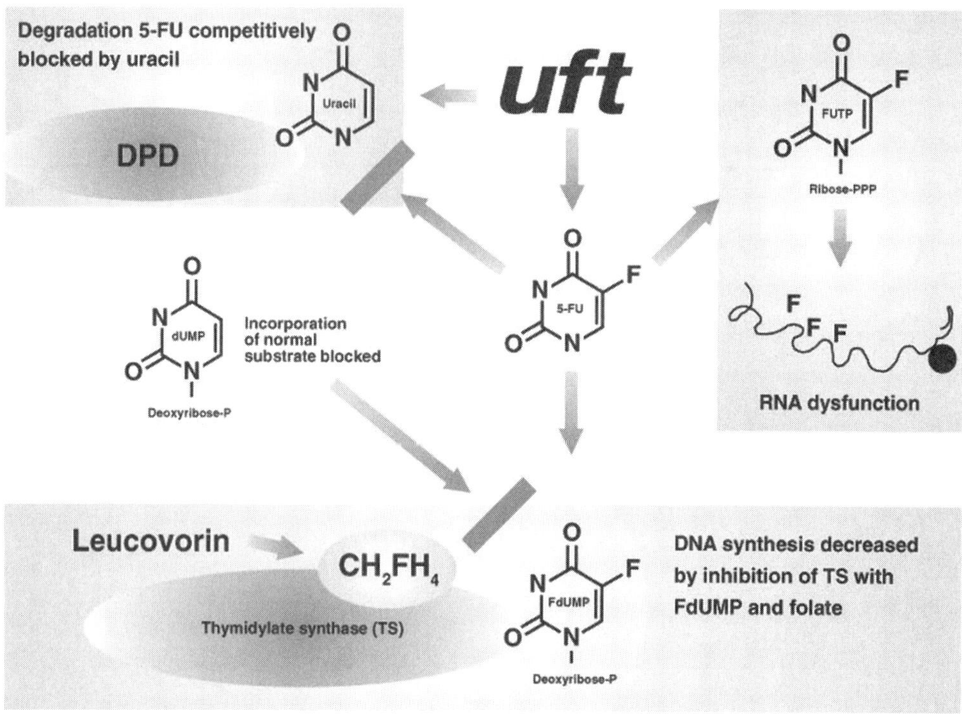

Fig. 1. The mechanism of action of UFT/LV.

More recent approaches to improve the therapeutic index of 5-FU have involved the following:

1. Study of 5-FU prodrugs.
2. The use of competitors of enzymes involved in the catabolism of 5-FU.
3. The adoption of oral drugs with an improved bioavailability profile.

These efforts have led to the development of tegafur-uracil (UFT). UFT represents one of the most comprehensive attempts to address the above issues; tegafur is a prodrug of 5-FU, uracil is a competitive inhibitor of 5-FU degradation, and both agents are well absorbed following oral administration.

2. DEVELOPMENT OF UFT (TEGAFUR-URACIL)

Tegafur (tetrahydrofuranyl-5-fluorouracil) was first synthesized by Hiller and colleagues in 1967. It is a prodrug of 5-FU and is metabolized to 5-FU in vivo, predominantly in the liver microsomes by the P-450 system, but also by thymidine phosphorylase and through spontaneous degradation. The activity of the 5-FU is mediated primarily by the two main metabolites: 5-fluoro-2′-deoxyuridine- 5′-monophosphate, which inhibits the enzyme thymidylate synthase, thereby inhibiting DNA synthesis of the tumor cell, and 5-flurouridine-triphosphate, which disrupts RNA synthesis (Fig. 1).

Tegafur has been developed as a drug for both intravenous and oral administration. It shows activity in a number of solid tumors, including metastatic colorectal cancer where objective response rates range between 11% and 25%.

Intravenous administrations of tegafur, however, have been characterized by a high incidence of neurological toxicity, in particular lethargy. This toxicity has been attributed to butyrolactone, a tegafur metabolite that can cross the blood-brain barrier. Bioavailability of oral tegafur has been shown to be more predictable than that achieved with 5-FU. However, bioavailability has proven to be somewhat problematic. In studies using doses similar to those administered intravenously (1000–1500 mg/m^2/d), tegafur has resulted in similar neurotoxicity, as well as gastrointestinal side effects, in approx 25% of the patients *(1–3)*.

Thus, tegafur has proven efficacy as a monotherapy for the treatment of metastatic colorectal cancer. However, at the doses required for maximum efficacy, tegafur is associated with a high incidence of dose-limiting neurotoxicity.

Uracil, a naturally occuring pyrimidine, is a competitive inhibitor of dihydropyrimidine dehydrogenase (DPD). This enzyme is responsible for approx 85% of 5-FU degradation. Uracil thus increases the amount of available 5-FU and ultimately results in increased RNA and DNA deregulation.

Fujii and collaborators in 1978 were the first to combine tegafur and uracil to produce UFT *(4)*. Comparative pharmacokinetic and pharmacodynamic UFT studies have revealed that substantially higher plasma 5-FU concentrations are achieved compared with tegafur alone. Preclinical studies have established a ratio of 1 mole of tegafur to 4 moles of uracil to be optimal. Although increased proportions of uracil increase the plasma and tissue concentrations of 5-FU (and thus enhance the antitumor effects), this also results in increased toxicity.

Importantly, following UFT administration, tumor concentrations were higher than normal tissue concentrations. This was attributed to the fact that tumors have higher levels of thymidylate synthase and lower levels of DPD than normal tissues. Thus, tegafur and uracil administered in combination have resulted in lowering the tegafur dosage and therefore toxicity, while at the same time maintaining the antitumor efficacy *(5)*.

3. CLINICAL APPLICATION OF UFT AS MONOTHERAPY

Early clinical development of UFT was conducted in Japan and focused exclusively on the oral administration of the compound. In initial trials conducted in almost 1000 patients, UFT was shown to have a broad spectrum of antitumor activity in several tumor types including colorectal, stomach, breast, and head and neck cancers *(6)*.

Three Phase II trials of single-agent UFT have been conducted in patients with metastatic colorectal cancer. Ota and collaborators pooled the results of the Phase II trials performed in Japan *(7)*; 80 of these patients had a diagnosis of colorectal cancer. UFT was administered at 400 to 600 mg/d (bid or tid) for at least 4 wk. A partial response was observed in 25% of the evaluable patients. Median survival time was 227 d (339 d in the responders).

These results were confirmed in a Phase II trial conducted in the United Kingdom in the late 1980s by Malik and colleagues *(8)*. Single-agent UFT at 600 mg/d (tid) was administered to 40 patients with metastatic colorectal cancer. A partial response was observed in 17% patients, but all except one responder relapsed with liver metastases. Median response duration was 22 wk.

A third study conducted in Spain utilized a more aggressive regimen of UFT at 800 mg/m^2/d for 21 d, with a 1-wk rest period in 35 patients *(9)*. A partial response was observed in 26% patients, with a median duration of response of 7 mo.

Administration of UFT at daily doses of 400 to 600 mg (bid or tid) resulted in a relatively low toxicity profile, with approx 30–40% of patients reporting anorexia, nausea and vomiting, diarrhea, epigastric pain, stomatitis, skin pigmentation, neurotoxicity, myelosuppression, or dizziness, of any grade of severity.

Table 1
Phase II Trials Evaluating UFT Plus LV in Advanced/Metastatic CRC

González Barón et al. (12)
- Phase II trial of 75 patients with advanced CRC
- Patients received oral UFT 195 mg/m^2 and iv LV 500 mg/m^2 on day 1, followed by oral UFT 195 mg/m^2 q 12 h and oral LV 15 mg q 12 h on days 2–14
- Objective response rate was 39% (95%, CI: 28–50%), with complete response in 9% of patients and a partial response in 29%
- Diarrhea (usually grade 1 or grade 2) was main toxicity; hematological toxicity was minimal

Feliu et al. (13)
- Phase II trial of 38 elderly patients (>70-yr-old) with advanced CRC
- Patients received oral UFT 195 mg/m^2 and iv LV 500 mg/m^2 on day 1, followed by oral UFT 195 mg/m^2 q 12 h and oral LV 15 mg q 12 h on days 2–14
- The objective response rate was 29% (95%, CI: 15–46%)

Abad et al. (14)
- Phase II trial that had 77 evaluable elderly patients (> 72 years)
- Patients received oral UFT 400 mg/d (fixed dose) plus folinic acid 45 mg/d, treatment was interrupted if grade 3 or 4 toxicity occurred
- Objective response was 16.9% (CR 5.2%, and PR 11.7%); median survival was 14.4 mo
- Toxicity was generally mild; 15.6% of patients had grade 3 nausea/vomiting, and 9.1% had grade 3 or 4 diarrhea

Pazdur et al. (15)
- 45 patients with metastatic CRC received oral UFT 300 mg/m^2/d plus LV 150 mg/day, administered in divided doses q 8 h for 28 d
- for 7 patients, initial dose included UFT 350 mg/m^2/d; reduced to 300 mg/m^2/d because of severe diarrhea in five of seven patients
- Objective response was 42.2%; median overall survival was 12.7 mo
- Treatment was well tolerated; adverse effects included diarrhea, vomiting, abdominal cramping, fatigue, minor oral mucositis, and rash

Sanchiz et al. (16)
- 52 evaluable patients with advanced rectal cancer received UFT 600 mg/m^2/d plus LV 90 mg/d for 14 d
- Partial response was seen in 70% of patients with no previous chemotherapy, and 22% of patients who had prior chemotherapy
- Median time to progression was 19.6 mo for patients with no previous chemotherapy, and 7.7 mo for patients with prior chemotherapy

4. PHASE I/II TRIALS OF UFT PLUS LV

Clinical development of UFT treatment as a single-agent has mostly been discontinued. This has been for two reasons. First, evidence for the positive biomodulation effects of leucovorin (LV) on fluoropyrimidines has become widely acknowledged, and has been confirmed in experimental models where UFT/LV has been compared to UFT alone. Second, the availability of oral formulations of LV has made an oral regimen of UFT/LV a realistic goal.

The UFT/LV regimen was developed in order to administer oral LV concomitantly with each dose of UFT. Initial studies were designed to develop the UFT/LV regimen examined dosing schedule. This consisted of UFT (bid) treatment for 14 d, repeated monthly, in combination with LV (UFT 500 mg/m^2 and low-dose LV 30 mg/d). This approach resulted in dose-limiting toxicities of diarrhea and stomatitis, and was brought into Phase II in metastatic colorectal cancer patients at a daily UFT dose of 390 mg/m^2.

Other approaches have also been tried, such as continuous daily doses of UFT in combination with daily low doses of LV. Using this regimen, diarrhea and vomiting were dose-limiting, and a regimen of UFT 400 mg/d (total dose) and LV 45 mg/d (total dose), given continuously, was proposed for Phase II *(10)*.

Finally, Camps and collaborators conducted a Phase I/II trial that included only patients with advanced colorectal carcinoma *(11)*. Doses of UFT were escalated from 200 to 500 mg/m^2/day accompanied by low-dose oral LV 15 mg/d bid, with the courses of treatment being repeated every 4 wk. A total of 22 patients were accrued, and dose-limiting toxicity was diarrhea. The recommended regimen for further studies was UFT 400 mg/m^2/day plus LV 30 mg/d, divided into two doses. One complete and five partial responses were obtained in this trial, with an objective response rate of 27% (95%, CI: 11–50%). Of note, all responses were seen at doses ≥300mg/m/^{2}/d of UFT and median response duration was 5 mo. Table 1 summarizes several other Phase II trials that evaluated UFT plus LV in patients with regionally advanced or MCRC.

Overall, objective responses to UFT/LV were observed in all the Phase II trials performed in previously untreated patients with MCRC. The level of activity observed appeared to be at least as good as that commonly seen with intravenously administered regimens of 5-FU/LV. Moreover, the reduction of the initial UFT dosage from 350 to 300 mg/m^2 appeared to increase the safety margins of the UFT/CF regimen, particularly at high oral LV doses, and did not seem to affect the efficacy in a meaningful way.

5. CLINICAL PHARMACOLOGY TRIALS

UFT in a dose range of 100–400 mg results in linear plasma exposures of tegafur, uracil, and 5-FU. In order to assess the pharmacokinetics of single- and continuous-dose UFT, patients with metastatic colorectal cancer initally received a single dose of UFT at either 100, 200, or 400 mg, accompanied by LV 25 mg orally, followed, after 7 d of rest, by treatment with UFT 300 mg/m^2 plus LV 75 mg/d. After single-dosing, the plasma concentrations of tegafur, 5-FU, and uracil rose rapidly, reaching peak plasma levels within 1–2 h. In contrast to tegafur, the plasma concentration of uracil and 5-FU then declined rapidly. However, 5-FU plasma concentrations remained detectable for 8 h after single 200- or 400-mg doses.

The steady-state plasma concentrations of tegafur, uracil, and 5-FU demonstrated a consistent peak and trough appearance during each dosing interval. In addition, peak plasma concentrations for tegafur, uracil, and 5-FU were consistent during the study, indicating that there was no significant accumulation of UFT. Continuous, although relatively low plasma 5-FU concentrations as compared with bolus 5-FU, were maintained during the 28-d treatment *(17)* (Fig. 2).

The addition of oral LV does not significantly change the plasma exposures of tegafur. In one study patients with metastatic colorectal cancer, who had previously received chemotherapy treatment, were randomized to receive either UFT 200 mg, LV 30 mg alone, or the combination for 8 d before being given UFT 300 mg/m^2 plus LV 90 mg. Both uracil and 5-FU plasma exposures were lower when UFT and LV were given together, as compared with UFT alone, but this was not significant. In addition, concurrent dosing of UFT with LV produced slightly higher plasma exposures of the two LV analytes (d, 1-citrovorum factor and 5-methyltetrahydrofolate), but, again, these differences were not significant.

The relative abundance of tegafur, 5-FU, and their metabolites has been investigated during UFT/LV therapy by magnetic resonance imaging (MRI). Seven days before starting UFT/LV, patients with metastatic colorectal cancer received a single intravenous dose of 5-

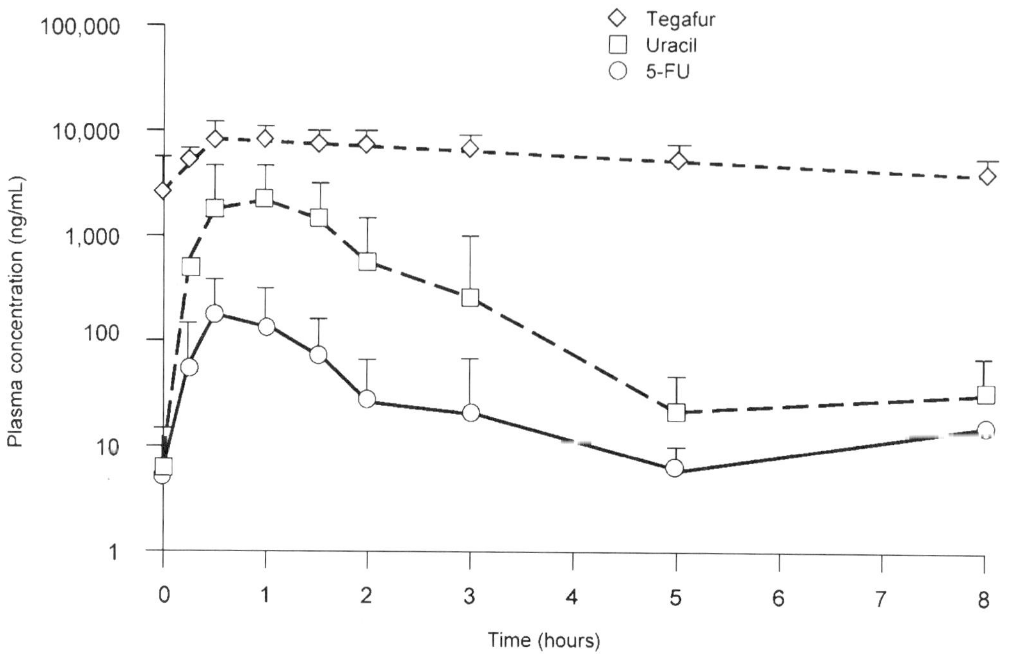

Fig. 2. Mean (SD) plasma concentration-time data for tegafur, uracil and 5-FU on d 8 of a 28-d treatment regimen.

FU 600 mg/m^2, without LV. Although peaks of tegafur and metabolites were detected in some patients, no 5-FU peaks could be assessed. Thus, although evidence of intratumoral uptake of fluoropyrimidines after UFT/LV administration has been established, their quantification throughout this investigational technique remains problematic.

The effects of a high-fat diet on the bioavailability of UFT/LV is currently under investigation. Patients were randomized on d 3 to receive therapy with or without a high-fat meal, and then crossed-over to the alternate arm. Subsequently, patients started receiving the standard regimen of UFT 300 mg/m^2 plus LV 90 mg. Data so far indicate that a high-fat meal reduces plasma levels of uracil and 5-FU and elevates plasma exposures of both LV analytes. Plasma levels of tegafur were not altered significantly. Thus, it appears that UFT/LV combination therapy should be taken at least 1 h prior to, or after, a meal. This dosing schedule was followed in the Phase III clinical studies.

All these trials utilized specific dosing lead-in periods that preceded the regular treatment regimen, which consisted of oral UFT 300 mg/m^2/d (tid) and oral LV 75 or 90 mg/d for 28 d followed by a 7-d rest period. This regimen was shown to have optimal bioavailability *(18)* and was selected as the regimen to be tested in Phase III trials.

6. PHASE III TRIALS OF UFT/LV IN PREVIOUSLY UNTREATED CRC

Two multicenter, randomized, open-label, Phase III trials have studied the efficacy and safety of oral UFT/LV in the treatment of 1196 patients with metastatic CRC who had received no previous chemotherapy.

One study *(19,20)* involved 816 patients with metastatic CRC treated in 85 centers in North America, Europe, and Israel. One group of patients was randomized to receive oral UFT (300 mg/m^2 d) plus oral LV (75 or 90 mg/d). Both agents were given in three separate

Table 2
Phase III Study Results

	Study	
	CA 146–011	*CA 146–012*
Number of patients treated		
UFT/LV	406/409 (99.3%)	188/190 (98.9%)
5-FU/LV	396/407 (97.3%)	185/190 (97.5%)
Treatment duration (weeks)		
UFT/LV	16.6	17.2
5-FU/LV	16.7	15.1
Median dose intensity of 5-FU (mg/m^{2}week)	452	418
Median (range) number of courses		
UFT/LV	3.5 (1–24)	3.0 (1–10)
5-FU/LV	4.0 (1–16)	3.0 (1–13)
Total number of courses		
UFT/LV	1648	728
5-FU/LV	1971	706
Anti-tumour response		
Objective clinical response[a]		
UFT/LV	12%	11%
5-FU/LV	15%	9%
Hazard ratio (survival); 5-FU/LV:UFT/LV	0.964 (95.6% CI 0.83–1.13)	1.144 (95% CI 0.92–1.42)

[a] Objective clinical response = complete and partial

doses every 8 h for 28 consecutive days, with cycles repeated every 35 d. The comparator group received 425 mg/m^2/d of 5-FU plus 20 mg/m^2/d of LV by rapid iv injection for five consecutive days, repeated every 28 d (the "Mayo regimen").

The other study *(21)* involved 380 patients with metastatic CRC treated in 47 centers in Europe, Canada, Israel, Australia, and New Zealand. Those randomized to receive UFT/LV received the same regimen as in the previous study, except that all patients were given 90 mg/d LV. The control group received repeat cycles every 35 d.

The efficacy of treatment was similar with both regimens (Table 2). In the first study, the UFT group had a response rate of 12% compared with 15% in the control group. The median time to progression was 3.5 mo in the UFT/LV group compared with 3.8 mo in the 5-FU group. Median survival of UFT-treated patients was 12.4 mo, compared with 13.4 mo in the 5-FU group.

In the latter study, the UFT group had a response rate of 11% compared with 9% in the control group. The median time to progression was 3.4 mo in the UFT/LV group compared with 3.3 mo in the 5-FU/LV group. Median survival of UFT-treated patients was 12.2 mo, compared with 10.3 mo in the 5-FU group.

It was concluded that these results showed equivalent survival in the two treatment groups. However, the safety profile was significantly better with UFT than with 5-FU. For instance, in the first and largest trial, 19% of the patients given 5-FU developed severe leukopenia and 13% had febrile neutropenia, compared with <1% and none, respectively, of patients receiving UFT. Similarly, stomatitis or mucositis occurred in 75% of 5-FU treated patients, and 19% suffered grade III–IV events, compared with 25% and 1% in the UFT group.

Oral treatment with UFT/LV had the additional advantage of greater patient preference. In a randomized, open-lable crossover trial, 37 patients with metastatic colorectal cancer received oral UFT (300 mg/m^2 tid) plus LV (90 mg/d) for 28 d followed by 7 d of rest, then IV 5-FU (425 mg/m^2) plus LV (20 mg/m^2 IV bolus), for 5 d followed by 3 wk rest. Overall, 84% patients who completed a therapy preference questionnaire indicated a preference for oral formulations of UFT therapy. The main reasons cited by patients included that the oral UFT was a pill (73%) and that it could be taken at home (69%) *(22)*.

7. FUTURE DEVELOPMENT OF UFT PLUS LV THERAPY

Anticancer drugs are often used in combination not only to improve therapeutic efficacy, but also to slow the development of resistance to the agents. UFT is being studied in combination with other new cytotoxic drugs and/or radiotherapy in order to improve the effectiveness of the treatment of metastatic CRC.

7.1. UFT Plus Irinotecan

Irinotecan (CPT-11, Campto, Camptosar) has been used in the treatment of metastatic CRC *(19)* with response rates of 14–31% *(23)*. Irinotecan exerts its anticancer action by inhibiting topoisomerase I, an effect that differs from that of 5-FU.

Several Phase I/II studies of the combination of UFT and irinotecan in metastatic CRC are in progress. A study in the UK has combined oral UFT/LV for 14 d with IV irinotecan on d 1 in 3 wk cycles *(24)*. The maximal tolerated dose was achieved with 250 mg/m^{2}d UFT plus 250 mg/m^{2}d irinotecan, together with 90 mg/d LV. Treatment at this dose level was well tolerated. One of 16 patients had a complete response, 3/16 had a partial response and 7/16 achieved stable disease.

In a different study using this combination treatment *(25)*, 4/13 patients had a partial response, 3/13 had a minor response, and 3/13 had stable disease (77% disease control).

In another study of advanced CRC *(26)*, UFT (250 mg/m^2/d for 3 wk) was combined with infusion of increasing doses of irinotecan on d 1, 8, and 15. Twelve of 18 patients achieved stable disease. The maximal tolerated dose of irinotecan was 110 mg/m^2. Adverse reactions were generally mild.

7.2. UFT plus Oxaliplatin

Oxaliplatin *(27)* is a platinum-containing compound with anticancer action attributable to DNA adduct formation not recognized by DNA mismatch-repair proteins. In nonrandomized phase II trials, response rates of about 10% have been observed *(28)*.

Douillard et al. *(19)* reported no dose-limiting toxicity with a UFT dose of 250 mg/m^{2}d plus LV (15 mg/d) for 14 d, together with 130 mg/m^2 oxaliplatin on d 1 of a 21-d cycle. Seven of nine patients achieved stable disease with this combination treatment.

In another study of patients with advanced CRC, a combination of UFT (300 mg/m^2/d) plus LV (15 mg/d) for 14 d was given together with oxaliplatin (85 mg/m^2) on d 1 and 14, in 28-d cycles *(29)*. Eighteen percent of the patients developed diarrhea and 9% had nausea/vomiting. There was no severe hematological toxicity.

7.3. UFT plus Radiotherapy

The combination of UFT/LV plus radiotherapy has been used in patients with operable rectal cancer. Oral UFT/LV was given three times daily for 5 d each week for 5 wk. During this time, the patients received full dose radiotherapy, followed by a rest period of 4–6 wk before surgery. Postoperatively, the patients received UFT/LV for 28 d every 35 d for four courses.

In one study, 18 patients with advanced rectal cancer received the combination treatment of UFT/LV plus radiotherapy *(30)*. Eleven patients had an operation after a median of 40 d. Two patients had a complete pathological response and 16 patients were alive after a median of 45 wk (range 17–84 wk). After a median follow up of 12 mo, 9/11 patients are still alive. The toxicity of the treatment was low, with no hematological adverse reactions and mainly grade I or II nonhematological toxicity. Only one patient had grade III diarrhea. It seems that high dose radiotherapy combined with UFT/LV downstages more than 50% of patients with inoperable rectal cancer and can produce pathologically complete responses with low toxicity.

In another study *(31)*, preoperative radiation therapy was given together with UFT/LV to 15 patients with rectal cancer and lymph node metastases (grade II/III). Oral UFT/LV (up to 350 mg/m^2/d) and radiotherapy were given for 5 d each week for 5 wk, followed by sphincter-preserving surgery 4–6 wk after the treatment course and, subsequently, by four 35-d cycles of UFT/LV. Pathological evaluation of the 14 resected specimens showed complete response in three patients and 10 achieved a partial response. These results are comparable with those of studies in which patients received preoperative radiotherapy with infusions of 5-FU *(32)*. The postoperative UFT/LV regimen was well tolerated, as in previous studies *(21,33)*.

8. CONCLUSIONS

Since its development over 40 yr ago, iv 5-FU treatment has remained a fundamental approach for the medical treatment of colorectal cancer. Now, the use of UFT and LV combination therapy represents an important step forwards in the treatment of colorectal cancer. Orally administered UFT/LV demonstrates a significant improvement in safety and patient tolerability, compared with standard iv 5-FU/LV treatment. Moreover, the reduced need for supportive care and less-frequent hospital-based treatment further support the improved profile of UFT/LV therapy.

UFT/LV is well suited for combination treatment regimens, such as with radiation therapy, and due to its low toxicity, for use in the adjuvant setting. Given the ongoing developments in the treatment of colorectal cancer, UFT/LV therapy is a future candidate for combination regimens with newer, nonfluoropyrimidine agents.

REFERENCES

1. Bjerkeset T, Fjosne HE. Comparison of oral ftorafur and intravenous 5-fluorouracil in patients with advanced cancer of the stomach, colon or rectum. *Oncology* 1986;43:212–215.
2. Palmeri S, et al. Oral tegafur in the treatment of gastrointestinal tract cancers: a phase II study. *Br J Cancer* 1990;61:475–478.
3. Ron IG, Lotan A, Inbar MJ, Chaitchik S. Advanced colorectal carcinoma: redefining the role of oral ftorafur. *Anticancer Drugs* 1996;7:649–654.
4. Fujii S, Ikenaka K, Fukushima M, Shirasaka T. Effect of uracil and its derivatives on antitumor activity of 5-fluorouracil and 1-(2-tetrahydrofuryl)-5-fluorouracil. *Gann* 1978;69:763–772.
5. Rustum YM. Mechanism-based improvement in the therapeutic selectivity of 5-FU prodrug alone and under conditions of metabolic modulation. *Oncology* 1997;54 Suppl 1:7–11.
6. Taguchi T. Experience with UFT in Japan. *Oncology (Huntingt)* 1997;11:30–34.
7. Ota K, Taguchi T, Kimura K. Report on nationwide pooled data and cohort investigation in UFT phase II study. *Cancer Chemother Pharmacol* 1988;22:333–338.
8. Malik ST, et al. Phase II trial of UFT in advanced colorectal and gastric cancer. *Br J Cancer* 1990;62:1023–1025.
9. Sanchiz F, Millia A. Tegafur (UFT) in advanced colorectal cancer, a phase II study. *Anticancer Res* 1988;8:1122.

10. Nogue Aliguer M, & Saigi Grau E. Tratamiento prologado con UFT y bajas dosis de leucovorin oral: estudio fase I. *Oncologia* 1992;15:114–116.
11. Camps C, Berrocal A, Vicent JM, et al. Phase I–II trial of Tegafur-Uracil and low dose leucovorin in advanced colorectal carcinoma. *Ann Oncol* 1994;5:56.
12. Gonzalez-Baron M, et al. Efficacy of oral tegafur modulation by uracil and leucovorin in advanced colorectal cancer. A phase II study. *Eur J Cancer* 1995;31A:2215–2219.
13. Feliu J, Gonzalez-Baron M, Ordonez A, & et al. Treatment of advanced colorectal cancer in the elderly with UFT-leucovorin: an active and few toxic scheme. *Ann Oncol* 1996;(Suppl 5):44.
14. Abad A, et al. A preliminary report of a phase II trial. UFT plus oral folinic acid as therapy for metastatic colorectal cancer in older patients. Spanish Group for the Treatment of Gastrointestinal Tumors (TTd Group). *Oncology (Huntingt)* 1997;11:53–57.
15. Pazdur R, et al. Phase II trial of uracil and tegafur plus oral leucovorin: an effective oral regimen in the treatment of metastatic colorectal carcinoma. *J Clin Oncol* 1994;12:2296–2300
16. Sanchiz F, Milla A. Tegafur-uracil (UFT) plus folinic acid in advanced rectal cancer. *Jpn J Clin Oncol* 1994;24:322–326.
17. Pazdur R. Phase I and pharmacokinetic evaluations of UFT plus oral leucovorin. *Oncology (Huntingt)* 1997;11:35–39.
18. Straw JA, Stapary D, Wynn WT. Pharmacokinetics of the diasteroisomers of leucovoriin after intraavenous an doral administration to normal subjects. *Cancer Res* 1994;44:3114–3119.
19. Douillard JY. A phase I study of oral uracil/tegafur (UFT) plus leukovorin (LV) combined with oxaliplatin in patients with metastatic colorectal cancer. 1999.
20. Douillard JY, Cunningham D, Roth AD, et al. A randomized phase III trial comparing irinotecan (IRI) + 5FU/folinic acid (FA) to the same schedule of 5FU/FA in patients (pts) with metastatic colorectal cancer (MCRC) as front line chemotherapy (CT). *Proc Am Soc Clin Oncol* 1999;18:233a.
21. Carmichael J, Popiela T, Radstone D, et al. Randomised comparative study of ORZEL ((oral uracil/tegafur UFT plus leucovorin (LV)) versus parenteral 5-fluorouracil (5-FU) plus LV in patients with metastatic colorectal cancer. *Proc Am Soc Clin Oncol* 1999;18:264a.
22. Borner M, Schoeffski P, de Wit R, et al. A randomised crossover trial comparing UFT + leucovorin (LV) and fluorouracil (FU) + LV for patient preference and pharmacokinetics in patients with advanced colorectal cancer. *Proc Am Soc Clin Oncol* 2000;19:191a.
23. Meropol NJ, Creaven PJ, Petrelli NJ. Metastatic colorectal cancer: advances in biochemical modulation and new drug development. *Semin Oncol* 1995;22:509–524.
24. Hill M, Twelves C, Cunningham D. A phase I/II study of oral uracil/tegafur (UFT) plus … or metastatic colorectal cancer (CRC). 2000.
25. Gravalos C, Garcia-Alfonso P, Castellanos D. Phase I trial of escalating doses of irinotecan (CPT-11) in combination with UFT/folinic acid (FA) in patients with advanced colorectal cancer (CRC). *Ann Oncol* 2000;11(Suppl 4):46.
26. Escudero P, Vicente A, Herrero et al. Phase 1–11 trial of irinotecan (CPT-11) over a short IV weekly infusion combined with a fixed does of UFT in second line advanced colorectal carcinoma (ACRC). ASCO. 2000.
27. Giacchetti S, Zidani R, Perpoint B, et al. Phase III trial of 5-fluorouracil (5-FU), folinic acid (FA), with or without oxaliplatin (OXA) in previously untreated patients (pts) with metastatic colorectal cancer (MCC). *Proc Am Soc Clin Oncol* 1997;16:229a.
28. Bleiberg H. Oxaliplatin (L-OHP): a new reality in colorectal cancer. *Br J Cancer* 1998;77 Suppl 4:1–3.
29. Garcia-Giron C, Feliu J, Vicent JM. Phase II trial of oxaliplatin-UFT-leucovorin (OXA-UFT-LV) combination in first line treatment of advanced colorectal cancer (ACC). n/a. 2000.
30. Pfeiffer P, Jakobsen A. Concurrent UFT/L-leukovorin and high-dose radiotherapy (60 Gy) in patients with locally advanced rectal cancer (LARC): a phase I/II trial. 2000.
31. Hoff PM, et al. Phase I study of preoperative oral uracil and tegafur plus leucovorin and radiation therapy in rectal cancer [In Process Citation]. *J Clin Oncol* 2000;18:3529–3534.
32. Janjan NA, et al. Tumor downstaging and sphincter preservation with preoperative chemoradiation in locally advanced rectal cancer: the MD Anderson Cancer Center experience. *Int J Radiat Oncol Biol Phys.* 1999;44:1027–1038.
33. Pazdur R, Doulliard J-Y, Skillings J, et al. Multicenter phase III study of 5-fluorouracil (5-FU) or UFT in combination with leucovorin (LV) in patients with metastatic colorectal cancer. *Proc Am Soc Clin Oncol* 1999;18:263a.

18 UFT in Elderly Patients with Colorectal Cancer

Albert Abad, MD, PhD, *and José Luis Manzano,* MD

CONTENTS

1. INTRODUCTION

Cancer is a disease of aging; at present 70% of cases occur in patients aged over 65 *(1)*. In general, however, there are few studies of elderly patients, and in most clinical trials, age over 72 has been exclusion criteria. Thus, elderly patients have not been analyzed in research, and patients between 65 and 72 have never been analyzed separately. There are data regarding the treatment for leukemia and lymphoma in the National Cancer Data Base *(2)* showing that survival by stage is worse in elderly patients and suggesting age-dependent biological differences in the cancer itself. Studies of the elderly are necessary so we can analyze these possibilities. Among the reasons for low or nonexistent participation by the elderly in clinical trials is the belief that older patients do not tolerate chemotherapy and the existence of concomitant medical conditions that may preclude certain treatments. Co-morbidities need to be considered as an objective reason for avoiding aggressive treatments. In the elderly population, 55% have three additional pathologies and 37% have one or two, while only 8% have cancer alone *(3)*. The pharmacokinetic changes associated with aging are also important. Volume of distribution is altered by increasing lipid-soluble drugs and decreasing water-soluble drugs; anemia and hypoalbuminemia increase the toxicity of the agents related to albumine or eritrocites; renal excretion can also decrease, thus increasing toxicity *(4)*. For these reasons, patients over 70 are often insufficiently staged and treated *(5)*. Survival decreases with age among patients with colorectal cancer (CRC); 5-yr overall survival is 47% in patients under 60 and 30% in patients over 60 *(6)*. Furthermore, in women older than 75, CRC is the second cause of cancer deaths *(2)*. It is clear that the cost of cancer care will have a major impact on our aging society. All of these factors prompted us to search for an alternative treatment that could be suitable for elderly patients with advanced CRC. The intravenous modulated bolus fluorouracil-based (5-FU) regimen has been the standard treatment for advanced CRC in the last 10 yr. The Meta-Analysis Group in Cancer showed

From: *Fluoropyrimidines in Cancer Therapy*
Edited by: Y. M. Rustum © Humana Press Inc., Totowa, NJ

an overall response rate of 19–23% and median survival of 10.7–11.5 mo *(7,8)* with this regimen, and we have obtained 19–26% and 10.6–14.3 mo *(9,10)*. An alternative to this regimen is the administration of 5-FU by continuous infusion (CI). Several studies have reported increased response rates with 5-FU CI; this could be related to higher dose intensity and to the short serum half-life of 5-FU, which does not exceed 11 min, a short period of time for cell exposure. Two comparative trials *(11,12)* have demonstrated the superiority of 5-FU CI in terms of response rate, toxicity, and time to progression compared to 5-FU bolus. Moreover, a meta-analysis of randomized trials comparing 5-FU CI with 5-FU bolus has shown that there is a small but significant improvement in survival *(13)*. Using a 48-h high-dose 5-FU CI (2–3.5 g/m2 48 h/wk) the TTD Spanish Group (Spanish Group for Treatment of Gastrointestinal Tumors) has obtained interesting results, with a response rate of 29–38% and 12–14 mo of median survival in patients with advanced CRC *(14–16)*. Nevertheless, 5-FU CI needs a subcutaneous port, a portable infusional pump, frequent hospital visits, and frequent complete blood counts, all of which make the treatment difficult in older patients. Several studies in Japan have demonstrated the activity of oral fluoropyrimidine UFT (tegafur plus uracil) in advanced CRC *(17–19)*. In Europe, Malik et al. obtained a response rate of 16.6% using UFT alone *(20)*. Recently in the United States and Europe, folinic acid modulation of UFT has shown good results with response rates of 42% and 39% *(21–22)*. The continuous oral administration of UFT simulates protracted 5-FU CI, making this oral therapy a possible substitute for intravenous chemotherapy.

2. CLINICAL EXPERIENCE

There have been only three published studies dealing specifically with patients treated with fluoropirimidine. The first study, by Feliu et al. *(23)*, included 38 patients older than 70 (median age, 74). All patients had measurable disease, and 65% had liver metastases. Treatment was intravenous folinic acid 500 mg/m^2 on d 1, oral folinic acid 15 mg every 12 h on d 2–14, and oral UFT 390 mg/m^2 on d 1–14. The treatment was repeated every 28 d for a minimum of four courses per patient. The median dose of UFT administered was 330 mg/m^2/cycle, 85% of the planned dose. The overall response rate was 29% (95% CI, 15–46%). Two patients achieved complete response (5%), 9 partial response (24%) and 17 stable disease (45%); more than 74% of patients had clinical benefit. No differences related to the metastasis location was shown. The median overall survival was 12.5 mo. Toxicity was acceptable. Grade 3–4 toxicity was only 3% nausea/vomiting, 10% diarrhea and 4% stomatitis.

The other two studies were carried out by the TTD Spanish Group, and their purpose was to examine whether continuous oral administration of UFT would provide an easy, nontoxic, and active treatment for elderly CRC patients. A total of 214 patients were included in two trials. The first TTD study included 106 patients older than 72 (median age, 74). All patients had measurable disease, and 56% had liver metastases. Treatment was as follows: UFT 400 mg/24 h in a fixed dose administered in two daily doses every 12 h continuously plus oral folinic acid 45 mg/24 h in three separate doses every 8 h continuously. If grade 3 or 4 toxicity appeared, treatment was withheld until recovery and patients resumed treatment at the same doses. The median time of treatment was 4 mo (range 1–23) and the median follow-up for the 106 patients was 16 mo (range 5–24). Responses included five complete responses (5%) and 12 partial responses (13%). Overall response rate was 18% (95% CI, 10%–27%). Disease was stable in 24 (25%) patients. In all, 41 (43%) patients had nonprogressive disease and 55 (57%) had progressive disease. Median time to disease progression was 5.6 mo, and overall survival was 13.7 mo. No differences in survival were observed between respon-

Table 1
Toxicity to Treatment in Elderly Patients

	Grade 1–2 (%)			*Grade 3–4 (%)*		
	Feliu et al.	*TTD 1*	*TTD 2*	*Feliu et al.*	*TTD 1*	*TTD 2*
Leukopenia	5	1	3	0	0	0
Thrombopenia	0	1	3	0	1	0
Nausea/V	8	23	39	3	6	6
Diarrhea	29	30	28	10	11	9
Mucositis	9	12	9	4	1	0
Alopecia	–	5	2	–	1	1

ders and stable patients (*p*=0.1). Toxicity calculated based on the maximum grade per patient was mild. Only one patient (1%) had grade 3 thrombocytopenia; 6 patients (6%) experienced grade 3 nausea/vomiting; 11 (11%) had grade 3–4 diarrhea; and 1 (1%) had grade 3 mucositis. Toxicity needed chemotherapy adjournment in 20 (20%) patients for a median 10-d delay per patient over the treatment period (range 1–48). The median UFT dose intensity was 400 mg/d as planned.

The second TTD study included 108 patients also older than 72 (median age, 76). All patients had measurable disease, and 65% had liver metastases. Treatment consisted of UFT 400 mg/m^2/24 h administered in two daily doses every 12 h continuously without folinic acid (nonmodulated UFT) until toxicity as in the first study. The median time of treatment was 4 mo (range 1–14) with a median follow-up of 14 mo (range 2–24.6). Five patients showed complete response (5%) and seven had partial response (8%). The overall response rate was 13% (95%CI, 6–20%). Forty-one patients had SD (45%) and 39 patients progressed (42%). The total number of patients with nonprogressive disease was 53 (58%). Median time to disease progression was 5 mo. Overall median survival was 11.8 mo. As in the first TTD study, no differences in survival were observed between responders and stable patients (*p*=0.09). Toxicity was also mild. No patients showed grade 3–4 hematological toxicity. Ten patients (9%) had grade 3–4 diarrhea and seven patients (6%) had grade 3–4 nausea/vomiting. Chemotherapy delay due to toxicity occurred in 32 (30%) patients for a median 10-d delay per patient (range 1–42). The median UFT dose intensity was 400 mg/m^2 *(24–26)* (Table 1 and 2).

3. DISCUSSION

The main purpose for using UFT in these studies was to evaluate the tolerance and benefits of an oral treatment in elderly CRC patients. In all patients, toxicity was mild and caused only a maximum of 11% grade 4 diarrhea. In the TTD studies, toxicity did not increase with modulated UFT compared with UFT alone, but it is important to emphasize that the dose intensity was originally higher in the UFT alone study. In the TTD experience with 5-FU CI, the maximum tolerable dose of 5-FU was 3.5 g/m^2/48 h/wk when used alone *(27)* and only 2.5g/m^2/48 h/wk when modulated with folinic acid *(14–16)*. Overall response rates in elderly UFT studies range from 13% to 29%. This is within the range found in the meta-analysis of randomized trials using either 5-FU modulated by folinic acid or 5-FU modu-

Table 2
Activity of UFT in Elderly Patients

	Feliu et al.	*TTD 1*	*TTD2*
No. patients	38	96	92
RR[a]	29%	17.7%	13%
No progresion	74%	43%	58%
S (m)[a]	12,5	13,7	12
Liver metastasis	65%	55%	68%

[a] RR: response rate; S: survival; m: months.

lated by methotrexate and 5-FU CI. If we compare these results with other phase II trials in the general population *(21,22),* the TTD studies have worse response rates but similar clinical benefit and overall survival. However, it should be pointed out that dose intensities in these general population studies are different. The dose intensity ranged from 8400 $mg/m^2/mo$ (300 $mg/m^2/d \times 28$ d) to 5460 $mg/m^2/mo$ (390 $mg/m^2/d \times 14d$). The dose intensity in the TTD fixed dose study ranged between 7500 $mg/m^2/mo$ over a body surface area of 1.6 m^2 to 6,650 $mg/m^2/mo$ over a body surface area of 1.8 m^2. Dose intensity in the TTD UFT alone study was 11,760 $mg/m^2/mo$. Dose intensity is therefore probably not the reason for the differences in response rate. Thus, while all regimens showed low toxicity, the low dose of UFT was shown to be as effective as more aggressive schemes, which is an important consideration when dealing with weak elderly patients with severe concomitant pathologies. A response rate of 12% has recently been reported in a phase III trial using oral modulated UFT at a dose intensity of 8400 $mg/m^2/d$ *(28).* In addition, Carmichael et al. *(29)* obtained a response rate of only 11% in a phase III trial comparing oral modulated UFT with modulated 5-FU/LV. However, UFT treatment achieved 43–74% SD. Patients with SD represent a sizable number of cases in CRC, and their prognosis for time to progression and survival is similar to that of patients with objective response. Overall survival in UFT studies was very good; median survival ranged from 11.8 to 13.7 mo, similar to that obtained using intravenous 5-FU.

The question remains as to the place of fluoropirimidines in the treatment of the elderly. In fact, there is no evidence that oral treatment is better tolerated by the elderly, nor is there a comparative study about the acceptance and toxicity of oral fluoropirimidines vs an intravenous regimen in the elderly population. Moreover, it is difficult to check the level of compliance with this treatment. On the other hand, it is not true that there has been no progress made in the treatment of CRC. The introduction of new drugs with new mechanisms of action, such as oxaliplatin and CPT-11, have allowed us to extend the possibilities of treatment in these patients. At the same time, the association of these drugs with 5-FU has notably increased the response rate, which reaches 50%, and survival *(30,31).* The increase in the response rate has also allowed us to increase the percentage of patients that can undergo a resection of liver metastases *(32).* Therefore, it seems that treatment with oral fluoropirimidines is recommendable in elderly patients, though age should not be a barrier to a more aggressive treatment when the goal is to obtain maximum remission, for example before liver metastasis resection.

REFERENCES

1. Monfardini S, Chabner B. Joint NCI-EORTC Consensus meeting on neoplasia in the elderly. *Eur J Cancer* 1991; 27:653–654.

2. Kennedy BJ. Cancer research and the aging population. *Oncol Issues* 2000; 15(1):20–28.
3. Yancik R and Ries LG. Cancer in the aged: an epidemiologic perspective on treatment issues. *Cancer* 1991; 68:2502.
4. Balducci L and Extermann M. Dificulties in treating older patients with cancer. *Oncol in Practice* 1998; 2:15–18.
5. Fentiman Ian S. Are the elderly receiving appropiate treatment for cancer? *Ann Oncol* 1996; 7:657–658.
6. Chapius PH, Dent OF, Fisher R, et al. A multivariate analysis of clinical and pathological variables in prognosis after resection of large bowel cancer. *Br J Surg* 1985; 72:698–702.
7. The Advanced Colorectal Cancer Meta-Analysis Project. Modulation of Fluorouracil by Leucovorin in Patients With Advanced Colorectal Cancer: Evidence in Terms of Response Rate. *J Clin Oncol* 1992; 10:896–903.
8. The Advanced Colorectal Meta-Analisis Project. Meta-analysis of randomized trials testing the biochemical modulation of fluorouracil by methotrexate in metastatic colorectal cancer. *J Clin Oncol* 1994; 12:960–969.
9. Abad A, Rosell R, Pastor MC, Barnadas A, Carles J, Ribelles N, et al. Sequential combination of methotrexate (MTX), 5-fluorouracil (FU), and high-dose folinic acid (FA) in advanced colorectal cancer: Double biochemical modulation. *Am J Clin Oncol* 1991; 14:393–396.
10. Abad A, Garcia P, Gravalos C, et al. Sequential methotrexate, 5-fluorouracil (5-FU), and high dose leucovorin versus 5-FU and high dose leucovorin versus 5-FU alone for advanced colorectal cancer. *Cancer* 1995; 5:1238–1244.
11. Aranda E, Diaz-Rubio E, Cervantes A, et al. Randomized trial comparing monthly low-dose leucovorin and fluorouracil bolus with high-dose 48-hour continuous infusion fluorouracil for advanced colorectal cancer: A Spanish Cooperative Group for Gastrointestinal Tumor Therapy (TTD) study. *Ann Oncol* 1998; 9:727–731.
12. de Gramont A, Bosset JF, Milan C, et al. Randomized trial comparing monthly low-dose leucovorin and fluorouracil bolus with bimonthly high-dose leucovorin and fluorouracil bolus plus continuous infusion for advanced colorectal cancer. *J Clin Oncol* 1997; 15:808–815.
13. The Meta-analisis Group in Cancer. Efficacy of intravenous infusion of fluorouracil compared with bolus administration in advanced colorectal cancer. *J Clin Oncol* 1998; 16:301–308.
14. Diaz-Rubio E, Aranda E, Camps C. A phase II study of weekly 48 hours infusion with high-dose fluorouracil in advanced colorectal cancer: an alternative to biochemical modulation. *J Infus Chemother* 1994; 4,1:58–61.
15. Aranda E, Cervantes A, Dorta J, et al. A phase II trial of weekly high dose continuous infusion 5-fluorouracil plus oral leucovorin in patients with advanced colorectal cancer. *Cancer* 1995; 76:559–563.
16. Aranda E, Cervantes A, Carrato A, et al. Outpatient weekly high-dose continuous infusion 5-fluorouracil plus oral leucovorin in advanced colorectal cancer. A phase II trial. *Ann of Oncol* 1996; 7:581–585.
17. Watanabe H, Yamamoto S, NaitoT. Clinical results of oral UFT therapy under cooperative study. *Jpn J Cancer Chemother* 1980; 7:1588–1596.
18. Murakami M, Ota K. Clinical results of UFT therapy for malignant tumors under cooperative study. *Jpn J Cancer Chemother* 1980; 7:1579–1586.
19. Ota K, Taguchi T, Kimura K. Report on nationwide pooled data and cohort investigation in UFT phase II study. *Cancer Chemother Pharmacol* 1988; 22:333–338.
20. Malik STA, Talbot D, Clarke PI, et al. Phase II trial of UFT in advanced colorectal and gastric cancer. *Br J Cancer* 1990; 62:1023–1025.
21. Pazdur R, Lassere Y, Rhodes V, et al. Phase II trial of uracil and tegafur plus oral leucovorin: an effective oral regimen in the treatment of metastatic colorectal carcinoma. *J Clin Oncol* 1994; 12:2296–2300.
22. Gonzalez-Barón M, Feliu J, de la Gándara I, et al. Efficacy of oral tegafur modulation by uracil and leucovorin in advanced colorectal cancer. A phase II study. *Eur J Cancer* 1995; 31A:2215–2219.
23. Feliu J, Gonzalez Baron M, Espinosa E, et al. Uracil and tegafur modulated with leucovorin: An effective regimen with low toxicity for treatment of colorectal carcinoma in the elderly. *Cancer* 1997; 10:1884–1889.
24. Abad A, Navarro M, Sastre J, et al. UFT plus oral folinic acid as therapy for metastatic colorectal cancer in older patients. *Oncology* 1997; supp 10:53–57.
25. Diaz-Rubio E, Sastre J, Abad A, et al. UFT plus or minus calcium folinate for metastatic colorectal cancer in older patients: Preliminary results. *Oncology* 1999; supp 3:35–40.
26. Abad A, Aranda E, Navarro M, et al. Two consecutive studies using oral UFT-based chemotherapy regimens in elderly patients with advanced colorectal cancer. *Rev Oncologia* 2000;2:154–158.
27. Diaz-Rubio E, Aranda E, Martin M, et al. Weekly high-dose infusion of 5-fluorouracil in advanced colorectal cancer. *Eur J Cancer* 1990; 26:727–729.
28. Pazdur R, Douillard JY, Skillings JR, et al. Multicenter phase III study of 5-fluorouracil (5-FU) or UFT in combination with leucovorin (LV) in patients with metastatic colorectal cancer. *Proc Am Soc Clin Oncol* 1999; 263 (abs 1009).

29. Carmichael J, Popiela T, Radstone D, et al. Randomized comparative study of Orzel (oral uracil/tegafur (UFT) plus leucovorin (LV)) versus parenteral 5-fluorouracil (5-FU) plus LV in patients with metastatic colorectal cancer. *Proc Am Soc Clin Oncol* 1999; 264 (1015).
30. Abad A, Navarro M, Sastre J, et al. Biweekly oxaliplatin (OXA) plus weekly 48 h continuous infusion (CI) 5 FU (TTD regimen) in first line treatment of advanced colorectal cancer (ACC). *Proc Am Soc Clin Oncol* 2000, 300.
31. Douillard JY, Cunningham D, Roth AD, et al. Irinotecan combined with fluorouracil compared with fluorouracil alone as first-line treatment for metastatic colorectal cancer: a multicentre randomized trial. *Lancet* 2000; 355:1041–1047.
32. Giacchetti S, Itzhaki, Gruia G, et al. Long-term survival of patients with unresectable colorectal cancer liver metastases following infusional chemotherapy with 5-fluorouracil, leucovorin, oxaloiplatin and surgery. *Ann Oncol* 1999; 10:663–669.

19 Clinical Trials of the Eniluracil/ 5-Fluorouracil Combination

Hedy L. Kindler, MD, and Richard L. Schilsky, MD

CONTENTS

1. INTRODUCTION

5-Fluorouracil (5-FU) is one of the most widely used drugs in cancer chemotherapy *(1)*. It is optimally delivered via continuous intravenous infusion *(2),* which is cumbersome, expensive, and prone to complications such as infection and thrombosis. When patients are offered a choice between agents that have equal efficacy and side effects, they overwhelmingly prefer oral chemotherapy *(3,4)*. Oral dosing of 5-FU over a prolonged period has the potential to mimic continuous infusion with less inconvenience and cost.

Unfortunately, oral administration of 5-FU has been hampered by its erratic and incomplete bioavailability, and by significant variability in its clearance, that can result in unpredictable toxicity and therapeutic failures *(1,5)*. The marked inter- and intrapatient variation in absorption of oral 5-FU is attributable to substantial variability in the activity of dihydropyrimidine dehydrogenase (DPD), the initial enzyme and the rate-limiting step in 5-FU catabolism *(6,7)*. Eniluracil (Ethynyluracil, 776C85, BW776, GW776, Glaxo-Wellcome, Research Triangle Park, North Carolina) is a mechanism-based, irreversible inhibitor of the enzyme DPD that was developed to facilitate predictable oral absorption of 5-FU by circumventing DPD catabolism in the intestinal mucosa and liver *(8)*.

From: *Fluoropyrimidines in Cancer Therapy*
Edited by: Y. M. Rustum © Humana Press Inc., Totowa, NJ

2. CLINICAL PHARMACOLOGY OF 5-FU AND THE ROLE OF DPD

5-FU is rapidly metabolized, with a plasma half-life of 5 to 20 min *(1)*. Sixty to 90% of an administered dose of 5-FU is catabolized in the liver and extrahepatic tissues, while only 10–20% is excreted unchanged in the urine *(9)*. The rate-limiting step in 5-FU catabolism is the reduction of 5-FU by the enzyme DPD to 5′,6′-dihydrofluorouracil. The subsequent metabolites formed are α-fluoroureidopropionic acid and-α-fluoro-β-alanine (FBAL) *(1)*.

DPD activity fluctuates in a circadian rhythm within individual patients *(10)*. Interpatient variability relates in part to genetic polymorphism, as an estimated 2–4% of the population is completely DPD deficient *(11)*. DPD is found principally in the liver, as well as in the intestinal mucosa, peripheral blood mononuclear cells, lung, kidney, and pancreas *(12)*. Hepatic metabolism of 5-FU by DPD accounts for most of its clearance *(13)*. DPD activity is elevated in solid tumors, which may contribute to drug resistance *(14,15)*.

3. PRECLINICAL PHARMACOLOGY OF THE ENILURACIL/FLUOROURACIL COMBINATION

Eniluracil is a uracil analog with an ethynyl substituent in the 5′ position. Porter and colleagues first described this mechanism-based, irreversible inhibitor of DPD when screening uracil analogs for DPD inhibitory activity *(8)*. Eniluracil inactivates DPD through covalent modification of an amino acid residue *(8)*. It is a potent inhibitor of DPD that binds to the enzyme with a K_m of 1.6 μM and inactivates it with a first-order rate constant of 20 min^{-1} *(14)*. The inactivation of DPD by eniluracil proceeds in two steps: eniluracil initially binds reversibly to the enzyme, then irreversibly inactivates it *(16)*.

The half-life of eniluracil in plasma is 4 h *(17)*. In rat liver extracts, eniluracil inhibits more than 99% of DPD activity within minutes of dosing. New DPD is resynthesized with a half-life of 63 h *(18)*. After a single dose of eniluracil, rat liver extracts are inhibited more than 96% in their ability to catalyze 5-FU degradation for up to 6 h *(19)*.

Although eniluracil is not cytotoxic by itself, it enhances the cytotoxicity of 5-FU when administered to cell lines expressing high levels of DPD *(20)*. Fischel treated a panel of human tumor cell lines with eniluracil and 5-FU. The combination produced a one- to five-fold enhancement of cytotoxicity compared with 5-FU alone; the degree of enhancement correlated with pretreatment DPD activity *(20)*.

Eniluracil is neither toxic nor active as an antitumor agent in animals, yet it potentiates the antitumor efficacy and improves the therapeutic index of 5-FU sixfold. Although single-agent 5-FU produces a response rate of 13% in animals with colorectal tumors, pretreatment with eniluracil followed by 5-FU yields a complete response rate of 100% *(21)*. Eniluracil is more effective than modulation of 5-FU with leucovorin in this tumor model *(21)*.

Eniluracil inhibits the formation of 5-FU catabolites that can potentially interfere with the antitumor activity of 5-FU or enhance its toxicity. It also decreases the formation of cardiotoxic and neurotoxic 5-FU metabolites, including 2-fluoro-3-hydroxy proprionic acid, α-fluoro-β-alanine, and fluoroacetate in rat liver *(22)*. More than 80% of a dose of 5-FU is converted into FBAL, a noncytotoxic, but neurotoxic catabolite with a prolonged half-life *(1)*. The neurotoxicity associated with high doses of 5-FU in dogs is not observed when eniluracil is coadministered *(23)*. Eniluracil may augment the antitumor activity of 5-FU in part by preventing the formation of 5-FU catabolites, such as 5-FUH_2 and FBAL, which attenuate its antitumor activity *(24,25)*. The enhanced response observed when 5-FU is given with eniluracil to rats is abrogated in the presence of 5-FUH_2 *(21,26)*. Eniluracil administration also increases the accumulation of active 5-fluorouridine mono-, di-, and triphosphates in both normal and tumor tissues *(24)*.

In animals, administration of eniluracil results in 100% bioavailability of orally administered 5-FU *(19)*. The addition of eniluracil prolongs the half-life of 5-FU from 9 to 100 min *(20)*. In mice and rats, eniluracil produces a significant increase in the elimination $t_{1/2}$ and the area under the plasma concentration time curve of 5-FU, and it significantly decreases variability in AUC values between animals. Eniluracil treatment also produces a more linear disposition of 5-FU, permitting better control of 5-FU levels in the therapeutic range *(19)*.

4. PHARMACOKINETICS AND METABOLISM

Eniluracil permits complete and rapid absorption of oral 5-FU with an approx 100% bioavailability in humans *(27)*. The bioavailability of an oral 5-FU dose of 10 mg/m^2 was 122% ± 40% (mean ± SD) in a phase I trial reported by Baker *(27)*. There was moderate interindividual variability in bioavailability (CV + 33%). While food intake delays absorption of 5-FU and significantly decreases the C_{max} values, the overall bioavailability of 5-FU is unaffected *(28)*.

Treatment with eniluracil substantially prolongs the half-life of 5-FU, and significantly reduces its clearance, but does not alter its volume of distribution *(17,27,29)*. The mean terminal half-life of 5-FU is 8–22 min. When 5-FU is combined with eniluracil, this becomes 4.4 and 4.5 h, after intravenous and oral administration, respectively *(27)*. The apparent volume of distribution (V_β) following an oral 5-FU dose of 10 mg/m^2 is 21.4 ± 5.9 L/m^2, the systemic clearance (Cl_{sys}) is 57.6 ± 16.4 mL/min/m^2 *(27)*. An intravenous bolus of 600 mg/m^2 of 5-FU produces an AUC of 5-FU which is only 15% greater than that obtained after a 20 mg/m^2 dose of oral 5-FU given with eniluracil *(29)*. Multiple daily dosing does not affect the pharmacokinetics of oral 5-FU *(27)*.

When Baker and colleagues evaluated the pharmacokinetics of a 28-d schedule of eniluracil with oral 5-FU, the mean terminal half-life of 5-FU was 4.5 h (SD 0.83 h), the apparent volume of distribution was 19 L/m^2 (SD 3 L/m^2), and the systemic clearance was 51 mL/min/m^2 (SD 13 mL/min/m^2) *(17)*. 5-FU pharmacokinetics become linear, with an almost twofold increase in C_{max} value, when the 5-FU dose increases from 1.0 to 1.8 mg/m^2. The AUC of 5-FU also increases linearly in proportion to dose. Steady-state concentrations of 5-FU are achieved within 1 wk *(17)*.

Eniluracil decreases the systemic clearance of 5-FU about 20-fold, from a range of values greater than the hepatic blood flow (1000–5000 mL/min/m^2) in the absence of eniluracil, to levels approaching the glomerular filtration rate (50–60 mL/min/m^2) *(27)*. In the presence of eniluracil, renal excretion of unchanged 5-FU becomes the primary pathway for its elimination *(27)*. About 77% of the administered 5-FU is excreted unchanged in the urine after 28 d of eniluracil treatment; <2% is excreted in the urine as FBAL *(17)*. There is a strong correlation between systemic clearance of 5-FU and the calculated creatinine clearance (r=74; p=0.009) and serum creatinine in eniluracil treated patients *(27)*.

Plasma uracil concentrations increase 24 h following eniluracil administration, and reach steady-state between three and 8 d. Steady-state concentrations of uracil average between 3000 and 4000 ng/mL after repeated eniluracil dosing, and are highest in patients who receive 10 or 20 mg of eniluracil twice daily. By contrast, in patients with normal DPD activity, plasma uracil concentrations are <100 ng/mL. Systemic clearance and the percentage recovery of unchanged 5-FU in urine are independent of eniluracil dose, once complete DPD inhibition is achieved. The greater the inactivation of DPD, the lower the urinary excretion of FBAL. Urinary excretion of FBAL is < 2% of the 5-FU dose in patients who receive 10–20 mg of eniluracil twice daily, suggesting that these doses produce maximal DPD inactivation *(17)*.

5. PHARMACODYNAMICS

Baker employed a sigmoidal E_{max} model (R^2=0.80) to describe the relationship between the AUC of 5-FU and the neutropenia observed following the administration of eniluracil and 5-FU on a 5-d schedule every 28 d *(27)*. This model was less predictive of the degree of thrombocytopenia (R^2=0.51). Interpretation of the pharmacodynamic findings is limited by the small number of patients and heterogeneity in the amount of prior myelosuppressive chemotherapy *(27)*. Similarly, Humerickhouse and colleagues observed an inverse correlation between absolute neutrophil count nadirs and average 5-FU plasma concentrations. They found no correlation with other toxicities *(30)*.

In a phase I trial of a 28-d schedule of eniluracil and 5-FU, Baker et al. observed a relationship between the worst grade of diarrhea during any course and 5-FU $C_{ss,min}$ values during the first course *(17)*. Patients who developed diarrhea ≥grade 3 had significantly higher mean $C_{ss,min}$ values (52 ng/mL) than those who did not (23 ng/mL, $p<0.0001$). Individuals who experienced grades 3 or 4 diarrhea during any course also had higher values for the AUC of 5-FU on d 2 of course 1 (702 ng/mL/h) than patients who experienced grades 0 to 2 diarrhea (413 ng/mL/h, $p<0.0001$). There was no correlation between any toxicity and 5-FU dose or C_{max} *(17)*.

There were two partial responses among the 36 patients in this phase I trial, and the relationship between 5-FU exposure and response was analyzed. The 5-FU $C_{ss,min}$ value of 69 ng/mL in one partial responder was the second highest value observed in the study. The other responder, who was in the cohort that received the lowest dose of 5-FU, 1.0 mg/m^2, had a 5-FU $C_{ss,min}$ value of 38 ng/mL, which was the highest value achieved at that dose level and the fifth highest level attained in the study *(17)*.

In a phase II trial of eniluracil, oral 5-FU, and leucovorin in patients with colorectal cancer, Meropol and colleagues determined that baseline creatinine clearance, but not serum creatinine, was inversely associated with severe toxicity (p=0.001), including neutropenia and diarrhea *(31)*. The mean baseline creatinine clearance for patients who experienced any grade 3, 4, or 5 toxicity was 88.5 mL/min, compared with 134.7 mL/min for those patients who developed toxicity less than or equal to grade 2 *(31)*.

6. PHASE I STUDIES

Three schedules of eniluracil plus 5-FU have been evaluated in phase I studies: daily for 5 d every 28 d, which mimics the Mayo Clinic bolus regimen of 5-FU; daily for 28 d every 35 d, which more closely parallels the continuous infusion schedule; and weekly for 6 wk every 8 wk, which simulates the weekly 24-h high-dose continuous infusion schedule. As expected, the maximum tolerated dose (MTD) of 5-FU administered with eniluracil is dramatically lower than the MTD of 5-FU as a single agent. The dose-limiting toxicity of the 5-d schedule is myelosuppression. Diarrhea is dose-limiting on the 28-d schedule. Both diarrhea and neutropenia are dose-limiting on the weekly schedule *(17,27,29,32)*.

6.1. Five-Day Schedule

Baker and colleagues conducted a phase I study in 12 patients with advanced solid tumors to determine the systemic disposition and absolute bioavailability of an oral 5-FU solution administered with eniluracil, and to assess the toxicity and pharmacokinetics of multiple-day dosing of this combination *(27)*. The study was divided into three periods. In periods 1 and 2, patients were randomly assigned to treatment with 5-FU 10 mg/m^2 on d 2 administered orally or intravenously with oral eniluracil, 3.7 mg/m^2, on d 1 and 2. In period 3, patients received escalating doses of 5-FU (10–25 mg/m^2/d on d 2–6), and eniluracil 3.7 mg/m^2 on d 1–7, every 28 d.

No hematologic toxicity was observed following a single intravenous or oral dose of 5-FU in combination with eniluracil in periods 1 and 2. Neutropenia was dose-limiting in period 3, precluding dose escalation of 5-FU above 25 mg/m^2/d for 5 d every 28 d with eniluracil 3.7 mg/m^2. Neutrophil nadirs occurred between d 8 and 29 (median d 20), and treatment delays were required in 8% of courses. Other toxicities included grade 1 nausea and vomiting following ingestion of oral 5-FU, and grade 1 and 2 diarrhea in 42% of patients. A possible potentiation of the effect of warfarin on the international normalized ratio (INR) was also noted. No antitumor responses were observed.

Schilsky and colleagues evaluated a 5 d schedule of eniluracil with 5-FU in a phase I trial in 65 patients with advanced solid tumors *(29)*. The study consisted of three periods. The first period determined the safety, pharmacokinetics, and pharmacodynamics of a 7-d course of eniluracil. In period 2, the effects of eniluracil on the pharmacokinetics of a single intravenous dose of 5-FU were assessed. Period 3 determined the MTD of intravenous and oral 5-FU, with or without leucovorin, which could be administered with oral eniluracil. An initial eniluracil dose of 3.7 mg/m^2 and doses fivefold above and fivefold below this were selected, based on preclinical data which suggested that 3.7 mg/m^2 was sufficient to inactivate DPD for 24 h. Thus, in period 1, cohorts of at least three patients received doses of 3.7, 18.5, or 0.74 mg/m^2 of eniluracil daily for 7 d. Once data from the first nine patients were analyzed, this was modified to a fixed daily dose of 10 mg, which provided an eniluracil dose of at least 3.7 mg/m^2 to patients with a BSA of up to 2.7 mg/m^2. After a 14-d washout period, each patient received the assigned dose of eniluracil daily for 3 d, with a single dose of bolus intravenous 5-FU, 10 mg/m^2, on d 2. After a second 14-d washout period, patients were administered the assigned dose of eniluracil daily for 7 d, with escalating doses of intravenous bolus 5-FU on d 2–6. After determination of the MTD of intravenous 5-FU plus eniluracil, oral leucovorin on d 2–6 was added at a dose of 50 mg/m^2. Finally, patient cohorts were treated with 50 mg eniluracil daily and oral 5-FU with or without leucovorin.

No toxicities were noted from eniluracil alone in period 1, or following the administration of eniluracil and a single dose of intravenous 5-FU in period 2. The principal and dose-limiting toxicity observed in period 3 was myelosuppression, mainly neutropenia, which was not cumulative. Hematologic toxicity of grade 2 or higher developed at 5-FU doses as low as 10 mg/m^2. Neutrophil nadirs occurred between d 16 and 24 with complete recovery in most patients by d 28. Five episodes of sepsis were documented in 207 cycles of chemotherapy. Nonhematologic toxicities were infrequent, and included grade 3 diarrhea in 5% of patients, and grade 2 mucositis in 3%. Other toxicities included anorexia and fatigue.

It is noteworthy that minor increases in the 5-FU dose produced significant increases in toxicity. For example, 20 mg/m^2 of 5-FU given with eniluracil and leucovorin was well tolerated; no patients experienced hematologic toxicity > grade 2. By contrast, of the six patients who were treated at a 5-FU dose of 25 mg/m^2 per day, only a 25% dose increase, four developed grade 4 neutropenia and one experienced grade 3 thrombocytopenia.

One partial response was noted, in a patient with metastatic colon cancer who had received prior adjuvant therapy with 5-FU and levamisole. The recommended phase II doses were eniluracil 10 mg/d with intravenous 5-FU 25 mg/m^2/d; eniluracil 10 mg/d with intra-

Table 1
Phase II Trials of the Eniluracil/Oral 5-Fluorouracil Combination in Patients with Metastatic Colorectal Cancer

Dose and schedule of Eniluracil (E) and 5-FU (F)	*No. of patients*	*Prior treatment*	*Response rate*	*Reference*
E: 11-11.5 mg/m^2 bid × 28d q 35d F: 1-1.15 mg/m^2 bid × 28d q 35d	55	No	25%	*(34)*
E: 20 mg qd × 7d q 28d F: 25 mg/m^2/d, days 2–6 OR E: 20 mg qd × 7d q 28d F: 20 mg/m^2/d, days 2–6 LV: 50 mg/d days 2–6	75	Yes	21% (no prior treatment) 0% (previously treated)	*(34)*
E: 50 mg qd × 7d q 28d F: 20 mg/m^2/d days 2–6	29	No	25%	*(35)*
E: 50 mg qd × 7d F: 20 mg/m^2/d days 2–6 LV: 50 mg/d days 2–6	60	No	13%	*(31)*

venous 5-FU 20 mg/m^2/d and leucovorin 50 mg/d; and eniluracil 50 mg/d with oral 5-FU 15 mg/m^2/d with leucovorin 50 mg/d.

DPD activity was measured in peripheral blood mononuclear cells. The enzyme was inactivated within one hour of eniluracil administration at all dose levels; this was sustained for up to 24 h after a single oral dose. DPD activity returned to values within a normal range 14 d after cessation of eniluracil treatment.

6.2. Twenty-eight-Day Schedule

The MTD, toxicities, and pharmacokinetics of eniluracil plus oral 5-FU administered twice daily for 28 d every 35 d were evaluated in a phase I trial conducted by Baker et al. in 36 patients with advanced solid tumors *(17)*. Oral 5-FU 1.35 mg/m^2 twice daily, and eniluracil 10 mg daily, were administered for 14, 21, or 28 d, followed by a 1 wk rest period. Eniluracil treatment began 1 d prior to 5-FU. Once the safety of a 28 d course was determined, escalated doses of oral 5-FU 1.35 to 1.8 mg/m^2 twice daily, and eniluracil 10 mg were administered twice daily for 28 d. They also evaluated doses of 5-FU 1.0 mg/m^2 twice daily with eniluracil 20 mg/m^2 twice daily. This is the recommended phase II dose.

The dose-limiting toxicity was diarrhea. Sixty-four percent of patients experienced grades 1 or 2 diarrhea, while 14% developed grades 3 or 4 diarrhea. Diarrhea developed during the third or fourth week of treatment and usually resolved prior to the initiation of the next cycle. Other nonhematologic toxicities included nausea and vomiting, flatulence, abdominal cramping, and anorexia. Grades 1 and 2 hand-foot syndrome occurred in 19% of patients; hand-foot syndrome of grade 3 or greater was not observed. Grade 1 and 2 mucositis developed in eight patients. Hematologic toxicity was infrequent. Two partial responses were noted, both in patients with colorectal carcinoma. Patient compliance was also monitored. An average of only two doses (range 1–3) were missed in 9 of 96 courses.

6.3. Weekly schedule

In order to simulate a weekly high-dose 24-h continuous infusion schedule of 5-FU, Grem and colleagues conducted a phase I trial in which oral 5-FU, leucovorin, and eniluracil were administered on a weekly schedule to patients with advanced solid tumors *(32)*. Patients were initially treated with one dose of 5-FU 2300 mg/m^2 by continuous infusion over 24 h on d 2, and leucovorin 15 mg po bid d 1–3, in order to provide a reference for plasma levels of 5-FU, α-fluoro-β-alanine, and uracil, and for DPD activity in peripheral blood lymphocytes. Two weeks later, patients began treatment with eniluracil 20 mg and leucovorin 15 mg both given po bid on d 1–3, and oral 5-FU at a starting dose of 15 mg po bid on d 2. None of the first three patients completed the planned weekly × 6 of 8 wk course owing to dose-limiting toxicities, which included neutropenia, diarrhea, and pulmonary embolus. When the schedule was altered to weekly × 3 of 4, three of six patients experienced dose-limiting toxicity in cycle 1 which included grade 3–4 diarrhea and grade 3 fatigue. The 5-FU dose was subsequently decreased to 10 mg/m^2 po bid. At that dose, one of three patients experienced grade 3 diarrhea *(32)*.

6.4. Renal Dysfunction

5-FU and eniluracil must be used cautiously in patients with renal impairment, since renal excretion is the primary elimination pathway of 5-FU in the presence of eniluracil. Punt and colleagues conducted a phase I study to evaluate the effect of renal impairment on the pharmacokinetics of 5-FU in the presence of eniluracil. Eight patients with normal renal function, defined as a creatinine clearance ≥50 mL/min, and nine patients with moderate renal impairment, who had a creatinine clearance < 50 mL/min initially, received eniluracil 50 mg po on d 1–3 and 5-FU 10 mg/m^2 po on d 2. Plasma was analyzed for eniluracil, uracil, and 5-FU, and urine was analyzed for α-fluoro-β-alanine. Patients subsequently received eniluracil 50 mg po on d 1–7 and oral 5-FU on d 2–6 every 4 wk. The patients with renal impairment demonstrated decreased clearance of eniluracil and 5-FU. A linear correlation between 5-FU clearance and creatinine clearance was noted in the patients with impaired renal function *(33)*.

Two other studies confirmed these findings. Baker et al. demonstrated a strong correlation between serum creatinine, calculated creatinine clearance, and 5-FU clearance in patients who received 5-FU with eniluracil *(27)*. Similarly, Meropol and colleagues observed an inverse association between baseline creatinine clearance and the development of severe toxicity *(31)*. Serum creatinine did not predict toxicity in this study, suggesting that it is important to utilize creatinine clearance when selecting patients for treatment *(31)*.

6.5. Effects on DPD in tumors

Ahmed administered eniluracil, 10 mg/m^2 twice daily for three d prior to colorectal tumor resection to assess the in vivo effect of eniluracil on DPD activity *(34)*. Mononuclear cells, colon tumors, and normal mucosa in treated and untreated patients were assayed pretreatment and on the morning of surgery for DPD activity, protein, and mRNA. Plasma uracil levels were determined as an indirect measure of DPD inhibition. DPD activity was not detectable in tumors or mononuclear cells in those patients who received eniluracil. Plasma uracil levels rose from a median of < 0.2 μmol/L before therapy to 27.62 μmol/L preoperatively, consistent with enzyme inactivation. DPD protein and mRNA and levels remained unchanged. These data suggest that synthesis of new DPD protein following eniluracil treatment is the rate-limiting step in the regeneration of DPD activity following discontinuation of eniluracil *(34)*. This trial is the only study that clearly demonstrates inactivation of DPD in human tumor tissue at clinical doses of eniluracil.

6.6. EU/FU in Colorectal Cancer

6.6.1. Phase II Studies

Mani and colleagues assessed the combination of oral 5-FU and eniluracil in 55 patients with previously untreated advanced colorectal cancer *(35)*. Eniluracil and 5-FU were administered in a 10:1 ratio. Initially, 5-FU was dosed at 1 mg/m^2 twice daily for 28 d every 35 d. Toxicities of grade 3 or greater were minimal: diarrhea in 16% of patients, mucositis in 4%, and hand-foot syndrome in 2%. Hematologic toxicities were minor; only 4% of patients developed grade 3 granulocytopenia. Owing to the limited toxicity observed in the first 28 patients, the 5-FU dose was escalated to 1.15 mg/m^2 and an additional 25 patients were treated. Although there were no significant differences in the incidence or severity of diarrhea, mucositis, or hand-foot syndrome between the two dose levels, patients who received the higher dose experienced greater malaise, fatigue, anorexia, nausea, and vomiting. The partial response rate was 25%, while 36% of patients had stable disease lasting a median of 29.6 wk. There was no difference in response rate between the two dose groups.

Schilsky and colleagues reported a multiinstitutional phase II trial in 75 patients with colorectal cancer who received oral 5-FU with eniluracil with or without leucovorin *(36)*. Patients were stratified by prior treatment: 24 patients received no prior treatment for metastatic disease, the remainder were refractory to intravenous 5-FU and leucovorin, defined as progression within 2 mo of therapy. All patients were administered 20 mg of eniluracil daily for 7 d every 4 wk. Oral 5-FU was given once daily on d 2–6. Patients received either 25 mg/m^2 of 5-FU without leucovorin or 20 mg/m^2 of 5-FU with 50 mg/d of oral leucovorin.

The 5-FU dose was rounded up to the nearest 5 mg in the first 20 patients. Owing to an unexpectedly high incidence of grade 4 neutropenia, the dose of 5-FU was rounded down to the nearest 5 mg in the remaining patients. Six of the first 20 patients were hospitalized for neutropenic sepsis. Of the 55 patients whose 5-FU dose was rounded down, only four patients developed neutropenic sepsis. Overall, grades 3–4 neutropenia developed in 54% of patients. Grades 3–4 thrombocytopenia were observed in 6% of patients. Nonhematologic toxicities were mild and included grades 3–4 diarrhea in 7%; hand-foot syndrome of grade 2 or greater did not develop. Five partial responses were observed in the previously untreated stratum for an overall response rate of 21% (17% for patients who received eniluracil/5-FU and 25% for patients who were treated with eniluracil/5-FU/LV). There were no responders among the patients who were refractory to intravenous 5-FU/LV treatment, however 30% had stable disease.

The North Central Cancer Treatment Group conducted a phase II study of 79 patients with previously untreated metastatic colorectal carcinoma. Patients received eniluracil 50 mg on d 1–7 and oral 5-FU 20 mg/m^2/d on d 2–6 every 28 d. The overall response rate was 25% (95% CI 17–37) and the median duration of response was 6.6 mo. The median survival was 11.3 mo. Twenty-six percent of patients experienced grade 4 neutropenia and 8% developed grade 4 diarrhea *(37)*.

The Cancer and Leukemia Group B reported a phase II study in 60 patients with previously untreated colorectal cancer. Patients received eniluracil 50 mg on d 1–7, oral 5-FU 20 mg/m^2 on d 2–6, and oral leucovorin 50 mg on d 2–6 of a 28-d cycle. Responses were observed in 13% of patients, including one complete response. The median survival was 12.6 mo. Eighty-five percent of patients developed toxicity of grade 3 or greater, and there

Table 2
Phase II Trials of Eniluracil and Oral 5-Fluorouracil in Patients with Other Malignancies

Disease	*No. of patients*	*Response rate*	*Reference*
Breast cancer			
untreated	33	52%	*(38)*
taxane/anthracycline refractory	35	11%	*(39)*
taxane/anthracycline refractory	40	16%	*(40)*
Head and neck cancer	28	26%	*(43)*
Hepatocellular carcinoma	35	0%	*(42)*

was one toxic death. Grade 4 neutropenia developed in 42% of patients, and febrile neutropenia in 20%. Grade 3 or 4 diarrhea was observed in 30% of patients *(31)*.

The Eastern Cooperative Oncology Group has completed a phase II study of eniluracil/5-FU given on a 28-d cycle every 35 d to patients with advanced colorectal cancer who had received no more than one previous treatment for metastatic disease. The results of this study are pending at this time.

6.6.2. Phase III studies

Two pivotal randomized multicenter phase III studies, one in the United States and one in Europe, compared eniluracil/5-FU on the 28-d schedule to intravenous 5-FU with leucovorin on the Mayo Clinic schedule of daily for 5 d every 28 d in patients with previously untreated metastatic colorectal cancer. The primary endpoint of the American trial was overall survival and 964 patients were randomized. Although no significant differences in median survival were observed (57.7 wk for EU/FU and 63.0 wk for FU/LV) and response rates were nearly identical (12.2% for EU/FU and 12.7% for FU/LV), the results did not meet the protocol-specified criteria for equivalence to FU/LV in overall survival *(37a)*. Based on these data together with inferior survival for EU/FU observed in the European trial, the sponsor has elected to discontinue further clinical development of eniluracil.

6.7. EU/FU in Other Solid Tumors

6.7.1. Breast cancer

Three phase II studies of eniluracil with 5-FU have been performed in patients with advanced breast cancer. Smith and colleagues reported a study in 33 previously untreated women with metastatic breast cancer who received eniluracil 10 mg/m^2 and oral 5-FU 1.0 mg/m^2 twice daily for 28 d every 35 d *(38)*. Sixteen partial responses were achieved in 29 assessable patients, for a 55% overall response rate, including responses in 40% of the 10 patients who had previously received adjuvant 5-FU. Treatment was well-tolerated: grade 3 neutropenia developed in 6% of patients, neutropenic sepsis in 3%, and grade 3 thrombocytopenia in 3%. The most common toxicity was grade 1 or 2 diarrhea; only one patient developed grade 3 diarrhea.

The same dose and schedule of eniluracil and 5-FU were evaluated in 35 patients with taxane and anthracycline-refractory metastatic breast cancer, defined as disease progression while receiving a taxane and an anthracycline, or relapsed within 6 mo of adjuvant anthracycline treatment. Partial responses were observed in 11%; progression-free survival was 30 wk. Hematologic toxicity was minimal. Grades 1 and 2 diarrhea developed in 41%. A second cohort of patients were treated at a higher dose level, eniluracil 11.5 mg/m^2 and oral

5-FU 1.15 mg/m²; these data have not yet been reported *(39)*. Another multicenter phase II trial in women with taxane and anthracycline-refractory breast cancer using the 28-d schedule achieved a 16% response rate and reported a mild toxicity profile *(40)*.

6.7.2. Pancreatic Cancer

A phase III study in pancreatic carcinoma that compared eniluracil and oral 5-FU to intravenous gemcitabine has also been completed. The primary endpoint of the trial is time to progression; the data have not yet been reported.

6.7.3. Hepatobiliary Cancer

There is inverse correlation between DPD activity and 5-FU sensitivity in some tumors *(14,15)*. Enhancement of 5-FU cytotoxicity by eniluracil occurs in vitro only in cell lines that express high DPD activity *(20)*. Thus, it may be possible to use a DPD inhibitor to overcome 5-FU resistance in tumors that overexpress DPD. This was the intent of a phase II multicenter study in hepatocellular carcinoma, a tumor with high DPD activity that does not respond to 5-FU *(42)*. Thirty-five patients with unresectable hepatocellular carcinoma who had received no more than one prior chemotherapy regimen received eniluracil 10 mg/m² and 5-FU 1 mg/m² bid for 28 d every 35 d. There were no grade 3 or 4 hematologic toxicities. Grade 3–4 diarrhea developed in 9% of patients. There were no partial or complete responders, however 24% of patients experienced stable disease ranging from 8 to 52 wk *(42)*.

6.7.4. Head and Neck Cancer

The National Institute of Canada Clinical Trials Group evaluated eniluracil and 5-FU on the 28-d schedule in 28 chemonaive patients with head and neck cancer recurrent after surgery or radiotherapy. The overall response rate was 26%, including two complete responses. Hematologic toxicity included grade 4 leukopenia in one patient, and grade 3–4 thrombocytopenia in two patients. There was one toxic death from bleeding in a patient with thrombocytopenia *(43)*.

6.7.5. EU/FU plus Radiation Therapy

Humerickhouse and colleagues conducted a phase I dose-escalation study to evaluate the safety and efficacy of eniluracil given with oral 5-FU in 13 patients who received concurrent radiation therapy for advanced or recurrent squamous cell carcinoma of the head and neck *(30)*. Eniluracil was given at a fixed dose of 20 mg/m² bid on days 1–7. Oral 5-FU and radiotherapy were given on d 2–6. The initial 5-FU dose was 2.5 mg/m² twice daily. Dose escalation of 5-FU was planned in 2.5 mg/m² increments. Cycles were repeated every 2 wk. One patient received once daily radiation in 2 Gy fractions; the remainder underwent hyperfractionated RT, using 1.5 Gy fractions bid.

The dose-limiting toxicity was cumulative myelosuppression, both neutropenia and thrombocytopenia, which developed during the fourth and fifth cycles of therapy after administration of 5-FU 5 mg/m² bid. The study was closed due to unacceptable toxicity, including two deaths, one from neutropenic sepsis in the fourth cycle and one from unknown causes. The absence of dose-limiting mucositis and dermatitis suggested that radiation sensitization did not occur. Of the six patients who were evaluable for response, there were three pathologic complete responses. DPD activity in peripheral blood mononuclear cells was assayed before treatment and at least once during therapy. All patients achieved complete or nearly complete inactivation of DPD. Plasma uracil concentrations, measured as an indirect assessment of DPD inactivation, were markedly elevated in all patients *(30)*.

Cohen and colleagues evaluated the safety and efficacy of eniluracil/5-fluorouracil with concurrent pelvic radiation for the preoperative treatment of patients with rectal adenocarcinoma in a phase I dose-escalation study *(44)*. Fifteen patients received 4500 cGy pelvic XRT in 25 daily 180 cGy fractions. Three cohorts of patients received escalating doses of 5-FU/eniluracil in a 10:1 ratio ranging from 6 to 10 mg/m^2 twice a day of eniluracil and 0.6 to 1.0 mg/m^2 twice a day of 5-FU. Dose-limiting toxicity consisting of grade 3 diarrhea in one patient and grade 4 diarrhea, dehydration, and abdominal pain in a second patient was observed at the third dose level, eniluracil 10 mg/m^2/d and 5-FU 1 mg/m^2/d. Other nondose-limiting toxicities included fatigue, nausea, vomiting, and cystitis. Tumor down-staging occurred in 11/13 patients who underwent surgery, including one pathological complete response. The recommended phase II dose of eniluracil/5-FU in combination with pelvic RT is 8 mg/m^2/0.8 mg/m^2 *(44)*.

Lee and colleagues conducted a phase I study to evaluate the administration of eniluracil/5-FU in combination with upper abdominal radiotherapy for patients with pancreatic or peri-ampullary adenocarcinoma in either the preoperative or palliative setting *(45)*. Patients received 4500 cGy of upper abdominal radiotherapy in 25 daily 180 cGy fractions, followed by three daily 180 cGy fractions to boost fields. Three cohorts of patients received escalating doses of eniluracil/5-FU in a 10:1 ratio, ranging from 6–10 mg/m^2/0.6–1.0 mg/m^2 orally twice daily. The only dose-limiting toxicity in the first nine patients was grade 4 neutropenia in one patient at the second dose level (8 mg/m^2/0.8 mg/m^2). Other toxicities included fatigue, anorexia, weight loss, nausea, vomiting, and diarrhea. Three of seven patients with potentially resectable disease underwent complete resection. There was one pathological complete response *(45)*.

7. CONCLUSION

Eniluracil permits reliable absorption of orally administered 5-FU, which provides convenience, safety, and potential cost savings to patients over continuous intravenous infusion. The combination has a predictable, mild toxicity profile and, in most settings, produces tumor responses comparable to those achieved with conventional iv 5-FU regimens. However, two recently completed large international phase III trials have demonstrated inferior survival for eniluracil/oral 5-FU compared with bolus 5-FU/LV in colorectal cancer and development of the eniluracil/5-FU combination has therefore been halted.

Eniluracil is rationally designed, specific inactivator of DPD. Extensive preclinical and clinical testing confirm that EU completely inactivates DPD in both tumor tissue and normal cells and markedly reduces the plasma clearance of 5-FU. Although the drug is a pharmacological success, it has failed to improve the efficacy of 5-FU in the clinic. Reasons for this are unclear but might range from poor patient compliance with an oral therapy regimen to infrequent overexpression of DPD in tumors as a basis for fluoropyrimidine resistance. The story of eniluracil illustrates the complexity and risk associated with development of new cancer therapeutics.

REFERENCES

1. Iyer L, Ratain MJ: 5-fluorouracil pharmacokinetics: causes for variability and strategies for modulation in cancer chemotherapy. *Cancer Invest* 1999;17(7):494–506.
2. Meta-analysis Group in Cancer: Efficacy of intravenous continuous infusion of fluorouracil compared with bolus administration in advanced colorectal cancer. *J Clin Oncol* 1998;16(1):301–308.
3. Liu G, Franssen E, Fitch MI, Warner E. Patient preferences for oral versus intravenous palliative chemotherapy. *J Clin Oncol* 1997;15(1):110–115.

4. DeMario MD, Ratain MJ. Oral chemotherapy: rationale and future directions. *J Clin Oncol* 1998;16(7):2557–2567.
5. Fraile RJ, Baker LH, Buroker TR, Horwitz J, Vaitkevicius VK. Pharmacokinetics of 5-fluorouracil administered orally, by rapid intravenous and by slow infusion. *Cancer Res* 1980;40(7):2223–2228.
6. Etienne MC, Lagrange JL, Dassonville O, et al. Population study of dihydropyrimidine dehydrogenase in cancer patients. *J Clin Oncol* 1994;12(11):2248–2253.
7. Diasio RB, Johnson MR: Dihydropyrimidine dehydrogenase: its role in 5-fluorouracil clinical toxicity and tumor resistance. *Clin Cancer Res* 1999;5(10):2672–2673.
8. Porter DJ, Chestnut WG, Merrill BM, Spector T. Mechanism-based inactivation of dihydropyrimidine dehydrogenase by 5- ethynyluracil. *J Biol Chem* 1992;267(8):5236–5242.
9. Heggie GD, Sommadossi JP, Cross DS, Huster WJ, Diasio RB. Clinical pharmacokinetics of 5-fluorouracil and its metabolites in plasma, urine, and bile. *Cancer Res* 1987;47(8):2203–2206.
10. Harris BE, Song R, Soong SJ, Diasio RB. Relationship between dihydropyrimidine dehydrogenase activity and plasma 5-fluorouracil levels with evidence for circadian variation of enzyme activity and plasma drug levels in cancer patients receiving 5-fluorouracil by protracted continuous infusion. *Cancer Res* 1990;50(1):197–201.
11 Diasio RB, Lu Z. Dihydropyrimidine dehydrogenase activity and fluorouracil chemotherapy. *J Clin Oncol* 1994;12(11):2239–2242.
12. Naguib FN, el Kouni MH, Cha S. Enzymes of uracil catabolism in normal and neoplastic human tissues. *Cancer Res* 1985;45:5405–5412.
13. Tateishi T, Watanabe M, Nakura H, et al. Dihydropyrimidine dehydrogenase activity and fluorouracil pharmacokinetics with liver damage induced by bile duct ligation in rats. *Drug Metab Dispos* 1999;27(6):651–654.
14. Etienne MC, Cheradame S, Fischel JL, et al. Response to fluorouracil therapy in cancer patients: the role of tumoral dihydropyrimidine dehydrogenase activity. *J Clin Oncol* 1995;13(7):1663–1670.
15. Beck A, Etienne MC, Cheradame S, et al. A role for dihydropyrimidine dehydrogenase and thymidylate synthase in tumour sensitivity to fluorouracil. *Eur J Cancer* 1994;10(22):1517–1522.
16. Rustum YM, Harstrick A, Cao S, et al. Thymidylate synthase inhibitors in cancer therapy: direct and indirect inhibitors. *J Clin Oncol* 1997;15(1):389–400.
17. Baker SD, Diasio RB, O'Reilly S, et al. Phase I and pharmacologic study of oral fluorouracil on a chronic daily schedule in combination with the dihydropyrimidine dehydrogenase inactivator eniluracil. *J Clin Oncol* 2000;18(4):915–926.
18. Spector T, Harrington JA, Porter DJ. 5-Ethynyluracil (776C85) inactivation of dihydropyrimidine dehydrogenase in vivo. *Biochem Pharmacol* 1993;46:2243–2248.
19. Baccanari DP, Davis ST, Knick VC, Spector T. 5-Ethynyluracil (776C85): a potent modulator of the pharmacokinetics and antitumor efficacy of 5-fluorouracil. *Proc Natl Acad Sci USA* 1993;90(23):11064–11068.
20. Fischel JL, Etienne MC, Spector T, Formento P, Renee N, Milano G. Dihydropyrimidine dehydrogenase: a tumoral target for fluorouracil modulation. *Clin Cancer Res* 1995;1(9):991–996.
21. Cao S, Rustum YM, Spector T. 5-Ethynyluracil (776C85): modulation of 5-fluorouracil efficacy and therapeutic index in rats bearing advanced colorectal carcinoma. *Cancer Res* 1994;54(6):1507–1510.
22. Arellano M, Malet-Martino M, Martino R, Spector T. 5-Ethynyluracil (GW776): effects on the formation of the toxic catabolites of 5-fluorouracil, fluoroacetate and fluorohydroxypropionic acid in the isolated perfused rat liver model. *Br J Cancer* 1997;76(9)1170–1180.
23. Davis ST, Joyner SS, Baccanari DP, Spector T. 5-Ethynyluracil (776C85): protection from 5-fluorouracil-induced neurotoxicity in dogs. *Biochem Pharmacol* 1994;48(2):233–236.
24. Adams ER, Leffert JJ, Craig DJ, Spector T, Pizzorno G. In vivo effect of 5-ethynyluracil on 5-fluorouracil metabolism determined by 19F nuclear magnetic resonance spectroscopy. *Cancer Res* 1999;59(1):122–127.
25. Cao S, Baccanari DP, Rustum YM, et al: ∞-fluoro-β-alanine. Effects on the antitumor activity and toxicity of 5-fluorouracil. *Biochem Pharmacol* 2000;59:953–960.
26. Spector T, Cao S, Rustum YM, Harrington JA, Porter DJ. Attenuation of the antitumor activity of 5-fluorouracil by (R)-5-fluoro- 5,6-dihydrouracil. *Cancer Res* 1995;55(6):1239–1241.
27. Baker SD, Khor SP, Adjei AA, et al. Pharmacokinetic, oral bioavailability, and safety study of fluorouracil in patients treated with 776C85, an inactivator of dihydropyrimidine dehydrogenase. *J Clin Oncol* 1996;14(12):3085–3096.
28. Janisch L, Mani S, Schilsky RL, et al. Phase I study to determine the effects of food on the absorption of oral 776C85 (776) Plus 5-fluorouracil (FU) in patients (pts) with advanced cancer. *Proc ASCO* (1998)17:224a.
29. Schilsky RL, Hohneker J, Ratain MJ, et al. Phase I clinical and pharmacologic study of eniluracil plus fluorouracil in patients with advanced cancer. *J Clin Oncol* 1998;16(4):1450–1457.

30. Humerickhouse RA, Dolan ME, Haraf DJ, et al. Phase I study of eniluracil, a dihydropyrimidine dehydrogenase inactivator, and oral 5-fluorouracil with radiation therapy in patients with recurrent or advanced head and neck cancer. *Clin Cancer Res* 1999;5(2):291–298.
31. Meropol NJ, Niedzwiecki D, Hollis D, Schilsky RL, Mayer RJ. Phase II study of oral eniluracil, 5-fluorouracil, and leucovorin in patients with advanced colorectal cancer. *Cancer* 2001;91:1256–1263.
32. Grem J, Harold N, Bi D, et al. Phase I and pharmacologic (PK/PD) study of weekly oral fluorouracil (FUra) given with eniluracil (GW 776C85) and leucovorin (LV) in patients (pts) with solid tumors. *Proc ASCO* 2000;19:173a
33. Punt CJ, Judson IR, Suttle AB, O'Callaghan ML, Ertel PJ, Beale P, Bryttan JM. Evaluation of the pharmacokinetics (PK) of eniluracil/fluorouracil after concurrent administration to patients with renal impairment. *Proc ASCO* 2000;19:192a.
34. Ahmed FY, Johnston SJ, Cassidy J, et al. Eniluracil treatment completely inactivates dihydropyrimidine dehydrogenase in colorectal tumors. *J Clin Oncol* 1999;17(8):2439–2445.
35. Mani S, Hochster H, Beck T, et al. Multicenter phase II study to evaluate a 28-day regimen of oral fluorouracil (5-FU) plus eniluracil in the treatment of patients with previously untreated metastatic colorectal cancer. *J Clin Oncol* 2000;18:2894–2901.
36. Schilsky RL, Bukowski R, Burris H 3rd, Hochster H, O'Rourke M, Wall JG, Mani S, Bonny T, Levin J, Hohneker J. A multicenter phase II study of a 5-day regimen of oral 5-flurouracil plus eniluracil with or without leucovorin in patients with metastatic colorectal cancer. *Annals of Oncology* 2000;11:415–420.
37. Goldberg RM, Kugler JW, Mahoney MR, et al. A Phase II trial of 7 days of oral 776C85 plus five days of 5-fluorouracil (5-FU) in patients (pts) with metastatic colorectal cancer (M-CRC): A North Central Cancer Treatment Group Study. *Proc ASCO* 2000;19:245a.
37a. Schilsky RL, Levin J, West WH, et al. A randomized open label phase III study of a 28 day oral regimen of eniluracil (776C85) plus 5-fluorouracil versus intravenous 5-fluorouracil plus leurovorin as first line therapy in patients with metastatic/advanced colorectal cancer. *J Clin Oncol* 2002;20:1519–1526.
38. Smith K, Johnston SR, O'Brien ME, et al. Llow dose oral 5-fluorouracil with eniluracil as first-line chemotherapy against advanced breast cancer: A phase II study. *J Clin Oncol* 2000;18:2378–2384.
39. Burris HA, Ravdin R, Gutheil J, et al. Eniluracil/5FU in anthracycline and taxane refractory breast cancer. *Proc ASCO* 1999;18:107a.
40. Rivera E, Chevlen E, Eckardt J, et al. A phase II open-label study to evaluate a 28-day oral regimen of 5-fluorouracil (5-FU) plus 776C85 for the treatment of patients with taxane and anthracycline resistant advanced breast cancer: preliminary results. *Proc ASCO* 1998;17:113a.
41. Jiang W, Lu Z, He Y, Diasio RB. Dihydropyrimidine dehydrogenase activity in hepatocellular carcinoma: implication in 5-fluorouracil-based chemotherapy. *Clin Cancer Res* 1997;3(3):395–399.
42. Benson AB, Mitchell E, Abramson N et al. A multicenter, phase II trial of oral eniluracil plus 5-FU in patients with inoperable hepatocellular carcinoma. *Proc ASCO* 1999;18:256a.
43. Knowling M, Browman G, Cooke A, et al. Phase II study of eniluracil (776C85) and oral 5-fluorouracil (5-FU) in patients with advanced squamous cell head and neck cancer (HNC). *Proc ASCO* 1999;18:396a.
44. Cohen DP, Lee CG, Anscher MS, et al. Phase I study of chemoradiation therapy with oral eniluracil (776C85)/5-Fluorouracil in patients with rectal adenocarcinoma. *Proc ASCO* 2000;19:261a.
45. Lee CG, Cohen DP, Petros WP, et al. Phase I/pharmacokinetic study of chemoradiation therapy with oral eniluracil (776C85)/5-Fluorouracil for pancreatic/peri-ampullary adenocarcinoma. *Proc ASCO* 2000;19:268a.

20 Discovery and Preclinical Pharmacology of Capecitabine

Hideo Ishitsuka, PhD

CONTENTS

1. INTRODUCTION

Cytotoxic drugs have been widely used for the treatment of cancer and will continue to play a major role in cancer chemotherapy at least throughout the next decade. However, the efficacy of cytotoxic drugs is still far from satisfactory for the treatment of many types of malignant diseases as they generally lack tumor selective activity. They act not only on cancer cells but also on rapidly growing normal cells, such as granulocyte progenitor cells in the bone marrow and cryptic cells in the intestinal mucosa, resulting in adverse events in these normal tissues. Consequently, such cytotoxic drugs could not be prescribed frequently for long periods or at a dose level sufficiently high to cure cancer. Bone marrow toxicity, whcih often results in opportunistic infections and thus limits the use of cytotoxic drugs particularly in the treatment of outpatients, is the most common problem in cancer chemotherapy with cytotoxic drugs. Intestinal toxicity is another adverse event of cytotoxic drugs, particularly when they are given orally. Oral administration of cytotoxic drugs leads to high local drug concentrations predominantly at the local sites, intestine and liver, and thus results in treatment-associated adverse effects of these organs. In addition, oral doses of cytotoxic drugs are in general larger than parenteral ones, because drugs given orally are often subjected to first-pass metabolic effects in the intestinal tract and liver. Dose reduction to spare such local organ toxicity would result in insufficient efficacy compared with that of parenteral administration.

Many cytotoxic drugs inhibit particular processes of the tumor cell. Not all tumor cells in cultures are susceptible to such cell-cycle-specific effects of cytotoxic drugs, and they should therefore be exposed to the drugs for longer periods beyond one cell cycle time. As a consequence, they should also be given more frequently to optimize the cytotoxic effects on

From: *Fluoropyrimidines in Cancer Therapy*
Edited by: Y. M. Rustum © Humana Press Inc., Totowa, NJ

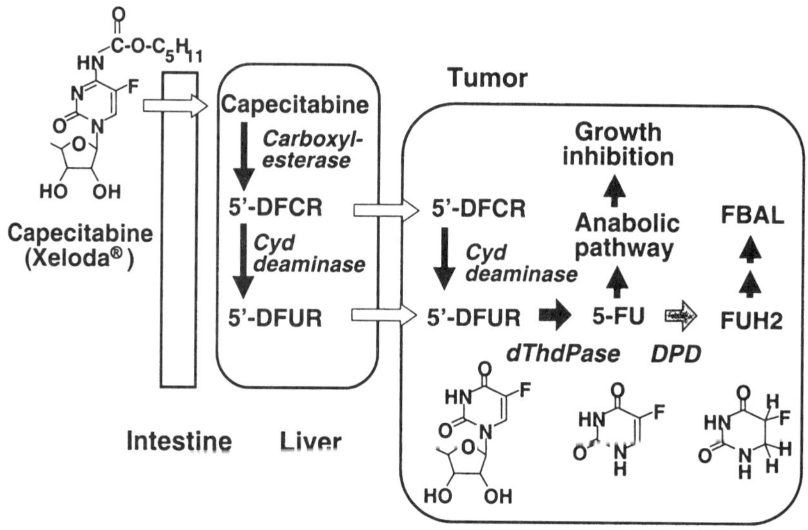

Fig. 1. Metabolic pathway of capecitabine.

tumor cells. However, they also act on normal tissues such as bone marrow and intestinal mucosa. This is the reason why they are given intermittently to avoid cumulative toxic effects on normal tissues. The most appropriate formulation for a frequent administration of anticancer drugs would be a tablet. It has been shown in clinical studies that cancer patients prefer oral treatment if it is as effective as parenteral treatment *(1)*.

Studies started in 1986 to design and synthesize orally available cytotoxic compounds that have a high tumor selective activity associated with little myelotoxicity or intestinal toxicity, and therefore could be safely given for daily oral treatment over prolonged time periods. Our strategy, specifically identifying new cytotoxic compounds with high tumor selective action, included the design and synthesis of a prodrug that generates the active cytotoxic component by enzymes preferentially located in tumors after oral administration. We previously developed a prodrug, 5′-deoxy-5-fluorouridine (5′-DFUR) (doxifluridine, Furtulon®), that is metabolized to the active drug 5-FU by an enzyme preferentially located in tumors *(2)*. It demonstrated better efficacy than 5-FU in many experimental tumor models *(2–4)* and is being prescribed in Japan, China, and Korea for the treatment of breast, colorectal, gastric, and other cancers. However, the efficacy of 5′-DFUR is not strictly tumor selective and caused intestinal toxicity when orally given at high doses *(5)*. We therefore tried to synthesize in a rational manner a novel fluoropyrimidine characterized by improved efficacy and safety profiles compared to those of 5′-DFUR and 5-FU. These studies enabled us to identify capecitabine (Xeloda®, N^4-pentyloxycarbonyl-5′-deoxy-5-fluorocytidine) (Fig. 1) with more improved efficacy and safety profiles over those of 5-FU, 5′-DFUR, and other fluoropyrimidines *(6–9)*. This chapter describes how capecitabine was designed and is effective in preclinical pharmacology studies.

2. DRUG DESIGN AND DISCOVERY OF CAPECITABINE

2.1. 5′-DFUR as a Lead Compound of Capecitabine

In 1976, Cook et al. synthesized 5′-DFUR *(10)*, which has shown higher antitumor activity at broader dose ranges than 5-FU and other fluoropyrimidines in many tumor models

(2–4). 5′-DFUR was identified as a prodrug that generates the active drug 5-FU through enzymatic conversion by pyrimidine nucleoside phosphorylases (PyNPase) *(2)*, which are preferentially located in tumor tissues *(6,11)*. Consequently, 5′-DFUR generates 5-FU efficiently in tumors *(12)*. PyNPase includes uridine phosphorylase (UrdPase) and thymidine phosphorylase (dThdPase), which predominantly exist as PyNPase in mice and human, respectively *(13)*. Oral 5′-DFUR (doxifluridine, Furtulon®) was developed in Japan and approved in 1987 for the treatment of breast, gastric, and colorectal cancer. The major drawbacks of oral 5′-DFUR therapy were its dose-limiting side effect, diarrhea *(14)*, and its insufficient oral availability. Passing through the intestine at high concentrations, 5′-DFUR causes intestinal toxicity through 5-FU generated by intestinal PyNPase *(5)*. 5′-DFUR may also cause myelotoxicity particularly when given at high doses, although the degree is generally mild and the incidence is low. We therefore tried to design and synthesize a novel oral fluoropyrimidine with a more pronounced tumor selectivity that can be given at high doses inducing a stronger cytotoxic effect and at the same time induce less toxicity than 5-FU and 5′-DFUR. Initial attempts focused on the synthesis of a 5′-DFUR precursor that passes through the intestine, is first metabolized to 5′-DFUR by enzymes located in the liver, and is ultimately converted to 5-FU by dThdPase in tumors.

2.2. 5′-DFCR Derivatives

To minimize the myelotoxicity and increase the tumor selective activity of 5′-DFUR, we selected 5′-deoxy-5-fluorocytidine (5′-DFCR) as a lead among many 5′-DFUR derivatives synthesized. 5′-DFCR is metabolized to 5′-DFUR by cytidine (Cyd) deaminase, the enzyme responsible for the metabolism of cytosine arabinoside (Ara C), an antileukemic cytotoxic drug, to the inactive molecule uracil arabinoside. The enzyme is highly expressed in the liver, kidney *(15)*, and solid tumors *(16)* of humans, whereas it is minimally expressed in immature, growing marrow cells and leukemic myeloblasts, compared to that in mature, normal granulocytes *(17)*. This unique localization of the enzyme explains the clinical efficacy of Ara C only in leukemia, and its dose-limiting adverse effect to the bone marrow. We confirmed the unique tissue enzyme localization *(6)* and low expression in the granulocyte progenitor cells from both human bone marrow and umbilical cord blood (unpublished). 5′-DFCR was thus selected as a potential lead compound based on the rationale that the specific tissue distribution of Cyd deaminase would result in the generation of 5′-DFUR at higher concentrations in liver and tumors but not in granulocyte progenitor cells. Capecitabine, a derivative of 5′-DFCR, was later demonstrated to show minimal myelotoxicity in clinical studies *(18,19)*.

2.3. N^4-Acyl-5′-DFCR Derivatives

Because certain levels of Cyd deaminase and dThdPase activities were found in the human intestinal tract *(6)*, it was hypothesized that 5-FU could be generated from 5′-DFCR to some extent within the intestinal mucosa and cause gastrointestinal toxicity (particularly diarrhea) when given orally. We therefore synthesized N^4-acyl-5′-DFCR derivatives that would pass as an intact molecule through the intestine and then be converted to 5′-DFCR by hepatic acylamidase *(5)*. Among them we selected N^4-trimethoxybenzoyl-5′-DFCR (galocitabine) that generated high levels of 5-FU in tumors as did 5′-DFUR, but much lower levels of 5-FU in the intestine than those by 5′-DFUR. In the human liver, however, it was not efficiently biotransformed to 5′-DFCR because of its very low susceptibility to the acylamidase. The development of this compound was therefore terminated at the clinical phase 2 study in Japan.

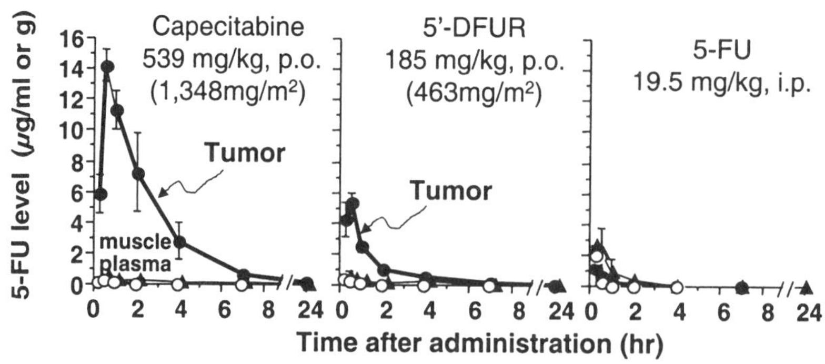

Fig. 2. Tumor-selective conversion of capecitabine to 5-FU in human colon cancer xenograft model set symbols as they appear. Capecitabine (1.5 mmol/kg, p.o.) and 5-FU (0.15 mmol/kg, ip) were given once at their MTD in multiple treatments to mice bearing the HCT116 human cancer xenograft. The averages of 5-FU concentrations in the plasma, the tumor, and the muscle, were plotted. Mean ± SD, $n=3$ per each time point. Tumor, ●; muscle, ▲, plasma, △.

2.4. N⁴-alkoxycarbonyl-5′-DFCR derivatives

We then synthesized a large series of N^4-substituted 5′-DFCR derivatives, which would be converted to 5′-DFCR by human and monkey hepatic enzymes, but not by intestinal enzymes *(20)*. In parallel, hepatic enzymes that catalyze the metabolic conversion to 5′-DFCR were investigated for rational drug design. These studies identified one particular series of 5′-DFCR derivatives, N^4-alkoxycarbonyl-5′-DFCR, which was converted to 5′-DFCR by an isozyme of the 60 kDa carboxylesterase family, which preferentially exists in the liver but not in the intestine in humans *(6)*. Among about a hundred N^4-alkoxycarbonyl-5′-DFCR derivatives synthesized, those that were chemically stable at acidic pH, susceptible to human hepatic carboxylesterase, and orally available in monkeys were selected. Capecitabine and N^4-hexyloxycarbonyl-5′-DFCR, which were moderately susceptible to the carboxylesterase (respectively, 20- and 60-fold more susceptible than galocitabine), yielded the largest AUC for 5′-DFUR in the plasma (5′-DFUR AUC four-fold higher than that by galocitabine) when given orally *(20)*. Both compounds were highly effective in human cancer xenograft models and demonstrated much less intestinal toxicity than 5′-DFUR in monkeys. Capecitabine was finally selected based on its pharmacokinetic profile in an exploratory human pharmacokinetic study.

3. TUMOR SELECTIVE DELIVERY OF THE ACTIVE 5-FU

Capecitabine selectively generates 5-FU in tumors as rationally intended. Therefore, it can be safely given at higher doses, which lead to higher 5-FU concentrations in tumors than is possible with either 5-FU or 5′-DFUR. When 5-FU (ip) was given at the maximum tolerated dose (in long-term treatment) to mice bearing the HCT116 human colon cancer xenograft, it yielded generally uniform concentrations of 5-FU in the plasma, muscle, and tumors (Fig. 2). In contrast, following the oral administration of capecitabine at equi-toxic doses, the amount of 5-FU in tumor tissue was considerably higher relative to the concentrations in the plasma or muscle: the intratumor AUCs for 5-FU were 114 to 209 greater than the plasma and muscle AUCs, respectively *(7)*. The administration of capecitabine (po) also resulted in a 5.5- to 36-fold and 2.8- to 4.3-fold higher AUC for 5-FU within tumors compared to 5-FU (ip) and 5′-DFUR (po) administrations, respectively, in four human cancer

Table 1
Antitumor Activity of Fluoropyrimidines in Human Cancer Xenografts[a]

Origin	Lines	Tumor Growth Inhibition (%) (Human cancer xenograft models) Capecitabine	5′-DFUR	5-FU	UFT
Colon	CXF280	96	77	57	66
	HCT116	101	72	39	33
	LoVo	78	61	17	52
	COLO205	61	53	35	42
	HT-29	34	22	27	46
	DLD-1	27	38	20	44
	WiDr	17	9	20	36
Gastric	GXF97	94	70	43	59
	MKN45	102	65	28	24
	MKN28	72	39	4	30
Breast	ZR-75-1	105	89	11	73
	MCF-7	77	72	9	45
	MAXF401	71	69	36	26
	MX-1	73	64	4	28
	MDA-MB-231	28	13	11	–5
Cervix	Yumoto	98	96	20	24
	ME-180	79	52	9	8
	SIHA	68	62	2	25
	HT-3	66	38	13	9
Bladder	Scaber	95	52	31	81
	T-24	5	11	1	18
Ovary	Nakajima	89	82	–16	40
	SK-OV-3	–11	4	5	–22
Prostate	PC-3	77	42	38	42
Susceptible lines (%)		18/24 (75)	15/24 (63)	1/24 (4.1)	5/24 (21)

[a] Capecitabine, 5′-DFUR, 5-FU, and UFT were administered orally at their MTD, daily or for 5 consecutive days/week, for 2–4 wk to BALB/c nu/nu mice bearing human cancer xenografts. Tumor size was measured, and tumor growth inhibition was calculated. Susceptible lines were defined as those whose growth was inhibited by more than 50%.

colon xenograft models studied (HCT116, COLO205, CXF280, and WiDr). This 5-FU generation in tumors at higher concentrations explains well why capecitabine was more effective than 5-FU in these and other tumor models (*see* subheading 4.1., Table 1) despite the fact that its active principal is the same, 5-FU. The tumor selective 5-FU delivery was later also demonstrated in a clinical pharmacodynamic study in colorectal cancer patients *(21)*.

The pharmacokinetic studies on capecitabine in patients demonstrated a rapid gastrointestinal absorption, followed by an extensive conversion into 5′-DFCR and 5′-DFUR, with only low systemic 5-FU levels as it was intended *(22)*. Among capecitabine and its metabolites, 5-FU showed the greatest level of cytotoxicity in cultures of human cancer cell lines, followed by 5′-DFUR and 5′-DFCR, whereas capecitabine showed only slight cytotoxic activity; their median IC_{50}s were 3.7, 67, > 1000, and > 1000 μ*M*, respectively (*n*=11 cell lines) *(6)*. The cytotoxic activity of 5′-DFCR was reduced by inhibitors of Cyd deaminase and dThdPase, whereas the activity of 5′-DFUR was diminished only by inhibitors of dThd-

Pase *(6)*. These results support the concept that 5′-DFCR becomes effective only after its conversion to 5′-DFUR by Cyd deaminase and then to 5-FU by dThdPase. By selectively generating high concentrations of 5-FU within tumor tissue through the noncytotoxic intermediates, capecitabine is expected to be more effective in the clinical setting than 5-FU and other fluoropyrimidines that are enzymatically activated to 5-FU in the liver, tegafur, and UFT (a fixed combination of tegafur and uracil, 1:4).

4. ANTITUMOR ACTIVITIES

4.1. *Efficacy of Capecitabine in Monotherapy*

Capecitabine is proved to be more potent and has a wider spectrum of antitumor activity than 5-FU, 5′-DFUR, or UFT against human cancer xenograft models of colon, breast, gastric, cervical, bladder, ovarian, and prostate cancer *(8)*. In these experiments, capecitabine administered orally at MTD was effective (defined as >50% growth inhibition) in 18 of 24 models (75%) and inhibited tumor growth by more than 90% in 7 models (Table 1). In contrast, 5′-DFUR was effective in 15 models (63%) and inhibited tumor growth by >90% in only one model. 5-FU and UFT were effective in one (4.1%) and five (21%) models, respectively. Neither of them inhibited the growth of any of the tumor models tested by more than 90%. Capecitabine thus showed activity against tumors that are resistant to 5-FU and UFT in vivo.

In similar experiments, capecitabine showed its antitumor activity in dose ranges much broader than those of 5-FU, 5′-DFUR, and UFT in mice bearing the human xenografts HCT116 and CXF280, which are, respectively, the intermediate and the highest level of susceptibility to fluoropyrimidines among various tumor models studied *(9)*. The therapeutic index (defined as the ratio of the lowest toxic dose to ED_{50}, the minimum dose inhibiting tumor growth by 50%) in the CXF280 model was 94 for capecitabine vs 2.7 for 5-FU when measured in the only model susceptible to 5-FU. The safety margin of capecitabine was also confirmed by comparing the ratio of the doses causing intestinal toxicity to those showing the minimum efficacy (ED_{50}) *(6)*. This ratio, measured in the HCT116 model, was 6.4 for capecitabine, compared to 1.5 for 5′-DFUR. Capecitabine was the only fluoropyrimidine demonstrating efficacy at doses associated with little or marginal myelosuppression (reduction of peripheral blood cell count) *(9)*.

4.2. *Mechanisms of Drug Sensitivity to Capecitabine*

4.2.1. Inefficient Conversion of 5′-DFUR to 5-FU by dThdPase in Tumors

The animal pharmacodynamic studies performed with human colon cancer xenografts that are either susceptible (HCT116) or refractory (WiDr) to capecitabine elucidated potential mechanisms of drug resistance *(7)*. Intratumoral concentrations of 5′-DFUR and 5-FU were measured at various times after oral administration of capecitabine. 5-FU levels in the refractory WiDr tumor were lower than those measured in the susceptible HCT116 tumor (4.8-fold lower AUC). In contrast, 5′-DFUR concentrations were higher (4.9-fold higher AUC). The molar ratio of the 5′-DFUR/5-FU AUC in the WiDr tumors was 11, as opposed to 0.47 in the susceptible xenograft (HCT116). These data suggested that 5′-DFUR is not efficiently converted to 5-FU by dThdPase in WiDr tumors, which could be the basis of drug resistance to capecitabine.

4.2.2. Increased Catabolism of 5-FU by the DPD Degradation Pathway

Another mechanism of drug resistance to capecitabine would be an increased catabolism of 5-FU by the dihydropyrimidine dehydrogenase (DPD) degradation pathway. This is one reported mechanism of 5-FU resistance *(23)*. High 5′-DFUR but low 5-FU levels were detected in the plasma after capecitabine administration *(22)*, while the efficacy of capecitabine appeared to mostly depend on the intratumoral generation of 5-FU *(7)*. Therefore, antitumor efficacy of capecitabine would mainly be affected by tumor levels of dThdPase and DPD, which, respectively, generate 5-FU from 5′-DFUR and catabolizes 5-FU to inactive molecules (Fig. 1). In preclinical studies with 24 human cancer xenograft models, tumor susceptibility to capecitabine therapy indeed correlated directly with dThdPase activity (p=0.0164) and inversely with DPD activity to some extent (p=0.125) *(8)*; however, it did not correlate with thymidylate synthase (TS) levels (unpublished data). The dThdPase/DPD ratio correlated best with the susceptibility of tumor cell lines to capecitabine (p=0.0015) *(8)*. Capecitabine retained its efficacy against tumors expressing relatively low concentrations of dThdPase, when DPD concentrations were low. In contrast, capecitabine was less effective in those tumors with higher levels of dThdPase activity associated with higher DPD levels. No similar correlation could be established between the efficacy of UFT (which is converted to 5-FU mainly in the liver) and the tumor levels of either enzyme. The correlation established for capecitabine supports the concept that its antitumor effects are mediated through 5-FU generated within tumors as opposed to 5-FU generated in peripheral tissues.

4.3. Optimization of Capecitabine Treatments

4.3.1. Rationale for Selection of Combination Partners

dThdPase is obviously the key enzyme responsible for the efficacy of capecitabine. Cell lines transfected with the human dThdPase gene became more susceptible to the intermediate metabolite 5′-DFUR *(24)*. The efficacy of capecitabine could therefore be enhanced by upregulating the expression of dThdPase. The inflammatory cytokines TNFα, IL-1α, and IFNγ were found to induce an increase in both dThdPase mRNA expression and enzyme activity in human cancer cell lines *(25)*. IFNα also enhanced dThdPase activity in human cancer cells *(26)*. Accordingly, these cytokines made tumor cells more susceptible to 5′-DFUR in cell cultures *(25)*. Moreover, some cytotoxic drugs, such as taxanes, cyclophosphamide, and mitomycin C, and X-ray irradiation also upregulated the activity of dThdPase in tumors and thereby enhanced the efficacy of capecitabine in human cancer xenograft models *(27–29)*. These cytotoxic drugs and X-ray irradiation simultaneously increased the tumor levels of human TNFα, which in turn upregulated dThdPase in the tumor cells in the cancer xenograft models. Interestingly, a similar dThdPase upregulation was not observed in the liver or intestine. The mechanism of this preferential effect on tumor tissues has not yet been fully clarified.

4.3.2. Combination Treatments with Other Agents

In combination with standard cytotoxic drugs, such as cyclophosphamide and methotrexate, cyclophosphamide and doxorubicin, taxol, taxotere, gemcitabine, and irinotecan, capecitabine was more effective than 5-FU in selected human cancer xenograft models (unpublished). The combination with capecitabine showed additive to synergistic efficacy in many xenograft models studied. Cao et al. also reported that capecitabine was also more effective than 5-FU against the human cecum cancer xenograft HCT-8 when used as a single agent or combined with leucovorin, but the efficacy potentiation was not associated with an increase in toxicity *(30)*.

4.3.3. Individualized Therapy with Capecitabine

As described in subheading 4.2.2., tumor susceptibility to capecitabine therapy correlated well with the dThdPase level and dThdPase/DPD ratio in tumor tissues. Despite a large interpatient variability of these enzyme levels, the dThdPase levels and dThdPase/DPD ratio are expected to impact on the individual drug response to capecitabine. Tumor levels of DPD are also reported to inversely correlate with the clinical response to 5-FU *(23)*. dThdPase and DPD as well as the ratio of their expression could therefore represent a promising factor for predicting efficacy with capecitabine treatment. In addition, dThdPase is identical with platelet-derived endothelial cell growth factor (PD-ECGF) with angiogenic activity *(31–33)*. dThdPase positive tumors were also reported to have poor prognosis *(34)*. However, clinical studies using adjuvant chemotherapy with doxifluridine (Furtulon®) suggested a survival benefit in those patients with high dThdPase levels *(35,36)*. A similar beneficial effect is expected with capecitabine.

5. ADDITIONAL CHARACTERISTICS OF CAPECITABINE

5.1. Antimetastatic Activity

Capecitabine and 5′-DFUR given orally were highly antimetastatic in a spontaneous metastasis model with Lewis lung carcinoma *(37)*, a highly metastatic mouse tumor, when given in the neoadjuvant setting. These drugs were only slightly more effective against the inoculated primary tumor than 5-FU in this tumor model *(9)*, whereas they were much more effective against spontaneous metastasis compared to 5-FU. Capecitabine, 5′-DFUR, and 5-FU all inhibited the formation of metastases at, respectively, 53-, 23-, and 4.4-fold lower doses than those needed for inhibiting the growth of the primary tumors. This preferential effect upon the formation of metastases was only weak for UFT and cyclophosphamide and not observed with doxorubicin, nimustine, and mitomycin C (unpublished observation).

The mechanism of this preferential effect of capecitabine and 5′-DFUR upon metastasis may stem from the upregulation of type IV collagenase, a metastatic factor, by intrinsic cytokines *(37)*. IFNγ, TNFα, and IL-1α, which are upregulators of dThdPase, increased levels of type IV collagenase by up to 12.2-fold in Lewis lung carcinoma cells, and made the tumor cells 4.6-fold more susceptible to 5′-DFUR in vitro. 5′-DFUR, but not 5-FU, induced lower levels of type IV collagenase at the primary tumor site in mice bearing Lewis lung carcinoma at low doses, which could only show antimetastatic activity. 5′-DFUR and capecitabine may selectively kill tumor cells exposed to intrinsic cytokines or other factors that upregulate dThdPase and a metastatic factor.

5.2. Anticachectic Activity

Mouse colon 26 causes progressive weight loss and physiological changes associated with cachexia when it grows to a certain size (1–2 g). Capecitabine and 5′-DFUR could reverse this progressive weight loss and improve hypoglycemia, hyperglucocorticism, and hepatic malfunctions, as well as inhibit tumor growth. This mechanism of action has not yet been clarified *(38)*. In contrast, cyclophosphamide, nimustine, and 2′-deoxy-5-fluorouridine (FUdR) were only minimally effective in reversing the weight loss. 5-FU, tegafur, cisplatin, doxorubicin, and mitomycin C were not active in this regard. Reversal of the weight loss was observed within 3 d following the administration of 5′-DFUR to cachectic mice with large tumor burdens even at doses that failed to inhibit tumor growth. The results suggest that 5′-DFUR reverses cachexia independently of its antiproliferative activity. In an additional cachexia model, mice bearing MAC-16 carcinoma, both capecitabine and 5′-DFUR reversed weight loss and lowered the proteolysis inducing factor *(39)*.

6. CONCLUSIONS

Capecitabine is a rationally designed cytotoxic drug so that it generates 5-FU preferentially within human tumors through three sequential enzymatic reactions *(6)*. The enzymes involved in the activation include a carboxylesterase isozyme located in the liver, Cyd deaminase preferentially located in the liver and many solid tumors, and dThdPase, the concentration of which is higher in tumor tissues than in healthy tissues. Capecitabine when given orally is therefore sequentially converted to 5-FU preferentially in tumors through the noncytotoxic intermediate metabolites 5′-DFCR and 5′-DFUR. Consequently, it can be safely given at higher doses, generated much higher levels of 5-FU in tumors than does 5-FU, and showed improved antitumor effects at broader dose ranges than do 5-FU, 5′-DFUR, and UFT. Capecitabine was later demonstrated to indeed given higher concentrations of 5-FU in human tumor tissues compared to adjacent healthy tissues in colon cancer patients. It has meanwhile established clinical efficacy in patients with metastatic breast and colon cancers *(21)*. The present approach for drug targeting that utilizes enzymes with unique tissue localization could also be useful for identifying new prodrugs with similarly improved efficacy and safety profiles as compared with current cytotoxic compounds.

Capecitabine, which is activated by enzymes in tumor tissues, has several unique characteristics not found in other anticancer drugs. The efficacy of capecitabine could be optimized further by selecting the most appropriate patient populations based on tumor levels of the enzymes, dThdPase and DPD, which, respectively, generate 5-FU and catabolizes it to inactive molecules. The susceptibility of tumor models to capecitabine correlated directly with dThdPase and, to some extent, inversely with DPD levels in tumors *(8)*. Retrospective clinical studies in breast and gastric cancer patients treated with 5′-DFUR (Furtulon®), the intermediate metabolite of capecitabine, also suggested that patients who had dThdPase positive primary tumors have a survival benefit from adjuvant chemotherapy with 5′-DFUR *(35,36)*. Such individualized therapy with capecitabine could further increase the antitumor efficacy of capecitabine and avoid unnecessary treatment in patients not suitable to this treatment due to low dThdPase and/or high DPD levels. Upregulating the enzyme dThdPase in tumors could also optimize the efficacy. In selected human cancer xenografts, several cytotoxic drugs, such as taxanes, and X-ray irradiation upregulated the enzyme activity in tumors and consequently enhanced the efficacy of capecitabine *(27–29)*.

Capecitabine and its intermediate metabolite 5′-DFUR demonstrated a preferential effect on pulmonary metastasis in tumor models *(9,37)* and reversed the abnormalities associated with cachexia in other tumor models *(38,39)*. Although the mechanisms of these actions have not yet been clarified, they may be associated with the characteristics of dThdPase, the enzyme essential for the bioactivation of 5′-DFUR to 5-FU. dThdPase is now known to be identical to PD-ECGF with angiogenic activity *(31–33)* and is upregulated by inflammatory cytokines, such as TNFα, IL-1α, and IFNγ *(25)*. These cytokines are often detected in tumor tissues, both in tumor cells and stromal cells, such as macrophages/monocytes. Selective effects of capecitabine and 5′-DFUR on these tumor and stromal cells exposed to the inflammatory cytokines may be associated with the antimetastatic and anticachectic activities. The low expression of Cyd deaminase, the enzyme necessary for the second step conversion of capecitabine to 5-FU, in granulocyte progenitor cells may also explain the low incidence of myelotoxicity seen in clinical trials with capecitabine. Thus, capecitabine has an efficacy and safety profile which clearly differs from that of 5-FU as a result of the unique characterization of the enzymes necessary for the conversion of capecitabine to the active component 5-FU.

REFERENCES

1. Liu G, Franssen E, Fitch MI, Warnew E. Patient preference for oral versus intravenous palliative chemotherapy. *J Clin Oncol* 1997; 15:110–115.
2. Ishitsuka H, Miwa M, Takemoto K, Fukuoka K, Itoga A, Maruyama HB. Role of uridine phosphorylase for antitumor activity of 5′-deoxy-5-fluorouridine. *Gann (Jpn J Cancer Res)* 1980; 71:112–123.

3. Bollag W, Hartmann HR. Tumor inhibitory effects of a new fluorouracil derivative: 5′-deoxy-5-fluorouridine. *Eur J Cancer* 1980; 16:427–432.
4. Uehara N, Baba H, Nitta K, et al. The therapeutic effects of orally administered 5′-deoxy-5-fluorouridine, 1-(2-tetrahydrofuryl)-5-fluorouracil and 5-fluorouracil on experimental murine tumors. *Jpn J Cancer Res* 1985; 76:1034–1041.
5. Ninomiya Y, Miwa M, Eda H, et al. Comparative antitumor activity and intestinal toxicity of 5′-deoxy-5-fluorouridine and its prodrug trimethoxy-benzoyl-5′-deoxy-fluorocytidine. *Jpn J Cancer Res* 1990; 81:188–195.
6. Miwa M, Ura M, Nishida M, et al. Design of a novel oral fluoropyrimidine carbamate, capecitabine, which generates 5-fluorouracil selectively in tumours by enzymes concentrated in human liver and cancer tissue. *Eur J Cancer* 1998; 34:1274–1281.
7. Ishikawa T, Utoh M, Sawada N, et al. Tumor selective delivery of 5-fluorouracil by capecitabine, a new oral fluoropyrimidine carbamate, in human cancer xenografts. *Biochem Pharmacol* 1998; 55:1091–1097.
8. Ishikawa T, Sekiguchi F, Fukase Y, Sawada N, Ishitsuka H. Positive correlation between the efficacy of capecitabine and doxifluridine and the ratio of thymidine phosphorylase to dihydropyrimidine dehydrogenase activities in tumors in human cancer xenografts. *Cancer Res* 1998; 58:685–690.
9. Ishikawa T, Fukase Y, Yamamoto T, Sekiguchi F, Ishitsuka H. Antitumor Activities of a Novel Fluoropyrimidine, N4-Pentyloxycarbonyl-5′-deoxy-5-fluorocytidine (Capecitabine). *Biol Pharm Bull* 1998; 21:713–717.
10. Cook AF, Holman MJ, Kramer MJ, Trown PW. Fluorinated pyrimidine nucleosides. 3. Synthesis and antitumor activity of a series of 5′-deoxy-5-fluoropyrimidine nucleosides. *J Med Chem* 1979; 22:1330–1335.
11. Kono A, Hara Y, Sugata S, Karube Y, Matsushima Y, Ishitsuka H. Activation of 5′-deoxy-5-fluorouridine by thymidine phosphorylase in human tumors. *Chem Pharm Bull* 1983; 31:175–178.
12. Suzuki S, Hongu Y, Fukazawa H, Ichihara S, Shimizu H. Tissue distribution of 5′-deoxy-5-fluorouridine and derived 5-fluorouracil in tumor-bearing mice and rats. *Gann (Jpn J Cancer Res)* 1980; 71:238–245.
13. Miwa M, Cook A, Ishitsuka H. Enzymatic cleavage of various fluorinated pyrimidine nucleosides to 5-fluorouracil and their antiproliferative activities in human and murine tumor cells. *Chem Pharm Bull* 1986; 34:4225–4232.
14. Taguchi T, Sakai K, Terasawa T, et al. Phase II study of 5′-DFUR (5′-deoxy-5-fluorouridine) by the Cooperative Study Group. *Gan To Kagaku Ryoho (Jpn)* 1985; 12:2179–2184.
15. Camiener GW, Smith CG. Studies of the enzymatic deamination of cytosine arabinoside – 1. Enzyme distribution and species specificity. *Biochem Pharmacol* 1965; 14:1405–1416.
16. Giusti G, Mangoni C, De Petrocellis B, Scarano E. Deoxycytidylate deaminase and deoxycytidine deaminase in normal and neoplastic human tissue. *Enzym Biol Clin* 1970; 11:375–383.
17. Chabner BA, Johns DG, Coleman CN, Drake JC, Evans WH. Purification and properties of cytidine deaminase from normal and leukemic granulocyte. *J Clin Invest* 1974; 53:922–931.
18. Blum JL, Jones SE, Buzdar AU, et al. Multicenter phase II study of capecitabine in paclitaxel-refractory metastatic breast cancer. *J Clin Oncol* 1999; 17:485–493.
19. Van Cutsem E, Findlay M, Osterwalder B, et al. Capecitabine, an oral fluoropyrimidine carbamate with substantial activity in advanced colorectal cancer: results of a randomized phase II study. *J Clin Oncol* 2000; 18:1337–1345.
20. Shimma N, Umeda I, Arasaki M, Murasaki C, et al. The design and synthesis of a new tumor-selective fluoropyrimidine carbamate, capecitabine. *Bioorg Med Chem* 2000; 8:1697–1706.
21. Schuller J, Cassidy J, Dumont E, et al. Preferential activation of capecitabine in tumor following oral administration to colorectal cancer patients. *Cancer Chemother Pharmacol* 2000; 45:291–297.
22. Mackean M, Planting A, Twelves C, et al. Phase I and pharmacologic study of intermittent twice-daily oral therapy with capecitabine in patients with advanced and/or metastatic cancer. *J Clin Oncol* 1998; 16:2977–2985.
23. Etienne MC, Cheradame S, Fischel JL, et al. Response to fluorouracil therapy in cancer patients: the role of tumoral dihydro-pyrimidine dehydrogenase activity. *J Clin Oncol* 1995; 13:1663–1670.
24. Haraguchi M, Furukawa T, Sumizawa T, Akiyama S. Sensitivity of human KB cells expressing platelet-derived endothelial cell growth factor to pyrimidine antimetabolites. *Cancer Res* 1993; 53:5680–5682.
25. Eda H, Fujimoto K, Watanabe S, et al. Cytokines induce thymidine phosphorylase expression in tumor cells and make them more susceptible to 5′-deoxy-5-fluorouridine. *Cancer Chemother Pharmacol* 1993; 32:333–338.
26. Tevaearai HT, Laurent PL, Suardet L, Eliason JF, Givel J-C, Odartchenko N. Interactions of interferon-alpha 2a with 5′-deoxy-fluorouridine in colorectal cancer cells in vitro. *Eur J Cancer* 1992; 28:368–372.
27. Sawada N, Ishikawa T, Fukase Y, Nishida M, Yoshikubo T, Ishitsuka H. Induction of thymidine phosphorylase activity and enhancement of capecitabine efficacy by taxol/taxotere in human cancer xenografts. *Clin Cancer Res* 1998; 4:1013–1019.
28. Endoh M, Shinbori N, Fukase Y, et al. Induction of thymidine phosphorylase expression and enhancement of efficacy of capecitabine or 5′-deoxy-5-fluorouridine by cyclophosphamide in mammary tumor models. *Int J Cancer* 1999; 83:127–134.

29. Sawada N, Ishikawa T, Sekiguchi F, Tanaka Y, Ishitsuka H. X-ray irradiation induces thymidine phosphorylase and enhances the efficacy of capecitabine (Xeloda™) in human cancer xenografts. *Clin Cancer Res* 1999; 5:2948–2953.
30. Cao S, Lu K, Ishitsuka H, Rustum YM. Antitumor efficacy of capecitabine against fluorouracil-sensitive and -resistant tumors. *Proc Am Soc Clin Oncol* 1997; 16:795.
31. Sumizawa T, Furukawa T, Haraguchi M, et al. Thymidine phosphorylase activity associated with platelet-derived endothelial cell growth factor. *J Biochem* (Tokyo) 1993; 114:9–14.
32. Moghaddam A, Zhang H-T, Fan TP, et al. Thymidine phosphorylase is angiogenic and promotes tumor growth. *Proc Natl Acad Sci USA* 1995; 92:998–1002.
33. Toi M, Hoshina S, Taniguchi T, Yamamoto Y, Ishitsuka H, Tominaga T. Expression of platelet-derived endothelial cell growth factor/thymidine phosphorylase in human breast cancer. *Int J Cancer* 1995; 64:79–82.
34. Takebayashi Y, Akiyama S, Akiba S, et al. Clinicopathologic and prognostic significance of an angiogenic factor, thymidine phosphorylase, in human colorectal carcinoma. *J Natl Cancer Inst* 1996; 88:1110–1117.
35. Toi M, Ohashi T, Takatsuka Y, et al. Selective effect of adjuvant 5′-deoxy-5-fluorouridine (5′-DFUR) treatment for thymidine phosphorylase positive tumors in primary breast cancer. *Proc Am Soc Clin Oncol* 1997;16:136a.
36. Ishii R, Takiguchi N, Oda K, Koda K, Miyazaki M. Thymidine phosphorylase expression is useful in selecting adjuvant chemotherapy for Stage III gastric cancer. *Int J Oncol* 2001;19:717–722.
37. Ishikawa T, Ura M, Yamamoto T, Tanaka Y, Ishitsuka H. Selective inhibition of spontaneous pulmonary metastasis of Lewis lung carcinoma by 5′-deoxy-5-fluorouridine. *Int J Cancer* 1995; 61:516–521.
38. Tanaka Y, Eda H, Fujimoto K, Tanaka T, Ishikawa T, Ishitsuka H. Anticachectic activity of 5′-deoxy-5-fluorouridine in a murine tumor cachexia model, colon 26 adenocarcinoma. *Cancer Res* 1990; 50:4528–4532.
39. Hussey HJ, Todorov PT, Field WN, et al. Effect of a fluorinated pyrimidine on cachexia and tumor growth in murine cachexia models. Relationship with a proteolysis inducing factor. *Br J Cancer* 2000; 83:56–62.

21 Capecitabine, A Tumor-Targeting Oral Fluoropyrimidine

Molecular Rationale and Clinical Validation

Dvorit Samid, PhD

CONTENT

1. INTRODUCTION: FLUROPYRIMIDINES IN CANCER MANAGEMENT

Fluropyrimidines have been a cornerstone in cancer management for the past five decades. The prototype pyrimidine analog, 5-fluorouracil (5-FU), interferes with pyrimidine biosynthesis and, consequently, with the synthesis and function of nucleic acids leading to tumor growth arrest and regression *(1)*. Consistent with its ubiquitous mechanism of action, 5-FU is active against a variety of solid tumors, including breast and colorectal cancer *(2,3)*. 5-FU proved effective in both the adjuvant and palliative settings when used alone or in combination with other treatment modalities (e.g., chemotherapy, radiotherapy). Owing its incomplete and unpredictable oral absorption, 5-FU must be administered by intravenous infusion, although patients prefer oral over intravenous palliative chemotherapy *(4)*. Continuous infusion of 5-FU is associated with complications due to use of indwelling vascular devices or pumps, and with severe dose-limiting gastrointestinal toxicities such as stomatitis, diarrhea, and mucosal ulceration. Myelosuppression can occur with bolus-dose regimens *(5)*. Limitations of 5-FU have prompted the development of several oral fluoropyrimidines. The first to obtain FDA's approval is capecitabine (N^4-pentyloxycarbonyl-5′-deoxy-5-fluorocytidine; Xeloda®, Roche Laboratories, Inc.) (Fig. 1).

Capecitabine is a fluropyrimidine carbamate rationally designed to generate 5-FU preferentially in tumor tissues. As such, capecitabine is not merely an oral prodrug of 5-FU, but rather a novel, tumor-targeting fluropyrimidine intended to maximize efficacy while sparing normal tissues. The unique molecular attributes of capecitabine provide the scientific rationale for its use alone and in combination with other treatment modalities. This chapter provides a brief overview of the molecular pathways, preclinical activity, and clinical experience that led to capecitabine approval for treatment of breast and colorectal cancer.

From: *Fluoropyrimidines in Cancer Therapy*
Edited by: Y. M. Rustum © Humana Press Inc., Totowa, NJ

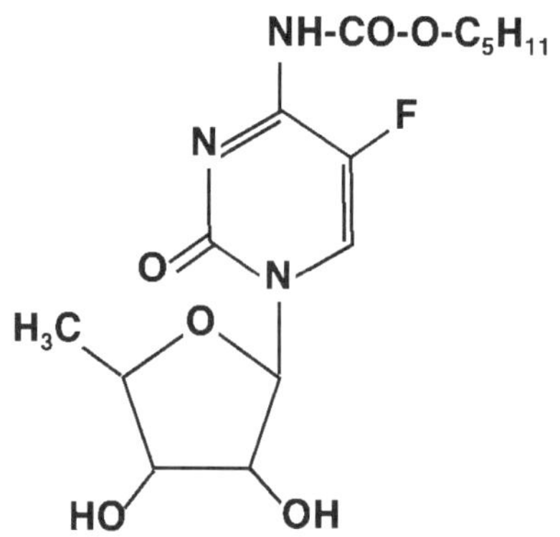

Fig. 1. Molecular structure of capecitabine (adapted from *Cancer Res,* 58, Ishikawa T, et al. Positive correlation between the efficacy of capecitabine and doxifluridine and the ratio of thymidine phosphorylase to dihydropyrimidine dehydrogenase activities in tumors in human cancer xenografts, p. 687, Copyright 1998, with permission from Elsevier Science.)

2. CAPECITABINE'S UNIQUE MOLECULAR PATHWAYS

2.1. Thymidine Phosphorylase (TP)-Mediated Conversion to 5-FU in Tumors

Capecitabine metabolism involves three enzymes: carboxylesterase, cytidine deaminase, and TP *(6)*. Carboxylesterase is almost exclusively confined to the liver and shows little variation in activity between normal and tumor tissue. Cytidine deaminase is expressed in the liver in a variety of solid tumors. TP, an enzyme with angiogenic and growth promoting properties *(7)*, shows the greatest differential expression between tumor and normal cells: Gene expression and enzyme activity are significantly higher in tumor tissues compared to surrounding normal tissue. The latter was documented in tissue samples obtained from the same patient for a range of solid tumor types, including breast, gastric, colorectal, cervical, uterine, renal, bladder, thyroid, and ovarian cancers (Fig. 2). The location of these enzymes would result in capecitabine passing intact through the gastrointestinal (GI) tract, thereby minimizing GI side effects. It would then be converted in the liver by carboxylesterase to 5′-deoxy-5-fluorocytidine (5′-dFCyd); subsequently by cytidine deaminase to 5′-deoxy-5-fluorouridine (5′-dFUrd) in the liver and tumor tissues; and finally by TP to 5-FU preferentially in tumors *(8)* (Fig. 3). Capecitabine and 5′-dFCyd have only weak cytotoxic actions at very high concentrations. Furthermore, the cytotoxicity of the interim metabolites, 5′-dFCyd and 5′-dFUrd, is suppressed by inhibitors of the enzymes that convert each to 5-FU, suggesting that the active metabolite is 5-FU.

TP-mediated activation of capecitabine results in the generation of higher 5-FU levels in tumor vs surrounding normal tissues or plasma. Indeed, tumor selectivity was demonstrated in animal models and confirmed in treated patients. Studies of mice bearing human colon cancer xenograft demonstrated that capecitabine administration results in 5-FU levels that are 114- to 209-fold higher in tumors compared to plasma, and 22-fold higher in tumors compared to muscle *(7)*. The molecular study in humans included 19 patients with colorectal cancer requiring surgical resection of their primary tumor and/or metastases. Patients received capecitabine 1250mg/m^2 twice daily for 5–7 d before surgery, and samples of tumor tissue, adjacent normal tissue, and blood were taken on the day of surgery 2–12 h after the last dose of capecitabine. The ratio of 5-FU concentration for primary tumor: healthy tissue was used as the primary marker of tumor selectivity. The concentrations of 5-FU were on average 3.2 times higher in primary colorectal tumor tissue than in adjacent healthy tissue

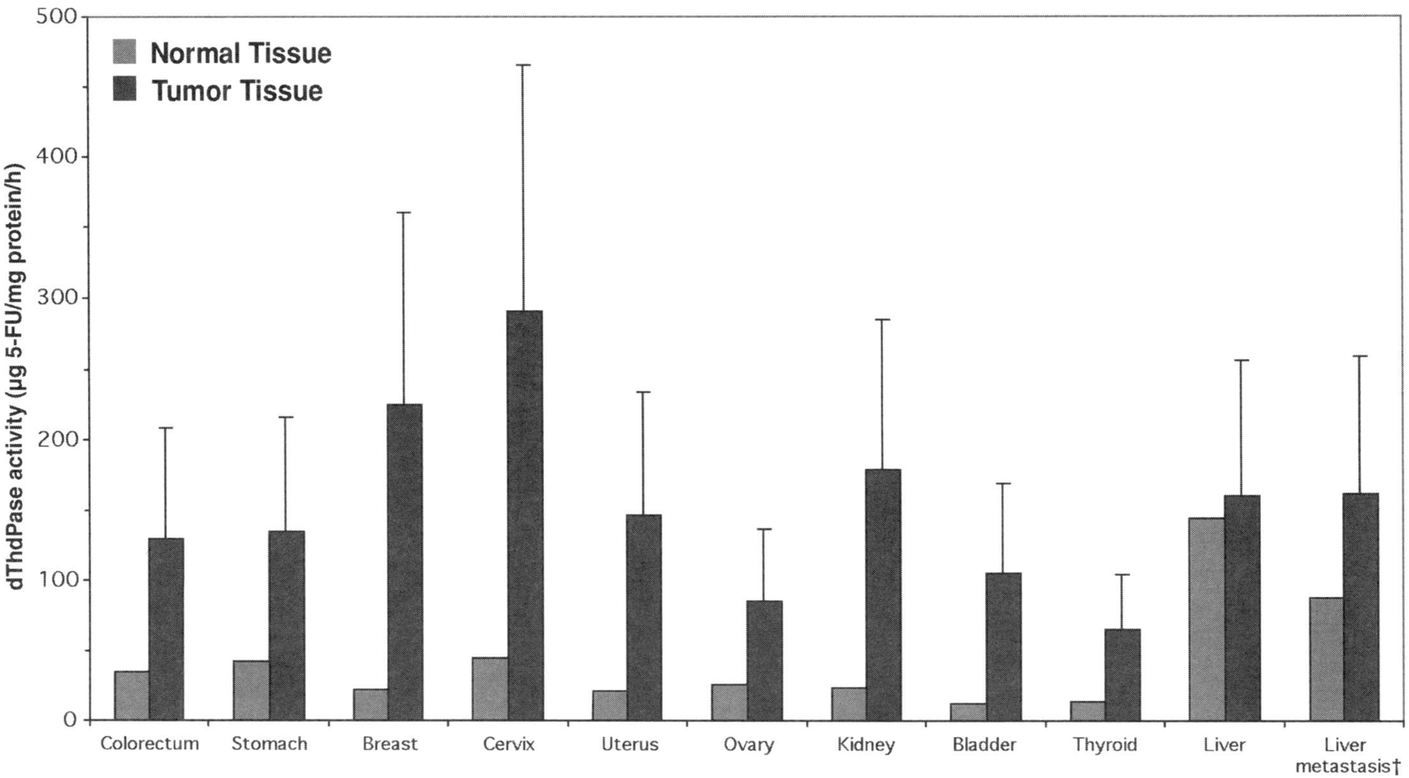

Fig. 2. Tissue distribution of thymidine phosphorylase in normal and tumor human tissue *(6)*. * $p<0.05$. † Metastasis of colorectal cancer. (Adapted from *Eur J Cancer, 34,* Miwa M, et al., Design of a novel oral fluoropyrimidine carbamate, capecitabine, which generates 5-fluorouracil selectively in tumours by enzymes concentrated in human liver and cancer tissue, p.1278, Copyright 1998, with permission from Elsevier Science.)

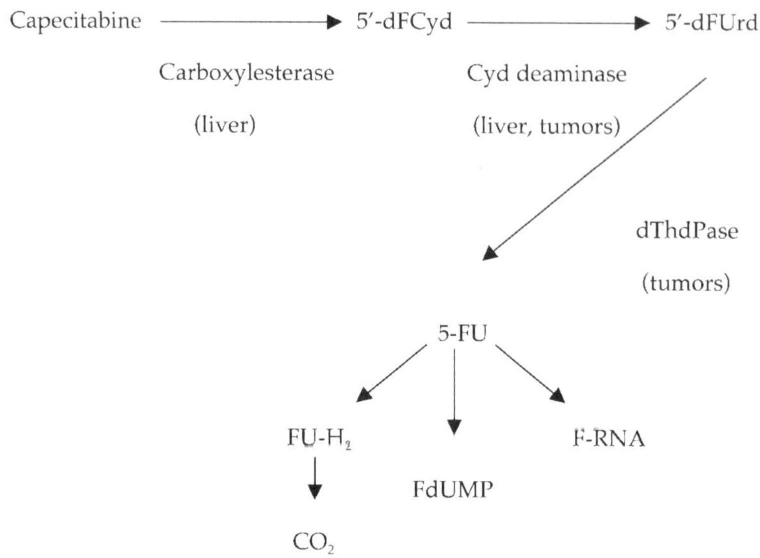

Fig. 3. Sequential metabolism of capecitabine *(6)*. (Adapted from *Eur J Cancer, 34,* Miwa M, et al., Design of a novel oral fluoropyrimidine carbamate, capecitabine, which generates 5-fluorouracil selectively in tumours by enzymes concentrated in human liver and cancer tissue, p. 1278, Copyright 1998, with permission from Elsevier Science.)

($p = 0.002$) and 21 times higher than in plasma. The results are consistent with the findings that, in colorectal tumors, TP activity was more than four times greater than in normal tissue (12.1 nmol/min/mg of protein vs 2.35 nmol/min/mg of protein, respectively). The tumor selectivity of capecitabine was compared retrospectively with that of iv 5-FU administered as either a bolus (500 mg/m^2) or continuous infusion (1000 mg/m^2 for 24 h) In contrast to capecitabine, following iv 5-FU administration the rations for 5-FU levels in tumor vs normal tissue or plasma were all close to 1, indicating lack of tumor selectivity.

The conversion of capecitabine to 5-FU is TP-mediated while 5-FU degradation is controlled by dihydropyrimidine dehydrogenase (DPD). A strong correlation was found between capecitabine's activity and the ratio of TP/DPD in tumor xenographs *(9)*. No such correlation between these biomarkers and response was detected for another oral fluoropyrimidine, uracil/tegafur (UFT), or with iv 5-FU. The correlation of TP/DPD ratio with capecitabine activity has potential implications to (a) prediction of tumor response and (b) rationale design of combination therapies. Exogenous stimuli that increase TP/DPD ratio in tumor tissues would be expected to enhance capecitabine's antitumor activity. Of interest is the fact that several antitumor therapies are capable of increasing TP expression in tumor tissues. These include taxanes (docetaxel and paclitaxel), mitomycin C, cyclophosphamide, vinblastine, cisplatin, gemcitabine, vinorelbine, and interferons. Increases of TP of 4–10-fold were observed in preclinical models within 7–8 d of treatment *(10),* and are thought to be mediated through induction of TNF-alpha. In addition to the chemotherapeutic and biological agents, radiotherapy has also been shown to enhance TP expression in tumor tissue in a number of human cancer xenografts, with single-dose irradiation resulting in a 13-fold increase in intratumoral TP activity noted within 9 d of treatment, whereas no upregulation was observed in healthy liver tissue *(11)*. TP upregulation by radiation is also thought to be mediated through induction of TNF-alpha. As would be expected, synergystic antitumor activity was documented in preclinical models when capecitabine was combined with TP-inducing chemotherapy or radiation. No such synergy was observed with iv 5-FU or oral 5-FU that does not depend on TP for conversion (e.g., UFT).

2.2. Bcl-2 Inhibition

Various agents may enhance capecitabine activity via TP upregulation, capecitabine, in turn, may improve activity of other agents (e.g., taxanes, platinum compounds, Topoisomerase inhibitors radiation) through inhibition of bcl-2, a key anti-apoptotic protein *(12–14)*. Preclincial studies documented up to 20-fold declines in bcl-2/Bax ratio expression, occurring within 1 wk of capecitabine treatment. No such effect on bcl-2 was achieved with iv 5-FU *(12)*.

What are the potential implications of bcl-2 inhibition by capecitabine? The normal physiological role of bcl-2 is to maintain microtubule integrity *(13)*; in tumor cells, bcl-2 prevents apoptosis. Taxanes, known to affect microtubule integrity, induce bcl-2 phosphorylation (which makes it inactive) with subsequent tumor apoptosis. Taxanes may not affect bcl-2 phosphorylation in cells that overexpress this protein. Using antisense technology, it was shown that inhibition of bcl-2 chemosensitizes to taxanes over and above the effects of taxane-induced phosphorylation of bcl-2 *(14)*. Therefore, capecitabine, an inhibitor of bcl-2, could significantly enhance taxane activity. This was confirmed both in preclinical models as well as in patients with breast cancer (see below). In addition to taxanes, numerous other anticancer therapies depend on effective tumor apoptosis, including platinum compounds, topoisomerase inhibitors, and radiation. Bcl-2 inhibition may be involved in capecitabine potentiation of efficacy of such treatments as well.

Taken together, the findings of capecitabine's unique molecular pathways may have important clinical implications, as they provide a strong scientific rationale for the design of new effective fluopyrimidine-based mono- and combination therapies.

3. ACTIVITY IN PRECLINICAL MODELS

3.1. Broad-Spectrum Activity with Increased Efficacy Compared to Other FPs

Capecitabine was shown to induce growth arrest and regression of human tumor xenographs of different origin, block metastatic spread, and prevent/reverse cachexia. Synergy was documented with other treatment modalities, particularly with those capable of TP upregulation, e.g., taxanes, cyclophosphamide, gemcitabine, vinorelbine, as well as with radiation *(10,11,15–18)*. Athymic mice bearing human cancer cell lines constituted the models for assessing the antitumor effects of capecitabine compared to 5-FU and other oral fluoropyrimidines, as well as the effects of capecitabine when used in combination with other chemotherapeutic agents. To assess the antimetastatic and anticachectic effects of capecitabine, athymic mice grafted with the Lewis lung carcinoma (LLC) cells or colon 26 adenocarcinoma cells were used, respectively. Effective antitumor action was defined as >50% growth inhibition. Capecitabine and the other oral fluoropyrimidines were administered orally, while 5-FU was administered through oral or peritoneal routes. Data from selected studies is reviewed below.

Ishikawa et al. studied the effects of 5-FU and various 5-FU prodrugs, including capecitabine, its intermediate metabolite, 5′-dFUrd (5′-deoxy-5-fluorouridine or doxifluridine), and UFT [comprised of 1-(2-tetrahydrofurl)-5-fluorouracil or tegafur and uracil in a 1:4 molar concentration] on tumor growth inhibition in 12 human cancer xenograft models. The latter included breast, colorectal, cervix, bladder, gastric, ovarian, and hepatoma *(8,15)*. All agents were used at their MTDs *(15)*. Capecitabine was effective in 75% (18/24) of xenograft models; it inhibited tumor growth by >90% in 29% (7/24) of the models. Doxifluridine (5′-dFUrd) was effective in 63% (15/24) of models and inhibited tumor growth by >90% in 4% (1/24) of the models. UFT was effective in 21% (5/24) of the models, while 5-FU was effective in 4.1% (1/24.) Both UFT and 5-FU inhibited tumor growth by no more than 90% *(15)* (Tables 2 and 3).

Table 1
Tumor Growth Inhibition (%) in Human Cancer Xenograft Models with Various Fluoropyrimidines *(16)*

Origin	*Cell lines*	*Capecitabine*	*5′-d FUrd*	*5-FU*	*UFT*
Colon	CXF280	96	77	57	66
	HCT116	101	72	39	33
	LoVo	78	61	17	52
	COLO205	61	53	35	42
	HT-29	34	22	27	46
	DLD-1	27	38	20	44
	WiDr	17	9	20	36
Breast	ZR-75-1	105	89	11	73
	MCF-7	77	72	9	45
	MAXF401	71	69	36	26
	MX-1	73	64	4	28
	MDA-MB-231	28	13	11	–5
Gastric	GXF97	94	70	43	59
	MKN45	102	65	28	24
	MKN28	72	39	4	30
Cervix	Yumoto	98	96	20	24
	ME-180	79	52	9	8
	SIHA	68	62	2	25
	HT-3	66	38	13	9
Bladder	Scaber	95	52	31	81
	T-24	5	11	1	18
Ovarian	Nakajima	89	82	–16	40
	SK-OV-3	–11	4	5	–22
Prostate	PC-3	77	42	38	42
Susceptible lines (%)		18/24 (75)	15/24 (63)	1/24 (4.1)	5/24 (21)

Table 2
Antitumor Actions with Capecitabine and 5-FU *(7)*

			Tumor volume change, mm³ (% tumor growth inhibition)							
			HCT116		*CXF280*		*COLO205*		*WiDr*	
Drug	*Route*	*Dose (mmol/kg/week)*	*qd × 7/week*	*qd × 5/week*	*qd × 7/week*	*qd × 5/week*	*qd × 7/week*	*qd × 5/week*	*qd × 7/week*	*qd × 5/week*
Vehicle	PO		1373	1188	1395	13	1413	1259	1373	887
Capecitabine	PO	10.5	191	–9	25	36	320	495	745	740
			(86)	(101)	(102)	(96)	(77)	(61)	(46)	(17)
5-FU	IP	1.05	1153	ND	228	ND	862	ND	907	714
			(16)		(84)		(39)		(34)	(20)
5-FU	PO	1.05	1056	728	ND	393	ND	813	927	ND
			(23)	(39)		(57)		(35)	(33)	

ND=Not done

Adapted from *Biochem Pharmacol, 55,* Ishikawa T, et al, Tumor selective delivery of 5-fluorouracil by capecitabine, a new oral fluoropyrimidine carbamate, in human cancer xenografts, p. 1093, Copyright 1998, with permission from Elsevier Science.

Table 3
Therapeutic Indices For Various Fluoropyrimidines Derived From Human HCT116 Colon Cancer and MX-1 Breast Cancer Xenografts *(6)*

	Therapeutic index			
	(TD/ED_{50})		*(TDi/ED_{50})*	
Drug	*HCT116*	*MX-1*	*HCT116*	*MX-1*
5-FU	NE	NE	NE	NE
UFT	NE	NE	NE	NE
5′-dFUrd	2.3	2.6	1.5	1.8
Capecitabine	6.4	3.4	>6.4	3.4

NE = Not effective

Adapted from *Eur J Cancer, 34,* Miwa M, et al., Design of a novel oral fluoropyrimidine carbamate, capecitabine, which generates 5-fluorouracil selectively in tumours by enzymes concentrated in human liver and cancer tissue, p. 1280, Copyright 1998, with permission from Elsevier Science.

Consistent with the increased efficacy of capecitabine over other FP's are findings of Miwa et al. who studied the effects of the same fluoropyrimidines in a human colon cancer and breast cancer xenograft model in order to determine their therapeutic indices *(6)*. Capecitabine demonstrated greater efficacy through a wider dosage range than the other fluoropyrimidines in both xenograft models. Two therapeutic indices were computed for the agents: One involving the ratio of the lethal toxic dose (TD) to the ED_{50} and the other involving the ratio of the minimum dose causing intestinal toxicity (TDi) to the ED_{50}. Both therapeutic indices were higher with capecitabine compared to the other fluoropyrimidines (*6*, and Table 3).

3.2. Antimetastatic Effect

Effect on tumor metastasis was examined using murine LLC as a model *(19)*. Both capecitabine and 5′-dFUrd demonstrated high antimetastatic activity, reducing pulmonary tumor nodules at dosages much lower than their toxic dosages *(19)*. High expression of uridine phosphorylase (a rodent gene similar to TP) may account for the antimetastatic effects of capecitabine in LLC. Inflammatory cytokines can upregulate the expression of type IV collagenase, an important factor in metastasis *(20,21)* as well as of uridine phosphorylase *(22)*. These inflammatory cytokines, known to up-regulate TP, may thus enhance the antitumor effects of capecitabine in tumor cells with high type IV collagenase activity.

3.3. Anticachectic Effect

In a study designed to assess the effects on cachexia of capecitabine, 5′-dFUrd, and 5-FU, Ishikawa et al. used a xenograft model involving mice with a large burden of colon 26 adenocarcinoma. Before administration of the fluoropyrimidines, the mice had experienced a progressive weight loss. Capecitabine as well as 5′-dFUrd but not 5-FU reversed this weight loss and improved physiological changes associated with the cachexia *(23)*. Proteolysis-inducing factor (PIF) is induced by certain tumors and is thought to contribute to the development of cachexia. Control mice bearing the murine adenocarcinomas MAC-18 and colon 26, and the human uterine carcinoma Yumoto evidenced cachexia and significant PIF levels in tumor, serum, and urine. However, those animals treated with 5′-dFUrd demonstrated an attenuation of cachexia and no evidence of PIF in tumor, serum, or urine *(23)*. Since 5′-dFUrd is a metabolite of capecitabine, it is likely that the same mechanism may be responsible for the anticachectic effects observed with capecitabine.

Table 4
Growth Inhibition with Capecitabine and 5-FU in Combination with Standard Chemotherapeutic Agents

Combination partners	*Human cancer xenografts*	*5-FU alone (%)*	*Capecitabine alone (%)*	*Partner alone (%)*	*5-FU + partner (%)*	*Capecitabine + partner (%)*
Cyclophosphamide/ Methotrexate	Breast Cancer					
	MX-1	–11	61	40	70	102
	MAXF401	52	77	48	64	89
	ZR-75-1	35	101	59	65	112
	H-62	24	61	36	50	92
	H-71	31	79	38	29	86
Cyclophosphamide/ Doxorubicin	Breast Cancer					
	MX-1	–11	61	67	104	105
	MAXF401	52	77	45	66	89
Paclitaxel	Breast Cancer					
	MX-1	14	51	109	109	109
	MAXF401	36	84	118	118	119
	ZR-75-1	1	105	93	94	125
	DU4475	–2	61	48	29	75
Docetaxel	Breast Cancer					
	MX-1	ND	38	36	ND	107
	ZR-75-1	ND	72	65	ND	111
Cisplatin	Gastric Cancer					
	MKN45	70	84	34	77	97

ND = Not Done

3.4. Antitumor Activity in 5-FU Resistant Tumors

Cao et al. studied the effects of capecitabine either alone and in combination with leucovorin in 5-FU-sensitive (ileocecal cancer line HCT-8) and 5-FU-resistant (ileocecal cancer line HCT-8/FU2h and colon cancer line C-26) tumors *(16)*.

Resistance to 5-FU was confirmed in athymic mice bearing the C-26 xenograft. Capecitabine demonstrated high antitumor activity in this xenograft model, resulting in complete tumor regression in 80% of the tumor models. Capecitabine demonstrated greater antitumor activity compared to 5-FU in the HCT-8 and HCT-8/FU2h xenografts, when both agents were used at their MTDs. Leucovorin potentiated the effects of capecitabine in HCT-8 but not in HCT-8/FU2h xenografts *(16)*.

3.5. Synergistic Activity (with TP-Inducing Drugs)

Sawada et al. studied the antitumor effects of capecitabine and other fluoropyrimidines (5′-dFUrd, UFT, and 5-FU) in combination with taxanes (paclitaxel and docetaxel) in colon cancer (WiDr) and breast cancer (MX-1) xenografts. The fluoropyrimidines were administered at their MTDs in the WiDr model, and at half their MTDs in the MX-1 model. The taxanes were administered across a range from one-eighth the MTD to the full MTD *(10)*.

In both xenograft models, the combination of capecitabine or 5′-dFUrd with either taxane resulted in synergistic activity, leading to tumor regression. The taxanes in combination with the other fluoropyrimidines resulted in additive activity (Table 4). The combination of capecitabine and either taxane did not result in increased toxicity *(19)*.

Endo et al. studied the antitumor activity of capecitabine and other oral fluoropyrimidines (5′-dFUrd and UFT) in combination with cyclophosphamide in a human breast cancer xenograft. The fluoropyrimidines were administered at 70% of their MTDs *(18)*. Cyclophosphamide in combination with either capecitabine or 5′-dFUrd demonstrated synergistic antitumor activity, resulting in tumor regression. Toxicity, as assessed by weight loss, did not appear to be synergistic with either drug combination *(18)*. Other TP-inducers including gemcitabine and vinorelbine also demonstrated synergistic activity with capecitabine.

3.6. Combination with Other Chemotherapeutic Agents

Three other studies assessed the effects of capecitabine compared to 5-FU when combined with standard chemotherapeutic agents and used in breast cancer and gastric cancer xenograft models. These agents were administered at their full MTDs or half of their MTDs. Capecitabine demonstrated greater efficacy compared to 5-FU, both as monotherapy and in combination with other chemotherapeutic agents (Table 4).

3.7. Capecitabine in Chemoradiation

Radiotherapy has been shown to upregulate TP *(11)*. In the WiDR colon and MX-1 mammary human cancer xenograft models, the combination of a single local X-ray irradiation with Xeloda was much more effective than either radiation or chemotherapy alone. In contrast, treatment with X-ray irradiation in combination with 5-FU showed no clear additive effects *(11)*.

4. CLINICAL EXPERIENCE-EARLY VALIDATION OF PRECLINICAL FINDINGS

Capecitabine is presently indicated in the United States for Breast and Colorectal Cancer, Mestastatic disease. In 1998, the drug was approved for use in anthracycline- and taxane-resistant metastatic breast cancer. The combination of capecitabine with docetaxel was subsequently approved (in 2001) for treatment of patients with metastatic breast cancer in whom anthracycline therapy has failed. That year capecitabine monotherapy was approved also as first-line treatment of metastatic colorectal cancer (CRC). The data serving as the basis for the above validate some of the hypotheses generated by the preclinical findings. Specifically, the approval as first-line treatment of metastatic CRC was based on capecitabine's superior anti-tumor activity and favorable safety profile compared to iv 5-FU/LV (Mayo regimen). The addition of capecitabine to docetaxel, a TP-inducer, offered patients with metastatic breast cancer a significant prolongation of survival compared to docetaxel alone. These and additional findings are consistent with the hypotheses generated by the pre-clinical data. Taken together, the data obtained thus far indicates that capecitabine has a broad-spectrum activity, is more active than iv 5-FU, is an attractive candidate for combination with other treatment modalities with a potential to manage tumor growth and prolong patient survival. The following is a brief review of key clinical trials with capecitabine, which served as a basis for approval in breast and colorectal cancer.

4.1. Monotherapy in Metastatic Breast Cancer—Phase II Trials

Four international phase II clinical trials were conducted to assess the therapeutic benefits of capecitabine in the setting of metastatic breast cancer. Two noncomparative trials involved patients who had failed previous treatment with paclitaxel or paclitaxel and/or docetaxel *(25,26)*. Based on the results of one of these studies *(25)*, capecitabine was approved in the United States, Switzerland, Canada, and 30 other countries for the treatment of patients with metastatic breast cancer that is either resistant to both paclitaxel and anthracycline-containing regimens or resistant to paclitaxel and further anthracycline therapy is not indicated. Capecitabine was administered in 3-wk cycles: a daily dose of 2510 mg/m^2 was given for 2 wk, followed by a 1-wk rest period. The primary endpoint was tumor response rate in patients with measurable disease. The tumor response rate was 20.0% (27/135) in one trial *(25)* and 24.6% (17/69) in the other *(26)*. These results were statistically significant according to 95% confidence intervals. Hand-foot syndrome, diarrhea, and nausea were the most common treatment-related adverse events. The majority of treatment-related side effects were rated as grade 1 (mild) or grade 2 (moderate) in intensity. Two open-label, randomized, comparative trials confirmed the benefits of using capecitabine in the setting of metastatic breast cancer *(27,28)*.

4.2. Capecitabine in Combination with Docetaxel for Metastatic Breast Cancer—Phase III Trial

Capecitabine and docetaxel show high single agent efficacy in metastatic breast cancer (mBC) and synergy in preclinical studies. An international phase III trial compared the efficacy and safety of capecitabine/docetaxel with single-agent docetaxel in anthracycline-pretreated patients with MBC. Importantly, results of the large open-label, randomized multicenter trial documented that addition of capecitabine to docetaxel results in 23% reduction in risk of death compared with docetaxel monotherapy. The study included 511 patients with metastatic breast cancer resistant to anthracycline-containing therapy or that has reoccurred after an anthracycline-based regimen. Patients were randomized to 21-d treatment cycles of either oral capecitabine 1,250 mg/m^2 twice daily, days 1–14, plus docetaxel 75 mg/m^2 day 1 (n = 255), or single-agent docetaxel 100 mg/m^2 day 1 (n = 256). After a minimum follow-up of 15 months, the combination regimen resulted in significantly superior efficacy compared with single-agent docetaxel, including objective tumor response rate (42% *v* 30%, p = .006), time to disease progression (TTP, hazard ratio = .652, p = .0001, median 6.1 *v* 4.2 months), and overall survival (hazard ratio = .775. p = .0126, median 14.5 *v* 11.5 months) Myalgia, arthralgia, and neutropenic fever/sepsis were more common with single-agent docetaxel, while there was a higher incidence of gastrointestinal side effects and hand-foot syndrome with combination therapy. The significantly superior TTP and survival achieved with the addition of capecitabine to docetaxel 75 mg/m^2 compared with single-agent docetaxel 100 mg/m^2, along with a manageable toxicity profile, indicate that this combination provides clear benefits to patients with metastatic breast cancer *(29)*. This combination is now being tested in the adjuvant and neoadjuvant settings with the aim to increase cure rate.

4.3. Monotherapy in Metastatic Colorectal Cancer Phase II and III Trials

An open-label, randomized phase II trial was conducted to evaluate the efficacy of three capecitabine drug regimens as first-line therapy in 109 patients with advanced and/or metastatic colorectal carcinoma *(30)*. The three regimens were as follows: capecitabine administered twice daily at 1331 mg/m^2/d as continuous therapy; capecitabine administered twice daily at 2510 mg/m^2/d as intermittent therapy; capecitabine administered twice daily at 1657 mg/m^2/d combined with a fixed dose of leucovorin as intermittent therapy. All three regimens demonstrated promising antitumor response activity. The intermittent regimen without leucovorin demonstrated the best results regarding time to disease progression as well as the best tolerability. This regimen was used in the subsequent phase III trials *(13)*.

Two open-label, randomized phase III trials compared capecitabine to the Mayo regimen (5-FU/leucovorin) in patients with metastatic colorectal cancer *(31,32)*. In the first trial involving 605 patients, capecitabine was associated with a 23.2% response rate compared to 15.5% for the Mayo regimen (p = 0.005). In the second trial involving 602 patients, capecitabine was associated with a 26.6% response rate compared to 17.9% with the 5-FU/leucovorin regimen ($p = 0.013$).

Because both studies had identical designs, the efficacy and safety data from both trials were pooled and analyzed *(33)*. In the pooled analysis, capecitabine was associated with a 25.5% response rate compared to 16.7% for the 5-FU/leucovorin regimen ($p \leq 0.0002$). Survival in the pooled population was equivalent in the two treatment groups. Capecitabine was associated with a significantly lower overall incidence of such common fluoropyrimidine toxicities as diarrhea, nausea, stomatitis, alopecia, and neutropenia.

5. SUMMARY AND PERSPECTIVES

Taken together, the data indicate that capecitabine is not simply a prodrug of 5-FU but rather a unique, tumor-targeting fluoropyrimidine. Its TP-mediated conversion to 5-FU at the tumor site and the generation of higher levels of 5-FU at the tumor site offer higher efficacy, broader activity, and favorable safety profiles. It also provides the rationale for combination with TP-inducers (e.g., taxanes, radiation). In addition, capecitabine's ability to block bcl-2 synthesis makes it an attractive candidate for in combination with apoptosis-dependent anti-tumor therapies (e.g., taxanes, radiation, platinum compounds). Indeed, the pre-clinical and clinical data obtained thus far indicate that capecitabine has a broad-spectrum activity, is more active than iv 5-FU, and significantly increases efficacy when added to other treatment modalities. Pivotal clinical trials led to the approval of capecitabine in the United States and Europe for front-line treatment of metastatic breast and colorectal cancer. Importantly, clinical data documented the ability of capecitabine to significantly extend patients' survival: addition of capecitabine to docetaxel in the treatment of patients with metastatic breast cancer after failure of anthracycline-containing chemotherapy results in 23% reduction in risk of death compared with docetaxel monotherapy. Clinical evaluation of the combination capecitabine and docetaxel was based on the scientific rationale of using a TP-inducer with synergic anti-tumor activity documented in pre-clinical models. The clinical experience, showing significantly superior efficacy of the combination over docetaxel alone, is consistent with the hypotheses generated by the pre-clinical data.

Moving forward, capecitabine is being evaluated in various tumor types, including those traditionally not treated with iv 5-FU. Its potential benefit is being examined both in the metastatic as well as the adjuvant and neo-adjuvant settings. Several of the ongoing and planned trials will be accompanied by molecular research aiming to identify biomarkers of clinical outcome. It is hoped that molecular correlates identified will guide future treatment design to maximize the therapeutic potential of capecitabine.

REFERENCES

1. Heidelberger C, Chaudhuari NK, Danenberg P, Mooren D, Gresbach. Fluorinated pyrimidines: a new class of tumor inhibitory compounds. *Nature* 1957; 179:663–666.
2. Meropol NK, Creaven PJ, Petrelli NJ. Metastatic colorectal cancer: advances in biochemical modulation and new drug development. *Semin Oncol* 1995; 22:509–524.
3. Bunnel CA and Winer EP. Oral 5-FU analogues in the treatment of breast cancer. *Oncology* 1998; 12(suppl 7):39–43.
4. Liu G, Franssen E, Fitch MI, Warner W. Patient preferences for oral versus intravenous palliative chemotherapy. *J Clin Oncol* 1997; 15:110–115.
5. Chabner BA, Allegra CJ, Curt GA, Calabresi P. Antineoplastic agents, in Hardman JG, Limbird LL, Molinoff PB, et al (eds): Goodman & Gilman's The Pharmacological Basis of Therapeutics. New York, NY, McGraw-Hill, 1996; 51:1233–1287.
6. Miwa M, Ura M, Nishida M, et al. Design of a novel oral fluoropyrimidine carbamate, capecitabine, which generates 5-fluorouracil selectively in tumours by enzymes concentrated in human liver and cancer tissue. *Eur J Cancer* 1998; 14:1274–1281.

7. Ishikawa T, Utoh M, Sawada N, et al. Tumor selective delivery of 5-fluorouracil by capecitabine, a new oral fluoropyrimidine carbamate, in human cancer xenografts. *Biochem Pharmacol* 1998; 55:1091–1097.
8. Modhaddam A, Zhang H-T, Fan T-P D, et al. Thymidine phosphorylase is angiogenic and promotes tumor growth. *Proc Natl Acad Sci* 1995; 92:998–1002.
9. Ishikawa T, Sekiguchi F, Fukase Y, Sawada N, Ishitsuka H. Positive correlation between the efficacy of capecitabine and doxifluridine and the ratio of thymidine phosphorylase to dihydropyrimidine dehydrogenase activities in tumors in human cancer xenografts. *Cancer Res* 1998; 58:685–690.
10. Sawada N, Ishikawa T, Fukase Y, Nishida M, Yoshikubo T, Ishitsuka H. Induction of thymidine phosphorylase activity and enhancement of capecitabine efficacy by Taxol/Taxotere in human cancer xenografts. *Clin Cancer Res* 1998; 4:1013–1019.
11. Sawada N, Ishikawa T, Sekiguchi F, Tanaka Y, Ishitsuka H. X-ray irradiation induces thymidine phosphorylase and enhances the efficacy of capecitabine (Xeloda) in human cancer xenografts. *Clin Cancer Res* 1999; 5:2948–2953.
12. Fujimoto-Ouchi K, Yasuno H, Tanaka Y. Schedule-dependency of antitumor activity in combination (Xeloda®) and docetaxel in breast cancer models. *Am Assoc Cancer Res* 2001; 42:86 (Abstract 463).
13. Haldar S, Basu A, Croce CM. Bcl2 is the guardian of microtubule integrity. *Cancer Res* 1997 Jan 15; 57(2):229–233.
14. Miayake H, Tolcher A, Gleave ME. Chemosensitization and delayed androgen-independent recurrence of prostate cancer with the use of antisense Bcl-2 oligodeoxynucleotides. *J Natl Cancer Inst* 2000; 92:34–41.
15. Ishikawa T, Fukase Y, Yamamoto T, Sekiguchi F, Ishitsuka H. Antitumor activities of a novel fluoropyrimidine, N4-pentyloxycarbonyl-5′-deoxy-5-fluorocytidine (capecitabine). *Biol Pharm Bull* 1998; 21:713–717.
16. Cao S, Lu K, Ishitsuka H, Rustum YM. Antitumor efficacy of capecitabine against fluorouracil-sensitive and -resistant tumors. *Proceedings of ASCO* 1997; 16:226a, (abstr).
17. Ishitsuka H. Capecitabine: preclinical pharmacology studies. *Invest New Drugs* 2000; 18:343–354.
18. Endo M, Shinbori N, Fukase Y, et al. Induction of thymidine phosphorylase expression and enhancement of efficacy of capecitabine or 5′-deoxy-5-fluorouridine by cyclophosphamide in mammary tumor models. *Int J Cancer* 1999; 83:127–134.
19. Ishikawa T, Ura M, Yamamoto T, Tanaka Y, Ishitsuka H. Selective inhibition of spontaneous pulmonary metstasis of Lewis lung carcinoma by 5′-deoxy-5-fluorouridine. *Int J Cancer* 1995; 61:516–521.
20. Liotta LA, Tryggvason K, Garbisa S, Hart I, Foltz CM, Shafie S. Metastatic potential correlates with enzymatic degradation of basement membrane collagen. *Nature* 1980; 284:67–68.
21. Nakajima M, Welch DR, Belloni PN, Nicolson GL. Degradation of basement membrane Type VI collagen and lung subendothelial matrix by rat mammary adenocarcinoma cell clones of differing metastatic potentials. *Cancer Res* 1987; 47:4869–4876.
22. Eda H, Fujimoto K, Watanabe S, Ura M, Hino A, Tanaka Y. Cytokines induce thymidine phosphorylase expression in tumor cells and make them more susceptible to 5′-deoxy-5-fluorouridine. *Cancer Chemother Pharmacol* 1993; 32:333–338.
23. Hussey HJ, Todorov PT, Field WN, Tanaka Y, Ishitsuka H, Tisdale MJ. Effect of a fluorinated pyrimidine on cachexia and tumour growth in murine cachexia models: relationship with a proteolysis inducing factor. *Br J Cancer* 2000; 83(1):56–62.
24. Ishikawa T, Fukase Y, Yamamoto T, Sekiguchi F, Ishitsuka H. Antitumour activities of a novel fluoropyrimidine, N4-Pentyloxycarbonyl-5-deoxy-5-fluorocytidine (capecitabine). *Biol Pharm Bull* 1998; 21:713–717.
25. Blum JL, Jones SE, Buzdar AU, et al. Multicenter phase II study of capecitabine in paclitaxel-refractory metastatic breast cancer. *J Clin Oncol* 1999; 17:485–493.
26. Blum JL, Buzdar AM, Dieras V, et al. A multicenter phase II trial of Xeloda™ (capecitabine) in taxane-refractory metastatic breast cancer (abstr). *ASCO* 1999; 18:403.
27. O'Reilly SM, Moiseyenko V, Talbot DC, Gordon RJ, Griffin T, Osterwalder. A randomized phase II study of Xeloda® (capecitabine) vs paclitaxel in breast cancer patients failing previous anthracycline therapy. *Proceedings of ASCO* 1998; 17:163a, (abstr).
28. O'Shaughnessy J, Moiseyenko V, Bell D, et al. A randomized phase II study of Xeloda® (capecitabine) vs CMF as first line chemotherapy of breast cancer in women aged≥55 years. *Proceedings of ASCO* 1998; 17:103a, (abstr).
29. O'Shaughnessy J, Miles D, Vukelja, et al. Superior survival with capecitabine plus docetaxel combination therapy in anthracycline-pretreated patients with advanced breast cancer: phase III trial results. *J Clin Oncol* 2002; 20:2812–2823.
30. Van Cutsem E, Findlay M, Osterwalder B, Kocha W, Dalley D, Pazdur R, et al. Capecitabine, an oral fluoropyrimidine carbamate with substantial activity in advanced colorectal cancer: results of a randomized phase II study. *J Clin Oncol* 2000; 18:1337–1345.

31. Hoff PM, Ansari A, Batist G, et al. Comparison of oral capecitabine versus intravenous fluorouracil plus leucovorin as first-line treatment in 605 patients with metastatic colorectal cancer: results of a randomized phase III study. *J Clin Oncol* 2001; 19(8):2282–2292.
32. Van Cutsem E, Twelves C, Cassidy J, et al. Oral capecitabine compared with intravenous 5-fluorouracil plus leucovorin (Mayo Clinic regimen) in patients with metastatic colorectal cancer: results of a large phase III study. *J Clin Oncol* 2001; 19:4097–4106.
33. Hoff P, et al. Capecitabine as 1st-line treatment for metastatic colorectal cancer: integrated results of 1207 patients from 2 randomized, phase III studies (abstr). *ESMO* 2000.

22 Capecitabine
A Rationally Developed Anticancer Drug

Daniel R. Budman, MD, FACP

CONTENTS

1. INTRODUCTION

The development of new anticancer agents has recently undergone a paradigm shift with greater understanding of the biologic processes involved in cell growth and the malignant phenotype. As a result, target-specific therapy has become the goal of drug design. The target can be a given organ, the tumor, the surrounding stroma, a given receptor, an enzyme, or a cellular pathway. The obvious goal of such an approach is to make the anticancer agent more selective and less toxic to the host with the goal of enhanced therapeutic effect. This approach may involve modification of an existing agent or the selection of new drugs through combinatorial chemistry or computer-aided design.

Modification of an existing agent, termed "retrometabolic drug design" *(1),* is an attractive approach to tumor targeting as it involves changing an effective agent into a prodrug, which is then activated at the target site by overexpression of enzymes by the target. Ideally, the prodrug would have little biologic activity on its own and would be selectively converted to the cytotoxic agent only at the tumor site. In addition, the resulting cytotoxic agent should have little systemic effects because drug concentration occurs mainly in the tumor. In clinical practice, this approach is not always evident with such a selective agent, perhaps because of the methods by which the dosage for further clinical development is chosen on the basis of phase I studies, which emphasize determining the dose range that demonstrates toxicity in the host.

This chapter describes the results of rationally "re-engineering" a fluoropyrimidine to a prodrug that takes advantage of tumor-selective expression of metabolic enzymes to target the disease and improve the therapeutic index of these agents.

From: *Fluoropyrimidines in Cancer Therapy*
Edited by: Y. M. Rustum

2. PRECLINCAL MODEL SYSTEMS

2.1. The First Attempt at Design of a Targeted Fluoropyrimidine—5′-DFUR

With the initial description of 5-fluorouracil (5-FU) dating back to 1957 *(2)*, the fluoropyrimidines are one of the oldest classes of cytotoxic agents studied in patients. However, drugs of this class have been limited by poor oral absorption, schedule-dependent effects on tumor, and no evidence of localization of the cytotoxic agent in tumor tissue compared to nonmalignant tissue. Prolonged infusions of 5-FU have been used clinically with some benefit, but are associated with marked intrapatient and interpatient variation in plasma levels, which may add to host toxicity *(3)*.

Overexpression of the enzyme pyrimidine nucleoside phosphorylase (thymidine phosphorylase in humans) was known to occur in many tumors and is also associated with the angiogenic phenotype *(4)*. Hence, this selective overexpression offers a potential approach to target tumor tissue by developing an agent that requires this enzyme for activation. In human primary breast tumors, 47% overexpressed this enzyme with 61% also showing expression of the enzyme in surrounding endothelial cells *(5)*. The initial attempt to target tumor tissue with this approach was the synthesis of the prodrug 5′-deoxy-5-fluorouridine (5′-DFUR) *(6)*. Initial studies suggested that this prodrug was not activated by bone marrow cells *(7)*, utilized the target enzyme for activation *(8)*, and generated higher levels of the cytotoxic metabolite 5-FU in tumor tissue than normal tissue *(9)*. As proof of principle, 5′-DFUR demonstrated a wide therapeutic index in murine model systems with marked superiority to 5-FU as an antitumor agent *(10)*. In a Lewis lung cancer murine system, 5′-DFUR inhibited pulmonary metastases at dosages 17-to 46-fold lower than the concentration needed to inhibit the primary tumor *(11)*. However, clinical trials of oral 5′-DFUR were limited by the unexpected appearance of dose-related diarrhea thus implying that tumor selectivity of activation was not achieved in man *(12)*. Further investigations have confirmed that thymidine phosphorylase is found in human intestinal tissue and thus is responsible for the conversion of 5′-DFUR to 5-FU in humans associated with toxicity *(13)*.

2.2. The Second Attempt to Achieve Tumor Selectivity—Capecitabine

An intensive search of enzymatic systems that are preferentially expressed in certain human organs lead to the findings of carboxyl esterase expressed in liver and hepatomas, cytidine deaminase in liver and many solid tumors, and reconfirmed the expression of thymidine phosphorylase in many tumors *(14)*. The differences in enzymatic expression can be from 10-to 80-fold in various tissues *(14)*. Hence, 5′-DFUR was "reversed engineered" to take advantage of the differential enzymatic expression in tissue with the hope of producing a relatively nontoxic prodrug. The goal of this approach was to develop an agent that would then be orally absorbed and converted in a variety of metabolic steps in normal organs to 5′-DFUR. The 5′-DFUR would then be activated to 5-FU in tumor tissue but less so in normal tissue. Capecitabine ((N-[1-(5-deoxy-β-D-ribofuranosyl)–5-fluoro-1,2,-dihydro–2-oxo–4-pyrimidiny1]–n-penty1–carbamate)) was the result of this effort (Fig. 1). This agent could be administered orally, would be inactive as a cytotoxic agent in intestinal tissue, absorbed, undergo metabolic conversion by carboxyl esterase in the liver, followed by deamination by cytidine deaminase, result in low systemic levels of 5′-DFUR, and then be activated by thymidine phosphorylase in tumor tissue (Fig. 2).

This approach has been validated in model systems as both capecitabine and the first metabolite of capecitabine (5′-DFCR, 5′-deoxy-5-fluorocytidine) are minimally cytotoxic *(14)*. In human xenograft systems, capecitabine treatment resulted in 5-FU concentrations

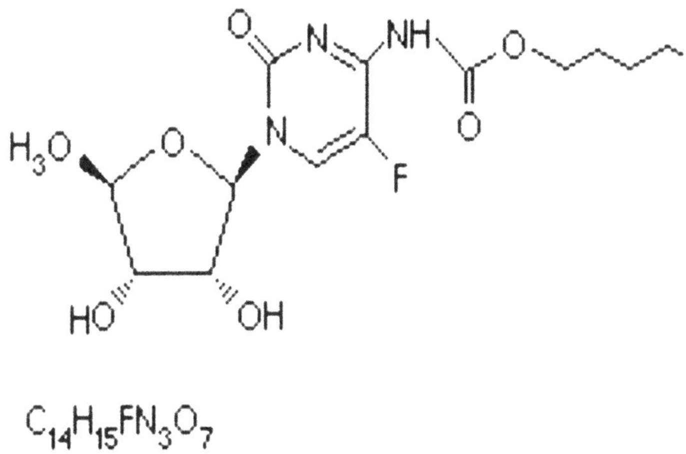

Fig. 1. Capecitabine.

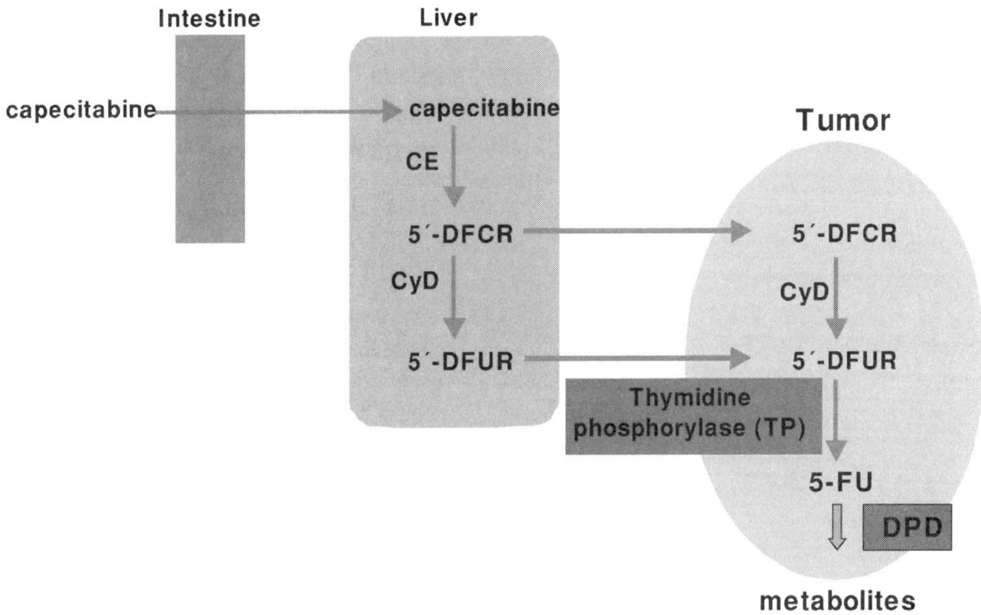

Fig. 2. Capecitabine's metabolic pathway in vivo.
5′DFCR = 5′-deoxy-5-fluorocytidine; 5′-DFUR = 5′-deoxy-5-fluorouridine; CyD = cytidine deaminase; CE = carboxylesterase.
DPD = dihydropyrimidine dehydrogenase.

over time that were 114–209-fold higher in tumor tissue than in plasma and offered a 20-fold advantage over 5-FU *(15)*. Capecitabine is more active in murine model systems than is either 5-FU or uracil with tegafur (UFT). The fluoropyrimidine-resistant WiDr tumor revealed poor conversion of the prodrug to 5-FU indicating one mechanism of resistance to this agent *(15)*. Additional mechanisms of resistance to capecitabine include enhanced degradation of drug in the tumor environs by the 5-FU metabolizing enzyme dihydropyrimidine dehydrogenase (DPD) *(16)*. The ratio of thymidine phosphorylase activity with DPD activity has been suggested as an index of whether or not a given tumor would be sensitive to capecitabine or 5′-DFUR *(16)*. These findings have potential clinical implications: determination of the amount of thymidine phosphorylase and DPD present in a tumor may prognosticate whether or not a patient will respond to capecitabine. Preliminary studies of this approach in human gastric cancer using an immunoperoxidase assay has suggested that the chance of response to 5′-DFUR corresponds to the degree of positive reaction of the assay for thymidine phosphorylase *(17)*. Japanese investigators have examined the ratio of thymidine phosphorylase to DPD in 241 human tumor tissue samples using an ELISA assay *(18)*. The ratio of these two enzymes was highest in esophageal, cervical, breast, pancreatic carcinomas, and hepatomas thus suggesting that these tumors should be clinically evaluated with capecitabine *(18)*.

2.3. Methods to Enhance Capecitabine Effect

Methods that increase expression of thymidine phosphorylase in either the tumor or the tumor-associated blood vessels would be expected to lead, after capecitabine treatment, to enhanced generation of cytotoxic metabolites in the tumor. Obviously, if DPD is also enhanced, there may be no gain in therapeutic index. Using the murine xenograft model of colon cancer, WiDr (a human cell line), investigators have demonstrated upregulation of thymidine phosphorylase in tumor tissue by prior exposure to docetaxel, paclitaxel, mitomycin C *(19)*, radiation *(20)*, and in Colo 205 tumors with interferon gamma *(21)*. These effects were accompanied by an increased therapeutic effect by capecitabine but not with 5-FU. Oral treatment with cyclophosphamide upregulated thymidine phosphorylase in human breast cancer xenografts without affecting normal tissue or enhancing DPD levels *(22)*. These effects seemed to be indirect and were associated with increased levels of human tumor necrosis alpha *(19)*. Inflammatory cytokines have also been noted to upregulate thymidine phosphorylase *(23, 24)*. In a human cancer xenograft system, irradiation of the animal upregulated the expression of thymidine phosphorylase in the tumor but not the host liver *(20)*. In the WiDr colon and MX-1 mammary xenograft model, radiation therapy combined with capecitabine was more effective than either modality alone suggesting another pathway for clinical evaluation *(20)*.

Initial data in humans of this approach to enhance the effect of capecitabine remains scanty and is just being reported. Eight patients with advanced breast cancer underwent biopsies of their tumors before and after treatment with docetaxel at 60 mg/m^2 for three cycles. Six of the patients demonstrated a significant enhancement in tumor expression of thymidine phosphorylase after taxane treatment *(25)*.

3. PHASE I STUDIES

As a single agent, capecitabine has been studied on three schedules in humans:

1. Continuous oral twice a day dosing *(26)*.
2. Oral twice a day dosing for 14 d with a 7-d rest period before restarting treatment *(27)*.
3. A fixed 60 mg dose of oral leucovorin with either the continuous or intermittent capecitabine schedule *(28)*.

In addition, a small pilot study of oral divided dose for 10 d has been reported *(29)*. The drug was administered within 30 min of a meal. On the continuous schedule, the maximum tolerated total dose was 1667 mg/m^2 per day with dose-limiting toxicities of hand-foot syndrome, abdominal pain, nausea/vomiting, diarrhea, and thrombocytopenia. Transient liver function abnormalities were also seen in approximately one-fifth of patients. The toxicities reversed upon discontinuance of treatment. Suggested phase II total dosing was 1331 mg/m^2 per day *(26)*. On the intermittent schedule, dose-limiting toxicity was seen at a total daily dose of 3000 mg/m^2 or greater with suggested phase II dosing of 2510 mg/m^2 and similar

Table 1
Phase I Trials in Combination with Other Agents

Second drug	*Second agent schedule*	*Phase II dose second agent Capecitabine (per day)*	*Reference*
Docetaxel Epirubicin	IV every 3 wk	75; 75 mg/m2 985 mg/m2	31
gemcitabine	IV Days 1 & 8	1000 mg/m2 1300 mg/m2	32
interferon	TIW sc	3MU 2000	37
Oxaliplatin	IV every 3 wk	130 mg/m2 2000 mg/m2	34
Paclitaxel	3-h infusion every 3 wk	175 mg/m2 1331 mg/m2	36
Paclitaxel	Weekly	60 mg/m2 2000 mg/m2	35

toxicities *(27)*. Recent reports of this intermittent schedule have suggested that a dose of 2000 mg/m^2 per day can be administered in patients with breast cancer with less toxicity and no loss of efficacy *(30, 31)*. The third trial with leucovorin established a phase II total daily dose of 1650 mg/m^2 with 60 mg of leucovorin *(28)*. Hand-foot syndrome is a common toxicity with this agent and usually occurs within the first two cycles of treatment *(32)*.

Phase I studies of capecitabine in combination with a variety of agents have been reported (Table 1). The majority of studies have noted toxicities either previously seen with capecitabine or with the second agent. A phase I study of this agent combined with docetaxel and epirubicin in untreated breast cancer patients with dose-limiting effects of nausea, vomiting, diarrhea, and leukopenia. Phase II capecitabine daily dosage in this triplet combination was 985 mg/m^2 per day *(33)*. A recent update of this triplet (administering docetaxel and epirubicin once every 3 wk) has noted an objective response rate of 91% in patients with metastatic breast cancer *(34)*. Combined with gemcitabine, given as a fixed dose of 1000 mg/m^2 on d 1 and 8 with capecitabine given daily for 14 d, dose-limiting toxicity was seen at 1600 mg/m^2 per day of capecitabine with a high response rate (33% PR) in inoperable pancreatic cancer *(35)*. Capecitabine as a 14-d treatment combined with irinotecan given as a weekly infusion has been shown to be feasible but has not reached maximum tolerate dosage *(36)*. Combined with oxaliplatin given as an intravenous infusion once every 3 wk and 14 d of capecitabine, dose-limiting toxicity as manifested by diarrhea was seen at dosages of 130 mg/m^2 and 2500 mg/m^2, respectively *(37)*. The drug has been studied in combination with either weekly paclitaxel *(38)* or once every 3 wk paclitaxel *(39)* with reversible neutropenia and cumulative diarrhea noted. Weekly docetaxel (36 mg/m^2) has been combined with capecitabine given daily (1250 mg/m^2 per day) from d 5 to 18 on a 21-d cycle with significant antitumor activity noted *(40)*. As with older fluoropyrimidines, capecitabine has also been combined with interferon *(41)*.

4. CLINICAL PHARMACOLOGY

Pharmacokinetic studies in the early phase I trials revealed that capecitabine is extensively metabolized in humans into 5′-DFCR and subsequently into 5′-DFUR. Systemic exposures to 5′-DFUR are approx 20-fold higher than the levels of 5-FU in the continuous dosing schedule *(26)* and 12-fold higher in the intermittent schedule *(27)*. Dose linear effects were seen over the dosing range studied with peak serum levels of parent drug seen within 1–2 h of ingestion. A recent study of ^{14} C-labeled capecitabine in six patients revealed a mean of 95.5% of label recovered in the urine with 84% recovered within the first 12 h *(42)*. Absorption was rapid and almost complete in this small sample size. A small trial of this agent in patients with hepatic dysfunction noted that although capecitabine levels increased 48% above patients without dysfunction, the levels of 5′-DFUR, 5-fluorouracil, and the metabolite α-fluoro-β-alanine (FBAL) were not significantly changed *(43)*.

The effect of concurrent administration of capecitabine with food revealed higher peak plasma concentration levels and shorter time to maximum peak plasma concentration for capecitabine, 5′-DFCR, 5′-DFUR, and 5-FU when given in a fasting state. However, there was little effect on the area under the plasma curve for 5′-DFUR implying that efficacy should not be compromised if the patient does not receive this agent in a fasting state *(44)*. Antacids do not affect absorption of this agent *(45)*, but the administration of warfarin with this agent should be avoided as it will increase the level of anticoagulation. Similar effects have been noted with 5-FU given with warfarin *(46)*.

The level of fluoropyrimidines in tumor tissue after administration of capecitabine has been studied in 19 patients with colorectal carcinoma. The patients received capecitabine at 1255 mg/m^2 per day for 5–7 d prior to surgery. At the time of surgical resection, the 5-FU concentrations in tumor and adjacent normal tissue were determined. A fourfold higher concentration of 5-FU was found in the tumor tissue validating the rational design of this drug *(47)*.

5. PHASE II–III STUDIES

Capecitabine was approved in the United States for the treatment of refractory breast cancer based on efficacy in a large phase II trial. The intermittent schedule was chosen for this study based on suggestions of a longer duration of response compared to the other phase I schedules in patients with colorectal carcinoma *(48)*. In the breast cancer phase II trial, entry requirements mandated that study subjects had to fail at least two but not more than three prior chemotherapeutic regimens. One of the treatment regimens had to contain paclitaxel. Of the 162 evaluable patients, the overall response rate was 20% (95% confidence limits 14–28%) with a median response duration of 8.1 mo. Grade 3–4 toxicities included hand-foot syndrome and diarrhea in approx 10% of patients *(49)*. As previously noted, a retrospective analysis suggested that efficacy could be maintained at a lower dosage of capecitabine, 2000 mg/m^2 per day, with less toxicity *(30)*.

The experience in colorectal carcinoma with this agent has also been positive. In the randomized phase II trial of this agent, patients were not allowed to have previous cytotoxic therapy except in the adjuvant setting. Patients were randomized to a continuous dosing schedule, intermittent, or intermittent with daily leucovorin. The overall response rate varied from 21% to 24% per arm with more toxicity in the arm receiving leucovorin *(48)*. Hence, the intermittent schedule was advanced to phase III studies in colorectal cancer.

Two large phase III trials in untreated, metastatic colorectal carcinoma have been reported in abstract form *(50,51)*. Both trials were international in scope with the SO14796 study involving Europe and Asia while the other study involved both North and South America. In both trials, identical entry criteria, response criteria, and treatment schedules were employed with a total of 1207 patients enrolled. Classical dosing of daily capecitabine for 14 d every 3 wk was compared to the "Mayo Clinic" regimen of 5-FU with leucovorin given for 5 d every month. Tumor response was evaluated every 6 wk after entry onto treatment. The combined

Table 2
Overall Response Rate of the Two Phase III Colorectal Carcinoma Trials

Response	*Capecitabine* *(n = 603)*	*5-FU/leucovorin* *(n = 604)*	
Investigator evaluated: PR + CR (%)	25.7	16.7	$p<0.001$
Stable disease	47.8	52.2	
Independent review: PR + CR (%)	22.4	13.2	$p<0.001$
stable disease	52.9	57.6	

results of the North American and international trials are shown in Table 2. Capecitabine at 2500 mg/m^2 per day was statistically equivalent to the older regimen with less leukopenia or hospitalizations. An independent review committee also measured response and toxicity. Capecitabine resulted in 14% serious adverse events (life threatening or leading to hospitalization) compared to 21% for 5-Fu with leucovorin. The results of these two studies imply that capecitabine can be substituted for 5-Fu/leucovorin as primary chemotherapy treatment for patients with metastatic colorectal carcinoma.

As a result, capecitabine is also being evaluated in other combination therapies for treatment of metastatic colorectal carcinoma. Large clinical trials with capecitabine combined with either irinotecan or oxaliplatin are awaited based on activity in the phase I studies *(36,37)*. Capecitabine has not been shown to have antitumor activity in colorectal carcinoma patients who have previously failed 5-FU *(52)*. Early phase II results have seen evidence of efficacy in advanced pancreatic carcinoma *(53)* and occasional responses in hepatocellular carcinoma *(54)*.

This drug has also demonstrated phase II activity in unresectable renal cell carcinoma with one patient having a partial response (8%) as third line treatment and 10 patients (83%) demonstrating disease stability after progressing on interferon treatment *(55)*. As metastatic renal cell carcinoma is a particularly drug-resistant tumor, the above results have led to capecitabine being combined with human interferon alpha 2a, recombinant human interleukin-2, and oral 13-*cis* retinoic acid. The combination resulted in two (7%) complete remissions and eight partial remissions (27%) with a median duration of response exceeding 8 mo. An additional 40% of the study patients had evidence of disease stability *(56)*. These interesting findings in which the cytokines may have both a direct effect on the tumor and perhaps an indirect effect by elevating thymidine phosphorylase levels needs to be confirmed.

6. Conclusions

Capecitabine represents a new approach of engineering a delivery system to bring the cytotoxic agent into contact with tumor tissue with the hope of lessening host toxicity. As such, the drug serves as a paradigm for anticancer drug development of future cytotoxics agents. Currently, this agent has shown activity in human tumors that have been previously demonstrated to respond to fluoropyrimidines. As capecitabine can be administered by the oral route and toxicity is manageable, the drug offers the convenience of oral dosing and the potential flexibility of many schedules of administration. The divided daily dose for 14 d every 3 wk has been best studied to date.

Methods to determine which patient will respond to this agent remain in early evaluation but include the potential of looking at intratumoral expression of both thymidine phosphorylase and DPD as a predictor of response. This drug offers potential synergy with radiation therapy and is now being added to conventional cytotoxic agents in the hope of improving the treatment of human malignancy.

REFERENCES

1. Bodor N, Buchwald P, Huang H-J. Computer-assisted design of new drugs based upon retrometabolic concepts. *SAR and QSAR in environmental research* 8. Amsterdam, Overseas Publishers Association, 1998; 41–92.
2. Heidelberger C. Fluorinated pyrimidines: A new class of tumor-inhibitory compounds. *Nature* 1957; 179:663–666.
3. Takimoto C, Yee L, Venzon D, et al. High inter- and intrapatient variation in 5-fluorouracil plasma concentrations during a prolonged drug infusion. *Clin Cancer Res* 1999; 5:1347–1352.
4. Moghaddam A, Zhang HT, Fan TP, et al. Thymidine phosphorylase is angiogenic and promotes tumor growth. *Proc Natl Acad Sci USA* 1995; 92:998–1002.
5. Fox SB, Westwood M, Moghaddam A, et al. The angiogenic factor platelet-derived endothelial cell growth factor/thymidine phosphorylase is up-regulated in breast cancer epithelium and endothelium. *Br J Cancer* 1996; 73:275–80.
6. Cook A, Holman M, Krammer M, Trown P. Fluorinated pyrimidine nucleotides. 3. Synthesis and antitumor activity of a series of 5′-deoxy-5-fluoropymidine nucleotides. *J Med Chem* 1979; 22:1330–1335.
7. Bollag W, Hartmann H. Tumor inhibitory effects of a new fluorouracil derivative: 5′- deoxy-5-fluorouridine. *Eur J Cancer* 1980; 16:427–432.
8. Ishitsuka H, Miwa M, Takemoto K, Fukuoka K, Itoga A, Maruyama H. Role of uridine phosphorylase for antitumor activity of 5′-deoxy-5 fluorouridine. *Gann* 1980; 71:112–123.
9. Suzuki S, Hongu Y, Fukazawa H, Ichihara S, Shimizu H. Tissue distribution of 5′-deoxy-5- fluorouridine and derived 5-fluorouracil in tumor bearing mice and rats. *Gann* 1980; 71:238–245.
10. De Cesare M, Pratesi G, De Braud F, Zuninno F, Stampino C. Remarkable antitumor activity of 5′-deoxy-5-fluorouridine in human colorectal xenografts. *Anticancer Res* 1994; 14:549
11. Ishikawa T, Ura M, Yamamoto T, Tanaka Y, Ishitsuka H. Selective inhibition of spontaneous pulmonary metastasis of Lewis lung carcinoma by 5′-deoxyfluorouridine. *Int J Cancer* 1995; 61:516–521.
12. Budman DR, Lichtman S. Investigational Drugs. In *The Chemotherapy Sourcebook* (Perry. M, ed.). Baltimore, Williams & Wilkins, 1996; 479–558.
13. Ninomiya Y, Miwa M, Eda H, et al. Comparative antitumor activity and intestinal toxicity of 5′-deoxy-5-fluoroуradine and its prodrug trimethoxybenzoyl-5′-deoxyflourocytidine. *Jpn Cancer Res* 1990; 81:188–195.
14. Miwa M, Ura M, Nishida M, et al. Design of a novel oral fluoropyrimidine carbamate, capecitabine, which generates 5-fluorouracil selectively in tumours by enzymes concentrated in human liver and cancer tissue. *Eur J Cancer* 1998; 34:1274–81.
15. Ishikawa T, Utoh M, Sawada N, et al. Tumor selective delivery of 5-fluorouracil by capecitabine, a new oral fluoropyrimidine carbamate, in human cancer xenografts. *Biochem Pharmacol* 1998; 55:1091–1097.
16. Ishikawa T, Sekiguchi F, Fukase Y, Sawada N, Ishitsuka H. Positive correlation between the efficacy of capecitabine and doxifluridine and the ratio of thymidine phosphorylase to dihydropyrimidine dehydrogenase activities in tumors in human cancer xenografts. *Cancer Res* 1998; 58:685–690.
17. Koizumi W, Saigenji K, Nakamaru N, Okayasu I, Kurihara M. Prediction of response to 5′-deoxy-5-fluorouridine (5′-DFUR) in patients with inoperable advanced gastric cancer by immunostaining of thymidine phosphorylase/platelet phosphorylase/platelet-derived endothelial cell growth factor. *Oncology* 1999; 56:215–222.
18. Mori K, Hasegawa M, Nishida M, et al. Expression levels of thymidine phosphorylase and dihydropyrimidine dehydrogenase in various human tumor tissues. *Int J Oncol* 2000; 17:33–38.
19. Sawada N, Ishikawa T, Fukase Y, Nishida M, Yoshikubo T, Ishitsuka H. Induction of thymidine phosphorylase activity and enhancement of capecitabine efficacy by taxol/taxotere in human cancer xenografts. *Clin Cancer Res* 1998; 4:1013–1019.
20. Sawada N, Ishikawa T, Sekiguchi F, Tanaka Y, Ishitsuka H. X-ray irradiation induces thymidine phosphorylase and enhances the efficacy of capecitabine (Xeloda) in human cancer xenografts. *Clin Cancer Res* 1999; 5:2948–2953.
21. Ishitsuka H, Ishikawa T, Fukase Y, Sawada N, Tanaka Y, Ouchi K, Yoshikubo T, Nishida M. Capecitabine and the dThdPase upregulators IFNgamma or Taxol showed synergistic activity in human cancer xenografts (Meeting abstract). *Proc Annu Meet Am Assoc Cancer Res* 1996; 37:2766a.
22. Endo M, Shinbori N, Fukase Y, Sawada N, Ishikawa T, Tanaka Y. Induction of thymidine phosphorylase expression and enhancement of efficacy of capecitabine or 5′-deoxy-5-fluorouridine by cyclophosphamide in mammary tumor models. *Int J Cancer* 1999; 83:127–134.

23. Eda H, Fujimoto K, Watanabe S, et al. Cytokines induce thymidine phosphorylase expression in tumor cells and make them more susceptible to 5′-deoxy-5-fluorouridine. *Cancer Chemother Pharmacol* 1993; 32:333–338.
24. Makower D, Wadler S, Haynes H, Schwartz EL. Interferon induces thymidine phosphorylase/platelet-derived endothelial cell growth factor expression in vivo. *Clin Cancer Res* 1997; 3:923–929.
25. Kurosumi M, Tabei T, Suemasus K, et al. Enhancement of immunohistochemical reactivity for thymidine phosphorylase in breast cancer cells after administration of docetaxel as neoadjuvant chemotherapy in advanced patients. *Oncol Rep* 2000; 7:945–948.
26. Budman DR, Meropol NJ, Reigner B, et al. Preliminary studies of a novel oral fluoropyrimidine carbamate: capecitabine. *J Clin Oncol* 1998; 16:1795–1802.
27. Mackean M, Planting A, Twelves C, et al. Phase I and pharmacologic study of intermittent twice-daily oral therapy with capecitabine in patients with advanced and/or metastatic cancer. *J Clin Oncol* 1998; 16:2977–2985.
28 Cassidy J, Dirix L, Bissett D, et al. A Phase I study of capecitabine in combination with oral leucovorin in patients with intractable solid tumors. *Clin Cancer Res* 1998; 4:2755–2761.
29. Bajetta E, Carnaghi C, Somma L, Stampino CG. A pilot safety study of capecitabine, a new oral fluoropyrimidine, in patients with advanced neoplastic disease. *Tumori* 1996; 82:450–452.
30. O'Shaughnessy J, Blum J. A retrospective evaluation of the impact of dose reduction in patients treated with Xeloda (capecitabine). *Proc Annu Meet Am Soc Clin Oncol* 2000; 19:400a.
31. Michaud L, Gauthier M, Woodlot J, et al. Improved therapeutic index with lower dose capecitabine in metastatic breast cancer. *Proc Annu Meet Am Soc Clin Oncol* 2000; 19:402a.
32. Abushullaih S, Saad E, Hoff P. Characterizing hand—foot syndrome caused by capecitabine. *Proc Annu Meet Am Soc Clin Oncol* 2000; 19:2403a.
33. Venturini M, De Mastro L, Merlano M, et al. Dose finding study of capecitabine in combination with docetaxel and epirubicin in prior untreated advanced breast cancer patients. *Proc Annu Meet Am Soc Clin Oncol* 2000; 19:419a.
34. Angiolini C, Venturini M, Del Mastro L, et al. Capecitabine in association with epirubicin and docetaxel as first line chemotherapy in advanced breast cancer: a dose finding study. *Breast Cancer Res Treat* 2000; 64:529a.
35. Herrmann R, Bornier M, Morant R, Roth A, Ludwig C, Bedoucha V. Combining gemcitabine and capecitabine in advanced pancreatic cancer. *Proc Annu Meet Am Soc Clin Oncol* 2000; 19:1038a.
36. Vanhoefer U, Mayer S, Harstrick A, et al. Phase I study of capecitabine in combination with a weekly schedule of irinotecan as first-line chemotherapy in metastatic colorectal cancer. *Proc Annu Meet Am Soc Clin Oncol* 2000; 19:1050a.
37. Diaz-Rubio E, Evans J, Tabernero J, et al. Phase I study of capecitabine in combination with oxaliplatin in patients with advanced or metastatic solid tumors. *Proc Annu Meet Am Soc Clin Oncol* 2000; 19:772a.
38. Elza-Brown K, Dees E, Wolff A, Carducci M, Donehower R. A phase I study of capecitabine and weekly paclitaxel in advanced solid tumors. *Proc Annu Meet Am Soc Clin Oncol* 2000; 19:921Ja.
39. Villalona-Calero M, Weiss G, Burris H, et al. Phase I and pharmacokinetic study of the oral fluoropyrimidine capecitabine in combination with paclitaxel in patients with advanced solid malignancies. *J Clin Oncol* 1999; 17:1915–1925.
40. Villalona-Calero M, Shapiro C, Otterson G, et al. Phase I study of weekly docetaxel in combination with capecitabine in patients with solid malignancies. *Breast Cancer Res Treat* 2000; 64:537a.
41. Olencki T, Pratt S, Budd G, Peereboom D, McClain D, Bukowski R. Phase I trial of capecitabine and subcutaneous interferon-alpha in renal cell carcinoma. *Proc Amer Soc Clin Oncol* 1999; 18:855a.
42. Judson I, Beale P, Trigo J, et al. A human capecitabine excretion balance and pharmacokinetic study after administration of a single oral dose of 14C-labelled drug. *Invest New Drugs* 1999; 17:49–56.
43. Twelves C, Glynne-Jones R, Cassidy J, et al. Effect of hepatic dysfunction due to liver metastases on the pharmacokinetics of capecitabine and its metabolites. *Clin Cancer Res* 1999; 5:1696–1702.
44. Reigner B, Verweij J, Dirix L, et al. Effect of food on the pharmacokinetics of capecitabine and its metabolites following oral administration in cancer patients. *Clin Cancer Res* 1998; 4:941–948.
45. Reigner B, Clive S, Cassidy J, et al. Influence of the antacid Maalox on the pharmacokinetics of capecitabine in cancer patients. *Cancer Chemother Pharmacol* 1999; 43:309–315.
46. Kolesar J, Johnson C, Freeberg B, Berlin H, Schiller J. Wafarin-5-FU interaction—aconsecutive case series. *Pharmacotherapy* 1999; 19:1445–1449.
47. Schuller J, Cassidy J, Dumont E, et al. Preferential activation of capecitabine in tumor following oral administration to colorectal cancer patients. *Cancer Chemother Pharmacol* 2000; 45:291–297.
48. Van Cutsem E, Findlay M, Osterwalder B, et al. Capecitabine, an oral fluoropyrimidine carbamate with substantial activity in advanced colorectal cancer: Results of a randomized trial. *J Clin Oncol* 2000; 18:1337–1345.
49. Blum JL, Jones SE, Buzdar AU, et al. Multicenter phase II study of capecitabine in paclitaxel-refractory metastatic breast cancer. *J Clin Oncol* 1999; 17:485–493.

50. Twelves C, Harper P, Van Cutsem E, et al. A phase III trial (SO14796) of Xeloda (Capecitabine) in previously untreated advanced/metastatic colorectal cancer. *Proc Annu Meet Am Soc Clin Oncol* 1999; 18:1010a.
51. Cox J, Pazdur R, Thibault A, et al. Phase III trial of Xeloda (Capecitabine) in previously untreated advanced/metastatic colorectal cancer. *Proc Annu Meet Am Soc Clin Oncol* 1999; 18:1016a.
52. Hoff P, Abbruzzese J, Medgyesy D, Thomas M, Carter S. A phase II study of Xeloda (capecitabine) in patients with metastatic colorectal cancer demonstrating progression on 5-FU therapy. *Proc Annu Meet Am Soc Clin Oncol* 2000; 19:993a.
53. Cartwright, T. A phase 2 trial of Xeloda (capecitabine) in advanced or metastatic pancreatic cancer. *Proc Annu Meet Am Soc Clin Oncol* 2000; 19:1026a.
54. Lozano R, Patt Y, Hassan M, et al. Oral capecitabine (Xeloda) for the treatment of hepatobilliary cancers (hepatocellular carcinoma, cholangiocarcinoma, and gallbladder cancer). *Proc Annu Meet Am Soc Clin Oncol* 2000; 19:1025a.
55. Wenzel C, Schmidinger M, Locker G, et al. Oral chemotherapy with capecitabine in the treatment of metastatic renal cancer failing immunotherapy. *Proc Annu Meet Am Soc Clin Oncol* 2000; 19:1457a.
56. Oevermann K, Buer J, Hoffmann R, et al. Capecitabine in the treatment of metastatic renal cell carcinoma. *Br J Cancer* 2000; 83:583–587.

23 Preclinical and Clinical Practice of S-1 in Japan

Tetsuhiko Shirasaka, PhD, and Tetsuo Taguchi, MD

CONTENTS

1. INTRODUCTION

Recently, there has been an increased demand more effective therapy cancer patients. To satisfy this demand, attempts have been made to develop novel drugs or to establish combination therapies with a new mechanism of action or a new concept in the field of chemotherapy. A number of anticancer chemical entities have been introduced into clinical practice since the discovery of 5-fluorouracil (5-FU) by Heidelberger et al. in 1957 *(1)*. However, none of the entities satisfied our demands, and concern about whether chemotherapy is effective against cancer is persistent. In this chapter, we provide a review on the history of cancer chemotherapy to date and concurrently refer to a novel oral anticancer agent, S-1, through a detailed description thereof from development to clinical results; the drug is proving preclinical theories in the clinical setting in Japan, validating the self-rescue concept (SRC)—a conceptual goal as a treatment modality that simultaneously has a dual action, i.e., enhancement of 5-FU effects and alleviation of 5-FU-induced adverse reactions, which we have groped for in the last 15 yr.

From: *Fluoropyrimidines in Cancer Therapy*
Edited by: Y. M. Rustum © Humana Press Inc., Totowa, NJ

2. HISTORY OF CANCER CHEMOTHERAPY AND REFLECTION THEREON

Originally, cancer chemotherapy started with nitrogen mustard, a derivative of poisonous gas yperite, a by-product in World War II. The pharmacological action of nitrogen mustard consists in cytotoxicities (e.g., leukopenia, diarrhea, and stomatitis) to the organism, and attempts were made to utilize these toxicities to obtain anticancer activity. Namely, the modality consisted in cancer therapy using toxicities to the organism that were inherent to nitrogen mustard. From the standpoint of establishing cancer chemotherapy that is ideally based on the premise that only the tumor should be attacked with the least damage to the organism, therefore, we cannot but consider that the approach was the tail wagging the dog (misoriented rescuing). A concept of high-dose chemotherapy, i.e., "an anticancer agent fails to be effective unless provoking considerable adverse reactions," still remains at present when half a century has elapsed since the introduction of nitrogen mustard.

The concept of high-dose chemotherapy seems to have been affected by the concept of total cell killing which Skipper et al. *(2)* proposed in 1964. The relevant concept, based on in vitro experiments, was successful to a certain extent in the treatment of leukemia. However, problems seem to have existed in the case of solid cancers. For example, a 10-g solid tumor contains approx 10^{11} tumor cells, and a tumor reduction rate of 99.9% would lead to complete response (CR) in the diagnostic imaging by computed tomography and roentgenography; however, 10^6–10^7 tumor cells still remain in that setting. High-dose chemotherapy causes more adverse reactions than antitumor effects, is restricted to short-term therapy, and fails in leading to the life-prolonging effect despite providing a certain level of response rate. Treatment is terminated due to adverse reactions even when CR is obtained in diagnostic imaging, which naturally leads to reproliferation of tumor cells. It is essential to reduce the number of cancer cells at least to 100–1000 in suppressing their proliferation by the immune ability of the host. To attain a life-prolonging effect, therefore, we must select not a short-term battle-type modality but "Fabian tactics" and long-term administration-type modality. For this purpose, it is crucial that an anticancer drug should have higher anticancer activity than that of conventional anticancer drugs and concurrently should provoke less adverse events. First of all, therefore, an attempt should be made to intentionally alleviate the adverse events from which the patient suffers most, to lessen the frequency of treatment rejection, and to allow long-term treatment.

We did not seek for a novel chemical entity as effector but attempted to explore a therapeutic modality with a dual action, i.e., enhancement of 5-FU effects and alleviation of 5-FU-induced adverse reactions, based on the theory of biochemical modulation of 5-FU, an anticancer drug whose mechanism of action and adverse reactions have been elucidated to the largest extent.

3. METABOLISM OF 5-FU

More than 40 yr have already elapsed since the discovery of 5-FU by Heidelberger et al. *(1)* in 1957. As shown in Fig. 1, their discovery resided in the finding that among nucleic acid bases uracil is most prone to aggregate in cancer cells. This discovery was very important and contributed much to his research thereafter. First, they synthesized 5-FU by replacing the position 5 of uracil with a halogen fluorine (F). As shown in Fig. 2, 5-FU has a structural formula similar to that of uracil. Therefore, 5-FU is anabolized and metabolized by the same enzyme for uracil via the same pathway, is converted to FdUMP through FUrd → FUMP → FUDP → FdUDP, forms a ternary covalent complex (5,10-CH_2FH_4-FdUMP-TS), inhibits dTMP synthase (TS), and suppresses the synthesis of DNA, thus exerting cytotoxic activity. Further-

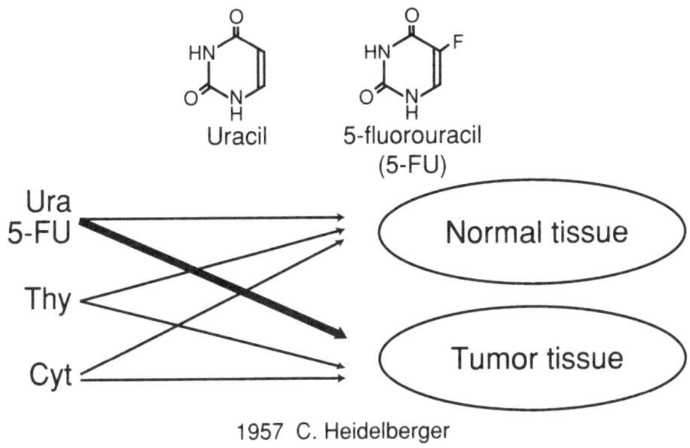

Fig. 1. Biological actions of uracil and 5-FU.

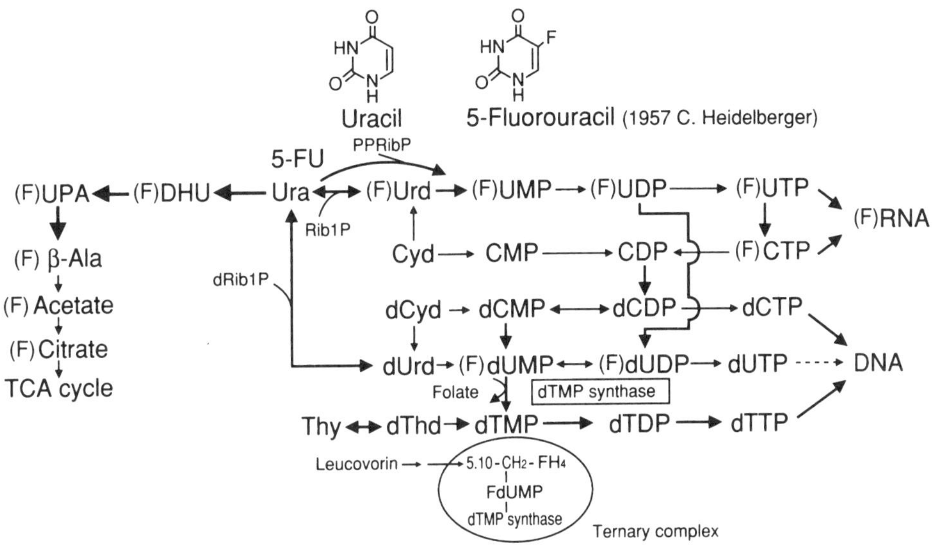

Fig. 2. Metabolism of pyrimidine nucleotides and 5-FU.

more, 5-FU is converted to (F)RNA through FUrd → FUMP → FUDP → FUTP, thus exerting cytotoxic activity due to the abnormal metabolism of RNA. In 1964, an in vitro study conducted by Skipper et al. *(2)* revealed that 5-FU is an antimetabolite with intense time dependency and reverified the propensity of 5-FU to aggregate in cancer cells that Heidelberger et al. had discovered. The abovementioned results readily allow us to presume that the optimal regimen for 5-FU is the long-term continuous intravenous infusion (CVI) method by which long-term contact with cancer cells is achieved. Summarizing Fig. 2, 5-FU, as shown in Fig. 3, is anabolized and metabolized to FdUMP in the organism, inhibits the synthesis of DNA, and shows cytotoxic activity in sorts of tissues. For example, 5-FU shows antitumor activity when converted to FdUMP in tumor tissue, exhibits gastrointestinal (GI) toxicities *(3)* when converted to FdUMP in the gastrointestinal tract, and indicates myelotoxicity when converted to FdUMP in bone marrow tissue *(4)*. On the other hand, more than 90% of 5-FU, which was administered to the organism is degraded by the action of dihydroxy pyrimidine dehydroge-

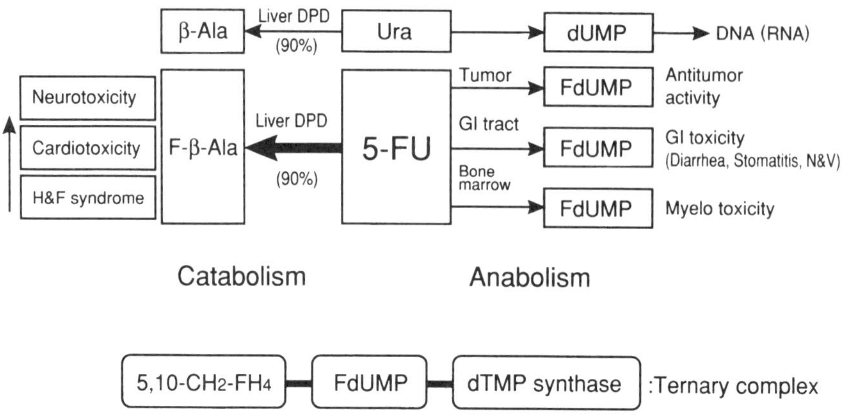

Fig. 3. Biological actions of 5-FU and Ura.

Table 1
Efficacy of 5-FU CVI Compared with 5-FU Bolus in Advanced Colorectal Cancer

Regimen	*Response rate (CR + PR) (%)*	*Adverse reactions (%) WBC (G3 + G4)*	*H & F.S*	*Authors*
Bolus (500 mg/m^2)	6.9 (6/87)	22	0	Lokich, JJ. (1989)
CVI (300 mg/m^2)	30.0 (26/87)	0	24	J. Clin. Oncol. 7:425
Bolus (400–500 mg/m^2)	13.9 (66/475)	31	13	Piedbois, P. (1998)
CVI (300–750 mg/m^2)	23.4 (113/483)	4	34	J. Clin. Oncol. 16:301

The incidences of nonhematological toxicities (e.g., diarrhea, N & V, and mucositis) were 14.0% and 13.0% for 5-FU bolus and 5-FU CVI, respectively.

nase (DPD) in the liver (E.C.1.3.1.2) and is excreted in the urine as F-β-Ala *(5)*. F-β-Ala has been elucidated to provoke neurotoxicity *(6–8)* and cardiotoxicity *(9)*. Dr. Diasio, Dr. Rustum, and other investigators discussed possible induction of the hand foot (HF) syndrome by degradation products of 5-FU at an ASCO meeting in 1997.

The results of recent studies on the regimen for 5-FU may be summarized by two papers. As shown in Table 1, the results of a controlled study on CVI and bolus administration *(10)* and of a meta-analysis *(11)* indicate that the a most efficacious administration schedule for 5-FU in the clinical setting is CVI, whose response rates were 23.4–30.0% and were superior to those (6.9–13.9%) by bolus administration. The dose-limiting factors (DLFs) for CVI are HF syndrome and GI toxicities, and myelotoxicity provoked by CVI is markedly less frequent as compared with bolus administration. Therefore, the concept of Heidelberger et al. was thus demonstrated by these clinical results.

4. INVENTION OF S-1

The optimal administration schedule for 5-FU in the clinical setting is CVI, whose DLFs are HF syndrome and GI toxicity *(10,11)*. These toxicities are intolerable to the patient. It is essential to alleviate these adverse reactions in incrementing drug tolerance and antitumor effect of 5-FU.

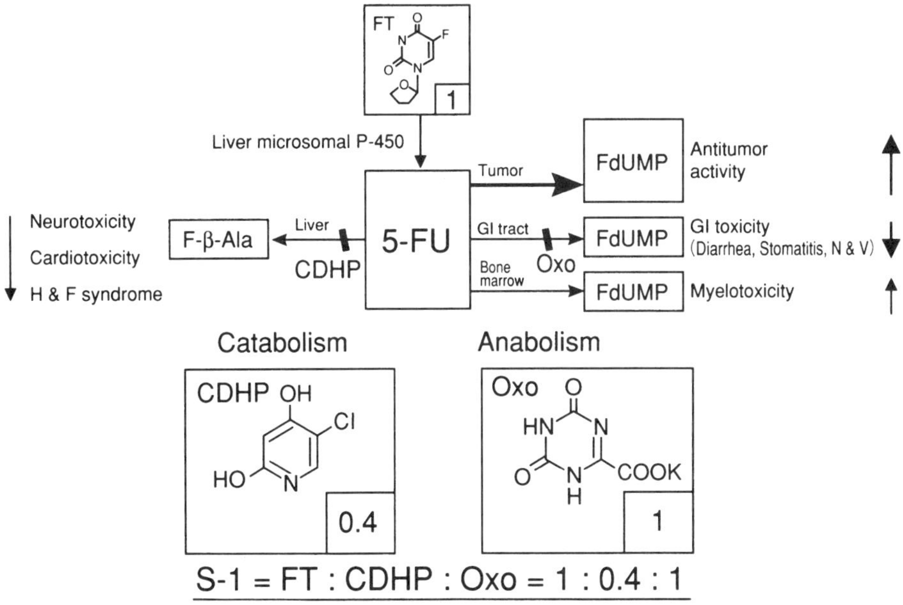

Fig. 4. Biological actions of S-1.

GI toxicities increase concurrently with enhancement of the antitumor effect of an anticancer agent. Diarrhea is attributable to 5-FU results from the impaired proliferation of mucous cells of the GI tract caused by DNA synthesis inhibition due to FdUMP, a product of anabolism and metabolism by 5-FU in mucous cells of the GI tract *(3)*. Therefore, we attempted to reduce GI toxicities caused by 5-FU without deteriorating the antitumor effect of 5-FU. In 1993, consequently, we discovered potassium oxonate, a chemical substance with alleviating activity on diarrhea attributable to 5-FU *(12)*.

We combined two modulators, i.e., a 5-FU-effect enhancer and a 5-FU GI toxicity-reducing agent, to an effector, FT *(13)* (tegaful is a prodrug of 5-FU) with good oral absorbability, persistent activity in the organism, and high safety; we thus invented a novel oral anticancer agent, S-1 (Fig. 4) *(14–16)*. We describe the actions of the two modulators below.

5. 5-FU EFFECT-ENHANCING ACTIVITY OF CDHP

As shown in Fig. 3, approx 90% of 5-FU administered to the organism is degraded by dihydroxypyrimidine dehydrogenase (DPD) (E.C.1.3.1.2), is excreted in the urine as F-β-Ala *(5)*, whereas the residual 10% is anabolized and metabolized, exerting antitumor activity and causing myelotoxicity and GI toxicities. To utilize 5-FU efficaciously, therefore, it is indispensable to block the degradation of 5-FU by DPD. We conducted enzymatic research on DPD inhibitors and consequently discovered 5-chloro-2, 4-dihydroxypyridine (CDHP) as a novel compound with inhibitory activity whose enzyme-inhibitory activity is potent and whose enzyme pattern shows reversible competitive inhibition *(17)*. As shown in Fig. 5, CDHP is a pyridine derivative with about a 200-fold inhibitory activity as compared with uracil that is contained in uracil and tegafur (UFT®); its inhibitory pattern is competitive *(17)*.

FT combined with CDHP and FT combined with uracil, whose inhibitory activity is 200-fold less potent as compared with CDHP, were administered orally to rats, and blood con-

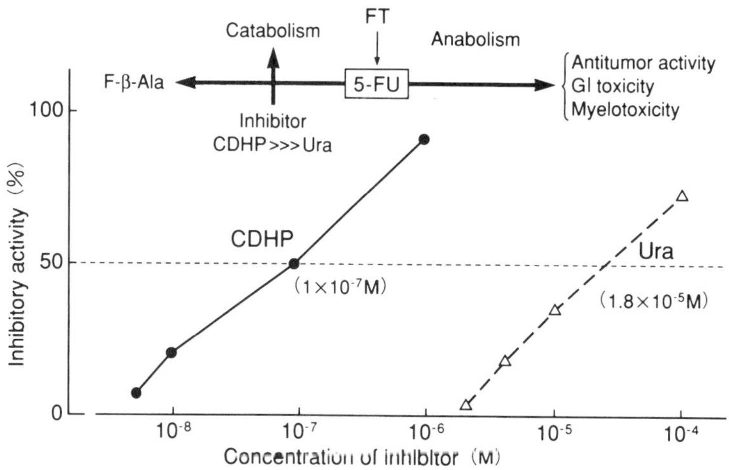

Fig. 5. Effects of inhibitors on 5-FU degradation.

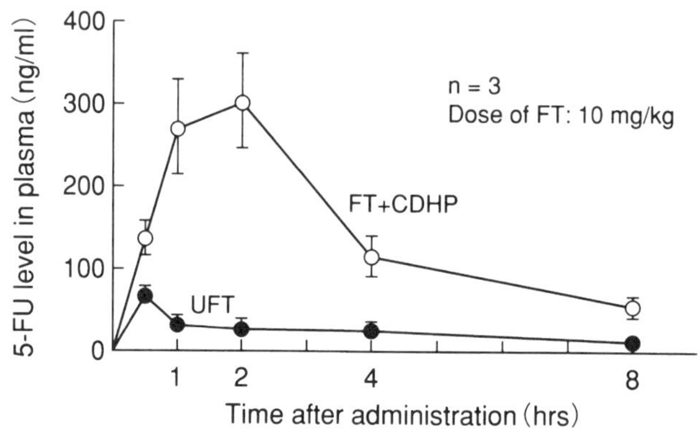

Fig. 6. 5-FU Levels in plasma after oral administration of FT + CDHP and FT + Ura (UFT) to rats.

centrations of 5-FU were examined. As shown in Fig. 6, consequently, the FT + CDHP combination group showed C_{max} of 300 ng/mL or higher; the values were markedly higher than C_{max} ($\leq$ 100 ng/mL) of the uracil group and allowed us to expect high anticancer activity. However, an increase in blood 5-FU concentration provokes higher incidences of myelotoxicity and GI toxicities, e.g., diarrhea and stomatitis. Therefore, exertion of a potent antitumor effect cannot be expected unless devising a scheme to reduce these toxicities.

6. OXO FOR REDUCTION OF 5-FU-INDUCED GI TOXICITIES

As shown in Fig. 3, the anabolism and metabolism of 5-FU occur in cells with active mitosis. Therefore, 5-FU is converted to FdUMP in the organism, mainly in tumor cells, mucous cells of the GI tract, and myelocytes. 5-FU shows antitumor activity in tumor cells and causes GI toxicities in mucous cells in the GI tract *(3)* and myelotoxicity in myelocytes *(4)*. Concurrently with elucidation of these mechanisms of action, attempts have been made to reduce adverse reactions and to increase drug tolerance and antitumor effects.

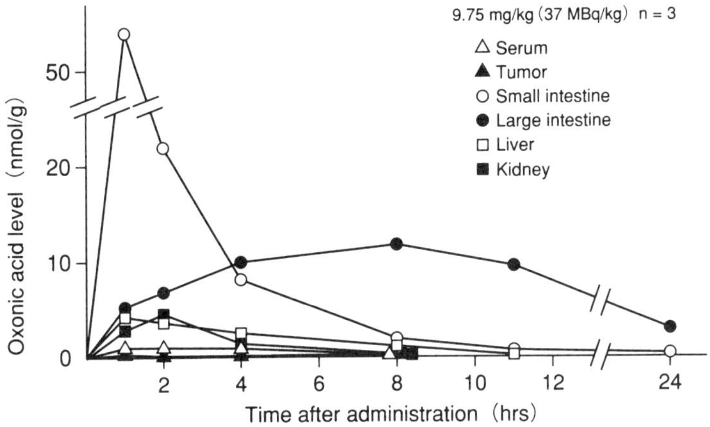

Fig. 7. [4] C-oxonic acid levels in blood and tissues of Yoshida sarcoma-bearing rats after oral administration of ^{14}C oxonic acid.

From 1979 to 1980, Schwartz et al. discovered cytotoxic activity of allopurinol (Allo), a potent xanthine oxidase inhibitor *(18);* they further reported that Allo and oxypurinol, a product of hydroxylation of Allo in the organism, inhibit the synthesis of FUMP from 5-FU in an in vitro system *(18–20)* and that these compounds, when combined with 5-FU in, reduce the cytotoxic effect of 5-FU *(18)*. Clinically, an attempt was made to reduce toxicities of 5-FU by the combination of 5-FU and Allo *(21,22)*. Consequently, toxicities of 5-FU were reduced and the total dose could be increased. However, the effects of 5-FU also lessened, and the objective failed to be accomplished. One admissible reason is that Allo, an oral agent with good absorbability, is rapidly hydroxylated to oxypurinol in the organism and that oxypurinol persists at high concentrations in the organism for a long term, also inhibiting the anabolism and metabolism of 5-FU in cancer cells and reducing the antitumor effect of 5-FU.

We explored a substance that inhibits orotate phosphoribosyltransferase (ORTC) (E.C.2.4.2.10), an enzyme that synthesizes FUMP from 5-FU, and that localizes in mucous cells of the gastrointestinal tract when administered orally. Consequently, we discovered potassium oxonate (Oxo) in 1993 *(12)*. In 1965 already, Granat et al. *(23)* reported that Oxo inhibits ORTC, the main pathway of phospholylation, and intended to discover the antitumor effect of Oxo as a single antitumor agent, without success.

As shown in Fig. 7, examination of Oxo distribution in organs after oral administration revealed that high concentrations of Oxo are distributed in the small intestine and large intestine and that a very low concentration of Oxo was distributed in the tumor *(12)*. This result suggested that Oxo, when administered orally, specifically inhibits the anabolism and metabolism of 5-FU in mucous cells of the GI tract and that the anabolism and metabolism of 5-FU are not inhibited because little Oxo exists in tumor cells, which is less prone to affect the antitumor effect of 5-FU.

7. PRECLINICAL STUDIES OF S-1

We invented a novel oral anticancer agent, S-1, as a combination drug of FT, CDHP, and Oxo at a molar ratio of 1:0.4:1 because of the following approaches:

1. To attain a balance between efficacy and toxicity of FT and two modulators, CDHP and Oxo.
2. Concurrent oral administration of the two modulators and FT is optimal *(14–16)*.

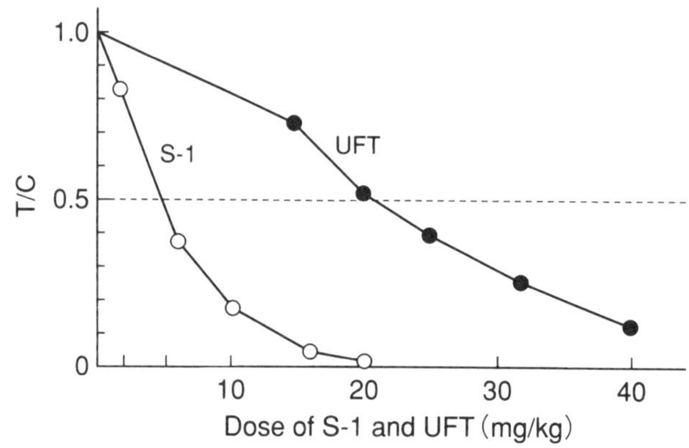

Fig. 8. Antitumor effect of S-1 and UFT on Yoshida sarcoma-bearing rats.

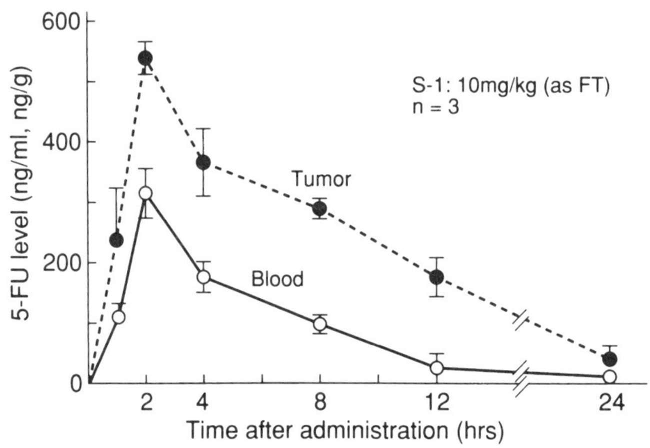

Fig. 9. 5-FU levels in blood and tumor after oral administration of S-1 in Yoshida sarcoma-bearing rats.

As shown in Fig. 5, a potent DPD inhibitor, CDHP, inhibits the degradation of 5-FU, which is released gradually from FT by the action of a P-450 drug-metabolizing enzyme (CYP2A6), thus increasing concentrations of 5-FU in the organism. Consequently, tumor concentrations of FdUMP also increase, thus enhancing the antitumor effect of S-1. On the other hand, FT was administered orally in combination with Oxo, an inhibitor of ORTC, which is an anabolizing enzyme for 5-FU. Consequently, FdUMP, a compound that is synthesized mainly in mucous cells of the GI tract, is reduced, and GI toxicities alleviated *(12)*.

We used an anticancer experiment system for Yoshida sarcoma and administered S-1 orally for seven consecutive days to examine the antitumor effect and tumor and blood concentrations of 5-FU. As shown in Fig. 8, consequently, S-1 showed a more potent antitumor effect as compared with that of UFT and indicated no tumor proliferation at all at an FT dose of 20 mg/kg. Furthermore, we administered S-1 orally at a dose of 10 mg/kg, an FT dose showing an T/C (Treatment/Control) value (≤ 0.5), to measure tumor and blood concentrations of 5-FU on a time-course basis. As shown in Fig. 9, consequently, T_{max} of 5-FU was 2 h in both blood and tumor. Blood concentrations of 5-FU persisted at 100 ng/mL or higher

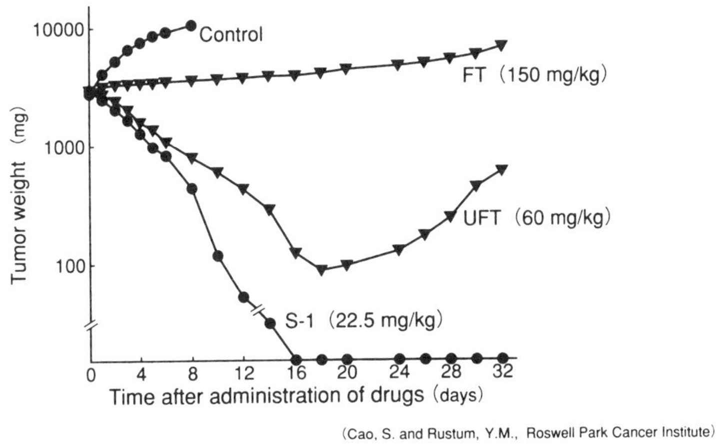

Fig. 10. Antitumor activity of S-1, UFT, and FT at MTD by po daily × 28 in rats bearing colon carcinoma.

Table 2
Toxicities of FT, UFT, and S-1 at MTD by 28-d Once-a-Day Oral Administration to Rats Bearing Colon Carcinoma

Drug	*Dose (mg/kg/day)*	*Incidence (%)* *Stomatitis*	*Incidence (%)* *Hair loss*	*MWL*
FT	150	75	100	−16.4 ± 2.5
UFT	60	42	100	−17.2 ± 5.8
S-1	22.5	0	0	−13.4 ± 3.1

MWL: Maximum weight loss

up to 8 h after administration, while tumor concentrations of 5-FU persisted to be 200 ng/mL or higher up to 12 h after administration. The results of these pharmacological studies validated the potent antitumor activity of S-1 *(24)*.

With the rat colon cancer implantation model, we administered S-1 orally for four consecutive weeks to examine the antitumor effect and adverse reactions of S-1 and to compare FT and UFT from the moment when the tumor weight after implantation became about 2 g. As shown in Fig. 10, a collaboration study with Roswell Park Cancer Institute *(25)* showed that 28-d oral administration of S-1 at an FT dose of 22.5 mg/kg caused the tumor to disappear on d 16 after administration, and the tumor did not reappear at least for 3 mo. The UFT group, in which UFT was administered orally for 28 consecutive days at an FT dose of 60 mg/kg, showed a transient reduction in tumor size; however, the tumor reproliferated and failed to disappear. The antitumor effect was markedly more potent in the S-1 group than in the FT and UFT groups. Furthermore, as shown in Table 2, the S-1 group showed no stomatitis and alopecia and exhibited the least adverse reactions, e.g., body weight loss *(25)*.

The usefulness of Oxo for nausea and diarrhea was examined in beagle dogs with high susceptibility to 5-FU. As shown in Table 3, the group, in which Oxo was removed from S-1, showed high incidences of nausea and diarrhea (7/11 and 10/11, respectively), while the

Table 3
Combination Effects of Oxonic Acid on Vomiting and Diarrhea after Oral Administration of FT Plus CDHP to Beagle Dogs

Drug	*Dose (mg/kg)*	*Duration (day)*	*Animal (n)*	*Vomiting (n)*	*Diarrhea (n)*
FT + CDHP (1:0.4)	6	5	11	7	10
S-1 [FT + CDHP + Oxo] (1:0.4:1)	6	5	11	1	1

Table 4
Response Rates in the Early Phase II Clinical Trial of S-1

Class of cancer	*R.R. (CR + PR/eligible patients)*	*Reference*
Stomach	53.6% (15/28)	K. Sugimachi et al. *(26)*
Colorectum	16.7% (5/30)	K. Sugimachi et al. *(26)*
Breast	40.7% (11/27)	T. Taguchi et al. *(27)*
Head & Neck	46.2% (12/26)	M. Fujii et al. *(28)*
NSCLC	12.5% (5/40)	M. Hino et al. *(29)*

R.R.: Responce Rate, CR: Complete Response, PR: Partial Response

Oxo-containing S-1 group showed marked improvement (1/11 and 1/11, respectively)*(24)*. These results suggested usefulness of Oxo in the clinical setting.

8. EARLY PHASE II CLINICAL TRIAL AND PHARMACOKINETIC STUDY OF S-1

The early phase II clinical trial of S-1 was conducted subject to patients with gastric cancer, colorectal cancer, head and neck cancer, breast cancer, and nonsmall cell lung cancer at a recommended dose of 50 mg/body, which was determined on the basis of the phase I clinical trial, with at least four courses, each of which consisted of twice-a-day (once each after breakfast and dinner), 4-wk consecutive oral administration and of 2-wk withdrawal. As shown in Table 4, S-1 showed high response rates, especially for stomach cancer, head and neck cancer, and breast cancer. As shown in Table 5, the incidence of adverse reactions ≥(G3) was 10% or below except neutropenia (10.8%) *(26–29)*.

The phase I and early phase II clinical trials are already completed, the results of which recommend the twice-a-day (once each after breakfast and dinner), 28-d consecutive oral regimen at a dose of 80 mg/m^2/d. Twelve patients were enrolled in this trial: five patients with gastric cancer, four with colorectal cancer, and three with breast cancer. As shown in Fig. 11, the pharmacokinetic parameters of 5-FU in plasma were as follows: C_{max}, 128.5 ± 41.5 ng/mL; T_{max}, 3.5 ± 1.7 h; AUC_{0-14}, 723.9 ± 272.7 ng/h/mL; and $t^{1/2}$, 1.9 ± 0.4 h. There were no fluctuations in pharmacokinetics nor any drug accumulation in the 28-d consecutive regimen. All patients showed plasma 5-FU concentrations of 60 to 200 ng/mL *(30)*. Since the pharmacokinetic parameters were nearly similar between S-1 administered orally and 5-FU given by CVI, we concluded that S-1 may improve the patient's quality of life.

Table 5
Early Phase II Clinical Trial of S-1

Class of toxicity	Grade 1	2	3	4	Incidence (≥ Grade 3) (%)
Leukopenia	35	30	6	3	5.4
Neutropenia	34	23	14	4	10.8
Thrombocytopenia	10	3	2	1	1.8
Anemia	17	36	11	0	6.6
Stomatitis	12	8	4	0	2.4
Nausea/vomiting	39	12	0	0	0.0
Diarrhea	17	6	5	2	4.2
Skin rash	32	11	0	0	0.0
Anorexia	30	28	6	0	3.6

Major toxicity (n = 167)

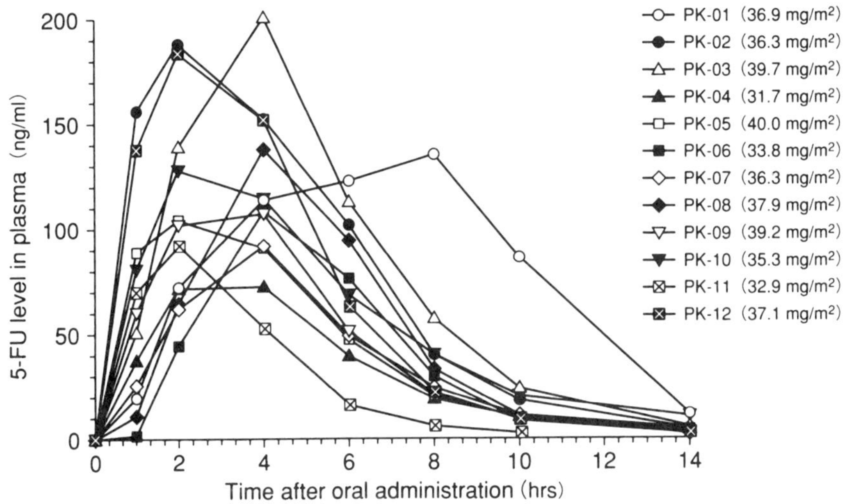

Fig. 11. Plasma concentrations of 5-FU after single oral administration of S-1.

9. LATE PHASE II CLINICAL TRIALS OF S-1 IN ADVANCED GASTRIC CANCER

According to the same schedule as that of the clinical pharmacological study, the late phase II clinical trial of S-1 was conducted subject to patients with advanced or recurrent gastric cancer at a dose of 40 mg/m^2, basically with four or more courses, each of which consisted of twice-a-day (once each after breakfast and dinner), 4-wk consecutive oral administration and of 2-wk withdrawal. The results of the late phase II clinical trials, which were reported by two groups, i.e., one of Sakata et al. *(31)* and another of Koizumi et al. *(32)*, are summarized in Table 6; the overall response rate was 44.6% (45/101). As shown in Fig. 12, the survival curve was based to consider that MST was 244 d. Adverse reactions of a total of 362 patients in the late phase II clinical trials are shown in Table 7; the incidence of adverse reactions (≥G3) was

Table 6
Response Rates in the Late Phase II Clinical Trial of S-1 (Gastric Cancer)

Group	*Patient registered*	*Patient eligible*	*Number of cases by response*						*Response rate (%)*
			CR	*PR*	*MR*	*NC*	*PD*	*NE*	
Group T	51	51	1	24	0	11	13	2	49.0
Group K	51	50	0	20	0	16	13	1	40.0
Total	102	101	1	44	0	27	26	3	44.6

CR: Complete Response, PR: Partial Response, MR: Minor Response, NC: No Change, PD: Progressive Disease, NE: Not Evaluated

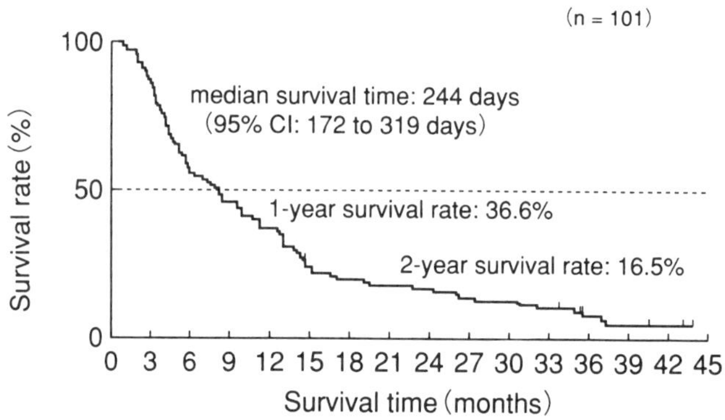

Fig. 12. Overall survival curve in gastric cancer of S-1 (late Phase II clinical trial).

Table 7
Late Phase II Clinical Trial of S-1

Class of toxicity	*Grade*				*Incidence (≥ Grade 3) (%)*
	1	*2*	*3*	*4*	
Leukopenia	95	93	5	2	1.9
Neutropenia	57	70	25	3	7.7
Thrombocytopenia	24	10	1	5	1.7
Anemia	56	55	15	1	4.4
Stomatitis	48	6	3	0	0.8
Nausea/Vomiting	64	23	3	0	0.8
Diarrhea	35	16	9	0	2.5
Skin rash	24	7	0	0	
Anorexia	62	32	14	0	3.9

Major toxicity (n = 362)

10% or below *(31,32)*. A high response rate of 53.6% (15/28), which Sugimachi et al. *(26)* had reported, was thus verified. The preclinical concept was demonstrated in the clinical setting, and S-1 is considered to be a novel drug which has reached the goal that we described previously. In January 1999, S-1 was given manufacturing approval from the Ministry of Health

Table 8
Response Rates in the Late Phase II Clinical Trial of S-1 (Colorectal Cancer)

Site of cancer	*Patient eligible*	*Number of cases by response*					*Response rate (%)*
		CR	*PR*	*NC*	*PD*	*NE*	
Primary cancer							
Colon	43	0	15	19	7	2	34.9
Rectum	19	0	7	9	1	2	36.8
Tatal	62	0	22	28	8	4	35.5*
Metastasis							
Liver	40	1	10	20	6	3	27.5
Lung	28	0	11	15	1	1	39.3
Others	14	1	4	4	2	3	35.7

CR: Complete Response, PR: Partial Response, NC: No Change, PD: Progressive Disease, NE: Not Evaluated
*: 95% confidence interval, 24.7%–47.9%

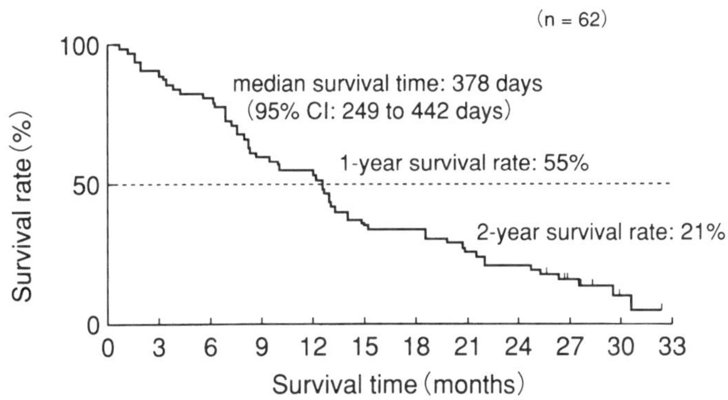

Fig. 13. Overall survival curve in colorectal cancer of S-1 (late Phase II clinical trial).

and Welfare of Japan through the priority review system, with an indication for advanced or recurrent gastric cancer. The late phase II clinical trials on other cancers (colorectal cancer, breast cancer, nonsmall cell lung cancer, and head and neck cancer) are in progress.

10. LATE PHASE II CLINICAL TRIAL OF S-1 IN COLORECTAL CANCER

The response rate of S-1 for colorectal cancer in the early phase II clinical trial was as modes at 16.7% (Table 4). However, the response rate was 25% in patients without prior chemotherapy, thus warranting further research on this disorder. The late phase II clinical trial of S-1 was conducted to evaluate the efficacy and toxicities in patients with metastatic colorectal carcinoma. Sixty-three patients with measurable metastatic colorectal carcinoma were enrolled in this clinical trial. None of the patients had received chemotherapy prior to this clinical trial, except the adjuvant setting. S-1 was administered orally at a standard dose of 80 mg/m^{2}d, twice daily for 28 consecutive days followed by 14-d withdrawal. This regimen was maintained until when the disease progressed, an intolerable toxicity developed, or the patient refused the drug. As shown in Table 8, the overall response rate was 35.5%. As shown in Fig. 13, the median survival time was 378 d. The main adverse reactions were

Table 9
Response Rates in the Late Phase II Clinical Trial of S-1 (Head and Neck Cancer)

Site of cancer	*Patient eligible*	*Number of cases by response*						*R.R.(%)*
		CR	*PR*	*MR*	*NC*	*PD*	*NE*	
Oral cavity	11		4		2	4	1	36.4
Nasopharynx	4		1		3			25.0
Oropharynx	12	2	4	1	3	1	1	50.0
Hypopharynx	6			1	2	2	1	0.0
Larynx	11	1	1		3	6		18.2
Nasal cavity/paranasal sinus	7	1	2		1	2	1	42.9
Salivary glands	5		1		4			20.0
Others (e. g., ear and trachea)	3				3			0.0
Total	59	4	13	2	21	15	4	28.8

CR: Complete Response, PR: Partial Response, MR: Minor Response, NC: No Change, PD: Progressive Disease, NE: Not Evaluated

myelosuppression and GI toxicities. The incidence of neutropenia (Grade 3 or 4) was 13%, where as the incidence of other adverse reactions was 10% or below. None of 53 outpatients required hospitalization due to adverse reactions *(33)*.

11. LATE PHASE II CLINICAL TRIAL OF S-1 IN HEAD AND NECK CANCER

This clinical trial was conducted to examine the antitumor activity and toxicities of S-1, in which 60 patients with head and neck cancer were enrolled. S-1 was administered at a dose of 40 mg/m^2d, with at least four courses, each of which consisted of twice-a-day (once each after breakfast and dinner), 28-d consecutive oral administration and of 14-d withdrawal; two courses were repeated every 6 wk unless the disease progressed. As shown in Table 9, there were four "complete response" cases and 13 "partial response" cases (response rate: 28.8%) among 59 evaluable cases. The adverse events that were assessed to be Grade 3 or higher were as follows: hemoglobinemia (6.8%); neutropenia (5.1%); leukopenia (1.7%); decreased RBC (3.4%); and anorexia, nausea/vomiting, stomatitis, and fatigue (1.7% each) *(34)*.

12. LATE PHASE II CLINICAL TRIAL OF S-1 IN BREAST CANCER

This clinical trial was conducted to examine the antitumor activity and toxicities of S-1. Eligibility required advanced and/or recurrent breast cancer which was verified by histopathological or cytological evidence. However, postoperative adjuvant chemotherapy for advanced or metastatic cancer, which was conducted six or more months prior to this clinical trial, was not counted as a regimen. S-1 was administered orally at a dose of 40 mg/m^2, with at least four courses, each of which consisted of twice-a-day (once each after breakfast and dinner) 28-d consecutive oral administration and of 14-d withdrawal; two courses were repeated every 6 wk unless the disease progressed. As shown in Table 10, there were six "complete response" cases and 28 "partial response" cases among 81 cases which were evaluable for response, with an overall response rate of 42.0%. As shown in Fig. 14, the median survival time was 910 d. The adverse events that were assessed to be Grade 3 or

Table 10
Response Rate in the Late Phase II Clinical Trial (Breast Cancer)

Site of cancer	*Patient eligible*	*Number of cases by response*							*R.R.(%)*
		CR	*PR*	*MR*	*L-NC*	*NC*	*PD*	*NE*	
Total	*81*	*6*	*28*	*4*	*4*	*19*	*12*	*8*	*42.0*
Metastasis									
Lung	28	1	8	3	2	6	5	3	32.1
Skin	25	7	6	1	0	5	2	4	52.0
Liver	6	–	1	0	0	2	1	2	16.7
Bone	15	0	4	0	2	4	0	5	26.7
Pleura	5	–	1	0	0	1	2	1	20.0
Lymph node	49	8	17	8	0	11	3	2	51.0

CR: Complete Response, PR: Partial Response, MR: Minor Response, L-NC: Long No Change, NC: No Change, PD: Progressive Disease, NE: Not Evaluated

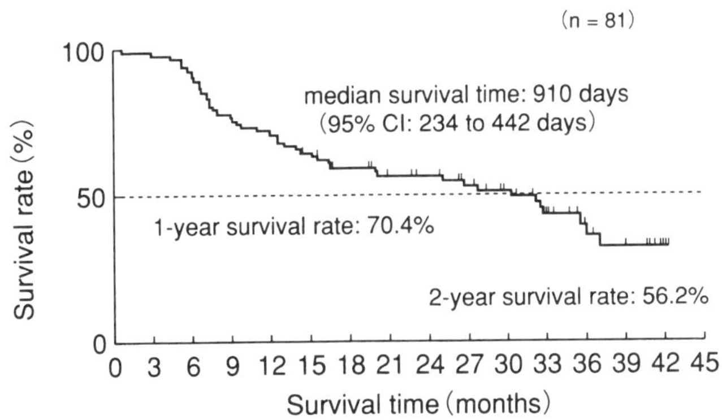

Fig. 14. Overall survival curve in breast cancer of S-1 (late Phase II clinical trial).

higher were as follows: neutropenia (8.6%); anorexia (4.9%); fatigue (3.7%); nausea/vomiting (1.2%); diarrhea (1.2%); and stomatitis (1.2%) *(35)*.

13. LATE PHASE II CLINICAL TRIAL OF S-1 IN LUNG CANCER

The objective of this clinical trial was to examine the antitumor activity and toxicity profile of S-1 in patients with stage IIIb or IV lung cancer who underwent no treatment prior to the onset of this clinical trial. Sixty-two patients were enrolled in this clinical trial, and 61 patients were treated with S-1. Fifty-nine patients were eligible for the analysis of response and toxicities. S-1 was administered orally at a dose of 40 mg/m^2, twice daily, i.e., once after breakfast and once after dinner. One course consisted of 28-d consecutive oral administration and of subsequent 14-d withdrawal. This regimen was repeated in four courses unless the disease progressed. Twenty-two patients with stage IIIb lung cancer and 37 patients with stage IV lung cancer were enrolled in this clinical trial. As shown in Table 11, the response rate per protocol set was 22.0% (13/59). As shown in Fig. 15, the median follow-up was 281

Table 11
Response Rates in the Late Phase II Clinical Trial of S-1 (NSCLC)

	Patient eligible	*Number of cases by response*						*Response rate (%)*
		CR	*PR*	*MR*	*NC*	*PD*	*NE*	
Type of NSCLC	*59*	*0*	*13*	*1*	*22*	*18*	*5*	*22.0*
Adenocarcinoma	38	0	10	1	13	11	3	26.3
Squamous cell carcinoma	20	0	2	0	9	7	2	10.0
Lage cell carcinoma	1	0	1	0	0	0	0	100.0

CR: Complete Response, PR: Partial Response, MR: Minor Response, NC: No Change, PD: Progressive Disease, NE: Not Evaluated

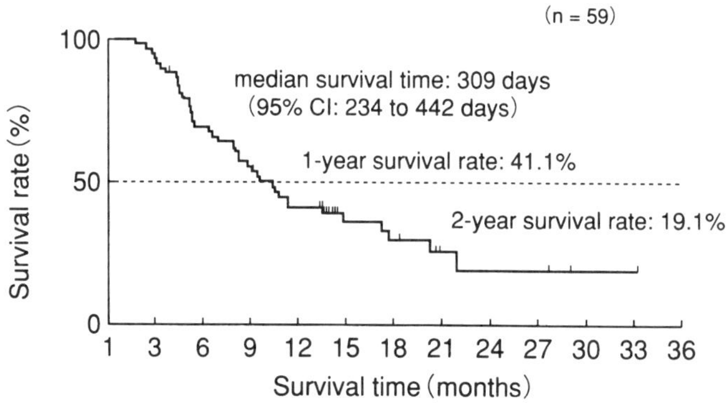

Fig. 15. Overall survival curve in NSCLC of S-1 (late Phase II clinical trial).

d (range: 50 to 994 d), and the median survival time was 309 d; 41.1% of patients were alive at year 1 of administration. In general, adverse reactions were mild in severity and were reversible. The adverse reactions which were assessed to be Grade 3 or higher were as follows: anemia (1.7%, 1/59); neutropenia (6.8%, 4/59); thrombocytopenia (1.7%, 1/59); proteinuria (1.7%, 1/59); anorexia (10.2%, 6/59); diarrhea (8.5%, 5/59); stomatitis (1.7%, 1/59); and fatigue (6.8%, 4/59). These results led us to consider that S-1 is effective against nonsmall cell lung cancer and its toxicities are tolerable to the patient. These results are based to consider that further research on the therapeutic benefits of S-1 in patients with nonsmall cell lung cancer is warranted *(36)*.

14. CONCLUSIONS

The therapeutical concept of conventional chemotherapy is that an anticancer drug fails to exert an antitumor effect unless adverse reactions develop to a certain extent. However, the development of adverse reactions preclude continuation of treatment, and treatment appears to have a considerable difficulty in contributing to life prolongation. Alleviation of the adverse reactions that provoke the greatest distress to patients, i.e., diarrhea, stomatitis, anorexia, and HF syndrome, and long-term treatment during which the patient can ingest meals by him/herself would not only improve QOL of the patient but also prolong the treatment period without a compliance decrease, exerting a life-prolonging effect. In this chapter, we explained in detail the preclinical and clinical profiles of S-1 in Japan as one of the approaches to the target, considering a therapeutic modality that is provided with a dual action consisting in enhancement of 5-FU effects and alleviation of 5-FU-induced adverse reactions as a goal SRC. We invented a novel oral anticancer agent, S-1, through the intentional devise of providing a drug with a dual action, i.e., enhancement of 5-FU effects and alleviation of 5-FU-induced adverse reactions. Consequently, the preclinical concept could be demonstrated in the clinical setting to a certain extent. In Japan, S-1 was given a manufacturing approval from the Ministry of Health and Welfare of Japan as a therapeutic agent for advanced/recurrent stomach cancer. Supplemental NDAs are under filing for breast cancer and head and neck cancer. Furthermore, the late phase II clinical trials of S-1 are in progress for colorectal cancer and nonsmall cell lung cancer. To establish the standard therapeutic modality for cancers, including gI cancers, in Japan, the conduction of clinical trials combining S-1 and other anticancer drugs is first expected in future.

van Groeningen et al. reported the results of European phase I study with the approximately same dose-schedule to the Japanese one, and the profiles of PK and toxicity were different from those of the Japanese *(37)*. 5-FU C_{max} and AUC were higher, and dose-limiting toxicity was diarrhea. One of the explanations for these differences may be the ethnic-related differences in the level and activity of a P-450 drug-metabolizing enzyme (CYP2A6), the converting enzyme of tegafur into 5-FU. The level and activity of CYP2A6 in Japanese were lower than those of Caucasians *(38)*. For further development of S-1 in Western countries, a more appropriate schedule in Western populations need to be studied.

REFERENCES

1. Dushinsky R, Pleven E, Heidelberger, C. The synthesis of 5-fluoropyrimidines. *J Am Chem Soc* 1957; 79:4559–4560.
2. Skipper HE, Schabel FM Jr, Wilcox WS. Experimental evaluation of potential anticancer agents. XIII on the criteria and kinetic associated with "curability" of experimental leukemia. *Cancer Chemother Rep* 1964; 35:1–111.
3. Houghton JA, Houghton PJ, Wooten RS. Mechanism of gastrointestinal toxicity in the mouse by 5-fluorouracil, 5-fluorouridine, and 5-fluoro-2′-deoxyuridine. *Cancer Res* 1979; 39:2406–2413.
4. Schuetz JD, Wallace HJ, Diasio RB. 5-Fluorouracil incorporation into DNA of CF-1 mouse bone marrow cells as a possible mechanism of toxicity. *Cancer Res* 1984; 44:1358–1363.
5. Fujii S, Shimamoto Y, Ohshima H, et al. Effect of the plasma concentration of 5-fluorouracil and the duration of continuous venous infusion of 5-fluorouracil with an inhibitor of 5-fluorouracil degradation on Yoshida sarcomas in rats. *Jpn J Cancer Res* 1989; 80:167–172.
6. Foenig, H, Patel, A. Biochemical basis for fluorouracil neurotoxicity–the role of Krebs cycle inhibition by fluoroacetate. *Arch. Neurol* 1970; 23:155–160.
7. Okeda, R, Shibutani, M, Matsuo, T, Kuroiwa T, Shimokawa, R, Tajima, T. Experimental neurotoxicity of 5-fluorouracil and its derivatives is due to poisoning by the mono-fluorinated organic metabolites, monofluoroacetic acid and alpha-fluoro-beta-alanine. *Acta Neuropathol* 1990; 81:66–73.
8. Akiba, T, Okeda, R, Tajima. Metabolites of 5-fluorouracil, alpha-fluoro-beta-alanine and fluoroacetic acid directly injure myelinated fibers in tissue culture. *Acta Neuropathol* 1996; 92:8–13.
9. Matsubara, I, Kamiya, J, Imai, S. Cardiotoxic effects of 5-fluorouracil in the guinea pig. *Jpn J Pharmacol* 1980; 30:871–879.
10. Lokich JJ, Ahlgren JD, Gullo JJ, Philips JA, Fryer JG. A prospective randomized comparison of continuous infusion fluorouracil with conventional bolus schedule in metastatic colorectal carcinoma: A Mid-Atlantic Oncology Program Study. *J Clin Oncol* 1989; 7:425–432.
11. The meta-analysis group in cancer: efficacy of intravenous continuous infusion of fluorouracil compared with bolus administration in advanced colorectal cancer. *J Clin Oncol* 1998; 16:301–308.
12. Shirasaka T, Shimamoto Y, Fukushima M. Inhibition by oxonic acid of gastrointestinal toxicity of 5-fluorouracil without loss of its antitumor activity in rats. *Cancer Res* 1993; 53:4004–4009.
13. Hilles S, Zhuk RA, Lidaks M. Analogues of pyrimidine nucleoside. N_1–(a Furanydil) derivative of natural pyrimidine bases and their antimetabolites. *Dokl Akad Nauk SSSR* 1967; 76:332–335.

14. Shirasaka T, Fukushima M, Shimamoto Y, Kimura K. Preclinical studies on S-1, a new oral tegafur plus modulators: Optimal molar ratio and antitumor activity. *Recent Advance in Chemotherapy. Proc 18th Int Congress Chemother* 1994; 927.
15. Shirasaka T, Shimamoto Y, Ohshimo H, et al. Development of a novel form of an oral 5-fluorouracil derivative (S-1) directed to the potentiation of the tumor selective cytotoxicity of 5-fluorouracil by two biochemical modulators. *Anti-Cancer Drugs* 1996; 7:548–557.
16. Shirasaka T, Nakano K, Takechi T, et al. Antitumor activity of 1M tegafur-0.4M 5-chloro-2,4- dihydroxypyridine-1M potassium oxonate (S-1) against human colon carcinoma orthotopically implanted into nude rats. *Cancer Res* 1996; 56:2602–2606.
17. Tatsumi K, Fukushima M, Shirasaka T, Fujii S. Inhibitory effects of pyrimidine, barbituric acid and pyridine derivatives on 5-fluorouracil degradation in rats liver extracts. *Jpn J Cancer Res* 1987; 78:748–755.
18. Schwartz PM, Handschumacher RE.: Selective antagonism of 5-fluorouracil cytotoxicity by 4-hydroxypyrazolopyrimidine (allopurinol) in vitro. *Cancer Res* 1979; 39:3095–3101.
19. Garewal HS, Ahmann FR, Alberts DS. Lack of inhibition by oxypurinol of 5-FU toxicity against human tumor cell lines. *Cancer Treat Rep* 1983; 67:495–498.
20. Schwartz PM, Dunigan JM, Marsh JC, Handschumacher RE: Allopurinol modification of the toxicity and antitumor activity of 5-fluorouracil. *Cancer Res* 1980; 40:1885–1889.
21. Kroener JF, Saleh F, Howell SB. 5-FU and allopurinol: toxicity modulation and Phase II results in colon cancer. *Cancer Treat Rep* 1982; 66:1133–1137.
22. Wooley PV, Ayoob MJ, Smith FP, et al. A controlled trial of the effect of 4-hydroxypyrimidine (allopurinol) on the toxicity of a single bolus dose of 5-fluorouracil. *J Clin Oncol* 1985; 3:103–109.
23. Granat P, Creasey WA, Calabresi P, Handschumacher RE. Investigations with 5-azaorotic acid, an inhibitor of the biosynthesis of pyrimidine de novo. *Clin Pharmacol Ther* 1965; 6:436–447.
24. Takechi T, Nakano K, Uchida J, et al. Antitumor activity and low intestinal toxicity of S-1, a new formulation of oral tegaful, in experimental tumor models in rats. *Cancer Chemother Pharmacol* 1997; 39:205–211.
25. Shirasaka T, Yamamitsu, Tuji A, Taguchi T. Conceptual change in cancer chemotherapy: from an oral fluoropyrimidine prodrug, UFT, to a novel oral fluoropyrimidine prodrug, S-1, and low-dose FP therapy in Japan. *Invest New Drugs* 2000; 18:315–329.
26. Sugimachi K, Maehara Y, Horikoshi N, et al. An early Phase II study of oral S-1, a newly developed 5-fluorouracil derivative for treating patients with advanced and recurrent gastrointestinal cancer. *Oncology* 1999; 57:202–210.
27. Taguchi T, Horikoshi N, Kinoshita H, Toge T, Takashima S. Early phase II study of S-1 in patients with advanced breast cancer *Proc Am Soc Clin Oncol* 1996; 15:121(#151).
28. Fujii M, Kanzaki J, Satake B, Baba S, Inuyama Y. Early phase II study of S-1 in patients with advanced head and neck cancer *Proc Am Soc Clin Oncol* 1996; 15:316 (#895).
29. Hino M, Kudoh S, Furuse K, et al. Early phase II study of S-1 in patients with non-small-cell-lung cancer Ann Oncol 1996; 7:105(#503).
30. Hirata K, Horikoshi N, Aiba K, et al. Pharmacokinetic study of S-1, a novel oral fluorouracil antitumor drug. *Clin Cancer Res* 1999; 5:2000–2005.
31. Sakata Y, Ohtsu A, Horikoshi N, Sugimachi K, Mitachi Y, Taguchi T. Late phase II study of novel oral fluoropyrimidine anticancer drug S-1 (1M tegafur-0.4M gimestat-1M otastat potassium) in advanced gastric cancer patients. *Eur J Cancer* 1998; 34:1715–1720.
32. Koizumi W, Kurihara M, Nakano S, Hasegawa K. Phase II study of S-1, a novel oral derivative of 5-fluorouracil, in advanced gastric cancer. *Oncology* 2000; 58:191–197.
33. Ohtsu A, Baba H, Sakata Y, Phase II study of S-1, a novel oral fluoropyrimidine derivativr, in patients with metastatic colorectal carcinoma. *Brit J Cancer* 2000; 83:141–145.
34. Endo S, Niwa H, Kida A. Late phase II study of S-1 in patients with head and neck cancer *Proc Am Soc Clin Oncol* 1999; 8:395a(#1526).
35. Sano M, Saeki S, Takashima S, et al. Late phase II study of S-1 in patients with advanced and/or recurrent breast cancer *Proc Am Soc Clin Oncol* 2000; 19:105a(#404).
36. Niitani H, Kawahara M, Segawa Y, Yoshimura A, Yoshimori K. Activity of S-1 in patients with non-small-cell lung cancer: Results from a phase II study *Proc Am Soc Clin Oncol* 2000; 19:510a(#1995).
37. van Groeningen CJ, Peters GJ, Schornagel JH, Gall H, Noordhuis P, de Vries MJ, Turner SL, Swart MS, Pinedo HM, Hanauske AR, Giaccone G. Phase I clinical and pharmacokinetic study of oral S-1 in patients with advanced solid tumous *J Clin Oncol* 2000; 8:2772–2779.
38. Shimada T., Yamazaki H., Guengerich F.P. Ethnic-related differences in coumarin 7-hydroxlation activities catalyzed by cytochrome P4502A6 in liver microsomes of Japanese and Caucasian populations *XENOBIOTICA* 1996; 26:395–403.

24 Preclinical and Clinical Practice of Low-Dose FP Therapy in Japan

Japanese Use of Low-Dose FP Therapy

Tetsuhiko Shirasaka, PhD, *Akihito Tsuji,* MD,
Susumu Yamamitsu, MD,
and Tetsuo Taguchi, MD

CONTENTS

1. INTRODUCTION

Cancer chemotherapy started with the treatment of leukemias with nitrogen mustards about 50 yr ago. The topsy-turvy concept of high-dose chemotherapy, "an anticancer agent would not be effective unless provoking considerable adverse reactions (misoriented approach)," still remains at present. High-dose chemotherapy provides relatively high response rates. However, the incidence of adverse reactions increases in proportion to dose increments in chemotherapy, which impedes long-term treatment. Therefore, it is difficult with chemotherapy to lead to life prolongation. To attain a satisfactory life-prolonging effect, not a short-term battle-type modality but "Fabian tactics" and long-term administration-type modality should be instituted. For this purpose, it is crucial that novel chemotherapy should not only have a higher anticancer effect as compared with that of conventional ones but also provoke less adverse reactions.

In the field of chemotherapy, many of attempts have been made to develop a novel drug with a new mechanism of action or concept and to establish combination chemotherapy with

From: *Fluoropyrimidines in Cancer Therapy*
Edited by: Y. M. Rustum © Humana Press Inc., Totowa, NJ

such a property. The fundamental concept for combination chemotherapy available to date has aimed to reduce the dose of each drug and to attain an additive effect. However, this approach adds adverse events as well and elicits concern about usefulness. From about 1988, we have attempted to explore, instead of seeking a novel compound as an effector, a therapeutic modality which is provided with a dual action, i.e., enhancement of 5-fluorouracil (5-FU) effects and alleviation of 5-FU-induced adverse reactions, based on the theory of biochemical modulation of 5-FU—an anticancer drug whose mechanism of action and adverse reactions were elucidated to the largest extent. Following a variety of devices, consequently, we invented therapeutic modalities that are intended to alleviate adverse reactions that afflict the patient most and that allow long-term treatment. In Chapter 23, we described in detail S-1, a novel oral anticancer agent as one of these modalities. In this chapter, we explain, as the second therapeutic modality, combination chemotherapy of 5-FU with cisplatin (CDDP) by which 5-FU is used as an effector and CDDP is used mainly as a modulator for 5-FU.

We provide herein explanations on the following two combination chemotherapies: 5-FU continuous venous infusion (CVI) + low-dose consecutive CDDP (low-dose FP therapy), a combination chemotherapy whose preclinical theory is being demonstrated in clinical practice in Japan through the theory of 5-FU biochemical modulation; and intermittent 24-h 5-FU (CVI) + low-dose consecutive CDDP (intermittent FP therapy).

The use of CVI, the optimal regimen for 5-FU which we described in the Chapter 23, constitutes the crucial key for the abovementioned two chemotherapies.

2. HISTORY OF EFFECT ENHANCEMENT AND ADVERSE REACTION ALLEVIATION

The fundamental concept of combination chemotherapy consists in a reduction of the doses of drugs whose mechanism of action differ among them and in an attempt to enhance their effects through their combination. One disadvantage of combination chemotherapy is the fact that not only the anticancer activity of a drug is enhanced but also its adverse reactions are potentiated. The ideal combination chemotherapy would not potentiate adverse reactions despite drug combination. To allow this, it is important to use drugs whose mechanism of action is explicit in an attempt to reduce their adverse reactions and to improve their dosing schedule.

5-FU, based on the theory of biochemical modulation, has been applied vigorously to clinical practice since the first half of the 1990s. A combination of 5-FU with methotrexate (MTX), a combination of 5-FU with leucovorin *(2)*, a combination of tegafur + uracil (UFT) with leucovorin *(3)*, and other combinations may be cited as such applications. All these approaches aim to enhance drug effects and have gained appreciation to a certain extent in clinical practice. However, these therapeutic modalities add drug adverse reactions due to the lack of a device to alleviate them and involve concern about their clinical usefulness. Durins the first half of the 1980s, on the other hand, allopulinol was used in combination with 5-FU as a modulator for alleviating activity on 5-FU-induced adverse reactions *(4,5)*. As described in detail in Chapter 23, the relevant combination alleviated 5-FU-induced adverse reactions and allowed increases in 5-FU dose. However, reductions in 5-FU effect also were observed simultaneously, and the combination exhibited no clinical usefulness.

3. THEORY OF LOW-DOSE FP THERAPY

We directed our attention to CDDP among the modulators for 5-FU and initiated our research 12 yr ago. According to the conventionally described mechanism of biological

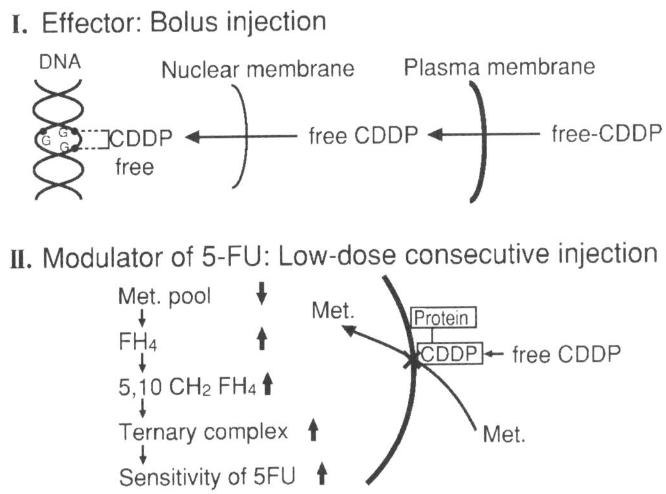

Fig. 1. Possible biological action of CDDP.

action as illustrated in Fig. 1, CDDP, which passes through the cell membrane and then the nuclear membrane, inhibits the DNA synthesis through coordinate bond with two guanine groups on the DNA chain. To reduce its toxicity, CDDP, which remains in the body, should be excreted by hydration for detoxication purpose. This usage is to apply CDDP as an effector. In 1983, Scanlon et al. *(6)* used cell lines in vitro and discovered a synergic cytotoxic effect in a combination of 5-FU with CDDP. They reported the following mechanism of action: CDDP inhibits the incorporation of methionine into cell, provoking an increase in intracellular reduced folate level—which, in turn, increases the formation of a ternary complex (5,10-CH_2FH_4 FdUMP-TS); the relevant formation enhances the cytotoxicity of 5-FU. We also conducted additional studies in vitro by using a variety of cells, without successful reverification. We presumed that the rationale for the failure was based on the fact that a large amount of folate in the medium that was used in the cell culture system in vitro made it difficult to precisely capture the CDDP-induced changes in intracellular folate level. For detailed examination, therefore, we used two in vivo cell lines allowing the precise measurement of changes in intrinsic folate level without the addition of extrinsic folate, i.e., ascites hepatoma in rats (Yoshida sarcoma) and ascites cancer in mice (P-388). In 1993, consequently, we elucidated the mechanism of action as illustrated in Fig. 2 *(7)*. The biochemical mechanism of synergy between 5-FU and CDDP was studied using transplantable tumors in rodents in vivo. Reduced folate—5, 10-methylenetetrahydrofolate (CH_2FH_4)—and its precursor tetrahydrofolate (FH_4) are the cofactors essential for the formation of a tight ternary complex of thymidylate synthase (TS) and 5-fluoro-2′-deoxyuridine-5-monophosphate (FdUMP) derived from 5-FU *(7)*. As shown in Table 1, intraperitoneal administration of CDDP (5 mg/kg) inhibited the incorporation of exogenous L-methionine into ascitic tumor cells. As shown in Table 2, the inhibited incorporation of L-methionine into cell also is observed with CDDP which has bound to proteins (data not shown). As shown in Table 3, the levels of CH_2FH_4 in Yoshida sarcoma and of P-338 cells transplanted into rats and mice showed two-to three-fold increases as compared with the levels in cells isolated from animals which had not been treated with CDDP *(7)*. Furthermore, the effect of CDDP on induction of the activity of methionine synthase, a synthase for methionine, was examined. As shown in Table 4, consequently, an about three-fold increase in methionine syn-

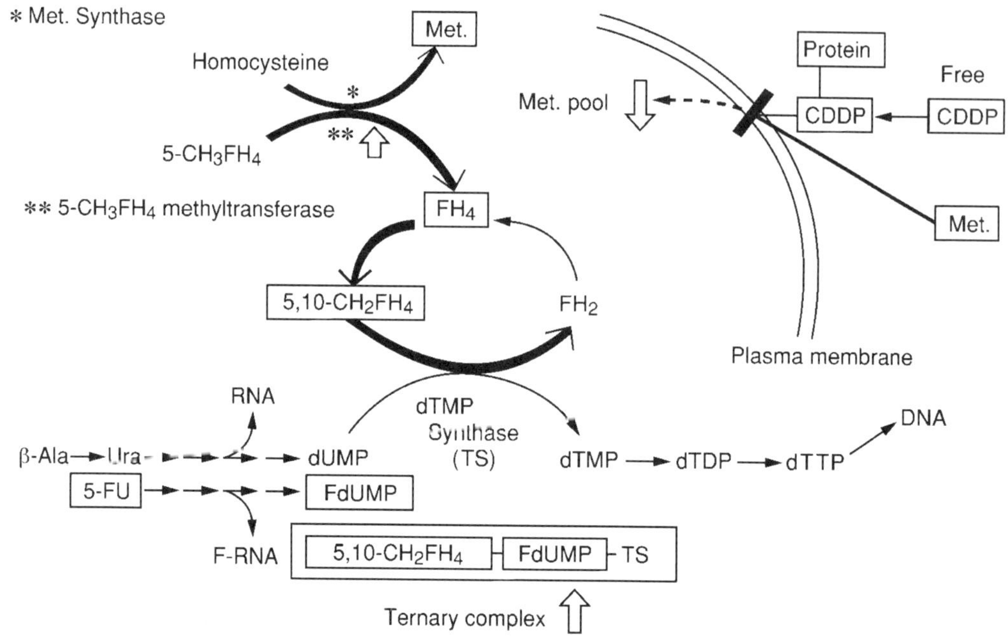

Fig. 2. Mechanism of biochemical modulation of 5-FU by CDDP.

Table 1
Uptake of L-Met into Ascitic Tumor Cells Isolated From Yoshida Sarcoma-Bearing Rats after Intra-Peritoneal Administration of CDDP

Dose of CDDP (mg/kg)	*Rats (n)*	*L-Met uptake (pmol/l × 10^{-7} cells/min)*	*% Inhibition*
Saline	4[a]	18.4 ± 2.9[b]	–
1.0	4	16.3 ± 0.3	11.4
2.0	4	15.8 ± 4.5	14.4
5.0	4	10.8 ± 1.9	41.3

[a] Rats were treated ip with CDDP on day 8 after the inoculation of Yoshida sarcoma cells.

[b] Tumor cells were incubated with 1 μM L-Met (18.5 KBq) for 10 min in the assay mixture. Data represent mean values ± SD.

thase activity induction was observed even in four-d consecutive administration of low-dose CDDP (1 mg/kg) *(8)*.

As shown in Table 5, intraperitoneal administration of CDDP on d 1 and continuous infusion of 5-FU from d 1 through d 6 showed a synergic effect in inhibiting tumor growth in Yoshida sarcoma-bearing rats. These results suggest that CDDP significantly enhances 5-FU cytotoxicity by inhibiting the intracellular L-methionine metabolism, increasing the intracellular reduced folate level in the mammalian tumor model in vivo *(8)*.

In addition, we demonstrated that CDDP, when administered at 1–8 mg/kg, increased the intracellular reduced folate level and elucidated that CDDP, when used in combination with 5-FU, shows sufficient effects by repeated administration at a low dose instead by single

Table 2
Uptake of L-Met into Human Colorectal Carcinoma Cells

		Cell lines			
		DLD-1		*HCT-15*	
CDDP (µg/mL)	*Albumin (mg/mL)*	*Met Uptake (pmol/1 × 10^7 cells/min)*	*% Control*	*Met uptake (pmol/1 × 10^7 cells/min)*	*% Control*
0	100	2.940	89.4	2.622	70.7
1.0	0	1.625	49.4	1.646	44.4
1.0	100	1.726	52.4	1.887	50.9
1.0	250	1.422	43.2	1.878	50.7

Uptake of Met
= Acid soluble + Acid insoluble
Medium: RPMI-1640
CDDP incubation time: 24 h
^{14}C-Met incubation time: 10 ± min

Table 3
Effect of Intra-Peritoneal Administered CDDP Administration on Intracellular Reduced Folates Levels in P388-Bearing Mice and Yoshida Sarcoma-Bearing Rats

		Reduced folate pool (pmol/2×10^7 cells)[a]	
Tumor cells	*CDDP (mg/kg)*	*CH_2FH_4*	*FH_4*
P388	–	0.075 ± 0.004	0.111 ± 0.004
	2.5	0.108 ± 0.013	0.172 ± 0.036
	5.0	0.152 ± 0.017	0.426 ± 0.200
Yoshida sarcoma	–	0.065 ± 0.004	0.190 ± 0.004
	5.0	0.139 ± 0.007	0.301 ± 0.055

Tumor cells were isolated from mice or rats at 24 h after the administration of CDDP. CH_2FH_4, 5,10-methylenetetrahydrofolate; FH_4 tetrahydrofolate

[a] Data represent mean values ± SD.

Table 4
Effect of Low-Dose Consecutive CDDP on Induction of the Methionine Synthase Activity in Yoshida Sarcoma Ascitic Cells (In Vivo)

(n = 5)

Durgs	*Route*	*Dose (mg/kg)*	*Duration (day)*	*Met. synthase activity (pmol/mg/min±SD)*
Saline	*ip*		days 5–8	47.0 ± 31.0
CDDP	*ip*	1.0	days 5–8	148.7 ± 60.1

Table 5
Antitumor Effect of the Combination of CDDP and Continuous Venous Infusion of 5-FU on Yoshida Sarcomas in Rats

FUra[a] (*mg/kg daily*)	*CDDP*[b] (*mg/kg*)	*Rats* (*n*)	*Tumor wt.*[b] (*g*)	*IR*[d] (*%*)	*Body wt. (g)*[c] *Start*	*End*
–	–	9	1.58 ± 0.43	–	236 ± 9	258 ± 11
–	5.0	8	1.11 ± 0.23	29.7	235 ± 9	234 ± 17
1.0	–	9	1.82 ± 0.81	0	239 ± 7	262 ± 11
1.0	5.0	8	0.40 ± 0.23	74.7	238 ± 7	212 ± 20
2.0	–	8	0.94 ± 0.18	40.5	239 ± 7	245 ± 13
2.0	5.0	8	0.07 ± 0.15	95.6	238 ± 7	204 ± 30

[a] 5-FU combined with a 10-fold molar ratio of CDHP (5 chloro-2, 4-dihydroxypyridine) (11.2 and 22.4 mg/kg, respectively) was continuously infused from day 1 to day 7.

[b] CDDP was injected ip on day 1 of the therapeutic periods (7 d).

[c] Data represent mean values ± SD.

[b] Inhibition rate of tumor growth.

administration at a high dose *(8,9)*. The results of the above mentioned preclinical studies evidenced the indirect action of CDDP as a modulator for 5-FU in addition to its direct action of acting as an effector.

Recently, we discovered that 5-FU and low-dose CDDP exhibited a synergic effect on Fas-Fas ligand-mediated apoptosis and that acridine orange stain identifies the fragmentation of DNA *(10)*.

We examined whether treatment of the T24 bladder cancer cell line with the combination of CDDP, 5-FU, and anti-Fas mono-clonal antibody (mAb) could overcome drug resistance. Cytotoxicity was determined in a day MTT assay. T24 cells were relatively resistant to the combination of CDDP, 5-FU, and anti-Fas mAb. The combination of these two drugs showed a synergistic effect in cytotoxicity. Moreover, treatment of T24 cells with the combination of CDDP (0.1—10 μg/mL), 5-FU (0.1–10 μg/mL), and anti-Fas mAb significantly enhanced their cytotoxicity, and synergism was thus achieved *(10)*. These findings suggested that chemoimmunosensitized cells required lower doses of CDDP and 5-FU, thus minimizing their toxicities in vivo and maximizing their potential therapeutic application in vivo.

4. CLINICAL PRACTICE OF LOW-DOSE FP THERAPY

We have reported clinical results of low-dose FP therapy since 1991 *(11–15)*. As described previously, CDDP acts as a modulator for 5-FU even when given by consecutive administration at a low dose. To examine the dose at which consecutive administration of CDDP is practicable, we initially repeated the following fundamental regimen: CDDP 15 mg/kg/d was administered by intravenous infusion over 1 h for 5 d followed by 2-d withdrawal (1-wk unit), with 4-wk administrations and 1-to 2-wk withdrawals. Consequently, about 20% of patients developed myelosuppression at wk 3–4 of treatment. Therefore, we reduced the dose of CDDP for further examination.

Consequently, we discovered the reference regimen as illustrated in Fig. 3. In this regimen by which low-dose CDDP (3 and 5 mg/m^2) was administered consecutively—five administrations (Monday through Friday) weekly and two withdrawals (Saturday and Sunday) to

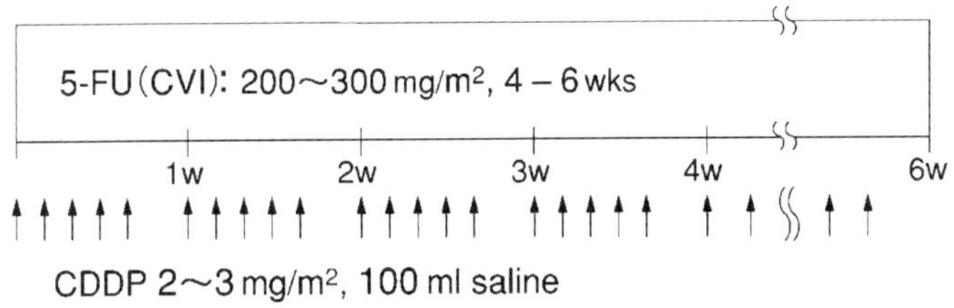

Fig. 3. Combination therapy of continuous 5-FU infusion with low-dose consecutive CDDP.

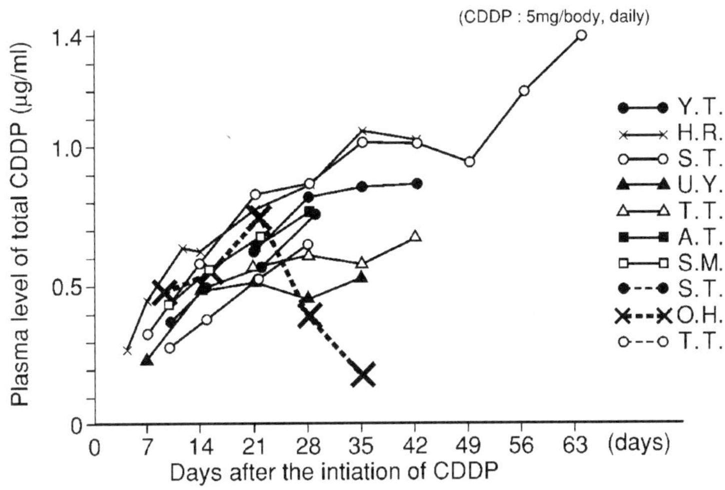

Fig. 4. Plasma level of total CDDP after daily injection of CDDP.

patients—the incidence of its adverse reactions lowered and no loss of its antitumor activity was observed. Furthermore, this regimen required no hydration.

As illustrated in Fig. 4, the plasma level of CDDP was 0.5 μg/mL at wk 2 of its daily administration to 10 patients at a dose of 5 mg/body, and this level was maintained for a long period, i.e., the plasma level of accumulated CDDP was higher than 0.5 μg/mL.

The clinical efficacy of the combination therapy is shown in Table 6. Recently, we synopsized and reported clinical results *(16)*. The overall response rate at Kochi Municipal Hospital was 55.0% (170/309), Although the population of patients examined was small, the response rates of CR + PR were as follows: About 63% for stomach cancer, 51.1% for colorectal cancer, and 63.3% for esophageal cancer. This regimen required no hydration. Little adverse reactions rated to be Grade II or higher were observed. Table 7 shows adverse reactions provoked by the combination of 5-FU with low-dose consecutive CDDP. The incidence of adverse reactions of Grade 3 rated to be higher was a few percent below.

Patients without pretreatment and patients who failed to respond to treatment with WHF *(17)* were treated with low-dose FP therapy, and differences in efficacy were examined. As shown in Table 8, a response rate comparable to the rate in the first treatment group, being as high as 60.7% (17/28), was obtained.

This therapeutic modality is consistently conducted on a nationwide basis in Japan. The nationwide questionnaire survey reported by Saji et al. *(18)* indicated response rates as high as 40–to 60% for the stomach cancer, esophageal cancer, colorectal cancer, cancer of the

Table 6
Efficacy in Combination Therapy of Continuous 5-FU Infusion with Low-Dose Consecutive CDDP

Type of cancer	*No. of patients*	*CR*	*PR*	*NC*	*PD*	*Response rate (%)*	*MST (day)*
Esophageal cancer	30	3	16	5	6	63.3	288
Stomach cancer	96	4	57	19	8	63.5	237
Colon cancer	88	2	43	33	8	51.1	420
Pancreatic cancer	32	0	8	16	8	25.0	210
Gallbladder cancer	22	0	13	5	2	59.1	165
Cholangiocarcinoma	17	0	7	6	4	41.2	231
Hepatocellular carcinoma	24	0	17	4	3	70.8	123
Total	309	9	161	88	39	55.0	

Table 7
Adverse Reactions in Combination Therapy of Continuous 5-FU Infusion
With Low-Dose Consecutive CDDP

	Grade				
	1	*2*	*3*	*4*	
Toxicity	*(No. of patients)*				*Incidence of ≥ G3 (%)*
Hematological	24	11	5	0	1.6
Leukopenia	3	3	1	0	0.3
Anemia	19	6	1	–	0.3
Thrombocytopenia	2	2	3	0	1.0
Nonhematological	69	31	7	2	3.2
Anorexia, nausea/vomiting	51	20	4	1	1.6
Stomatitis	4	3	1	0	1.0
Diarrhea	1	2	2	0	0.3
Pigmentation	1	1	–	–	
H & F	4	1	–	–	
Creatinine	5	3	–	1	0.3
Malaise	2	–	–	–	
Total					15/309 (4.9%)

head and neck, lung cancer, breast cancer, hepatic cancer, and uterine cervical cancer. The incidence of adverse reactions rated to be Grade 3 or higher was 10% or below. This therapeutic modality, which provided response rates that exceeded the rates attained with conventional combination therapies and caused less intense adverse reactions, may be considered to be highly useful for cancer patients.

5. THEORY OF TOXICITY ALLEVIATION BY THE INTERMITTENT ADMINISTRATION OF 5-FU UTILIZING A DIFFERENCE IN CELL CYCLE

From 1963 to 1965, Lipkin et al. *(19)* and Clarkson and Ota et al. *(20)* investigated the cell cycle (T_G) of human normal and tumor cells and reported the changes to be described

Table 8
Response Rates in Patients Without Prior Chemotherapy and Patients Treated with WHF Therapy for Advance/Recurrent Colorectal Cancers

	No. of patients	*CR*	*PR*	*NC*	*PD*	*Response rate (%)*
Patients without prior therapy	60	1	30	24	3	51.7
Patients treated with WHF therapy	28	1	16	7	4	60.7
Total	88	2	46	31	7	54.5
Reasons of shifting from WHF therapy to low-dose FP therapy						
(1) Newly appeared lesion in extrahepatic areas	4	0	3	0	1	75
(2) PD of hepatopathy	9	0	4	4	1	44.4
(3) (1) + (2)	10	1	5	3	1	60
(4) Others	5	0	4	0	1	80
Total	28	1	16	7	4	60.7

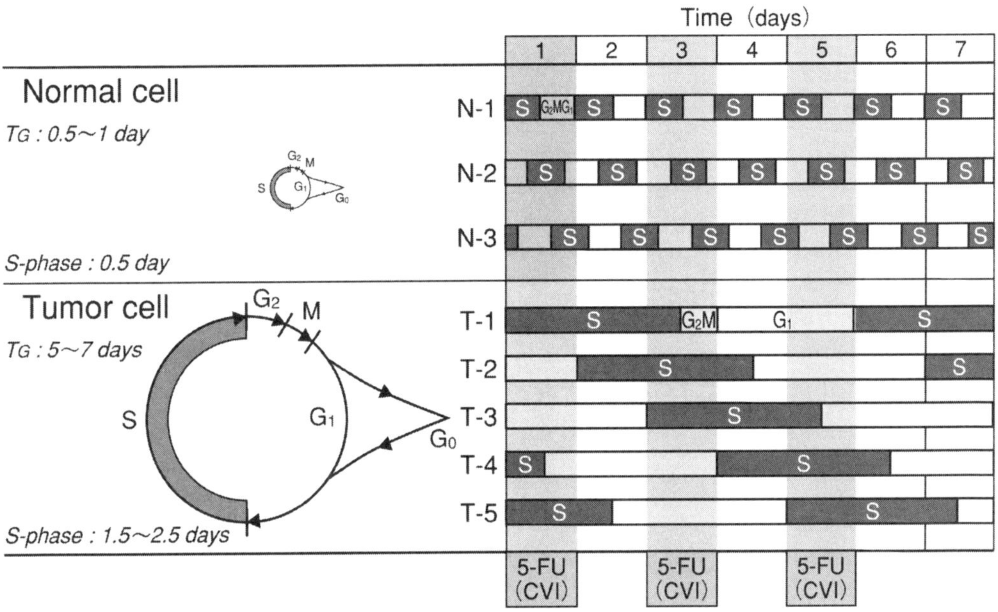

Fig. 5. Cell cycle of normal and tumor cells in vivo.

below. Namely, they administered ^{3}H-dThd to examine T_G and discovered that T_G was longer for tumor cells than for normal cells (bone marrow and gastrointestinal mucosa), being 5–7 d and about 0.5–1.5 d, respectively. This discovery was of crucial importance and elicited much interest in those days. As illustrated in Fig. 5, 5-FU is a typical drug among highly dose-dependent antimetabolites and is considered to act in the S phase of the cell cycle only *(21)*. In humans, an overt difference exists in terms of T_G of normal and tumor cells. This difference in cell cycle suggested possible preservation of effects and alleviation of adverse reactions. Therefore, we used cells with a short cell cycle and cells with a long

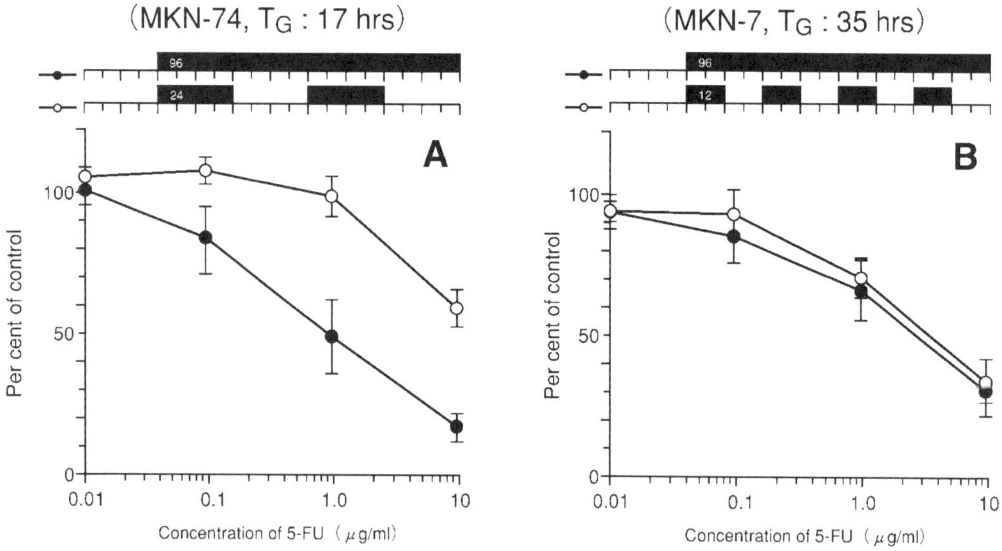

Fig. 6. Comparison of cytotoxic activity of 5-FU continuous and intermittent regimens with the colony formation assay.

cell cycle in the in vitro system, considering them as the normal cell model and the tumor cell model, respectively, in an attempt to examine a difference in cytotoxic effect according to the regimen for 5-FU. Namely, we used a stomach cancer cell line with a short T_G (MKN-74; T $_G$: 17h) as the model of normal cells (e.g., mucus cells and bone marrow cells) and used the 96-h consecutive contact method of 5-FU and the intermittent contact method by which 5-FU was administered repeatedly every 24 h to compare their cytotoxicity. As illustrated in Fig. 6A, the intermittent contact method showed a marked decrease in cytotoxicity for the gastric cancer cell with a short T_G On the other hand, we used a stomach cell line with a long T_G (MKN-74; $_G$: 35h) as the model of tumor cells and used the 96-h consecutive contact method of 5-FU and the intermittent contact method by which 5-FU was administered repeatedly every 12h to compare their cytotoxicity. As shown in Fig. 6B, 5-FU was shown to maintain its cytotoxic activity even by repetition of intermittent contact *(16)*. Review of treatment with 5-FU, as illustrated in Fig. 5, indicates that nearly half of normal cells (e.g., mucus cells and bone marrow cells) are rescued by withdrawal every 24 h because their cell cycle is short and that cytotoxicity of tumor cells is maintained even by withdrawal every 24 h because the cell cycle of tumor cells is long, leading to incomplete rescue. Therefore, the intermittent contact method allows us to expect a cytotoxic effect of 5-FU that is comparable to or better than that attained by the long-term contact method. The above mentioned results led us to presume possible alleviation of adverse reactions without reduction in cytotoxic activity when 5-FU is given by intermittent (every 24 h) administration at a high dose rather than by long-term intravenous infusion.

6. CLINICAL PRACTICE OF INTERMITTENT FP THERAPY

In the 1996 Congress of Japan Society for Cancer Chemotherapy, we proposed, instead of consecutive administration (CVI) of 5-FU, a combination chemotherapy consisting in intermittent administration of 5-FU (5-FU: 750–1000 mg/body/day; administration by 24-h CVI:

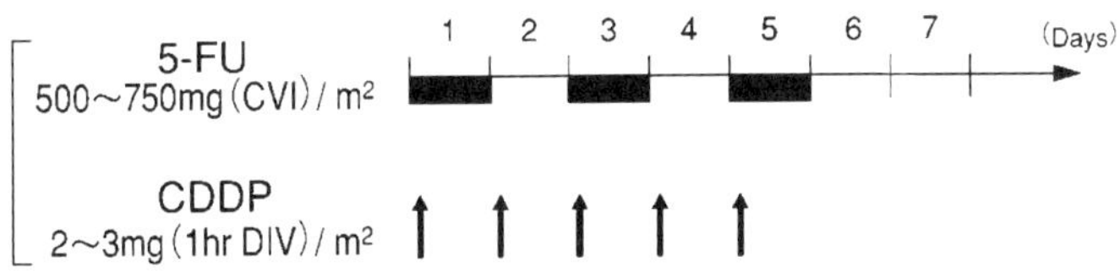

Fig. 7. Combination therapy of intermittent 24-hr continuous 5-FU infusion with low-dose consecutive CDDP.

Table 9
Response Rates in Combination Therapy of Intermittent 24-h Continuous 5-FU Infusion with Low-Dose Consecutive CDDP

	No. of patients	*Lesion evaluated*	*CR*	*PR*	*NC*	*PD*	*R.R. (%)*
Esophageal cancer	5	4	1	1	2		50.0
Stomach cancer	16	11	2	4	5		54.5
Colon cancer	22	16		9	6	1	56.3
Rectal cancer	15	12		5	6	1	41.7
Pancreatic cancer	7	7	1	1	4	1	28.6
Hepatocellular carcinoma	3	3		1	1	1	33.3
Breast cancer	5	2		1	1		50
Lung cancer	6	5	1	4			100
Others	4	2		1	1		50
Total	83	62	5	27	26	4	51.6

Monday, Wednesday, and Friday; and withdrawal: Tuesday, Thursday, Saturday, and Sunday) and consecutive administration of low-dose CDDP (CDDP: 3–5 mg/body/d; administration: Monday, Tuesday, Wednesday, Thursday, and Friday; and withdrawal: Saturday and Sunday). The fundamental schedule is illustrated in Fig. 7. As shown in Table 9, which shows its effects, as well as in Table 10, which shows adverse reactions, this therapeutic modality deserves attention because of its beneficial effects even on breast cancer and pancreatic cancer, in addition to different cancers of the gastrointestinal tract. The overall response rate in this therapeutic modality was as high as 51.6% (32/62). However, little adverse reactions, e.g., diarrhea and stomatitis, were observed; the incidence of adverse reactions rated to be Grade 3 or higher was 10% or below, and the incidence of myelotoxicity rated to be Grade 3 or higher also was 10% or below. The response rate in this therapeutic modality was as high as 50.0% (14/28) for Stage IV colorectal cancer. Among 14 patients in whom PR was attained, a response period of 0.5–1 yr was observed in nine (64.3%). There were no non-hematological adverse reactions afflicting the patient most, which were rated to be Grade 3 or higher (0/83). The above mentioned results indicate that this therapeutic modality markedly improved gastrointestinal toxicities without losing its effects. Furthermore, this modality improved myelotoxicity as well and is considered to allow long-term treatment.

Results of three clinical trials of 5-FU and *l*-LV are available as the clinical results for advanced and recurrent colorectal cancer in Japan *(22–24)*. Comparison of these results with the results obtained with S-1*(25),* low-dose FP therapy, and intermittent FP therapy show, as

Table 10
Adverse Reactions in Combination Therapy of Intermittent 24-h Continuous 5-FU Infusion with Low-Dose Consecutive CDDP

Toxicity	*Grade* 1	2 (*No. of patients*)	3	4	*Incidence of ≥ G3 (%)*
Hematological (83 cases)					
Leukopenia	22	24	4	0	4.8
Anemia	22	22	2	0	2.4
Thrombocytopenia	11	2	0	0	0
Nonhematological (83 cases)					
Anorexia	15	6	0	0	0
Nausia/vomiting	6	2	0	–	0
Stomatitis	6	4	0	0	0
Diarrhea	3	1	0	0	0
Rash	5	0	0	0	0
Alopecia	1	0	0	–	0

detailed in Table 11, that low-dose FP therapy and intermittent FP therapy caused lower incidences of adverse reactions than those of the relevant clinical trials of 5-FU and *l*-LV in terms of their effects and adverse reactions. Therefore, usefulness of these therapeutic modalities was suggested. In particular, intermittent FP therapy was superior to other therapies in terms of the response rate, survival period, and response period, although it showed longer time required to reach PR; concurrently, intermittent FP therapy markedly improved the incidence of adverse reactions. Therefore, we consider that intermittent FP therapy would become the fundamental therapeutic modality in future.

7. POINTS FOR THERAPY

We have described two combination therapies of 5-FU with low-dose consecutive CDDP as the therapeutic modalities that are gentle to patients. Treatment of cancer patients at precise doses and with a correct regimen are considered to be more useful treatment for them. We below three points for therapy on the basis of accurate and valid information which we have obtained from a number of medical institutions in Japan.

1. The regimen of 5-FU and CDDP constitues the key for continuous FP therapy. The regimen of 5-FU consists in the conduction of 24-h CVI of 5-FU (250 to 350 mg/body) for 4 wk. From Monday through Friday at wk 4–6, CDDP (3–5 mg/body), previously dissolved into 100 mL of saline, should be administered by CVI for about 1 h via a route that differs from another used for 5-FU. The regimen should be repeated, with cycles of 4–6 wk. In the case that the administration of CDDP is impracticable on a daily and ambulatory basis due to circumstances at the relevant medical institution, CDDP can be administered at a dose of 5–10 mg/body on a twice-weekly basis (Monday and Thursday or Tuesday and Friday). Laboratory tests should be conducted every week to check any changes, especially myelotoxicity.
2. The regimen of 5-FU and CDDP constitutes the key for intermittent FP therapy. The regimen of 5-FU consists in the intermittent administration (administration on Monday, Wednesday,

Table 11

Efficacy and Adverse Reactions in Clinical Studies on Advance and Recurrent Colorectal Cancers

	Efficacy				*Adverse reaction (≥ G3)*			
Chemotherapy	*Response rate (%)*	*MST (days)*	*Response period (days)*	*Time required to PR onset (days)*	*Diarrhea (%)*	*Leuko-penia (%)*	*Thrombo-cytopenia (%)*	*References*
(1) 5-FU+I-LV								
Nationwide collaborative study in Japan	32.4 (12/37)	375	90	62	30	15	0	*(22)*
East Japan collaborative study	30.0 (21/70)	297	90	42	12	20	7	*(23)*
West Japan collaborative study	32.8 (21/64)	384	118	49	19	8	1.5	*(24)*
(2) Late phase II study of S-1	35.5 (22/62)	378	78	36	1.6	4.8	8.1	*(25)*
(3) Low-dose FP therapy	51.1 (45/88)	362	150	52	1.1	0	1.1	*(16)*
(4) Intermittent FP therapy	50.0 (14/28)	485	159	77	0	0	0	*(16)*

and Friday) of 5-FU (750–1000 mg/body) by 24-h CVI for 4–6 wk. From Monday through Friday at wk 4–6, CDDP (3–5 mg/body), previously dissolved into 100 mL of saline, should be administered by CVI for about 1 h via a route that differs from another for 5-FU. The regimen should be repeated, with cycles of 4–6 wk. In the case that the administration of CDDP is impracticable on a daily and ambulatory basis due to circumstances at the respective medical institution, CDDP can be administered at a dose of 5–10 mg/body on a twice-weekly basis (Monday and Thursday or Tuesday and Friday). Laboratory tests should be conducted every week to check any changes, especially myelotoxicity.

We describe below the points for therapy which are shared between the two therapeutic modalities described in Items 1 and 2.

3. In the case of finding no abnormalities, the cycle should be repeated two or three times, followed by 4- to 6-wk withdrawals. The dose should be reduced when finding any adverse event rated to be Grade 2. The dose of 5-FU only should be reduced, considering 70% of the dose as a reference value. Withdrawal should be conducted when finding any adverse event rated to be Grade 3 or higher, and administration should be resumed after recovery of laboratory values. A decrease in white blood cell count during repeated cycles (e.g., a decrease in white blood cell count from about 7000/mm^3 at the onset of treatment to about 3500/m^3 during treatment) leads us to consider an increase in total blood platinum level. Therefore, the daily dose of CDDP should be reduced to 2–3 mg/body.

8. CONCLUSIONS

The therapeutical concept of conventional cancer chemotherapy has been, "no adverse reaction, no effect." However, the development of an adverse reaction precludes the conduction of long-term treatment, and cancer chemotherapy would involve great difficulty in contributing to life prolongation. Allowance of long-term treatment which enables the patient to eat through alleviation of adverse reactions which are most unendurable for the patient, e.g., diarrhea, stomatitis, anorexia, and HF syndrome, will not only improve QOL of the patient but also prolong the treatment period without lowering patient compliance, thus leading to life prolongation.

In this chapter, we explained the theory and practice of the following two therapeutic modalities as the therapies which are at the position of SRC that is provided with a dual action, i.e., effect enhancement and adverse reaction alleviation, and which are prevailingly used in Japan:

1. A combination therapy (low-dose FP therapy) of continuous 5-FU (CVI) with low-dose consecutive CDDP, using CDDP as a modulator for 5-FU.
2. A combination therapy (intermittent FP therapy) of intermittent (administered on Monday, Wednesday, and Friday) 5-FU (CVI)—utilizing a difference in cell cycle between normal cells (e.g., gastrointestinal mucus cells and bone cells) and tumor cells, with low-dose consecutive CDDP.

Regarding the clinical results, the low-dose FP chemotherapy showed an overall response rate which was as high as 55.0% (170/390) for solid tumors, exhibited an incidence of adverse reactions rated to be Grade 3 or higher, being as low as 3.2 (10/309), and allowed the conduction of long-term treatment. Furthermore, intermittent FP therapy maintained the effects of low-dose FP therapy and showed a further lower incidence of adverse reactions; therefore, its clinical usefulness was suggested. Namely, intermittent FP therapy showed an overall response rate which was as high as 51.6% (32/62) for solid cancers and exhibited a long response period; in particular, the therapy showed a response rate which was as high as

50.0% (14/28) for Stage IV colorectal cancer. Among 14 patients in whom PR was attained, 9 (64.3%) had a response period which lasted from half a year to one year. There were no nonhematological adverse reactions afflicting the patient most, which were rated to be G3 or higher (0/83). Therefore, intermittent FP therapy improved gastrointestinal toxicities, allowed the conduction of long-term treatment and was suggested to possibly become a therapeutic modality which leads to life prolongation. We are eagerly willing that these two therapeutic modalities be examined internationally as potential standard therapeutic modalities for advanced and recurrent solid cancers.

REFERENCES

1. Cadman E, Heimer R, Benz C. The influence of methotrexate pretrearment on 5-fluorouracil metabolism in L1210 cells. *J Biol Chem* 1981; 25:1695–1704.
2. Grem JL, Hoth DF, Hamilton JM, King SA, Leyland-Jones B. Overview of current status and future direction of clinical trials with 5-fluorouracil in combination with folinic acid. *Cancer Treat Rep* 1987; 71:1249–1264.
3. Pazdur R, Lassere Y, Rhodes V, et al. Phase trial of uracil and Tegafur plus oral leucovorin. An effective oral regimen in the treatment of metastatic colorectal carcinoma. *J Clin Oncol* 1994; 12:2296–2300.
4. Kroener JF, Saleh F, Howell SB. 5-FU and allopurinol: Toxicity modulation and Phase II results in colon cancer. *Cancer Treat Rep* 1982; 66:1133–1137.
5. Wooley PV, Ayoob MJ, Smith FP et al. A controlled trial of the effect of 4-hydroxypyrimidine (allopurinol) on the toxicity of a single bolus dose of 5-fluorouracil. *J Clin Oncol* 1985; 3:103–109.
6. Scanlon KJ, Safirstein RL, Thies H, Gross TB, Waxman S, Guttenplan JB. Inhibition of amino acid transport by *cis*-diaminedichloroplatinum (II) derivatives in L-1210 murine leukemia cell. *Cancer Res* 1983; 43:4211–4215.
7. Shirasaka T, Shimamoto Y, Ohshimo H, Saito H, Fukushima M. Metabolic basis of the synergistic antitumor activities of 5-fluorouracil and cisplatin in rodent tumor models *in vivo. Cancer Chemother Pharmacol* 1993; 32:167–172.
8. Araki H, Fukushima M, Kamiyama Y, Shirasaka T. Effect consecutive lower-Dose cisplatin In enhancement of 5-fluorouracil cytotoxicity in experimental tumor cells *in vivo Cancer Lett* 2000; 160:185–191.
9. Omura K, Misaki T, Hasimoto T, et al. Change in folate concentration in Yoshida sarcoma after administration of leucovorin or cisplatin. *Cancer Chemother Pharmacol* 1995; 35:183–187.
10. Mizutani Y, Wu XX, Yoshida O, Shirasaka T, Bonavida B, Chemoimmunosensitization of the T24 human bladder cancer line to Fas-mediated cytotoxicity and apoptosis by cisplatin and 5-fluorouracil. *Oncol Rept* 1999; 6:979–982.
11. Kondo K, Murase M, Kodera Y, et al. Feasibility study on protracted infusional 5-fluorouracil and consecutive low-dose cisplatin for advanced gastric cancer. *Oncology* 1996; 53:64–67.
12. Chung Y, Yamashita Y, Matsuoka T, et al. Continuous infusion of 5-fluorouracil and low dose cisplatin infusion for the treatment of advanced and recurrent gastric adenocarcinomas. *Cancer* 1997; 80:1–7.
13. Sasaki K, Hirata K, Takasaka H, et al. Combination chemotherapy of continuous infusion 5-FU and CDDP for advanced colorectal cancer. A Sapporo Cancer Study (SACS) trial. *Proc Am Soc Clin Oncol* 1997; 16:269a(#955).
14. Chung S, Yamashita Y, Inoue T, et al. Continuous 5-FU and low-dose cisplatin for advanced and recurrent gastric cancers. *Proc Am Soc Clin Oncol* 1999; 16:285a(#1011).
15. Kondo K, Kataoka M, Ichihara, T, et al. Neoadjuvant chemotherapy for metastatic gastric cancer with 5-fluorouracil and repeated low-dose cisplatin. *Proc Am Soc Clin Oncol* 1997; 16:294a(#1046).
16. Shirasaka T, Yamamitsu, Tsuji A, Taguchi T. Conceptual change in cancer chemotherapy: From an oral fluoropyrimidine prodrug, UFT, to a novel oral fluoropyrimidine prodrug, S-1, and low-dose FP therapy in Japan. *Investigational New Drugs* 2000; 18:315–329.
17. Saji S, Aiba K, Araki H, et al. Current status of low-dose CDDP•5-FU therapy for solid malignant tumor-Nationwide questionnaire survey- *Jpn J Cancer Chemother* 1997; 24:1892–1900.
18. Lipkin M. Sherlock P, Bell B, Cell proliferation kinetics in the gastrointestinal tract of man Cell renewal stomach, ileum, colon, and rectum. *Gastroenterology* 1963; 45:721–729.
19. Clarkson B, Ota K, Ohkita T, O'Connor A, Kinetics of proliferation of cancer cell in neoplastic effusions in man *Cancer* 1965; 18:1189–1213.
20. Skipper HE, Schabel FM Jr, Wilcox WS. Experimental evaluation of potential anticancer agents, XIII On the criteria and kinetic associated with "Curability" of experimental leukemia. *Cancer Chemother Rep* 1964; 35:1–111.

21. Sugano K, Ota K, Taguchi T, et al. Early phase trial of *l*-leucovorin and 5-fluorouracil in advanced colorectal cancer. *Jpn J Cancer Chemother* 1995; 22:627–637.
22. Yoshino M, Ota K, Kurihara M, et al. Late phase trial of high-dose *l*-leucovorin and 5-fluorouracil in advanced colorectal carcinoma. *Jpn J Cancer Chemother* 1995; 22:785–792.
23. Konishi K, Yabushita K, Taguchi T, et al. Late phase trial of *l*-leucovorin and 5-fluorouracil in advanced colorectal cancer. *Jpn J Cancer Chemother* 1995; 22:925–932.
24. Ohtsu A, Baba H, Sakata Y, et al. Phase II study of S-1, a novel oral fluoropyrimidine derivative, in patients with metastatic colorectal carcinoma. *Brit J Cancer* 2000; 83:141–145.

Index

D

E